PRIMARY CARE PEDIATRICS

PRIMARY CARE PEDIATRICS

A Symptomatic Approach

Steven P. Shelov, M.D.
Associate Professor of Pediatrics

Andrew P. Mezey, M.D.
Associate Professor of Pediatrics

Chester M. Edelmann, Jr., M.D.
Professor of Pediatrics
All of Albert Einstein College of Medicine
New York, New York

Henry L. Barnett, M.D.
Medical Director,
The Children's Aid Society
New York, New York
Professor Emeritus of Pediatrics
Albert Einstein College of Medicine
New York, New York

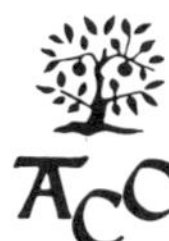

APPLETON-CENTURY-CROFTS Norwalk, Connecticut

Copyright © 1984 by Appleton-Century-Crofts
A Publishing Division of Prentice-Hall, Inc.

All rights reserved. This book, or any parts thereof, may not be used or reproduced in any manner without written permission. For information, address Appleton-Century-Crofts, 25 Van Zant Street, East Norwalk, Connecticut 06855.

84 85 86 87 88 / 10 9 8 7 6 5 4 3 2 1

Prentice-Hall International, Inc., London
Prentice-Hall of Australia, Pty. Ltd., Sydney
Prentice-Hall Canada, Inc.
Prentice-Hall of India Private Limited, New Delhi
Prentice-Hall of Japan, Inc., Tokyo
Prentice-Hall of Southeast Asia (Pte.) Ltd., Singapore
Whitehall Books Ltd., Wellington, New Zealand
Editora Prentice-Hall do Brasil Ltda., Rio de Janeiro

Library of Congress Cataloging in Publication Data
Main entry under title:

Primary care pediatrics.

  Bibliography: p.
  Includes index.
  1. Children—Diseases—Diagnosis.   2. Symptomatology.
I. Shelov, Steven P. [DNLM: 1. Pediatrics. 2. Primary
health care. WS 100 P952]
RJ50.P74   1983   618.92   83-9960
ISBN 0-8385-7897-7

Cover and text design: Lynn Luchetti
Production: Carol Pierce

PRINTED IN THE UNITED STATES OF AMERICA

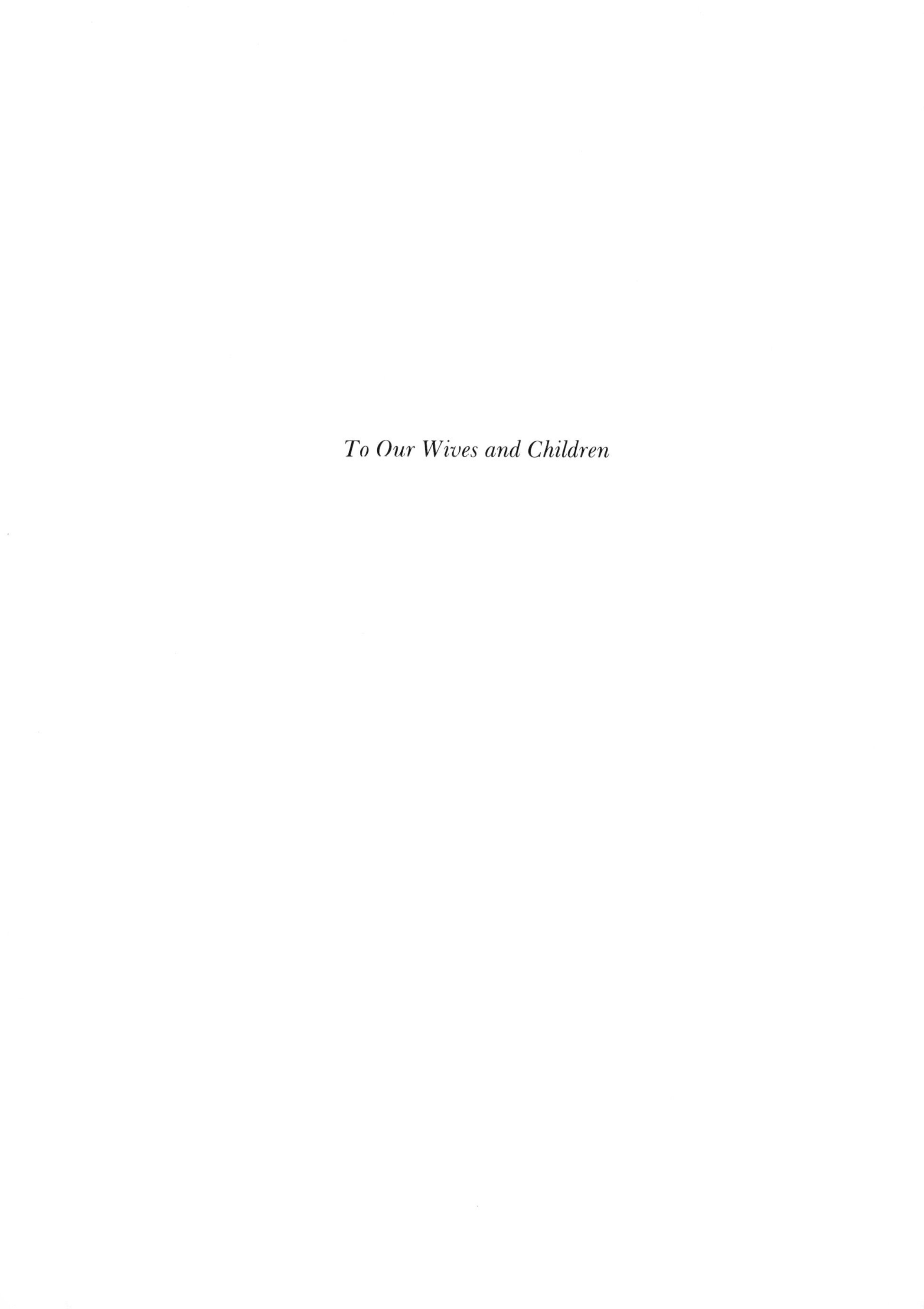

To Our Wives and Children

Contents

Contributors

HENRY L. BARNETT, M.D.
Professor Emeritus of Pediatrics
Albert Einstein College of Medicine

MARC BESTAK, M.D.
Assistant Professor of Pediatrics
Albert Einstein College of Medicine

MARGERY A. BOECK, M.D., PH.D.
Assistant Professor of Pediatrics
Albert Einstein College of Medicine

LOUIS BORGENICHT, M.D.
Assistant Professor of Family Medicine
University of Utah
Salt Lake City, Utah

**FRANCES M. CERULLO, M.A. SPECIAL
EDUCATION**
Principal Associate in Pediatrics
Albert Einstein College of Medicine

MICHAEL I. COHEN, M.D.
Professor and Chairman of Pediatrics
Albert Einstein College of Medicine

JANNA COLLINS, M.D.
Assistant Professor of Pediatrics
Albert Einstein College of Medicine

SUSAN M. COUPEY, M.D.
Assistant Professor of Pediatrics
Albert Einstein College of Medicine

ELLEN F. CRAIN, M.D., PH.D.
Assistant Professor of Pediatrics
Albert Einstein College of Medicine

DAVID L. DIAMOND, M.D.
Assistant Clinical Professor of Pediatrics
Albert Einstein College of Medicine

GABRIEL DINARI, M.D.
Chief, Pediatric Gastroenterology
Assistant Director, Department of
Pediatrics
Beilinson Medical Center, Israel

HAROLD DINER, D.D.S.
Professor of Dentistry (Pedodontics) and
Dental Director
Rose F. Kennedy Center
Albert Einstein College of Medicine

CHESTER M. EDELMANN, JR., M.D.
Professor of Pediatrics
Albert Einstein College of Medicine

BERNARD FISH, M.D.
Assistant Professor of Pediatrics
Albert Einstein College of Medicine

LEWIS FRAAD, M.D.
Professor of Pediatrics
Albert Einstein College of Medicine

JEFFREY GERSHEL, M.D.
Assistant Professor of Pediatrics
Albert Einstein College of Medicine

JOY GLASER, M.D.
Assistant Professor of Pediatrics
Albert Einstein College of Medicine

DAVID GOLDSMITH, M.D.
Assistant Professor of Pediatrics
Albert Einstein College of Medicine

RUTH L. GOTTESMAN, ED.D.
Associate Professor of Pediatrics
Albert Einstein College of Medicine

S. HAHM, M.D.
Assistant Professor of Pediatrics
Albert Einstein College of Medicine

PAUL HARRIS, M.D.
Assistant Professor of Pediatrics
Albert Einstein College of Medicine

CAROL LEICHER, M.D.
Pediatric Neurologist
Hartford Hospital
Rockville, Connecticut

NATHAN LITMAN, M.D.
Assistant Professor of Pediatrics
Albert Einstein College of Medicine

ANDREW P. MEZEY, M.D.
Associate Professor of Pediatrics
Albert Einstein College of Medicine

WALTER M. ROSENFELD, M.D.
Assistant Professor of Pediatrics
Albert Einstein College of Medicine

PAUL SAENGER, M.D.
Associate Professor of Pediatrics
Albert Einstein College of Medicine

MARCOS SASTRE, M.D.
Pediatric Dermatologist
Quincy, Massachusetts

S. KENNETH SCHONBERG, M.D.
Associate Professor of Pediatrics
Albert Einstein College of Medicine

STEVEN P. SHELOV, M.D.
Associate Professor of Pediatrics
Albert Einstein College of Medicine

MARILYN B. SILVER, PH.D.
Assistant Professor
Department of Otorhinolaryngology
Albert Einstein College of Medicine

RUTH E. K. STEIN, M.D.
Associate Professor of Pediatrics
Albert Einstein College of Medicine

FREDERICK WANG, M.D.
Assistant Professor of Ophthalmology
Albert Einstein College of Medicine

ESTHER H. WENDER, M.D.
Associate Professor of Pediatrics
Albert Einstein College of Medicine

Preface

This new pediatric text has several well-defined purposes that in combination distinguish it from other books currently available. Originally, the idea for such a book was conceived by Henry L. Barnett, the first Chairman of the Department of Pediatrics of the Albert Einstein College of Medicine of Yeshiva University. He used as his role model of the primary care pediatric practitioner, Lewis M. Fraad, a unique individual who has inspired literally hundreds of pediatric residents, pediatric generalists, and pediatric specialists over the last forty years. The focus of the book therefore, is on the primary care of infants and children. Its organization and structure are determined by this central purpose, and also by the fact that it is closely related and extensively cross-referenced to a comprehensive textbook of pediatrics, the 17th edition of *Pediatrics*, edited by Abraham M. Rudolph. Thus, the present book is not intended to be encyclopedic in its coverage, nor does it include extensive discussions of the etiology and pathogenesis of diseases of infants and children. Rather, the conditions included have been selected because they represent most of those for which children are brought to the pediatric primary care practitioner. Most of the conditions are those for which the primary care practitioner is the true "specialist," even though primary care is increasingly concerned with diseases for which hospital based "system specialists" have evolved. Consequently, the more common of these are included in the discussion.

An additional important aspect of this text is that it discusses childhood illnesses in terms of presenting symptoms since most primary medical care is sought because of symptoms rather than for diseases.

It is with pleasure and a true sense of appreciation that we acknowledge the contribution to this book made by Lois Ceriani, Eileen Foley, Grace Bonaro, and Jean Massaro. We thank them for their invaluable secretarial support in preparing this manuscript.

We are grateful to Robert E. McGrath for his guidance and encouragement during the preliminary stages of this text. Finally, we thank our editors at Appleton-Century-Crofts, Carol Pierce and Mary K. Cowell, for their invaluable assistance in completing this project.

Steven P. Shelov
Andrew P. Mezey
Chester M. Edelmann, Jr.
Henry L. Barnett

New York City

Introduction

The content of pediatric practice has undergone numerous changes since pediatrics was established as a separate academic discipline by the appointment of Abraham Jacobi as Clinical Professor of Diseases of Children at the College of Physicians and Surgeons of Columbia University in 1870. By 1950, the initial role of the practicing pediatrician had shifted in large part from the diagnosis and treatment of acute, severe, episodic illnesses to one in which treatment of mild illnesses, advice on behavioral and feeding problems and provision of preventive measures occupied an increasing proportion of time. These aspects of child care continue to occupy a major share of the time of the practicing pediatrician as well as the family practitioner and pediatric nurse practitioner.

It appears that we are now in the process of another shift in the role of the pediatric practitioner. An increasing proportion of the medical care sought for infants and children, as has always been true for adults, is for complex chronic illnesses, mostly of unknown causes. The primary disease in these illnesses usually involves specific systems and pediatric system specialists have evolved to meet the more complex diagnostic and therapeutic needs of these patients.

This shift in one aspect of medical care of children has made pediatric practitioners increasingly uneasy about their ability to handle complex chronic illnesses, especially if several years have elapsed since completion of their training. However, we believe that the primary care pediatric practitioners are better prepared to care for these children with complex chronic illnesses than they realize. The first encounter of these patients is usually with them and they should also be able to provide continuing principal care, either alone or in consultation with system specialists.

The purposes of this book, therefore, are twofold: to present a symptom approach and differential diagnosis of conditions for which the primary care practitioner is the specialist and, second, to describe the body of knowledge needed by the primary care practitioner to care for patients with complex chronic illnesses of specific systems. An approach is made also, not attempted previously to our knowledge, toward defining for each of the latter conditions how much of the differential diagnosis and treatment can be confidently done by the primary care practitioner and when referral to a pediatric system specialist is indicated. The source of additional information needed by the pediatric primary care practitioner in the continuing care of children with complex chronic illnesses after consultation with system specialists is indicated through the cross-references with the 17th edition of *Pediatrics,* edited by Abraham M. Rudolph.

It is anticipated that this new text will serve to fulfill an unmet need of medical students, pediatric residents, pediatric primary care physicians, family practitioners, and pediatric nurse practitioners. To provide the material in the most useful and practical manner, each chapter will be constructed following a similar format. The format will entail the following:

- Statement of the problem, physical finding or symptom encountered by the primary care practitioner.
- How frequently this problem is seen by the practitioner.
- Questions that would be most important to ask to better understand the significance of this finding or symptom.
- How these questions might be asked.
- Essentials of the physical examination that must be done to lead toward an accurate diagnosis.
- Elements in the history that would reassure you as to the non-serious nature of the complaint or finding. Historical elements the practitioner should explore with further work-up including laboratory investigation, or more detailed examinations.
- Essentials of this further examination or laboratory investigation.
- Results that would be reassuring, and the results that would confirm the more serious diagnosis.
- Determining the major diagnosis(es) to be considered in terms of the essential elements of history and physical examination.
- Determining diagnostic considerations that should be seen by a consultant, and those that can and should be managed by the primary care practitioner. How diagnostic situations managed by the practitioner would be evaluated, using laboratory or x-ray, and how the situation would be therapeutically managed. In those diagnostic situations which need consultation the following points should be considered:
  - At what point a consultant/specialist should become involved.
  - What questions the primary practitioner should ask the specialist.
  - Minimum amount of historical information, physical findings, and laboratory data required by the specialist.
  - Information the practitioner should expect from the specialist with respect to further work-up, prognosis, family management, management of medication, future intervals for return visit.

Obviously there will be some chapters in which it will not be either possible or appropriate to follow this outline so narrowly; but the overall purpose is to provide a useful, logical presentation of a symptom oriented approach for the pediatric primary care practitioner.

PART I

General Approach of the Pediatrician to Children and Families

ONE

The Approach to the Normal Newborn

Andrew P. Mezey

For most families, the birth of a child is a joyful, miraculous event. The culmination of pregnancy is, in truth, the beginning of the nuclear family. It triggers a series of events that herald the start of a fantastic adventure. The need to nurture, to love, and to be loved is present in all of us. A child gives us the opportunity to fulfill those needs while experiencing vicariously another's childhood. Those of us who have raised children and have experienced the joys and sorrows that necessarily accompany that process know that a newborn child is the most precious of treasures. Pediatric practitioners must keep this concept clearly in mind in order to deal successfully with the needs and concerns of parents.

THE PRENATAL INTERVIEW

A model for a meeting between the pediatric practitioner and the near term woman and her husband has evolved. This prenatal interview is usually for parents of a first child. The future parents choose a pediatric practitioner and make an appointment for an interview a month or so prior to the expected delivery date. This process is facilitated if parents are encouraged by the obstetrician or midwife, but they know about the availability and advisability of such an interview through word of mouth. It is also valuable for the practitioner to talk to childbirth preparatory groups, during which the concept of an individual prenatal visit can be introduced.

How does one conduct the interview, where and when does it take place, what subjects are covered, and what purpose does it serve? Whenever possible, the visit should be at the beginning or the end of office or clinic hours. It is almost impossible to concentrate on the content of the interview in the middle of the bedlam that generally occurs in a busy pediatric practice during the office session. It is a more valuable experience for the expectant parents when the practitioner is relaxed and not worrying about what is going on in the waiting room. We have found it enjoyable to have the interview at the end of an office session. It is a good way to decelerate after a 3 or 4 hour stretch of a busy practice. Perhaps more importantly, the parents can both be present if they can be seen late in the afternoon. Since many women now work until very late into their pregnancies, it is a more convenient time for them as well as for the father.

Why bother? Is anything accomplished? Are there any measurable outcomes? No systematic evaluations of the effectiveness of such interviews have been done to our knowledge. Nevertheless, as in so many aspects of practice, we accept, even without validation, that the prenatal interview is valuable and that the time is worth spending. The interview makes a statement about the kind of care the pediatrician believes the infant and family should receive. It also permits the pediatrician to gain an impression about the parents and the type of care they are seeking. Finally, it facilitates the beginning of a trusting relationship between the two. Unlike visits for other purposes, the time allotted for the prenatal interview cannot be less than 30 minutes.

What is discussed? The easiest way to start, after introductions are made, is to take a formal history.

Maternal and Paternal Age.

Maternal and Paternal History. This should include medications, past and present, occupational history, and social history.

History of the Present Pregnancy. This should include questions about previous pregnancies, planning for and ease of conception, amount of weight gain or loss, time of onset and quality of fetal movements, blood type and Rh group, and any problem, such as hypertension, proteinuria, glycosuria, bleeding, vomiting, febrile illnesses, or rashes. If an amniocentesis is indicated, has it been performed? If it has not, why not? If it has, what are the results?

Family History. This should include questions about parents, siblings, and siblings' children, religion, race, and illnesses of genetic origin. Very often people will mention allergic symptoms in nieces, nephews, or siblings. On requestioning, they will acknowledge some allergies in themselves that they had neglected to mention earlier.

Childbirth Classes. Many couples attend childbirth classes, and this information should be obtained. At the least, it means that the father will be present throughout labor and delivery. In general, it means that the parents will be informed about the birthing process. In fact, they may have elected to have the delivery occur in a birthing room rather than a delivery suite. The pediatric practitioner may want to discuss these issues with the parents to learn more about them or to uncover some misconceptions or to answer questions about parent-infant bonding. This is an opportunity to discuss concerns around the possibility of a cesarean section and its effects on the postpartum course.

Preparations for the Baby's Arrival. This should include questions about what support there will be from family, friends, or a live-in helper. One should ask whether or not the infant will be in the parents' room. This line of questioning often gives the practitioner insights into attitudes and concerns that might otherwise not be elicited. A woman who is confident about her ability to handle herself in the postpartum period will answer questions differently from one who is deeply concerned about her ability to cope. Even the novice interviewer, structuring the situation this way, probing in areas where problems are evident, will find it easy to get much important information quickly. If necessary, another interview may be needed prior to the delivery.

Fears and Anxieties. The unknown is always a source of fear and anxiety; it is magnified greatly in anticipating the birth of an infant. Concerns about the health of the infant, especially about congenital defects, are probably universal. If the facts learned from a thorough history warrant, a reassuring statement can be made that there is no evidence for increased fetal risk. Risk factors uncovered during the interview should be discussed openly. Misconceptions, usually exaggerating the importance of a specific incident, are very common. Ignoring them serves as a source of unnecessary anxiety. Most concerns are dispelled relatively easily, but they must be identified before anything can be done about them. A parent may have been treated for gonorrhea at one time and be concerned about the effect on the fetus, confusing something he or she might have heard in relation to syphilis as applying to other venereal diseases. Another parent may be concerned that the pregnancy was unplanned and that an initial ambivalence may have an adverse effect on the infant's personality. This kind of concern may need to be explored further in another appointment. Some women might mention that they have a special problem enduring pain and express concern about the effects of analgesia or anesthesia on the baby. The patient should be encouraged to discuss this problem with her obstetrician. Reinforcement of information given by the obstetrician relating to maternal medications, smoking, and alcohol can be made at this point. Sexual intercourse in the terminal weeks of pregnancy has been reported to be associated with an increased risk of prenatal infection and is an appropriate area of concern. Medications, smoking, and alcohol as teratogens are discussed in a later section.

Parents frequently ask where information about infant care can be obtained. The subjects vary from questions about equipment, such as type of crib, type of carriage, clothing, cloth versus disposable diapers, bottle sterilizers, ointments, powders, and bathing accessories, to temperature of the home, air conditioners, pets, siblings, and grandparents. The answers to these and other questions are somewhat subjective but are answered in a later section on the newborn. Other parenting information, relating to day-to-day management is best given after the baby is born, since it needs to be tailored to the specific situation. However, the main thing the parents need to hear is that the pediatric practitioner is interested and will be available to provide the advice.

Discussion of Feeding. The major question in this area is the choice between breast and bottle feeding; and most women will have already made up their minds. Breast feeding is undergoing a renaissance, and the majority of women coming to private offices and clinics either will have decided to nurse their infants or can be encouraged to do so. There are, however, some who have no desire to breastfeed. In any case, it is worthwhile inquiring about the reason for their decision, whether pro or con.

If one listens carefully, valuable insight into the parents' feelings can be gained. The discussion of breastfeeding is a good example of this process. For example, the small-breasted woman may believe incorrectly that she will be unable to produce enough milk. Another woman's mother or friend may have told her about a breast infection she got because she or someone she knew breastfed. Some people are concerned about what nursing will do to the size and shape of their breasts. A woman who wants to go back to work shortly after delivery may not realize that she can nurse once or twice a day and continue to work. The father of the infant may have concerns about his role if the infant is breastfed. He should be included in the conversation, and his opinion should be actively sought. Whatever the reason for choosing one method or the other, to the sensitive pediatric practitioner the answers will shed light on feelings and concerns that encompass the total experience of giving birth.

For the woman who, for any number of reasons, has decided definitely not to breastfeed, it is important to support that decision rather than to adopt a punitive attitude that will make her feel guilty. Though there is increasing evidence that human milk is physiologically better suited to the human infant than cow milk and may protect against some infections, infants can and do thrive very well, both physically and emotionally, on formulas. In families where there are multiple caretakers or where conditions exist that might make nursing very difficult or where the desire to nurse is just not there, formula feeding is very satisfactory.

Pediatrician's Role. The interview ends with an explanation of the role of the pediatrician during the postpartum period in the hospital. Most hospitals require that the attending physician perform a physical examination on the baby within the first 24 hours. A discharge examination is generally required within 24 hours of discharge. In actual practice this conforms to the usual 3 day hospital stay; a child born during the day is seen by the next morning. If everything is normal, the next visit is 48 hours later, and the child is discharged. If there are any problems, either at the time of birth or later, this schedule is adjusted appropriately. This process is explained to the parents, and they are given a description of the physical examination of a newborn. Finally, the parents should be told that the pediatric practitioner is available by telephone, both pre- and postpartum. If the practitioner likes what he or she is doing and shows concern for the expectant parents, the prenatal interview should be a source of comfort to them, as well as an educational experience.

PREGNANCY AND ITS OUTCOMES

While most pregnancies are not associated with an increased risk to the fetus, it is important for the pediatric practitioner to be familiar with factors associated with potential problems and what, if anything, can be done about them (Table 1). These problems are usually handled by the obstetrician. Howev-

er, the pediatric practitioner may become involved when decisions must be made concerning four major aspects of prenatal care (Table 2).

Amniocentesis

This procedure is relatively safe and has become much more common in the past several years. Amniocentesis has a success rate of about 95%, a risk of 0.5–1% fetal loss if done at 15–16 weeks gestation, with about 3 weeks required to obtain the results of karyotyping. Other studies may yield quicker results. The main indications are maternal age, heritable diseases, and Rh incompatibility.

Maternal Age. Since many women have postponed having children until after they are 30 years of age, they are likely to be 35 or more by their second pregnancy. Age 35 is considered to be an age when the risk of an abnormal conception, as judged by the incidence of chromosomal disorders, is greater than the risk of amniocentesis. The incidence of trisomy 21 is about 1.5% between 35 and 39 years and about 2.5% between 40 and 45 years.

Heritable Diseases. A large number of heritable diseases (over 50) can now be diagnosed prenatally by examination of amniotic fluid. The most common of these are chromosomal abnormalities, neural tube defects (5% chance of recurrence after a first affected infant), adrenogenital syndrome, and hemoglobinopathies.

Rh Incompatibility. The incidence of erythroblastosis fetalis secondary to Rh incompatibility has decreased markedly since 1969 when passive immunization with Rh (D) immune globulin became available. Fortunately, it has become an uncommon reason for performing an amniocentesis. When done, it is used as a guide for judging the degree to which the fetus has been affected

TABLE 1. RISK FACTORS IN PREGNANCY

Maternal		Fetal	
History of habitual abortion	Primigravida >35 years	Cardiac disease	Multiple gestation
Polyhydramnios	Age <18 years	Chronic hypertension	IUGR
Prolonged gestation	Second and third trimester bleeding	Renal disease	Premature rupture of membranes
Preeclampsia	Thyroid disorders	Macrosomia	Abnormal presentation
Diabetes mellitus	Collagen disease	Abruptio placentae	Amnionitis
Hematologic disorder	History of stillbirth	Placenta previa	Abnormal fetal heart rate
History of premature labor	History of incompetent cervix	Erythroblastosis fetalis	Meconium in amniotic fluid
History of intrauterine growth retardation (IUGR)	History of uterine surgery	Abnormal	
History of premature deliveries	Grandmultiparity		
Viral or bacterial infection	Drug abuse		
Gastrointestinal disorder	Malnutrition		
Malignant disease	Pulmonary disorder		

by the Rh incompatibility. Decisions can then be made for either early delivery or intrauterine transfusions.

Maternal Infection

Any infection during the course of a pregnancy poses a potential risk to the fetus or newborn. A number of illnesses have well-defined syndromes associated with them, although the actual incidence is not clear. Examples of these diseases are shown in Table 3.

TABLE 2. PRENATAL AREAS OF CONCERN TO PEDIATRICIANS

Amniocentesis
    Advanced maternal age
    Heritable diseases
    Rh incompatibility with sensitization
Maternal infection
Maternal medications
Complications of delivery

Congenital rubella is avoidable simply by determining the immune status of women as they enter their childbearing years. If the results of antibody titers show no immunity, rubella vaccine should be given and pregnancy delayed for 3 months after vaccination. If a pregnant woman is exposed to rubella, antibody titers should be drawn and the immune status determined. If the woman is immune, nothing further need be done. If she is not immune, repeat titers should be drawn after 2–3 weeks even if no disease symptoms occur. If there has been evidence of rubella infection, termination of the pregnancy must be considered. This decision should be based on the acceptability of termination of the pregnancy by the parents, the stage of pregnancy when the infection occurred, and the stage of pregnancy when the decision is made. The earlier in pregnancy rubella occurs, the more seriously affected the infant will be. A more complete discussion of the

TABLE 3. MATERNAL INFECTIONS THAT POSE RISKS TO THE FETUS OR NEWBORN

Illnesses	Period of Risk	Effect
Rubella	First 16 weeks	Rubella syndrome: cardiac, eyes, brain, hearing
Varicella	Near term	Neonatal varicella, often fatal
Hepatitis B	Last trimester	Neonatal hepatitis
Cytomegalovirus	Throughout	Hepatosplenomegaly, microcephaly, chorioretinitis with primary infection
Toxoplasmosis	Throughout	Hepatosplenomegaly, chorioretinitis, microcephaly or hydrocephalus
Syphilis	Last two trimesters	Stillbirth, rash on palms and soles, snuffles, osteomyelitis, splenomegaly, jaundice, rhagades, CSF pleocytosis
Mumps	?	? Endocardial fibroelastosis
Herpes simplex	Late pregnancy	Microcephaly, retinopathy, encephalitis, hepatitis
Chlamydia	Intrapartum	Conjunctivitis, pneumonia
Group B streptococcus	Late pregnancy and intrapartum	Sepsis, meningitis, pneumonia, respiratory distress

various manifestations of the rubella syndrome can be found in *Pediatrics*, 17th ed.

If a mother develops varicella within 2 weeks of delivery, the infant will develop neonatal varicella. This is a potentially fatal infection, although most infants will survive. Prematures are at greater risk than are full term infants.

Hepatitis B is transmissible from the mother to the infant in the third trimester. Specific recommendations about the use of hepatitis B immune globulin have been made and can be found in *Pediatrics*, 17th ed. When the infant is affected, the infection is generally mild and usually results in an asymptomatic state with only minimal changes in liver function tests. However, the infant may become a chronic carrier of hepatitis B surface antigen.

Cytomegalovirus and toxoplasmosis can both be associated with severe infections in the infant. In most instances in the United States, the illnesses are asymptomatic. Untreated syphilis, however, generally causes serious illness in the newborn. This is an illness in which the diagnosis is relatively easy to make and where specific and very effective therapy exists.

Mumps is a preventable disease, since there is a live attenuated vaccine with approximately 98% efficacy that is now part of the routine immunization procedure for children. Since it was only introduced in 1968, there are women who have not been immunized and who have not had clinical mumps. Mumps skin testing is a reliable means for assessing immunity, but the antigen may not be readily available. Therefore, since there are no adverse reactions to the vaccine, immunization against mumps in nonpregnant women of childbearing age is indicated if there is any questions about susceptibility.

Genital herpes simplex infection is considered to be an indication for cesarean section at term in order to prevent infection of the newborn during a vaginal delivery.

Chlamydia trachomatis is a microorganism carried in the genital tract. The most common manifestation of the disease in the newborn is an inclusion body conjunctivitis which is easily treated with sulfonamide eyedrops. There may also be a benign pneumonia with a characteristic staccato cough, diffuse rales, tachypnea, and no fever. Characteristically, the infant does not appear ill despite symptoms and signs of pneumonia. At present it is unknown whether treating mothers harboring *Chlamydia* is necessary or effective.

Group B streptococcus has become a serious cause of morbidity and mortality in infants. Carrier states among pregnant females are high, and it is difficult to to eradicate the organism from the genital tract. Controversy exists over prophylactic treatment of newborns with penicillin to prevent group B streptococcal infections.

Maternal Medications

It is reasonable to state that pregnant women should, if possible, take no medications during pregnancy. Many medications have definite associations with abnormalities in the fetus, and many others have possible associations. As a general rule, the earlier a medication is given in pregnancy, the more likely it is to produce major congenital defects. This fact can be used when weighing the risks of using medications. (Table 4).

There are numerous other medications that have been shown to affect the fetus. Parents should be aware that any medications might have harmful effects on the fetus. Abnormalities may take many years to become manifest, as seen with diethylstilbestrol (DES). These warnings must not be permitted to persuade women that necessary medications, such as insulin in an insulin-dependent diabetic, be discontinued.

ROLE OF THE PEDIATRIC PRACTITIONER AFTER DELIVERY

Most infants, whether delivered vaginally or by cesarean section, will be healthy and vigorous and have an uneventful stay in the hospital. If the delivery has been uncomplicated and the infant appears normal to the delivery and nursery personnel, the first visit by the

TABLE 4. MATERNAL MEDICATIONS AND THEIR POTENTIAL EFFECTS ON THE FETUS AND CHILD

Drug	Effect
Alcohol	Fetal alcohol syndrome: (IUGR, short stature, microcephaly, blepharophimosis, midface hypoplasia, cardiac defects)
Phenytoin (Dilantin)	Fetal phenytoin syndrome: hypertelorism, hypoplastic nails, cardiac defects, possible mental retardation
Trimethadione	Fetal trimethadione syndrome: short nose, upward slanted eyebrows, cardiac defect, mental retardation
Coumadin, warfarin	Bleeding in the fetus
Corticosteroids	Possible cleft palate
Androgenic steroids	Masculinization of the female fetus
Iodides, methimazole, propylthiouracil	Thyroid goiter
Stilbestrol	Increased potential for early development of adenocarcinoma of vagina
Thalidomide	Phocomelia
Nicotine (smoking)	Intrauterine growth retardation
Heroin, morphine, methadone	Withdrawal syndrome: sneezing, vomiting, diarrhea, irritability, seizures

pediatrician should be during the first 24 hours. A history should be obtained from the chart, from the mother, and from the nursing staff, and the physical examination should be complete. A physical examination is required within 24 hours of discharge. It can be less complete than the admitting examination but should definitely include reassessment of skin for jaundice and attention to the cardiopulmonary status, abdomen (including the umbilicus), hips, and eyes. At present the average length of hospital stay after a vaginal delivery is 3 days and after a cesarean section 7 days. We recommend at least two visits for a normal, vaginally delivered infant and a minimum of four visits for an infant delivered by cesarean section. If the infant is premature or if there are ongoing or new medical problems, visits should be made at least once daily. The mother should be seen at each visit. See Tables 5 and 6 for areas to be assessed on the admission and discharge visits.

At the admission visit, several areas must be discussed with the mother. Parents need to be told that the infant is normal, that the heart and lungs are fine, that fingers and toes are normal, that the eyes are brown or blue, that the molding of the head will go away, that the genitalia are normal. Birth marks, no matter how minor, should be described. If there is a problem, such as forefoot adduction or hip click, or a potential problem, such as ABO incompatibility, it must be discussed. Although anxiety may be aroused, it is better

**TABLE 5. ADMISSION VISIT:
AREAS TO BE DISCUSSED**

Introduction and review of pregnancy and
  family history
Description of findings
Discussion of feeding—breast vs bottle
Encourage other questions
Information regarding time of next visit
Information regarding availability by telephone

TABLE 6. DISCHARGE VISIT

Encourage questions
Discussion of feeding technique
Discussion of infant care
Plans for follow-up

to be forthright in a sensitive way. Most people would prefer to be prepared than to be surprised, and the informative practitioner will generally be seen as thoughtful, thorough, and concerned. The parents should then be encouraged to ask questions, especially if this is the first encounter. Since most people will have made a decision about breast or bottle feeding before delivery, the choice of method will not be an issue. However, reasons for the decision provide insight into other attitudes, and the technique of feeding should be reviewed. A closing statement about the time of the next visit and about your availability between visits is very reassuring for the parents.

The discharge visit should be longer than the initial one, for much has occurred since that time, and the orientation of the parents has shifted from the delivery of the infant to the care of the infant. The visit starts with the physical examination, preferably in front of the parents, either in the mother's room or in the nursery. The examination provides a convenient setting for discussion of any concerns the parents have. It is more useful to ask what these are rather than to launch into a lecture on the care of the newborn. Listening to what is asked, and especially how it is asked, will indicate how comfortable the parents are about taking the infant home. Parents who ask detailed questions about very specific situations and who are unwilling to break off the conversation are telling you that the prospect of caring for the child frightens them. Rather than to keep answering each question in detail, it is better to close the conversation after a reasonable length of time by making some general care statements but with reassurance that most of the questions will answer themselves. The interview should end with a statement that you will be in touch with them daily for a while. A 10 minute conversation by telephone for the first few days will usually be all that is necessary to allay much of the anxiety. If it is not, further exploration of the causes of parental concern is necessary, since other more serious factors need to be considered. Postpartum depression, internal family dissensions, or loss of financial security are some examples of stressful situations that may lead to an inability to cope effectively with the newborn infant.

Most often the discharge visit goes smoothly, with the parents feeling comfortable about their ability to care for the infant. During the physical examination, the practitioner should ask the parents if they have any concerns about the infant's condition. In addition, anything the parents might not have noticed should be discussed. During the course of the examination, some positive statements should be made about the infant. We have been impressed with how often someone has told us several years later how much that kindness meant to them at the time. The visit should end with a review of some previously discussed subjects, breast or bottle feeding, visitors, going outdoors, vitamins, when to call in, and when to come in for the first visit.

All pediatric practitioners develop a set of biases about the care of newborns based on a variety of experiences. Our own include encouraging breastfeeding, allowing infants out of the house immediately, even in the winter, eliminating formula sterilization if the water supply is safe, cornstarch powders rather than talc-based ones, the lack of need for ointments and lotions unless specifically indicated, avoiding smoking or holding hot liquids when tending the infant, use of approved car seats, and comforting the infant as often as is needed without worrying about spoiling the infant.

Nursing mothers should be allowed to feed their infants frequently. This means every 2 hours or so during the daytime. They should also be advised that the length of time at each breast should begin with a few minutes the first day and gradually increase 1 or 2 minutes each day. Within 6–8 days, one should be nursing for 10 minutes on the first breast and until the infant falls asleep or seems satisfied on the second breast. This regimen is based on the knowledge that 90% of the obtainable milk comes during the first 10 minutes of nippling. Nursing longer than this on the first breast is inefficient and unnecessary. Starting with only a few minutes at each breast and increasing the time slowly avoids the problem of cracked and tender nipples. Mothers literally see stars when they nurse with sore nipples. As mentioned above, frequent feedings are encouraged if indicated by the infant's needs (as often as every 1½–2 hours). This practice does not increase the incidence of nipple breakdown but does allow the infant to feed at its own schedule and does increase milk production. If difficulties arise, the parents should be encouraged to telephone, even when this means calling after office hours. Since an effective alternative to nursing exists (formula feedings), it is very important that maximum support for the nursing mother be available. Parents may ask how they will know if the infant is receiving enough milk from the breast to grow properly. This question is difficult to answer since, in truth, it is difficult to be certain of the adequacy of the milk supply without weighing the infant. However, our policy has been to ask parents not to use a scale. We prefer to use close contact to determine whether the infant needs to be seen prior to 3 weeks of age, the usual time for the first visit. Most parents will find this regimen acceptable, especially since they are asked to phone in routinely 2–3 days after discharge from the hospital to chat and to make an appointment.

It should be recognized that there are

ingrained lay practices involving newborns which are usually not taught in residency training programs. These include the belief in the absolute need for sterilization of formula, keeping the baby in the house for 3 weeks, the need for daily baths, the need for baby lotions, ointments, or oils, and the need for baby powders. There is no need for formula sterilization if the water supply is safe, although there is a need for basic hygiene. Despite this, even physicians and nurses will insist on sterilizing the formula, especially with the first infant, despite their intellectual acceptance of the explanation for its being unnecessary. Arguments over sterilization should be avoided and the parents' wishes accepted in a nonjudgmental fashion. Keeping an infant indoors for 3 weeks is another example of an accepted practice that has no basis in fact. Some general guidelines for temperatures are described for parents stressing a need for a lack of extremes, either hot or cold. Daily baths for infants are also unnecessary but frequently done, almost as a ritual. We tell parents that keeping the infant clean can be accomplished without daily baths, suggesting that they bathe the infant in a sink or tub only when it is indicated, e.g., after a large and runny stool. In the same vein, the routine use of oils, ointments, or lotions is discouraged. The infant with cracked and dry skin or with seborrhea may need baby lotions, but oils are avoided. Ointments can be used to protect the infants diaper area when the skin has become abraded from loose bowels. Powders may be used routinely with clean diapers as prophylaxis against skin macerations. If powder is used, cornstarch-based ones are preferred since talc-based powders are irritating when inhaled.

Vitamins A, C, and D are not prescribed for formula-fed infants since all commercial preparations are supplemented with vitamins. For breastfed infants vitamins are recommended, since the quantities of vitamins A, C, and D vary in human breast milk and may not be adequate to meet the infant's needs. Iron supplementation is not necessary for the breastfed infant for the first 6 months of life, while iron-containing formula should be prescribed for the bottle-fed infant. We do not believe that the small amount of iron contained in formula (13 mg per quart) causes constipation. Fluoride, if not supplied in the drinking water, should be offered to the bottle-fed infant, the recommended dose being 0.5 mg per day. For breastfed infants, fluoride should be prescribed regardless of its presence in the water supply, since levels in breast milk are almost always low and are not adequate for dental caries prophylaxis. This recommendation can be modified if the breastfed infant is consuming large quantities of fluoride-supplemented water.

The type of crib or carriage bought is a matter of personal preference as long as it is safe. Consumer guides are helpful in pointing up the pros and cons. Grandparents, siblings, and pets should be retained since they are generally not hazardous to the newborn's health. Cats have been accused of smothering infants though we have never seen this happen and, frankly, do not believe it to be true. Clothing should be appropriate for the ambient temperature. Air conditioners are wonderful in the summertime, for parents as well as for infants, and cloth diapers offer no advantage over disposable ones except for wiping the furniture or placing under infants' heads.

By the time the discharge visit is over, the parents should be comfortable with the information they have received. The practitioner's concern for the welfare of the parents and the infant should have been communicated and a bond formed between all concerned. The next great adventure, that of rearing this little being, begins.

BIBLIOGRAPHY

Brunell PA: Prevention and treatment of neonatal herpes. Pediatrics 66:806, 1980

______. Varicella-zoster interactions in pregnancy. JAMA 199:315, 1967

Cooper LZ: Congenital Rubella in the United States, *in* Kingsman J and Gershon AA (eds) Infections of the Fetus and the Newborn Infant. AR Liss 1975

Klauss MD, Diaz-Rossello J: Breast feeding, 1980. Pediatr Rev 1:289, 1980

Milunsky A: Prenatal genetic diagnosis. Pediatr Rev 1:283, 1980

Smith DW: Fetal drug syndromes: Effects of ethanol and hydantoins. Pediatr Rev 1:165, 1979

Stagno J: Congenital toxoplasmosis. Am J Dis Child 134:635, 1980

Cross-Reference to *Pediatrics,* 17th ed.

TWO

Caring for Children with Chronic Illness

Ruth E. K. Stein

Children with chronic illness represent an increasing proportion of the pediatrician's practice. Epidemiologic studies suggest that at least 6% and perhaps as many as 20% of American children have a chronic condition,[1] defined as one that lasts 3 or more months in a given year or that requires at least 1 month of hospitalization.[2] These estimates exclude primary behavioral or psychiatric problems and show that the incidence of chronic illness increases with the age of the child.

The primary care pediatrician, referred to in this chapter as the pediatrician, has three alternatives when confronted with a child with a chronic medical problem. The first is to adopt a hands-off approach and refer the child for total management to the subspecialist. Although this approach assures the most technologically sophisticated care for the specific condition, there is considerable evidence that it provides less than adequate overall pediatric health care.[3–5] Divorcing the pediatrician from a role in the care of children with chronic problems may also lead to fragmentation of the care of children within the family unit. This alternative seems highly undesirable, therefore, from the perspective of the patient, the family, and the pediatrician.

The second alternative is for the pediatrician to manage the case entirely on his or her own. In an era of increasing technologic sophistication and with the complexity of many chronic diseases, this approach denies necessary expertise to the patient who could benefit from the depth of clinical experience of the specialist. This omission is especially serious if the illness is an uncommon one.

The third alternative, and the one that we espouse, is joint management by the pediatrician and the appropriate subspecialist(s). It is the underlying assumption of this chapter that the care of chronically ill children properly belongs with the pediatrician, working closely with the appropriate subspecialist(s) and that their combined efforts provide the optimal care for children with chronic illness and for their families.

The success of this approach is dependent on several essential elements. First, the pediatrician must have a sense of his own role and the contribution that he can make. As a corollary of this, the subspecialist must accept the limitations of his role and not attempt to provide aspects of care for which the pediatrician is more skilled.

Second, the division of responsibilities between the pediatrician and the subspecialist must be defined in order to assure that aspects of care are not missed by each. Criteria must be established which the pediatrician and subspecialist will use for involving each other.

Finally, both subspecialists and primary care pediatricians must be aware that there are many issues that are common to all children with chronic health problems, regardless of the type of chronic illness they have, and that these common issues and concerns need to be addressed and are as important to the child and family as those issues specific to an individual disease.

The discussion that follows will describe these elements and outline specific aspects of care provided by the pediatrician. While this chapter focuses primarily on children with serious chronic illness, the principles of management apply also to children with less serious disease.

THE ROLE OF THE PEDIATRICIAN

In order for the pediatrician to be effective in providing care to a child with a chronic illness, he must come to terms with his own discomfort. The pediatrician often has the mistaken idea that he has little to offer in the care and management of a chronically ill child.[6] This is far from the truth. He must have a clear idea of aspects of the child's care that are appropriately in his domain as a primary care specialist. Unlike the treatment of a patient with an acute disease, the main considerations and issues may not be entirely medical,[7] and hence it is even more essential to provide total comprehensive health care rather than only technologic medical care. As a primary care specialist and as a professional knowledgeable about the strengths of the child and the family, the pediatrician is in an ideal position to help define the needs of the family and to provide the necessary continuity of care. The fundamental task that the family has in raising a child with a chronic condition is that of integrating medical, social, and psychologic factors; the pediatrician is in the best position to help the family with this complex challenge.

Diagnosis and Evaluation

Regardless of the nature of the chronic medical condition or the context in which it is recognized, the pediatrician plays a critical role in informing the family and must be direct and honest with them. Allmond et al.[8] have stressed the importance of "respecting the event" and of creating an open pattern of communication. It is best not to overload the family with extensive information at a time when they can only react emotionally. Rather, it is helpful to provide an opportunity in the very near future for further discussion. It is imperative to assure the family of the continuing availability and support of the pediatrician. Understanding the need for frequent contacts is often the first tangible evidence of this availability and support. The sensitivity and honesty with which a pediatrician conveys information is appreciated by the family even years later and is often cited by them as an important aid in coping with the problem.

Whenever possible, it is preferable to provide information to both parents jointly. This minimizes the likelihood that information provided will be misinterpreted and avoids the temptation of one parent's protecting the other. Giving information separately to each parent may create a serious impediment to the parents' mutual trust and support at a time when these are most needed.

In those instances in which the diagnosis depends on future clinical developments, the pediatrician can play an important role in preparing the family for further tests and for referral to the subspecialist. In addition, the pediatrician may help by coordinating diagnostic studies and anticipating the nature of the information the family may ultimately hear. This situation is particularly common in the case of a child with developmental delay, in which situation the pediatrician may experience and share concerns over a period of time prior to making a definitive diagnosis. Parents may become distrustful if their concerns have been negated, only to be confirmed later, and report that they prefer having a pediatrician deal honestly with them, even when the physician must admit that he is not able to give definitive answers. Sharing uncertainty is often difficult for the pediatrician, but it is valued by families and important in building a trusting and lasting relationship.

Explanation and Interpretation

It is difficult to appreciate the number of times it may be necessary to provide information and explanations about a child's condition before it is understood and integrated by the parents. When family members are emotionally upset by the information they are receiving, they may fail totally to hear explanations. Moreover, different levels of understanding are appropriately incorporated by the family at different stages of the child's illness. One method that may be extremely helpful is to ask parents on a follow-up visit to relate to the pediatrician the things that were discussed at the last visit. Gaps or distortions suggest areas requiring further review.

The pediatrician plays an important role in translating the medical explanation into its effects on everyday life in order to help in concrete planning. For example, the family of a diabetic child may have been told that the symptoms of hypoglycemia may be induced by exercise, especially when insulin is peaking, but they may still require explanation that afterschool sports activities are a time of increased vulnerability for this problem.

The family may need help in explaining the illness to the patient and his siblings. Families may be caught off guard if they are not prepared to expect questions and to anticipate the need to provide answers. In giving advice, the pediatrician should use his knowledge of normal child development and of the young child's concrete and magical thinking. It is also useful to anticipate the questions that may be raised by friends and relatives. Parents should be encouraged to give honest, simple answers to questions, rather than to get themselves into complicated patterns of deception. This approach must be balanced against their desire to protect themselves from prying and unwarranted interference in their privacy.

Assistance in Monitoring the Illness

Plans should be made for the pediatrician to monitor the chronic condition jointly with the subspecialist, even when highly technologic and toxic treatments are involved. Involving the pediatrician reduces the overall cost of care to the family and makes practice more satisfying to both the pediatrician and subspecialist.[9,10]

An essential aspect of monitoring illness is continued education of the family in preventing avoidable problems, controlling symptoms, and carrying out treatments. Much assistance can also be provided in adjusting to the course of the illness. This joint participation in ongoing management of a child with chronic illness minimizes the probability of overlooking important aspects of care.

Coordination of Care

A frequent concern of families of children with chronic health problems is the lack of a single identified professional with overall responsibility for directing care. It has been suggested that the ". . . ultimate responsibility for coordination remains with the physician. The actual tasks involved can be assigned to an allied professional or trained lay assistant."[11] Families of chronically ill children are often asked to interact with a large number of professionals and systems, for both the medical and psychosocial issues, and they need and want a single person to coordinate the many demands for their time and energy. They may receive conflicting professional advice and appreciate help in sorting it out.

These needs can usually be met directly by the pediatrician.

On some occasions the pediatrician may find it necessary to assist in obtaining a second opinion or consultation. The judicious use of consultation may be helpful to a family struggling with a difficult decision or confronted with upsetting information.

In coordinating care it is helpful to know that the guilt and anger of chronically ill children and their families is sometimes directed to professionals. These reactions must be recognized by the pediatrician when they occur so that the family can be helped to acknowledge their feelings as normal and so that the pediatrician can continue to work effectively with the family.

As the coordinator of the child's overall health care, the pediatrician performs many other important functions. By remaining the central person, he helps to balance general and special health needs of the child and to balance the family's overall priorities with the child's needs. These are not always identical. When there is conflict among these factors, the pediatrician can help maintain a perspective and shape a long-range plan. During periods of hospitalization or surgical intervention, he may serve as an important member of the care team. His role is central in preparing the family for different phases of care. Perhaps most helpful of all is the pediatrician's ability to build on and encourage the strengths and coping of the child and family, whom he often knows better and longer than any of the other health care personnel.

Listening to Concerns

Surveys have shown that the most remarkable gap in services provided to chronically ill children and their families is the lack of someone who listens to their concerns. Many of the suggestions described above are of little help if they do not address the main concerns and preoccupations of the family. Unexpressed worries and fears are frequently a source of great anxiety and of inappropriate guilt. It may seem extravagant in a busy practice to set aside a special appointment for the family of chronically ill children to talk with the physician. However, a few minutes devoted directly to such concerns may be an efficient use of time, allowing the physician to avoid irrelevant tangents arising from unverbalized fears. One effective method of eliciting these concerns is to suggest that relatives, neighbors, and friends often raise questions and television and magazines suggest information that the family would like to clarify or discuss to determine its relevance to their child's situation. Frequently, it is easier for a parent or child to express a concern, particularly one highly charged emotionally, if it can be raised as someone else's question. Consistent attention of the pediatrician to these issues during casual visits may be more effective than devoting one long conference to them. Each contact is able to build on the base of the previous one.

Provision of Direct Services for Health Care Maintenance

Many parents, preoccupied by a serious health problem, overlook the need for regular check-ups to provide immunization, do routine screening, monitor growth and development, assess nutrition and dentition, and evaluate overall adjustment and school performance. These areas are sorely neglected in the care of chronically ill children, whose need for a periodic comprehensive reassessment and for many concrete services is even more pressing than that of a well child. The pediatrician has particular expertise in these general areas, and providing these services is important. When the pediatrician is uncertain about specific issues concerning the effect of the chronic medical problem on normal growth and development or preventive measures, he should not hesitate to consult with the appropriate subspecialist.

Care of Intercurrent Illnesses

Children with chronic medical problems get the usual intercurrent illnesses at least as frequently as well children, and these episodes usually are treated by the pediatrician. However, as discussed below, the pediatrician should also be knowledgeable about any special risks related to the underlying chronic illness. Parents of chronically ill children often have anxiety about whether an intercurrent condition will affect the child's underlying condition, even in instances in which there are no special risks. Evidence of this is amply demonstrated by Levy[12] in studies of pediatric emergency room visits, in which it was found that as many as one third of the visits were prompted by parental concerns related to a previous illness or perceived vulnerability. Unless these issues of "second agendas" are addressed, families tend to be dissatisfied with the care and worried that the physician did not appreciate the child's special problem.

Questions of Genetic and Familial Risks

Parents of children who have a chronic condition are almost universally concerned about the possibilities that other members of their family may develop the illness. Even in the absence of a familial risk, each parent tends to blame him or herself, as well as the other parent, for the child's condition. Moreover, it is not uncommon for parents subconsciously to want to replace the chronically ill child with a normal one, in order to demonstrate their adequacy as parents capable of producing a normal child. It is important, therefore, to discuss genetic or familial risks in a forthright and supportive manner with the best available information. When there is a recognized genetic pattern of transmission, it is necessary to help the family deal with their guilt and to stress that they did not choose to have genes that caused a problem in their offspring. As children approach adolescence, parents often are concerned about the reproductive potential of their chronically ill child, as well as the possibility of their other children producing a child with the same condition. All of these issues require discussion.

Advice on Childrearing

A common reaction of parents of a chronically ill child is to give them extra attention and overprotect them. This well-intentioned behavior serves to confuse the child and may delay normal psychologic and social development. There are many aspects of such behavior that the pediatrician is in an ideal position to discuss.

Parents need help in knowing what their child is competent to do and in encouraging appropriate activities and independence. They should be urged to help develop interests and abilities in compensatory areas in which the child can experience gratification. Current information suggests that problems of adjustment may be as frequent and severe in children with only minimal or absent functional limitations as in those with obvious deficits. Therefore, the pediatrician should be concerned with providing advice on childrearing and assistance in normalizing child development in the most marginally ill children as well as in those with severe or overwhelming problems.

COORDINATION WITH SUBSPECIALISTS

There must be a clearly designated plan for coordination between the pediatrician and the pediatric subspecialist. A number of studies have shown that there are large portions of total care that are not met by either provider alone. The pattern of significant gaps in services received by children with ongoing health problems suggests a generalized problem. For example, less than 20% of children with arthritis or birth defects had most areas of service covered adequately.[4] In another survey,[5] it was demonstrated that one third of children in subspecialty clinics, selected because of frequent visits, had no source of primary care, 60% had other perceived health needs, and 38% had problems that they had never discussed with a medical provider.

These trends have been documented also in our studies of urban children with a wide array of chronic conditions.[13] More importantly, they do not appear to be influenced by demographic or social factors or the degree of disability.[5]

The following is an outline of steps that may be helpful in coordinating care between the primary care pediatrician and the pediatric subspecialist.

The Referral Process

At the time a referral is made to a subspecialist, it is useful to discuss the referral process directly with the parent and to set the tone for good communication among the subspecialist, the referring pediatrician, and the family. The pediatrician should offer to be in direct contact with the subspecialist. The majority of families welcome this type of communication, especially when it can be demonstrated that unnecessary duplication of tests and procedures may be avoided by transfer of information between physicians. Parental consent for transfer of information should be obtained. It is helpful if the referring physician indicates the nature of his questions and concerns and gives some indication of whether he is requesting a consultation, joint continuous management, or, in rare instances, a complete transfer of care to the subspecialist. If the referring physician and the consultant see their roles differently, it is important to clarify the nature of their respective responsibilities with one another and with the family.

Outlining a Plan

A mechanism should be established to communicate the result of the initial consultation and, if additional procedures are indicated, to outline the steps that will be taken in the diagnostic work-up. It should be determined which physician will help to coordinate necessary procedures and who will communicate the arrangements and interpret the results to the family.

Once the nature of the condition is clarified, the frequency of visits with the subspecialist should be discussed. The components of care should be outlined specifically between the two physicians to determine which physician will provide each. Guidelines should be delineated for regular monitoring of the patient and should include the subspecialist's recommendations. In many instances, it may be possible to delegate the responsibility for monitoring the patient to the pediatrician, with less frequent visits to the subspecialist. This process works extremely well in those circumstances in which the pediatrician and subspecialist agree on the criteria for reinvolvement of the subspecialist. It is appropriate to define symptoms and laboratory test results that would warrant further evaluation by the subspecialist and to discuss signs and symptoms of complications that might be anticipated or require special attention. It is useful to review any precautions related to preventive procedures (e.g., withholding of live vaccines from immunosuppressed children) and signs of toxicity (e.g., cataracts in children taking steroids).

When the pediatrician is unfamiliar with the subspecialist's advice, it may be initially embarrassing to ask for a review of the plan of treatment and the prognosis. An overriding principle should be that if the information is not clear to the practitioner, it is most certainly not clear to the family and deserves further exploration. Both physicians feel most comfortable when they are sure that the patient's best interest will be served by such discussions.

Establishing Mechanisms of Communication

The subspecialist and pediatrician should determine the most practical way to communicate with one another, whether by phone, in person, through written transfer of information, or a combination of these mechanisms. When such communication exists, the pediatrician can play an important role in clarifying information and explanation for the family. Moreover, regular communications enable subspecialist and pediatrician to be consistent in their interpretation of information to the family. Without direct communication, it is extremely difficult to sort out the important misconceptions and denial on the part of the parents or patient.

Whenever the family has contact with the subspecialist, it is extremely helpful for him to share the content of the visit directly with the pediatrician, so that the two doctors are working with the same information. In addition, the pediatrician may find it useful to ask the family to share information with him about the visit to the subspecialist. This may provide an opportunity for the family to ask questions and obtain clarification about issues that were unclear at the time of the consultation. If obvious answers are not available, it is appropriate to suggest a follow-up contact with the subspecialist for further clarification.

It is also important to recognize that there may be occasional problems in communications between the pediatrician and the subspecialist. One of the reasons for this, which may be overlooked, is that some families respond to their imposed dependency on health professionals by becoming hostile or by exercising a degree of control through establishing conflict among the professionals. In such instances, the family may complain to each physician about the behavior of other professionals involved in the child's care. The provider coordinating care must be aware of this risk and help to recognize this situation when it occurs, rather than become a participant in the conflict. While this situation may create an initial impulse on the part of the pediatrician to withdraw from the situation and to let the family manage the care on their own, it should be recognized as one of many normal reactions of the family to a stressful situation. If this behavior can be seen as a signal of distress, it becomes easier for the physicians to talk with one another in order to help the family obtain the services they need. On some occasions, it may be useful for the physicians to meet together with the family and to demonstrate their unwillingness to be drawn into a conflict that is harmful for the child.

Periodic Reassessment

In situations in which joint management continues over many years, it is useful to have regular contact between the involved physicians. The subdivision of care may need periodic reassessment as the abilities and needs of the child, family, and physicians change over time. Sometimes changes occur in the distribution of responsibilities without deliberate decisions by the respective physicians. In order to avoid repetition or default in important areas of service, it is best to review the respective roles at regular intervals. In addition, such discussion of the child's management provides the pediatrician with continuing education and understanding of the special problems that may arise in a particular case. It also helps to increase the pediatrician's confidence in the adequacy of his care. Finally, it provides a high standard of care for the chronically ill child by ensuring that the primary practitioner's expertise is included in all phases of the treatment.

PROBLEMS COMMON TO ALL CHILDREN WITH CHRONIC ILLNESS

Much of the literature in pediatrics has focused on the differences between children with individual diseases rather than the common issues faced by all children with chronic illness and by their families. While only the minority of chronic conditions produce significant functional limitations or need for intensive medical care, virtually all are of significant concern to the family. The concerns are often addressed directly or indirectly to the pediatrician. From a perspective of primary care, both in treatment and in the prevention of secondary handicaps, there is often great similarity in the needs and services required. These are the very areas in which care has been most lacking in the past and in which the pediatrician is the legitimate expert. In light of this, it seems useful to suggest an outline that primary care pediatricians can use in focusing on special needs of children with chronic medical problems and their families.

Understanding and Anticipating the Normal Reaction to Illness

Regardless of the diagnosis, a family confronted with information about a serious chronic condition in their child is likely to respond immediately with a sense of shock and denial. This reaction is usually followed fairly quickly by grief, anger, and often depression. In many instances, the family experiences bereavement and mourns the loss of a normal child, even when there is no threat of death. During this period, their focus may be on getting through the next 24 hours rather than on long-term planning, and they may be unable to incorporate much of the information that is given to them. At times the anger is directed toward professionals, and it may be difficult for the pediatric staff to deal with it, particularly when they share the family's discouragement with their inability to solve or reverse the problem. During this period, it is especially important for the pediatrician to understand these reactions and not to feel personally threatened or defensive. Reactive responses to the family's anger and accusations result only in a battle with the parents and interfere with their ultimate ability to use the services that are needed. With time, the family begins to accept the reality of the illness and is able to move on to areas of concrete planning for short- and long-range needs and the issues of normalizing their lives within the context of the special health problem. The more overwhelming emotional reactions are often reactivated during exacerbations of the illness.

Certain critical developmental stages also seem particularly fraught with risk for reactivation of intense emotional feelings. These include the beginning of independent functioning of the toddler, school entry, the end of latency, and early adolescence. It appears that during these times families become more intensively aware of functional limitations, special needs, and differences between the child with a chronic medical problem and normal children. It is extremely useful to help families by acknowledging their feelings and expressing confidence that these are normal reactions for which they need not have additional guilt.

Effect on the Family

The presence of a chronic illness in a child has significant effects on all members of the family. Initially, it may cause major disruption and disequilibrium, often resulting in social isolation of the family members and restriction of normal lifestyles. Families with the most marginal function appear to be the ones most likely to experience severe disruption. The pediatrician should be able to assist families through the period of disequilibrium and to help them move toward a stage of reorganization and normalization of family life. This function is particularly important in view of the observation that overall family function appears to be an important predictor of long-range adjustment of the chronically ill child.[14]

There are many aspects of family life in which the pediatrician can assist the family. Offering an opportunity to discuss some of the demands that the illness is placing on the family and supporting them in dealing with difficult problems can be of great help. An informed professional can also assist by translating the specific therapeutic regimen into a manageable form and distinguishing between unnecessary rigidity and important medical priorities.

Ultimately, the pediatrician can help the family achieve a degree of control by increasing their competence in managing the condition and in handling mild fluctuations. The family will feel less vulnerable and dependent if allowed to play an active role in choosing among alternative approaches. In addition, they may benefit a great deal from the physician's confidence in their ability to cope.

It is important that the pediatrician, who may have more frequent contact with the child's mother, include the father whenever possible. A small gesture on the part of the pediatrician in reaching out to him can result in a significant change in the father's role in relationship to the child's illness and to the family.

Another primary responsibility of the pediatrician is to recognize the potential effect of the child's illness on healthy siblings in the family. Siblings may have significant adverse personal consequences as a result of the stress the illness places on them and the family. It is extremely important for the pediatrician to help by encouraging the family to use appropriate supports and by suggesting that a serious medical problem may create stress for other members of the family who may need extra assistance. If families think it is unusual for family members to need counseling, they are more likely to experience an additional sense of failure when it is recommended. Assistance may be provided directly by the pediatrician or through referral.

Encourage Self-care and Health Knowledge

The primary care pediatrician should have a continuous role in teaching the families of children with chronic illness to assume increasing responsibility and to decrease their dependence on the health care system. This process must be done with a clear understanding of the illness and its risks, but it is an important step in normalizing life. The parents should be encouraged to share responsibility with the child within the limits of his capabilities. Ultimately, the patient should become as independent and self-sufficient as possible. Assisting the child in developing an age-appropriate sense of mastery is a fundamental task of childrearing, which is as important in the family dealing with a child with a special condition as it is in raising a normal child.

Schooling and Future Planning

One of the primary tasks of childhood is participating in school activities. Failure to integrate a child with a chronic illness into an appropriate school placement may lead to excessive absenteeism and to secondary educational and social consequences and handicaps for the child. Under Public Law 94-142 the health care provider and the school system share responsibility for planning necessary educational resources in the "least restrictive" environment. Schools are often ill equipped to accept children with primary medical, rather than primary educational, needs. Parents deserve realistic information about schools, the degree of functional limitation imposed by the child's chronic condition, and the level of participation the child can handle. Many school personnel are hesitant to include a chronically ill child in a classroom and may be unnecessarily restrictive. A telephone call from the physician, with the permission of the parent, often alleviates unwarranted restrictions and fears on the part of the school personnel and improves their understanding of the real versus fictitious issues. Liaison with the school staff may be necessary throughout the child's school years, and as the child reaches adolescence, both school and parents may need assistance in allowing the youngster to reach appropriate independence. In order to plan realistically for the future, parents should have ongoing information and opportunity to ask questions and participate with the pediatrician and school personnel.

Knowledge of Community Supports and Resources

Many families of chronically ill children experience significant economic difficulties on the basis of their children's health-related needs and expenses. The pediatrician and subspecialist can be of great assistance in referring the family for appropriate assistance and familiarizing them with special resources. These include eligibility for special benefits under federal, state, and local programs, such as the Crippled Children's Program of Maternal Child Health or Medicaid programs. Some legislation is categorical, that is, it depends on the presence of certain diagnostic labels, while other programs are based on financial eligibility or on the presence of functional limitations. The pediatrician and subspecialist should familiarize themselves with local eligibility requirements and referral procedures for special benefits in the areas of health, education, and social services.

In addition, many communities have resources that provide support and counseling services. Parents' groups and special disease-oriented programs, such as local chapters of private foundations (e.g., March of Dimes), and of disease-based programs, such as Cystic Fibrosis, Juvenile Diabetes, or Hemophilia foundations, provide many opportunities for families to deal with practical problems of raising a child with serious chronic illness and to reduce their sense of social isolation. Many states and cities have directories of such facilities. Families who have had to work out solutions to practical problems in the community are often eager to serve as a resource to help other families of children with similar needs. The pediatrician can be extremely helpful in introducing such families to one another but should do so only after obtaining the permission of the families in order not to violate their confidentiality and privacy.

SUMMARY

The primary care pediatrician has many critical roles to play in helping to maintain the integrity of a child with a chronic medical problem. He must help the family to maintain a sense of equilibrium and to adjust to a life that is responsive to the child's medical and health care needs but is not totally dominated and orchestrated by it. Goals of management should be to help the child and family adjust to the illness and to maximize the health and potential of the child. The pediatrician is an important member of the team and must work closely with the subspecialist, the family, and the patient. He is in an optimal position to help to prevent unnecessary physical and psychologic handicaps as a result of the illness. The pediatrician cares for a large number of families, many of whose children have some ongoing medical problems, and he is in an ideal position to anticipate questions, universalize feelings, support strengths, encourage coping, and provide honest and patient counsel. In situations in which "care" rather than "cure" can be offered, the pediatrician plays an essential role with the family and the subspecialist in helping to maximize health for the child and his family unit.

REFERENCES

1. Ireys HT: Health care for chronically disabled children and their families. Select Panel on the Promotion of Child Health, Better Health for our Children: A National Strategy, Vol IV. Washington, DC, US Government Printing Office, 1981, pp 321–353

2. Pless IB, Pinkerton P: Chronic Childhood Disorder: Promoting Patterns of Adjustment. Chicago, Year Book, 1975

3. Kanthor H, Pless IB, Satterwhite B, Myers G: Areas of responsibility in the health care of multiply handicapped children. Pediatrics 54:779, 1974

4. McAnarney EB, Pless IB, Satterwhite B, Friedman S: Psychological problems of children with chronic juvenile arthritis. Pediatrics 53:523, 1974

5. Palfrey J, Levy JC, Gilbert KL: Use of primary care facilities by patients attend-

ing specialty clinics. Pediatrics 65:567, 1980

6. Green M, Haggerty RJ (eds): Ambulatory Pediatrics - II. Philadelphia, Saunders, 1977

7. Lefton E, Lefton M: Health care and treatment for the chronically ill: toward a conceptual framework. J Chronic Dis 32:339, 1979

8. Allmond BW Jr., Buckman W, Gofman HF: The Family Is the Patient—An Approach to Behavioral Pediatrics for the Clinician. St. Louis, Mosby, 1979

9. Kisker CT, Strayer F, Wong K, et al.: Health outcomes of a community-based therapy program for children with cancer—a shared-management approach. Pediatrics 66:900, 1980

10. Strayer F, Kisker CT, Fethke C: Cost-effectiveness of a shared-management delivery system for the care of children with cancer. Pediatrics 66:90, 1980

11. Pless IB, Roghmann KJ: Chronic illness and its consequences: observations based on three epidemiologic surveys. J Pediatr 79:351, 1971

12. Levy JC: Vulnerable children: parents' perspectives and the use of medical care. Pediatrics 65:956, 1980

13. Stein REK, Jessop DJ, Riessman CK: Health care services received by chronically ill children. Am J Dis Child. 137:225, 1983

14. Pless IB, Satterwhite B: Health and illness: chronic illness. In Haggerty RJ, Roghmann KJ, Pless IB (eds): Child Health and the Community. New York, Wiley, 1975

Cross-Reference to *Pediatrics,* 17th ed.

THREE

The Recurrently Ill Child

Louis Borgenicht

The Family: A unit composed not only of children, but of men, women, the occasional animal, and the common cold.

Ogden Nash

The problem of the always sick or recurrently ill child is a common and often frustrating one, producing anxiety for practitioners and families alike. The basis of concern is that the child who suffers from what seems to be an excessive share of the usual childhood diseases has some underlying chronic, organic medical condition that predisposes him to recurrent illness. In the majority of patients, this is not the case, and the affected patient is merely reflecting the normal spectrum of childhood illness.

Given the frequency of the problem and limited medical resources, it is essential that practitioners develop a systematic approach to the recurrently ill child. This chapter, limited to preschool and school-aged children who suffer from recurrent, minor illnesses (primarily respiratory and gastrointestinal) but who enjoy normal good health during the intervening illness-free periods, is structured to incorporate such a systematic approach (Table 1).

FREQUENCY OF THE PROBLEM

Most practitioners concur with statements found in the major pediatric texts that 50–60% of patient visits in early childhood are because of acute problems. The majority of these are respiratory and gastrointestinal infections and are self-limited, requiring little intervention. The fact that approximately 10% of a general pediatric population will develop some chronic disorder by age 15 (the majority of these being allergic) puts this into clearer perspective. Most children do not become seriously ill from life-threatening or handicapping problems.

The sources of morbidity for the average child vary with age and season. Normal children are protected against most infectious illnesses by placentally transmitted maternal antibody during the first 6 months of life. As children expand their social and school contacts, their risk of contracting one of the usual childhood diseases naturally increases. The peak incidence for common respiratory illness is at 2–4 years of age. Gastrointestinal illnesses follow a similar pattern but peak at ages 5–7.

Acute respiratory problems tend to occur in the late fall and early winter, whereas gastrointestinal problems are more variable in occurrence. Exacerbations of allergies, of course, may develop at any time, depending on the allergen and a number of other factors.

Several studies corroborate these gener-

**TABLE 1. THE WORK-UP OF THE
RECURRENTLY ILL CHILD:
A SIMPLIFIED WORKSHEET**

History:
    Age of onset
    System involved
    Location involved
    Type of infection
    Response to treatment
    Frequency of problem
Parental Expectation:
    What is normal to them?
    What were parents' pediatric problems?
Environmental Factors:
    Family stress
    Overcrowding
    Allergic environment
    Dryness
Psychosocial Factors:
    What is family's illness story?
    Is this a vulnerable child?

al comments, e.g., Dingle, and Roghman. Hill provides a concise summary:

It has been estimated that such children (patients who suffer from recurrent infections) have an average of six respiratory infections per year; it is not unusual, however, for them to have as many as twelve in a year. If one assumes that prodrome, illness, and convalescence takes approximately two weeks for each infection, then a child can be sick 12–24 weeks (3–6 months) a year and still be within the range of normal.

GENERAL APPROACHES TO THE DIAGNOSIS OF THE RECURRENTLY ILL CHILD

History

A number of general questions will help the practitioner to evaluate a child with recurrent illness.

What are the parents' expectations about illness in their child? What is a normal amount of illness to them? What are the history and pattern of illnesses in the family up to this point? Answers will provide a sense of the specific and general concerns and how the family is coping with the current problem.

What were the parents' problems during childhood? Often similar patterns of illness are repeated in subsequent generations for a variety of complex and poorly understood reasons.

Is the recurrently ill child viewed as a "vulnerable child?" If so, why? Is this child a "nonmedically vulnerable" child (one with no evidence of organic illness that might have sensitized the family)? One may need to do more factual counseling with families in this latter category.

Are there environmental factors of relevance? Family stress? Overcrowding? An allergic environment? Dry climate? Some of these factors may be modifiable.

What has the family done about the problem? What are their expectations from you now? Specific answers will permit more specific responses.

Physical Examination

The severity and general physical impact of any problem, particularly a recurrent one, may be assessed best by an examination of the child's growth. Although significant chronic illness disturbs growth more than do simple, acute, self-limited infectious problems, a prolonged series of recurrent illnesses can impede growth. A child with 6 months of otitis media may temporarily plateau on the growth curve. Weight may be disproportionately affected. In the child with chronic debilitating disease, all growth parameters are affected, and the change persists.

Observation of family interaction in the examination room may permit the practitioner to assess the emotional impact of the problem. Behavioral cues may help clarify how the recurrently ill child is perceived by the parents. Their degree of frustration and occasional inability to tolerate behavioral infractions may be evident from casually noting family responses during the course of the patient's visit.

Laboratory Examination

Two relatively nonspecific laboratory tests, a complete blood count (CBC) and erythrocyte sedimentation rate (ESR), may be indicated to give the practitioner a general guideline about the health status of the child. Anemia is readily detected, and an elevated ESR may suggest an inflammatory or infectious process. Occasionally, the incidental finding of eosinophilia is helpful in pursuing the possibility of allergic or parasitic disease.

SPECIFIC APPROACHES TO THE DIFFERENTIAL DIAGNOSIS

Immunologic Problems

Despite the fact that the most common clinical entities causing recurrent illness are respiratory and gastrointestinal, many practitioners are concerned initially with the possibility that the child may have an immunodeficiency disorder. Accurate information about the frequency of clinically significant immunodeficiency disease is lacking in the current literature. The most common immunodeficiency problem is hypogammaglobulinemia A, with an estimated prevalence of 1 in 700. However, most individuals with this immunoglobulin disorder are asymptomatic. Only 60–70 cases of clinically significant immunodeficiency states are diagnosed in the United States per year. These figures, however, may reflect laboratory insensitivity in identifying immunologic abnormalities rather than the true frequency of certain disorders. Iatrogenic immunodeficiency disorders may become more significant over the next few years as serious illnesses (e.g., juvenile rheumatoid arthritis, lymphoma, nephrotic syndrome) are treated with steroids and other potent chemotherapeutic agents. Acquired secondary immunodeficiency problems are more common in certain patients (e.g., those with sickle cell anemia) who become asplenic either functionally or from surgery.

History. Certain aspects of a child's past history should raise one's index of suspicion about the possibility of an immunologic problem.

- Has there been a series of unusually severe infections (e.g., meningitis, pneumonia, abcesses)? Was the infection an unusually severe presentation for a usually less problematic organism (e.g., an infant who developed staphylococcal sepsis from what appeared to be uncomplicated skin infection)? These may be associated with disorders of cell-mediated immunity.
- Was the infection caused by an uncommon infectious agent? Immunoglobulin deficiency disorders may be manifested by repeated infections with common organisms. Problems of cell-mediated immunity may predispose the patient to infection with uncommon agents (e.g., *Pneumocystis carinii*).
- Did the child have problems with neonatal hypocalcemia? Certain immunologic problems, such as thymic hypoplasia (with an associated disorder of the parathyroid gland), can present as neonatal hypocalcemia.

Although the inheritance of many immunologic disorders is unclear, some have delineated inheritance patterns (e.g., panhypogammaglobulinemia). In any event, a detailed family history of recurrent infection and even parathyroid, thyroid, or adrenal problems may clue the practitioner into looking closer at possible immune system dysfunction.

Physical Examination and Laboratory Findings. Some immunologic disorders, such as thymic hypoplasia, are associated with characteristics facies or other physical findings. In most, however, the findings are nonspecific. Some helpful features are shown in Table 2.

Respiratory Problems

History. Particular aspects of the past history are relevant in evaluating a child with recurrent respiratory problems.

- How old was the child at the onset of the problem? Serious infections at an early age, before frequent peer contacts occur, may indicate an underlying chronic disorder (e.g., cystic fibrosis, immune disorder).
- Was the problem localized to one specific anatomic area (e.g., right middle lobe of the lung, sinuses)? Anatomic factors, such as impinging lymph nodes or vascular structures, may predispose to infections in a localized area.
- What were the specific infecting agents (e.g., viral, bacterial, unclear), and what is the frequency of the problem? A significant

number of lower respiratory problems may be allergic in origin, yet be labeled "pneumonia" or "bronchopneumonia." Bronchial plugging in different areas of the lung may lead to atelectasis and secondary infection. Some allergists feel that a second radiographic diagnosis of pneumonia in a year's time should lead to a full investigation for allergy. A family history of allergy or cystic fibrosis is important to ascertain. Social history will determine if there are others in the household with whom the child may trade infectious agents. Close contacts that the child may have outside the home (e.g., day care center, nursery school) may be important.

A detailed, chronologically precise history of present illness is extremely helpful.

- Are there symptoms of allergy, such as runny nose, itchy nose or eyes, sneezing,

TABLE 2. PHYSICAL EXAMINATION AND LABORATORY FINDINGS IN CHILDREN WITH POSSIBLE ORGANIC ETIOLOGY FOR RECURRENT ILLNESS

Parameter	Finding/Test	Significance/Comment
Physical examination	Hepatosplenomegaly, persistent seborrheic or eczematoid rashes, conjunctivitis, failure to gain expected weight, chronic candidiasis	Separately or in combination may indicate problem of the immune system
	Chest pain/x-ray	Abnormal cardiac shadow, possible spontaneous pneumothorax, size of thymus
Laboratory	CBC and differential	Detect neutropenia associated with certain cell-mediated disorders
	Immunoelectrophoresis	Compare with age-related values to detect specific immunoglobin abnormalities
	Nitroblue tetrazolium test	Tests better done by consultant
	Candida, streptokinase/streptodornase, tetanus skin test, isohemagglutinin titers, polio, diphtheria, tetanus titers in previously immunized child	

swollen eyes, constant throat clearing? These are all suggestive of atopic problems. The clearing of the throat may be evidence of postnasal drip or sinus drainage on a partially allergic basis. Is there a night time or early morning cough? Asthma may be a consideration.

- Was there an episode of aspiration? An infant with a tracheoesophageal fistula or, more commonly, reflux, may be prone to aspiration with feeding. The possibility that a foreign body has been aspirated and has lodged in the lower respiratory tract is a concern in the 2–4 year old.
- Has there been unilateral nasal discharge (e.g., yellow-green and foul-smelling)? A foreign body lodged in a nostril should be considered.
- What specific medications have been used (e.g., decongestants, antihistamines, antibiotics)? The response of a patient to both the efficacy and the side effects of most medications used to treat upper respiratory infections symptomatically tends to be very individual and idiosyncratic. One can plan future therapy on the results of past treatment.

Physical Examination and Laboratory Findings. Allergy is associated with a number of moderately specific physical and laboratory findings. These are summarized in Table 3.

Management. Most recurrent respiratory problems can be handled well by the primary practitioner, and symptomatic management of recurrent upper respiratory infections (URI) is a keynote of most daily practices. Recurrent otitis media requires a more careful approach. Follow-up of every episode with pneumatic otoscopy is a necessity. After three episodes of otitis in a 6-month period, or with unremittent otitis requiring several courses of antibiotics, a tympanogram should be obtained. If the results suggest abnormal mid-dle ear function, referral should be made to an otolaryngologist. (See Chapter 8.) The primary practitioner may be able to gain some time before referring by a number of pharmacologic maneuvers:

1. A trial of different antihistamines or decongestants for persistent serious otitis media. Although the efficacy of these preparations is hotly debated, an empirical trial of antihistamines might be efficacious. Weekly follow-up and changing of medications is necessary.
2. A trial of prophylactic antibiotics may help the child who is having repeated episodes of otitis. The drugs of choice are sulfisoxazole or trimethoprim/sulfmethoxazole daily for 2–3 months or more. (See Table 2 in Chapter 8.)

Allergic problems can be readily handled by the practitioner without referral to the specialist in the majority of cases. The diagnosis, which is based primarily on the history and physical, can be done easily by the primary care practitioner. Special attention must be paid to instituting environmental controls over the allergenic household; e.g., plastic covers over mattresses, nonallergenic pillows and curtains, no rugs, no pets, and marked attempts to decrease dust. These efforts are often more useful than any pharmacologic therapy. Bronchodilators (even for simple nighttime cough) and antihistamines are the mainstays of therapy.

Gastrointestinal Problems
History. The past history of gastrointestinal problems is important to obtain.

- How old was the child at the onset of the problem? Chronic nonspecific diarrhea (a diagnosis of exclusion) often starts in infancy.
- How long do the symptoms (e.g., pain or diarrhea) last, and are they affected by any therapeutic interventions? Many families

TABLE 3. PHYSICAL EXAMINATIONS AND LABORATORY FINDINGS IN CHILDREN WITH POSSIBLE ALLERGIC ETIOLOGY FOR RECURRENT ILLNESS

Parameter	Finding/Test	Significance/Comment
Physical examination	Clear, watery rhinorrhea; pale, boggy, swollen, nasal turbinates	Allergic rhinitis
	Swelling, redness of periorbital tissues	
	Conjunctival redness	
	Dark vascular rings below eyes	
	"Allergic salute" (upward wiping of nose with hand)	
	Expiratory wheezing (pre- or post-exertion)	Asthmatic bronchitis
	Kyphotic or barrel chest	
	Prolonged expiratory phase	
	Distended abdomen with thin extremities	Cystic fibrosis with possible intrinsic liver disease or pulmonary hyperinflation
	Variable auscultatory findings	
	Clubbing of fingers	
	Hepatomegaly	
Laboratory	Throat culture	Detect beta-hemolytic streptococci
	Chest x-ray (PA/lateral)	Detect chronic respiratory disease and anatomic anomalies
	Sputum cultures, tracheal aspirates, nasopharyngeal cultures	Determine bacterial etiologies
	Nasal smear	Eosinophils suggest allergy
	Sinus films (even a simple Water's view)	Sinusitis a possibility
	Sweat chloride	Elevated in cystic fibrosis
	Viral cultures	Costly and less routine

will have tried a series of dietary manipulations (changing diets as frequently as every 12 hours) to alleviate the problem and may expect miraculous cures.

- Are the symptoms related to diet? Dietary intolerances or allergies may be suggested.
- Has there been exposure to unsafe water supplies either at home or during travel? Infectious agents, such as *Salmonella, Shigella, Giardia lamblia,* and *Campylobacter,* are possibilities.

- Has growth been affected? True failure to thrive indicates more serious pathology than a minor recurrent gastrointestinal problem.
- Have urinary tract infections (UTI) been a problem? Urinary infections can masquerade as a recurrent gastrointestinal problem, with diarrhea or abdominal pain. Obtaining documentation of urinary infections from past medical records is essential. This may necessitate reviewing records

from previous practitioners to ascertain details of urine cultures, treatment, and evidence of whether the infection was in the upper or lower tract.

Family History. A family history of cystic fibrosis, gastrointestinal disease, nervous stomach, or irritable bowel is relevant. Chronic, nonspecific diarrhea tends to occur in families with a history of gastrointestinal problems. The 10% of school-aged children who may develop recurrent, nonspecific (functional) abdominal pain often have positive family histories for either gastrointestinal disease or gastrointestinal symptomatology. In only 10% of these children, however, can a definable organic cause for the pain be found.

Social History. Social history may reveal sources of family stress and disruption that a child with gastrointestinal symptoms tends to reflect through his symptoms. The abdomen is an easy target area for a child to focus on. It is essential that the practitioner obtain a sensitive understanding of family dynamics. In dealing with the child with a primary symptom of recurrent abdominal pain, important information may be gleaned by determining the family's response to the problem. Does the patient attend school when pain occurs? Does the pain occur more during times of stress? What kind of attention is given to the patient when in pain?

Present History. If there is vomiting and diarrhea, how frequent is it? A parent's perception of diarrhea and vomiting may be very different from the practitioner's. Strictly speaking, diarrhea refers to liquid stools occurring with greater than normal frequency. Vomiting is the forceful emptying of stomach contents and must be differentiated from spitting up or the secondary vomiting that may follow an episode of coughing.

• Has there been any blood or mucus in the stool? If so, infectious or inflammatory

bowel disease is a possibility. Do the stools float or smell unusually foul? If so, malabsorption should be considered.

Clinical Findings and Laboratory Data. Some of the characteristic findings on physical examination or laboratory testing are shown in Table 4.

Management. Recurrent gastrointestinal problems can be handled easily by the primary practitioner. Dietary manipulation is usually all that is necessary, and drug therapy rarely is needed or advisable. Viral gastroenteritis is treated with clear liquids (Pedialyte or Lytren in the bottle-feeding infant). UTIs presenting as diarrhea are treated with specific antibiotics. Chronic nonspecific diarrhea is more of a management problem because dietary manipulations seem to have little effect. Various pharmacologic approaches have been tried to little avail. Reassurance of the family that the disorder is simply "something to be coped with" and that it usually stops by the age of 3 often serves a useful purpose. A specific parent education sheet about this problem is helpful.

APPROACHES TO THE FAMILY

General

Once the determination has been made that the child does not have underlying chronic disease, the practitioner can begin to assist the family in its understanding of the problem and its ability to cope. Families with such children tend to utilize medical services sooner in any given illness and with greater frequency than do other families. Parents may be chronically anxious because they perceive their child as sicker than normal and may have an inordinate fear of early symptoms or signs of minor illness. They may feel that their child may have a unique suscep-

TABLE 4. PHYSICAL EXAMINATIONS AND LABORATORY FINDINGS IN CHILDREN WITH POSSIBLE ORGANIC GASTROINTESTINAL ETIOLOGY FOR RECURRENT ILLNESS

Parameter	Finding/Test	Significance/Comment
Physical examination	Nonspecific abdominal examination	Functional problems, gastroenteritis
	Impressive tenderness	Inflammatory bowel disease
	Intra-abdominal mass	Tumor
	Arthritis	Ulcerative collitis
	Erythema nodosum	Regional enteritis
	Edema	Malnutrition
	Ascites	Malabsorption syndromes, liver disease
	Tissue wasting	Malabsorption syndromes
Laboratory findings	Stool ova	Infectious etiology (further details in Chapter 7)
	Stool parasites	"
	Stool culture	"
	Stool fat, pH, reducing substance	Evidence of malabsorption; may be temporarily present following gastroenteritis
	Sweat chloride	Elevated in cystic fibrosis

tibility. An almost hypochondriacal dependency may develop between parent and child as a result of this unresolved anxiety. These families suffer from a significant degree of social disruption by having to adjust family activity and operations around the reality of an ill child. Parents may miss work, have their social and personal life disturbed, and suffer the increased emotional demands of the caretaking role. The ill child may miss school and be unable to participate in normal play activities. Healthy children in the same family may look on their ill sibling as privileged and may seek parental attention in unusual ways. Family stress is often the result of such dynamics, manifested both in intrafamily function and between health provider and family.

Within the family, certain definable conditions exist simply as a result of parental response to illness in a child. Parental guilt (e.g., "Did we do something wrong?" "Am I not taking care of my child properly?") may arise.

Many practitioners have a natural response to allay this parental guilt about minor illnesses. Recently, some have suggested that this may not be a totally valid approach. Herzog states that guilt may be an "unconscious process whereby people choose to blame themselves rather than admit that illness may be caused by mere chance and that nothing can be done to control it."[9] Parental anger because of time lost from work or other activities may develop and often be directed at the child. Finally, parental anxiety (present with any illness in a child but certainly exacerbated by illness in a recurrently ill child) may heighten the general emotional tension in the family and may further preclude the parent's ability to view the situation realistically.

Similarly, the intrafamily stress affects relationships with the family's health care practitioner. Some families present a demanding posture with which one has to deal. This is manifested by a number of behaviors and attitudes, such as provider shopping, searching for magic cures (e.g., tonsillectomy, alternative therapies, gamma globulin therapy), and persistent demands for antibiotics. Other families, in an effort to relieve some of the responsibility and perhaps guilt, form closely dependent attachments to a practitioner who is willing to listen to their concerns. The practitioner, then, is confronted with a difficult clinical and behavioral situation. He may share the parents' anxiety that the child is not within the range of normal and thus need to deal with both his anxiety and theirs.[10] Furthermore, the actual clinical management of such families is time consuming and demanding for the busy practitioner.

The Therapeutic Relationship

The degree of success that the practitioner may have with a family of a recurrently ill child can be measured by the nature of the trusting therapeutic relationship that evolves between the family and the practitioner. Open communication with the family is a necessity, and the reassurance that the provider will seek appropriate consultative assistance when the need arises is central to this issue. Very specific concerns and anxieties should be addressed as specifically as they are offered. The parents of a child with cervical adenitis, for example, who finally blurt out that they are worried that their child has leukemia should be told the facts of the situation. Sloughing over their misapprehension may lead to dissatisfaction on all levels. A number of leading, open-ended questions may assist in the quest to determine family concerns:

- What did you think the problem was?
- How serious did you think the problem was? Why?
- If there was one thing I could do for you, what would it be?
- What are you unable to do because of the illness?

A second way in which the therapeutic relationship can be set up is by the provider making a commitment either to see or to speak with the family every time the child becomes ill. This intense contact need last only for a short period of time (a few months). It serves not only to cement the provider's relationship with the family but also permits the physician to develop some understanding of the family's illness pattern.

Finally, the provider may need to discourage magical thinking on the part of the family. This does not mean that alternative approaches to these problems should necessarily be discouraged or demeaned but rather that they should be accepted as part of the general armamentarium for the family, assuming they are not harmful. Unrealistic thinking usually relates to the need for antibiotics to treat viral infections, tonsillectomy to cure upper respiratory infections, and the need for gamma globulin to help a susceptible child.

Education and Counseling

Certain educational and counseling issues must be dealt with as an adjunct to management. Clarification of past history is essential to remove inaccurate diagnoses from consideration in the general care of the child. An example of this is a child who carries a diagnosis of rheumatic heart disease on an uncertain basis.

Comprehensible language should be used in discussions with the family. Recent work has suggested that inadvertent or unclear comments by practitioners during the course of a visit may result in iatrogenically induced parental anxiety about the health of a child.[11] This can be well understood in connection with the concept of the vulnerable child, a notion first promulgated in 1964 by Green et al.[12] The authors studied families of 25 children who had recovered from a major, life-threatening illness early in life but who manifested separation difficulties (often abdominal pain before school), infantilization by parents, bodily overconcerns, and school underachievement in ensuing years. Their approach to the management of the problem is similar to the suggestions made here, and a review of the original article is worthwhile.

Conceptual issues that many families may not be familiar with need to be mentioned. The first of these is the notion of the natural history of disease. Useful catch phrases are: "Medicine is not an exact science." "Illnesses, especially acute ones, evolve" (e.g., URIs may develop into otitis). "Most children get better by themselves."

The second notion, often more difficult for parents to accept is that a transient baseline level of illness for a circumscribed period of time may be normal for a large number of children. Useful phrases are: "Some children just have a bad year of otitis." "The diarrheal episodes will usually stop by the age of 3" (used in conjunction with chronic nonspecific diarrhea). "Six to twelve colds per year may be normal." Retraining the family to adopt these views requires the equanimity of a philosopher, since they suggest that an overall laissez-faire view of illness be adopted. This is not easy for families that may be more used to an active, interventionist approach by health care providers.

Self-reliance

A final element in the approach to families with a recurrently ill child is getting the family to become largely self-reliant. Just as they have learned to trust your medical judgment initially, after a term of trial and much reassurance, they may be able to trust their own. They may be able both to assess medical problems realistically and to treat them logically. This takes time, perseverance, and education. There are two key elements in this area.

Intrafamily Dynamics. Making the family sufficiently aware of intrafamily dynamics so that it can adjust various roles with any given episode of illness. For example, the parental caretaker who is extremely close to a recurrently ill child may not be the best person to minister to the child's needs. The parent's anxiety may exacerbate the symptoms and the situation in general, and the overinvolved parent may need to give up the caretaking role temporarily.

Pediatric Self-care. The child can actually assume a large degree of responsibility for his own problems. The average preschool or school-aged child can do a lot more for himself than either the family or the practitioner expects. The asthmatic 4-year-old boy who awakens in the middle of the night coughing to the point of vomiting may awaken his parents for help and then spend the remainder of the evening with them. As this happens on subsequent evenings, the behavior (regardless of its organic base) gets reinforced. When the practitioner suggests that the child can handle his secretions himself by "coughing into a bowl by the bedside" and then "going back to sleep in his own bed," the child agrees. Other positive reinforcement is given: "I am sure you are old enough now to handle some of your problems yourself." Reassurance of the availability of parental aid if needed is also given: "Your parents will be in their room in case you are having problems that you cannot handle." A 2-week trial is suggested. Parents and practitioner are surprised 1 week later when not only has the behavior ceased but also the symptoms have abated. Pediatric self-care is not a fantasy. The concerned practitioner can promote it through skill, interest, commitment, and dealing directly with the child as well as the parents.

CONSULTATIVE EVALUATION OF THE RECURRENTLY ILL CHILD

General

Consultation with specialists serves an important role in both management and diagnosis. The practitioner's readiness to utilize a consultant to either corroborate a diagnosis or to suggest appropriate therapy may further garner a family's trust. It matters little whether the consultation is obtained primarily for the needs of the primary practitioner or because of a specific request from the family. The practitioner who responds to the question of a consultation in a non-threatened manner does much to improve his status with the family. It is important, however, for specific questions to be addressed to the consultant, for the practitioner to clarify the purpose of the consultation (i.e., evaluation, therapeutic suggestions, or assumption of care), and to follow up with the family shortly after the visit to the consultant. It is reasonable to ask the family to phone you 1–2 days after they have seen the consultant so that you can obtain some information even before a formal letter arrives and so that you can determine what they have learned from the specialist.

Respiratory Problems

The allergist is probably the most sought after consultant for the child who suffers from recurrent respiratory infections. Parents may wonder whether their allergic child needs shots. The practitioner may wonder whether a child's predilection to recurrent respiratory problems has a partially allergic basis. A few specific questions should be asked once the decision has been made to seek consultative help.

- Is part of this child's problem allergic in nature? If the practitioner feels unsure about the answer to this question, a second opinion is in order.
- Is this child on appropriate therapy for the problem? For the child already diagnosed as allergic but who has not responded to environmental controls and pharmacologic management, immunotherapy may be indicated. This use of the allergist should be considered only after the practitioner feels he is at a therapeutic dead end. A pulmonary specialist is consulted only rarely unless one has evidence for an anatomic problem,

such as recurrent localized pneumonia, chronic severe pulmonary disease, or suspicion of a tracheoesophageal fistula.

Gastrointestinal Problems

The child who suffers from recurrent bouts of GI symptoms (especially diarrhea) for which one can find no overt cause probably merits a consultation with a gastroenterologist. Again specific questions need to be asked:

- Is the problem suggestive of an anatomic, metabolic, or malabsorptive disorder?
- Is further evaluation necessary?
- Does the child have chronic, nonspecific diarrhea? A certain number of these children may require radiographic studies and even a biopsy before the benign diagnosis of nonspecific diarrhea can be considered with confidence. The family may also need short-term counseling from a qualified behavioral specialist familiar with this disorder.

Immunologic Problems

Referrals to allergists or clinical immunologists are rare because most significant immune disorders are uncommon. The patients who have clinically important immunologic problems should probably be followed conjointly by the specialist and the primary care practitioner.

SUMMARY

It is reasonable to expect a moderate number of patients in any practitioner's practice to be recurrently ill children. Their families are forced to cope with minor, usually self-limited illnesses on a continual basis. Thus, the stresses attendant to any illness in a child may become cumulative.

The challenge to the practitioner comes from having to apply his clinical as well as behavioral acumen to a situation on a recurring basis. An ultimate goal may be to decrease the continual need for intervention or assistance by the practitioner, placing some of the responsibility back on the family. This can be achieved through trust and understanding. In elemental terms the task may be simply that of getting the family to accept Ogden Nash's definition of The Family as a fact of life.

BIBLIOGRAPHY

Brewster AB: Chronically ill hospitalized children's concepts of their illness. Pediatrics 69:355, 1981

Carey WB, et al.: Avoiding pediatric pathogenesis in the management of acute minor illness. Pediatrics 49:553, 1972

Davidson M, et al.: The irritable colon of childhood (chronic nonspecific diarrhea syndrome). J Pediatr 69:1027, 1966

Dingle: Cleveland Family Study. 1964

Gardner R: The guilt reactions of parents of children with severe physical diseases. Am J Psychol 126:636, 1969

Green M, et al.: Reactions to the threatened loss of a child: a vulnerable child syndrome. Pediatrics 34:58, 1964

Herzog DB, et al.: Unexplained disability: diagnostic dilemma and principles of management. Clin Pediatr 20:761, 1981

Hill H: Evaluating the patient with recurrent infection. South Med J 70:230, 1977

Jones JF, et al.: Recurrent bacterial infections in children. Pediatr Rev 1:99, 1979

Levy J: Vulnerable children: Parents' perspectives and the use of medical care. Pediatrics 65:956, 1980

Roghman: Child Health Diary Study. 1975

Wald ER, et al.: Acute maxillary sinusitis in children. N Engl J Med 304:749, 1981

Cross-Reference to *Pediatrics,* 17th

Abdominal Pain	p 941	Gastrointestinal Problems	pp 547, 615
Allergy	Chapter 12	Immunologic Problems	Chapter 10
Education and Counseling	pp 79–80	Respiratory Illness	p 595

Part II

Major Presenting Symptoms of Acute Illness

FOUR

Abdominal Pain

Steven P. Shelov and Lewis M. Fraad

The child with abdominal pain presents an important diagnostic challenge to the pediatric practitioner. Studies in both the United States and Europe have shown that abdominal pain accounts for a significant percentage of all illness in children. In Apley's series, 1 of every 9 unselected school-aged children interviewed in person with their mothers had a complaint of recurrent abdominal pain. Other studies have indicated even higher percentages. Given this high rate of occurrence, what proportion of these children have an identifiable organic etiology for their pain? It is generally agreed that most, in fact, are not organic in origin. Nevertheless, the pain is real. The challenge, then, is to distinguish the child with abdominal pain secondary to an organic etiology from those with no organic etiology and to understand how to evaluate and manage both situations.

ACUTE ABDOMINAL PAIN

The child who presents with the abrupt onset of abdominal pain may have a number of underlying disturbances. The most common are listed in Tables 1, 2, and 3.

Nonsurgical Organic Causes

The majority of these conditions can be diagnosed by a careful history and physical examination, with some specific laboratory studies.

The first five entities, gastroenteritis, urinary tract infection, streptococcal pharyngitis, pneumonia, and regional enteritis, are described in Chapters 7, 31, 18, 6, and 10, respectively. Some other major nonsurgical causes are briefly described here.

Henoch-Schönlein Purpura (Anaphylactoid Purpura). This illness, which is seen most commonly in children 4–15 years of age, often presents with a triad of symptoms. Crampy abdominal pain, described by Henoch, is often the initial complaint. This is usually followed by the onset of arthralgia, described by Schönlein, and a hemorrhagic rash, which often occurs on the buttocks and then progresses to the lower extremities. Renal involvement, often heralded by hematuria, frequently accompanies this symptom complex.

Henoch-Schönlein syndrome is a generalized vascular disorder, consisting of a vasculitis of the arterioles and capillaries. The etiology is unclear, but it appears to be a hypersensitivity phenomenon (hence the name anaphylactoid). Occasionally, a preceding bacterial infection has been implicated, or the condition has seemed to be related to a specific food or drug, but no characteristic allergic history has been implicated.

The illness usually subsides over a period of 4–6 weeks. The vast majority of children make an uneventful and complete recovery.

TABLE 1. NONSURGICAL ORGANIC CAUSES OF ACUTE ABDOMINAL PAIN

Most Common	Less Common
Gastroenteritis	Hepatitis
Streptococcal pharyngitis	Pancreatitis
Urinary tract infection	Diabetes mellitus
Pneumonia	Pelvic inflammatory disease
Regional enteritis	
Henoch-Schönlein purpura	
Mesenteric lymphadenitis	
Sickle cell crisis	
Lead poisoning	
Acute toxic ingestion	

The major sequela is the development of chronic nephritis, which may go on to renal failure. Therapeutic intervention is controversial and dependent on the severity of the symptoms. Short-term steroid therapy (prednisone 1–2 mg/kg) has been recommended for children with severe arthralgia or unremitting abdominal pain. A prompt symptomatic response provides good evidence against the presence of a surgical problem, such as an intussusception. Steroid therapy, however, does not seem to alter the ultimate course.

Mesenteric Lymphadenitis. Mesenteric lymphadenitis is a poorly defined entity in which a child presents with symptoms of acute abdominal pain, often following an upper respiratory infection. The physical examination may suggest appendicitis, with occa-

TABLE 2. SURGICAL CAUSES OF ACUTE ABDOMINAL PAIN

Acute appendicitis	Regional enteritis
Intussusception	Abdominal mass
Ulcer disease	Trauma

TABLE 3. ORGANIC ETIOLOGIES OF RECURRENT ABDOMINAL PAIN

Parasitic disease *Giardia lamblia*	Regional enteritis
Biliary colic	Abdominal epilepsy
Tuberculous mesenteric adenitis (in endemic areas)	Aerophagia
	Lactose intolerance
Peptic ulcer disease	Defined emotional causes

sional localization of the pain to the right lower quadrant. Signs of localized or diffuse peritonitis are not present. In children in whom the diagnosis of acute appendicitis could not be ruled out, resulting in performance of a laparotomy, histologic examination of the lymph nodes has demonstrated nonspecific hyperplasia. The appendix is normal. No etiology has been determined, although a number of viruses have been isolated.

Sickle Cell Crisis. The child with sickle cell disease may present with a variety of different clinical manifestations. Painful crisis as a result of tissue hypoxia, due to small, thrombo-occlusive events occurring at terminal blood capillaries, is the most common of these. There is usually bone pain, crampy abdominal pain, and lower back pain. The abdominal pain may be extremely severe, with vomiting, generalized abdominal tenderness, and even rigidity, mimicking a surgical condition. The accompanying laboratory results, however, are usually diagnostic, with a hematocrit of 15–25% and sickle cells on smear or a positive sickle cell test.

Once the diagnosis is made, management includes hospitalization, transfusion (if crisis is severe or hematocrit is low enough), rehydration, and appropriate medication for pain.

Lead Poisoning. A child with pica who ingests small amounts of lead-containing paint or plaster may develop the clinical symptomatology of plumbism. Characteristically, these children are 1–4 years of age, are anorectic, somewhat apathetic, and hyperactive; they have some degree of incoordination and subtle loss of learned skills and complain of abdominal pain of varying severity, with sporadic episodes of vomiting. If the ingestion of lead continues, this clinical condition can deteriorate to a full-blown encephalopathic picture. Careful questioning may reveal that the child has pica. Management includes removal of the child from the lead-containing environment and hospitalization for chelation therapy.

Surgical Causes of Acute Abdominal Pain

The surgical etiologies are important to diagnose promptly; usually immediate intervention is required.

Appendicitis. In 1889, McBurney wrote:

In every case the seat of greatest pain, determined by the pressure of 1 finger, has been exactly between an inch and a half and 2 inches from the anterior superior spinous process of the ileum on a straight line drawn from that process to the umbilicus.

The child does not always present with such localized findings, but it is remarkable how often McBurney's point is the site of the inflammatory process. The course is usually acute, over a 24-hour period of time, with pain first described in the midumbilical region and then shifting to the right lower quadrant. Anorexia usually accompanies the gradual onset of pain, and over the ensuing 12–18 hours vomiting often begins. The physical examination usually elicits more localized pain at this time, as the peritoneum is now locally inflamed. Further progression may result in perforation of the appendix and, after a quiet period of several hours, full-blown peritonitis. Occasionally, the perforation becomes walled off, in which case the diagnosis may be difficult to establish.

Other Etiologies. The other major surgical causes of abdominal pain usually present with gastrointestinal bleeding and are discussed in Chapter 10.

RECURRENT ABDOMINAL PAIN (RAP)

Once it is determined that the child's abdominal pain is not an isolated episode but is a recurring or chronic condition, a different series of causes must be considered.

Organic Causes

Though infrequent as causes of recurrent abdominal pain, certain organic etiologies must be included as possibilities. Among the organic causes (Table 3) in older children is regional ileitis, discussed in Chapter 10. In developing countries, the most frequent cause of recurrent abdominal pain is massive worm infestation. Although less common in the US, parasitic disease still must be considered. In certain sections of the country, especially the far west, the water supply has become contaminated with *Giardia lamblia*, a well-recognized cause of recurrent abdominal pain.

Occasionally, recurrent abdominal pain is due to biliary colic, even in a child without hemolytic disease. Where tuberculosis is prevalent, tuberculous mesenteric adenitis must be considered. Peptic ulcer disease may cause recurrent abdominal pain (See Chapter 10.) The symptoms in children are similar to those in the adult, although sometimes the presentation is more atypical, especially in young children. Recurrent urinary tract infections, particularly in girls, are a frequent cause of recurrent abdominal pain. A controversial entity, which some feel does not exist, is abdominal epilepsy. One of the difficulties in making this diagnosis is that 10% of children with recurrent abdominal pain have abnormal electroencephalograms, as do 10% of normal children.

Some children with recurrent abdominal pain have aerophagia. The importance of this finding is not the diagnosis of aerophagia per se but why the child finds it necessary to swallow air throughout the day.

Levine and his associates[3] from the Boston Children's Hospital found among a group of white children with recurrent abdominal pain a number with secondary lactase deficiency. When milk was removed from the diet, most of these children lost their abdominal pain. Several groups, including ours, have failed to duplicate these findings by eliminating milk. It is our impression, therefore, that lactase deficiency is not a frequent cause of recurrent abdominal pain, certainly not in white children.

Emotional stress can trigger recurrent episodes of abdominal pain, although the precipitating events are often hard to determine. Such circumstances as a death in the family, illness or death of a sibling, new teacher, new school, new neighborhood, or pregnancy in the family may provide clues as to why the child is suffering from abdominal pain. Merely by having a close, nonjudgmental relationship with the child, the pediatrician may achieve a therapeutic effect even without understanding the underlying psychodynamics.

Nonorganic Causes

The etiologies for recurrent abdominal pain described thus far can be found as causes of recurrent abdominal pain in only a small percentage of children. For example, in the British series, only 8 of 100 and, in our series, 3 of 50 had one of these diagnoses. Recurrent abdominal pain most often is a functional condition, as described by Apley. He defined recurrent abdominal pain as 3 bouts of pain severe enough to affect the child's activities over a period of not less than 3 months. The attacks often have continued for a year preceding the examination. In 1,000 unselected British schoolchildren, the incidence of recurrent abdominal pain increased in males and females with advancing age. The overall incidence was 10.8% (girls 12.3%, boys 9.5%). In girls the peak occurred at 9–11 years, in boys at 12–13 years. The reason for the difference in age is presumed to be the earlier onset of adolescence in girls.

Apley followed 30 children from 5 to 20 years, hospitalizing them and evaluating them completely. By the end of this follow-up period, only 9 were symptom free. In another 9 new symptoms developed, mostly severe headaches with stress. In 12 children abdominal pain persisted throughout. Of the 30 children, 1–3 had typical migraine, 15 had headaches and other symptoms, and 13 had variable neurotic manifestations.

In our practice, we have followed 17 patients closely, only 2 of whom were hospitalized. Ten to twenty-seven years after the diagnosis was made, 5 of these children are entirely well. Of the other 12, 3 have developed migraine headaches, 3 have occasional vomiting and headache with stress or illness, 1 has recurrent peptic ulcer, and 2 have recurrent abdominal pain as adults and frequent headaches with any type of stress. Apley found, as we did, that the problem often clears up for a period of time in childhood and then recurs in adolescence and later in adult life.

Occasional vomiting was found in two thirds of the children in the British series and in half of the children we have followed. Headache was present in one fifth of both series. Elevated temperature occurs but is rare.

The physical examination is usually nonspecific. Apley found two thirds of the children to have pain in the region of the umbilicus and the epigastrium. As a general rule, the more central the pain, the less likely it is that there is an organic etiology. Conversely, the more peripheral the pain, the more likely it is to be organic. There are, however, striking exceptions.

THE APPROACH TO THE DIFFERENTIAL DIAGNOSIS

History

The history is important in differentiating between acute abdominal pain and recurrent abdominal pain. Tables 4 and 5 list the historical features characteristically seen in the common nonsurgical and surgical etiologies for acute abdominal pain. Careful questioning should reveal how recently the pain began, if anything improves or aggravates it, if there is anything else associated with the pain (sore throat, diarrhea, cough, vomiting, anorexia, fever), if the child can localize the pain (common in appendicitis, more vague in other entities), and if there is any genitourinariy discharge.

In children with recurrent abdominal pain there is a sixfold increase in familial incidence, particularly in the mother. In addition, there is significantly more peptic ulcer disease, migraine headaches, and serious psychiatric problems in the parents. The past history of the child frequently is positive for headaches, even though headaches in children under the age of 7 or 8 are unusual. Finally, children with the RAP syndrome often have episodes of vomiting with stress and with illness.

Physical Examination

Tables 4 and 5 summarize the positive physical findings in surgical and nonsurgical causes of acute abdominal pain. There are few positive physical findings in children with the classic recurrent abdominal pain picture. Some investigators have described a vague tenderness on examination, but most have found none. Some investigators feel that an important part of this syndrome involves an autonomic imbalance, evidenced, for example, by a slower decrement in the pupil dilation response to cold pressure test than in normal children. One study showed a markedly positive rectosigmoid motility response to prostigmine as compared to normal children. Another group found delayed transit time and a high percentage of children with constipation.

Laboratory Tests

Tables 4 and 5 indicate the abnormal laboratory findings in surgical and nonsurgical causes of acute abdominal pain. The practitioner should use the laboratory sparingly to investigate children who present with signs and symptoms characteristic of recurrent abdominal pain. A CBC, ESR, PPD, stool for ova and parasites and reducing-substances, and perhaps lactose elimination and rechallenge test are usually indicated and may serve to uncover an organic etiology. However, only in 5% of patients will these investigations yield fruitful results. In the remainder, all tests will be normal. The challenge is to avoid an excessive and invasive work-up in an effort to establish a specific (organic) etiology.

MANAGEMENT

A number of conditions require surgical intervention. These children should be managed jointly by the pediatrician and the surgeon. Nonsurgical causes of acute abdominal pain should be managed either by the pediatrician alone or in conjunction with an appropriate consultant. Table 6 provides some guidelines.

How should a pediatrician manage the child with recurrent abdominal pain once an organic etiology has been ruled out? How intensively should the average pediatrician conduct psychotherapy? Does simple relationship psychotherapy do any harm? It is

TABLE 4. CHARACTERISTICS OF NONSURGICAL ORGANIC CAUSES OF ACUTE ABDOMINAL PAIN

Cause	Characteristic History	Frequently Found Physical Findings	Frequently Found Laboratory Results
Gastroenteritis	Acute onset, vomiting often in beginning, diarrhea	Diffuse, nonlocalized tenderness, rectal examination NL	Viral: often nl WBC, stool culture ($-$) Bacterial: $\uparrow$ or $\downarrow$ WBC (salmonellosis), stool culture ($+$)
Streptococcal pharyngitis	Sore throat, fever 1–2 days, nausea	Reddened tonsils, purulent exudate, tender adenopathy	$\uparrow$ WBC, ($+$) throat culture for group A β-hemolytic streptococci
UTI	Dysuria, frequency, suprapubic pain, male or female, preschooler common age	Slight suprapubic tenderness, if febrile or upper tract involvement may have flank tenderness	Nl or $\uparrow$ WBC, urine culture >100,000 col/HPF
Pneumonia	Cough, fever, upper quadrant pain	Rales at right or left base	Chest x-ray ($+$) (usually RLL or LLL), $\uparrow$ WBC with shift to left
Henoch-Schönlein purpura	URI for several days, crampy abdominal pain, pain in joints, rash over buttock or lower extremities	Petecchial rash on buttocks, legs, diffuse abdominal tenderness	NL CBC, platelets; stool, urine ($+$) for heme
Sickle cell crisis	Hx of sickle cell disease, pain in extremities or chest, often simultaneous	Pallor, tachycardia with heart murmur, distended abdomen without decreased bowel sounds, diffuse tenderness	S-S preparation ($+$) or HCT 20–25, positive Hb electrophoresis, Reticulocyte count variable
Hepatitis	Jaundice, exposed to known case, malaise, anorexia	RUQ tenderness, hepatomegaly	$\uparrow$ SGOT, SGPT, bilirubin (direct fraction), alkaline phosphatase, should test for Hb_SAg or specific hepatitis antibody
Pancreatitis	Acute onset, midepigastric pain, vomiting, pain might be boring in type	Mid- to upper epigastric tenderness	$\uparrow$ Amylase, ($+$) sonogram
Diabetes mellitus	Polyuria, polydipsia, weight loss, ($+$) family history	Abdominal distention, decreased bowel sounds, mild diffuse tenderness	Glucosuria, ketonuria, $\uparrow$ blood glucose, Nl or $\downarrow$ pH

TABLE 5. CHARACTERISTICS OF SURGICAL CAUSES OF ACUTE ABDOMINAL PAIN

Cause	Characteristic History	Frequently Found Physical Findings	Frequently Found Laboratory Results
Acute appendicitis	1 day Hx of intermittent midepigastric pain, migrates to more localized RLQ area, pain becomes more persistent, anorexia then followed by vomiting	Periumbilical tenderness or localized RLQ pain, occasional pain in RLQ when palpate LLQ, tender on rectal examination	↑ WBC (13,000–15,000), left shift, often (+) KUB for appendicolith
Intussusception	Age 2 mo–1 yr, severe crampy, colicky pain, bursts of crying out, legs drawn up followed by quiescent periods, occasional change in sensorium	Diffuse tenderness, paucity of bowel in RLQ, RQ, sausage mass in midepigastrium, bloody stool	Stool (+) for blood, diagnostic KUB shows paucity of gas in RLQ and sausage mass in R to midepigastrium, barium enema is diagnostic and curative in 85%
Ulcer disease[a]			
Regional enteritis[a]			

[a]See Chapter 10.

our feeling that if the physician is comfortable in the somewhat more passive, slower role of the psychotherapist, this approach can be effective.

It is important to establish from the beginning that the physician is interested in all aspects of the child, not just the possible organic causes of abdominal pain. As the practitioner begins to see a child with recurrent abdominal pain, questions are asked about the child's social life, family life, school life, in an age-appropriate manner. Once this questioning proceeds, the pediatrician may be surprised to find that the child is extremely grateful for the interest shown by this nonjudgmental professional. What emerges often is much more pertinent to the child's symptoms than a myriad of laboratory tests.

It is wise to remember that emotional components can set in motion many of the same patterns of response that the body utilizes against physical, chemical, or bacterial attack. Canon recognized this 60 years ago, and George Engel further developed this concept. The role of depression in lowering body defenses or in preparing the ground for organic injury is well accepted. Whether in recurrent abdominal pain or in any other condition in which emotions play an important role, physicians who treat symptoms by giving prescriptions are not effective. The practitioner who manages such patients must learn the value of listening and providing guidance.

Some prepubertal children with hypochondriacal tendencies use abdominal pain as an escape from problems that seem overwhelming or too difficult to solve. The presenting symptoms are often determined by which symptom is more effective in manipulating parents. In the older child one encounters problems of puberty: issues of sexuality or related areas, onset or delay in menstruation, masturbation, or fear of masturbation. Even if the practitioner does not delve deeply into the details of these prob-

TABLE 6. GUIDELINES FOR MANAGEMENT OF ABDOMINAL PAIN

Nonsurgical Cause	Appropriate Management	Consultant Used
Gastroenteritis	Rehydrate if necessary Clear liquids and advance feeding slowly Antibiotics only if shigella or salmonella <3 mo of age	Pediatrician alone
Streptococcal pharyngitis	Antibiotics (see Chapter 18)	Pediatrician alone
UTI	Antibiotics (See Chapter 31)	Pediatrician alone
Pneumonia	Antibiotics (See Chapter 6)	Pediatrician alone
Henoch-Schönlein purpura	Steroids if abdominal pain intractable	Pediatrician alone
Sickle cell disease	Transfuse with packed cells, consider hypertransfusion if multiple and frequent crises	Hematologist and pediatrician
Lead poisoning	Chelate if level and FEP in class III	Pediatrician
Toxin ingestion	Depending on type of toxin	Pediatrician
Hepatitis	Isolate patient	Pediatrician

lems, the physician must know that there are age-related problems and discuss them in that context. Using the third person, "I know children of your age who. . . ." rather than the first person is less threatening to the child and easier for the pediatrician and permits a nonjudgmental approach. Treating children with recurrent abdominal pain provides an opportunity for the child to present a host of potentially troubling or worrisome concerns. It is often the key to the locked inner emotions that are important to understand if true mastery over them and elimination of the symptom is to result. Does an understanding of these emotional issues lead to better mental health in adulthood? I do not know, but, most emphatically, these issues must be addressed. One should not just give aspirin but try to understand and discover the problems of the child. What is needed is not "don't worry, you will outgrow it," but (1) rational reassurance, (2) an attempt to understand what goes on in school and in the family, (3) evaluation of the emotional development of the child, and (4) a clear statement that you, the practitioner, are available and can be de-

pended on. A small minority of children need referral to psychiatrists.

A few typical cases of recurrent abdominal pain may serve to put the problem into proper prospective. A child came to us a number of years ago. He was allegedly an American Indian. His father, along with many other American Indians, worked on the iron work in skyscrapers. The family was well off and lived in a pleasant neighborhood. The child had had his appendix out in another hospital, but he had continued to have recurrent abdominal pain. A psychiatrist felt that the boy was having pregnancy fantasies because a favorite aunt had died in childbirth. It finally was determined that this child was not an American Indian at all but a light-skinned black. The family was posing as American Indians. Only after working with a sensitive black pediatrician was the child able to accept and understand his problem. Such problems as these are often more important than the purely emotional.

Another child seen by us had been to three physicians and had had an upper GI series and two intravenous pyelograms. She was a slim, short, 11-year-old girl who was a year younger than her classmates in the seventh grade. Every day another buxom child would announce that she had just menstruated, and our patient, with a brassiere full of nylon stockings, felt that she would never mature. When she was reassured that she, too, would mature, the abdominal pain disappeared. We have seen at least four children within the past few years with similar difficulties. The important thing is for the practitioner to know and to share with the patient and family the age-appropriate concerns of the child.

Finally, a faculty member's child with recurrent abdominal pain was brought to us with an enormous list of laboratory reports. The parent, a basic scientist, felt that the child's condition resulted from abnormalities in intestinal enzymes. The child was a delightful 11-year-old who attended a very strict school in New York. In addition, she was given ballet lessons, was being groomed to be a champion skater, and on Saturdays took Spanish lessons. When the child was given a sensible program, enough for one or one and a half children, the abdominal pain went away and did not return.

The examples are numerous and continuous. The important thing is that one must address oneself to the whole child. History taking must be broadened from the beginning to include psychologic and social factors. Proper management of the symptoms involves a relationship with the child in the context of his or her environment.

BIBLIOGRAPHY

Apley J: The Child with Abdominal Pain, 2nd ed. London, Blackwell, 1975

Apley J, et al.: Pupillary reaction in children with recurrent abdominal pain. Arch Dis Child 46:337, 1971

Barr RG, Watkins B, Levine MD: Recurrent abdominal pain (RAP) of childhood due to lactose intolerance: a prospective study. N Engl J Med

Kopel FB, et al.: Comparison of rectosigmoid motility in normal children, children with recurrent abdominal pain, and children with ulcerative colitis. Pediatrics 39:539, 1967

Longino LA: Appendicitis in childhood—a study of 1358 cases. Pediatrics 22:238, 1958

McBurney C: NY J Med 50:679, 1889

Shrand H: Acute abdominal pain. J Fam Prac 2:131, 1975

Winter ST: Recurrent abdominal pain in children. Clin Pediatr 15:771

Cross Reference to *Pediatrics,* 17th ed.

FIVE

Anemia

Jeffrey Gershel

Anemia is one of the most common laboratory abnormalities that practitioners encounter in the infant and child. The incidence of anemia cannot be determined precisely, since not all children are screened. It is estimated, however, that at least 10% of 9–19-month-old infants and 5% of 2-year-old children have iron deficiency. These percentages seem to be higher among low socioeconomic groups. The increase in survival of very low-birth-weight and of sick newborns and the increased frequency of pregnancy in teenagers have probably resulted in a further increase in iron deficiency anemia, the extent of which is not known. Anemia is sufficiently common, however, that screening for this abnormality should be performed in infants between 9 and 12 months of age, in preschool children, and in children at about 12 years of age.

DEFINITION AND CLASSIFICATION

Anemia is defined as a reduction per unit volume of blood in (1) the number of erythrocytes (RBCs), (2) the quantity of hemoglobin, or (3) the volume of packed red cells. These values are age dependent, as shown in Table 1. The major consequence of anemia is a reduction in the oxygen-carrying capacity of the blood, the end result being tissue hypoxia.

The causes of anemia can be grouped under three headings:

1. Failure to produce RBCs (aregenerative anemia)
2. Loss of RBCs (blood loss anemia)
3. Destruction of RBCs (hemolytic anemia)

Since the relative importance of each of these categories varies with the age of the patient, the differential diagnosis of anemia is age dependent. Therefore, separate consideration is given to anemia in the newborn and anemia in the infant and child.

ANEMIA IN THE NEWBORN

Etiology

As can be seen in Table 2, anemia in the newborn is caused by disease in each of the three major categories. The most common cause is blood loss, which can occur in association with such obstetric complications as placenta previa or abruptio, delivery by cesarean section, or fetal-maternal or twin-twin transfusion. In each case, the newborn does not receive the usual placental transfusion of blood. After delivery, blood loss is caused most often by excessive phlebotomies for laboratory tests without sufficient replacement. Other common causes include disseminated intravascu-

TABLE 1. AGE-DEPENDENT HEMATOLOGIC VALUES

| | Hemoglobin (gm/dl) | | MCV (fl) | | Hematocrit (%) | MCHC | Reticulocytes (%) |
| | Median | Lower Limit | Median | Lower Limit | Median | Median | Median |
Age (yr)							
0.5–2	12.5	11.0	77	70	36	33	0.8
2–5	12.5	11.0	79	73	37	33	1.0
5–9	13.0	11.5	81	75	38	33	1.0
9–12	13.5	12.0	83	76	39	33	1.0
12–14							
Female	13.5	12.0	85	77	39	34	1.0
Male	14.0	12.5	84	76	41	34	1.0
14–18							
Female	14.0	12.0	87	78	40	34	1.0
Male	15.0	13.0	86	77	44	34	1.0
18–49							
Female	14.0	12.0	90	80	42	34	1.0
Male	16.0	14.0	90	80	47	34	1.0

Adapted from Dallman PR, Siimes MA: J Pediatr 94:26, 1979.

lar coagulation with subsequent bleeding and blood loss into a large cephalohematoma.

Second in frequency as a cause of anemia is hemolysis, the most common etiology being hemolytic disease of the newborn (isoimmunization). (See Chapter 14.) The administration of RhoGAM (anti-Rh antibody) to Rh-negative women within 72 hours of delivery or abortion has led to a marked decrease in cases of Rh hemolytic disease of the newborn. Since the introduction of RhoGAM, most cases of hemolysis have been secondary to ABO incompatibility, usually with the mother's blood being type O and the baby's being B or A. Cases of Rh incompatibility continue to occur, especially in older women or in those who underwent first trimester abortion without subsequently receiving RhoGAM.

Other causes of hemolysis include bacterial sepsis and transplacentally acquired infections, such as toxoplasmosis, rubella, cytomegalovirus, herpes simplex, and syphilis.

Underproduction is the least frequent cause of anemia in the neonatal period. It results usually from iron deficiency caused by prior blood loss without sufficient transfusions, since the newborn's iron stores are almost totally contained in his erythrocytes. Other rare causes of anemia in the newborn include congenital hypoplastic anemia (Diamond-Blackfan syndrome) and congenital leukemia.

Differential Diagnosis

The history and physical examination often provide the correct diagnosis so that the temptation to proceed immediately with laboratory tests should be resisted.

History.

Blood Loss. Were any obstetric procedures performed, e.g., amniocentesis? What were the details of the labor and delivery, including length of gestation, method of delivery, birth weight, and single or multiple gestation (how are the other offspring doing)? Any obstetric manipulation or complication raises the possibility of excessive antenatal or perinatal blood loss.

TABLE 2. ETIOLOGY OF ANEMIA IN THE NEWBORN

Blood Loss	Hemolysis
Iatrogenic	Isoimmunization (ABO, Rh)
Obstetric complications	Congenital red blood cell defects
Cord hematoma or rupture	Enzyme deficiency (glucose-6-phosphatase
Placental incision, previa, or abruptio	dehydrogenase, pyruvate kinase)
Malformations of the placenta and cord	Membrane abnormality (hereditary sphero-
Aberrant vessels	cytosis or elliptocytosis)
Velamentous insertion	Acquired red blood cell defects
Communicating vessels in multilobed placenta	Drug
Occult hemorrhage (antenatal)	Toxin
Fetomaternal	Infection
Twin to twin	Disseminated intravascular coagulation
Internal hemorrhage	Microangiopathic hemolytic anemias
Intracranial	*Failure of Production*
Cephalohematoma	Congenital hypoplastic anemia
Retroperitoneal	Congenital leukemia
Ruptured liver or spleen	

What drugs did the mother take during the last trimester that might cause a coagulopathy (warfarin, aspirin) or thrombocytopenia? Was the baby sick, requiring multiple blood tests or transfusions? Most postnatal blood loss is iatrogenic in origin. Was the baby desperately ill, suggesting bacterial sepsis with resultant disseminated intravascular coagulation (DIC)?

Hemolysis. Were there any previous stillbirths that might have been secondary to erythroblastosis caused by ABO or Rh incompatibility?

Did the mother have a rash, viral syndrome, or veneral disease during the pregnancy? These suggest a transplacentally acquired infection, which often results in hemolysis. Did the baby suffer neonatal jaundice that might have been secondary to hemolysis?

Is there a family history of splenectomy or gallstones? This might indicate a familial hemolytic disorder, such as hereditary spherocytosis.

Decreased Production. Did the clinical circumstances suggest blood loss, as discussed above? This might lead to iron deficiency if inadequate replacement of iron was not given (via blood transfusion or oral supplementation).

Physical Examination. A well-appearing, vigorous baby usually is not suffering from a serious illness, such as sepsis, acute blood loss, or massive hemolysis, whereas severe anemia may be associated with pallor, respiratory distress, murmur, or a gallop rhythm.

General. Generalized edema suggests erythroblastosis secondary to blood group incompatibility. The unusual presence of lymphadenopathy in the newborn should alert the practitioner to congenital leukemia.

Skin. The presence of petechiae, purpura, or bleeding from puncture sites or the umbilicus suggests a bleeding diathesis. Hemolysis is the most common cause of severe or prolonged jaundice.

HEENT. A large cephalohematoma may be of significance as a site of blood loss. A bulging fontanelle can be caused by an intraventricular hemorrhage. Microcephaly, chorioretinitis, and cataracts suggest intrauterine infection. A cleft palate and webbed neck may be seen in congenital hypoplastic anemia. Low set ears can occur in association with congenital leukemia.

Abdomen. A tender or rigid abdomen might be due to necrotizing enterocolitis, which can lead to DIC. Hepatosplenomegaly is usually associated with hemolytic disease of the newborn or intrauterine infection.

Neurology. An abrupt change in neurologic status can signify an intracranial bleed.

Extremities. Deformities of the thumb are sometimes seen in congenital hypoplastic anemia.

Laboratory Examination. A complete blood count, with RBC morphology, white blood count and differential, reticulocyte count, and platelet count, is mandatory. Further testing, including infant and maternal blood types and Coombs tests, and serum bilirubin levels in the infant may be required to make a specific diagnosis. The typical laboratory findings in the most common causes of neonatal anemia are summarized in Table 3.

Blood Loss. Acute blood loss is manifested by reticulocytosis of greater than 10% (Fig. 1), in conjunction with normochromic, normocytic red blood cells. The Coombs test is negative, while the total bilirubin is usually <12 mg per dl.

Chronic antenatal blood loss is manifested by a reticulocytosis with a hypochromic, microcytic smear. Once again, the Coombs and bilirubin tests are normal. If fetomaternal transfusion is suspected, a Kleihauer-Bethke stain on the mother's blood will document the presence of fetal hemoglobin.

If a bleeding diathesis is suspected, prothrombin and partial thromboplastin times should be obtained. Disseminated intravascular coagulation is indicated by a prolongation of both, along with thrombocytopenia and elevated levels of fibrin-split products in serum. In the case of maternal drug-induced thrombocytopenia, these clotting studies are normal.

Hemolysis. The hallmark of a hemolytic disorder is a marked reticulocytosis (up to 40%). The serum bilirubin usually is elevated (indirect >12 mg%), while the smear reveals polychromasia. With ABO incompatibility, the indirect Coombs is positive (direct is variable), and the smear is remarkable for microspherocytosis. In Rh incompatibility, both direct and indirect Coombs tests are positive. The smear reveals anisocytosis and polychromasia, but no microspherocytes are seen.

Direct hyperbilirubinemia along with hemolysis suggests intrauterine infection or bacterial sepsis. The Coombs tests are negative, but fragmented RBCs may be seen on the peripheral smear.

Coombs-negative hemolytic anemia occurs in association with RBC membrane defects; the characteristic morphology is seen on the smear. Specific assays can be performed for RBC enzyme deficiencies.

Underproduction. This category is manifested by a reticulocyte count that is less than 2%. Iron deficiency causes hypochromic, microcytic RBCs; the WBC and platelet counts are normal. In congenital leukemia, lymphoblasts and thrombocytopenia are present.

Management
Blood Loss. If the degree of blood loss has been small, early institution of iron replacement is the only treatment required. Ferrous sulfate, 6 mg/kg/day of elemental iron, in three divided doses, should supply adequate iron to achieve a normal hematocrit. Afterwards, 2 mg/kg/day is continued as a maintenance dose. Side effects include constipation, diarrhea, and darkening of stool color.

The newborn who has suffered major blood loss, causing symptoms or resulting in a

TABLE 3. LABORATORY FINDINGS IN ANEMIA IN THE NEWBORN

Diagnosis	Reticulocyte Count	Serum Bilirubin	Mother's Blood Type	Baby's Blood Type	Indirect Coombs	Direct Coombs	Blood Smear and RBC Morphology
Rh incompatibility	Increased	Increased	Rh positive	Rh negative	+	+	Polychromasia
ABO incompatibility	Increased	Increased	O	A or B	+	+/−	Microspherocytes
Acute blood loss	Increased	Normal	Any	Any	−	−	Normal
Chronic blood loss	Increased	Normal	Any	Any	−	−	Microcytic/hypochromic
Intrauterine infection	Increased	Increased	Any	Any	−	−	Anisocytosis
Disseminated intravascular coagulation	Increased	Increased	Any	Any	−	−	Fragmentation
Membrane defect	Increased	Increased	Any	Any	−	−	Characteristic morphology
Enzyme deficiency	Increased	Increased	Any	Any	−	−	Anisocytosis
Iron deficiency	Decreased	Normal	Any	Any	−	−	Microcytic/hypochromic
Diamond-Blackfan syndrome	Decreased	Normal	Any	Any	−	−	WBC, platelet normal
Congenital leukemia	Decreased	Normal	Any	Any	−	−	Mycloblasts

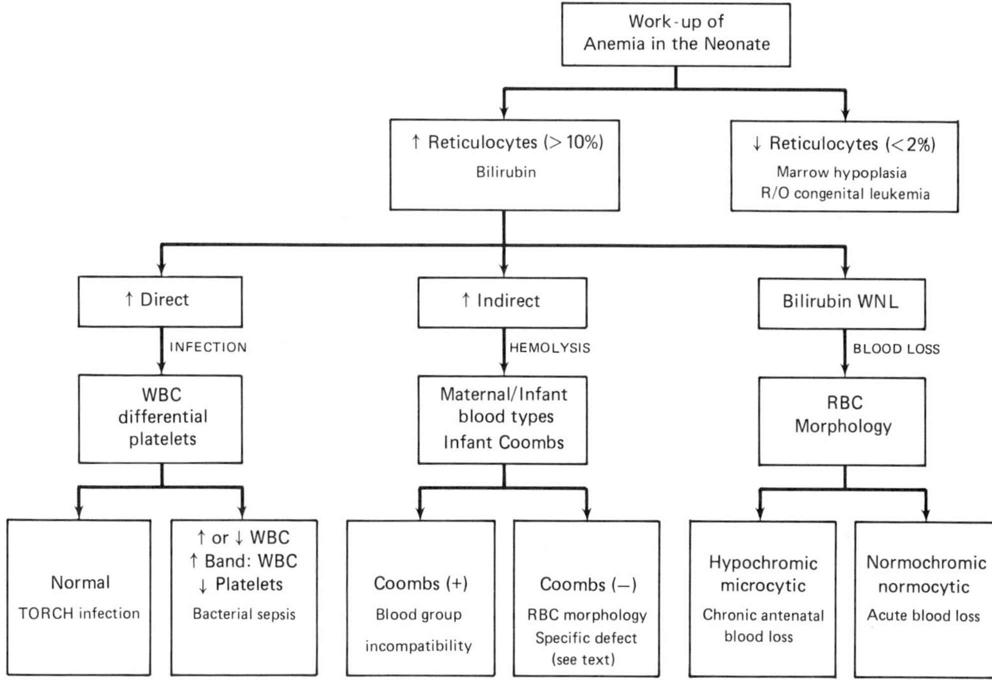

Figure 1. Work-up of anemia in the neonate.

hematocrit of 25%, should be transfused with packed red cells (10 ml/kg). In a dire emergency, unmatched O-negative blood may be used.

Hemolysis. The treatment of major hemolysis secondary to blood group incompatibility is the performance of an exchange transfusion, which should be supervised by a neonatologist or a pediatrician who has experience with the procedure. When the diagnosis of erythroblastosis fetalis has been made in utero, the neonatologist should be prepared to perform an exchange transfusion in the delivery room.

The infant with a less severe degree of hemolysis may be managed by the general practitioner after consultation with a neonatologist. At 1 week of age, a hematocrit and reticulocyte count should be performed to ascertain the degree of anemia and the bone marrow response. Ongoing hemolysis, as indicated by a fall in hematocrit to less than 20% in the face of a reticulocytosis greater than 10%, demands weekly repetition of the blood tests. A substantial drop in hematocrit, such that the patient is symptomatic (cardiac gallop, tachypnea, heart failure), requires admission to the hospital for a partial exchange transfusion, under the supervision of a neonatologist or hematologist. These infants do not require iron supplementation.

Newborns with congenital RBC enzyme or membrane defects should be referred to a hematologist for proper follow-up. If G-6-PD deficiency is diagnosed, the most important issue is to instruct the family to avoid exposure to possible oxidants (Table 4).

Hemolysis secondary to acquired red blood cell defects requires treatment of the primary cause (e.g., antibiotics for infection, discontinuation of drugs, heparin and fresh frozen plasma for DIC). Transfusions of packed cells are given as required to keep the hematocrit above 25% and to keep the infant asymptomatic.

TABLE 4. OXIDANTS THAT CAN CAUSE HEMOLYSIS IN PATIENTS WITH G-6-PD DEFICIENCY

Antipyretics/Analgesics
  p-Aminosalicylic acid
  Phenacetin

Antibiotics
  Salicylazosulfapyridine (Azulfidine)
  Sulfanilamide
  Sulfisoxazole (Gantrisin)

Antimalarials
  Chloroquine (Aralen)
  Primaquine
  Quinacrine (Atabrine)
  Quinine

Nitrofurans
  Nitrofurantoin (Furadantin, Macrodantin)
  Nitrofurazone

Miscellaneous oxidants
  Ascorbic acid (vitamin C, high doses)
  Chloramphenicol (Chloromycetin)
  Diabetic ketoacidosis
  Dimercaprol (BAL)
  Fava bean
  Isoniazid (INH)
  Nalidixic acid (NegGram)
  Naphthalene (mothballs)
  Methylene blue
  Probenecid
  Quinidine
  Vitamin K (water-soluble)

Underproduction. A newborn with the diagnosis of congenital hypoplastic anemia or congenital leukemia should be referred to a pediatric hematologist. Iron-deficiency anemia, encountered after the newborn period, is treated with oral supplementation, as described above. A follow-up hematocrit is obtained in 2 or 3 weeks to document the efficacy of treatment and compliance.

ANEMIA IN INFANTS AND CHILDREN

Etiology

The various causes of anemia in infancy and childhood are summarized in Table 5. The vast majority of cases are caused by nutritional iron deficiency. Dietary iron deficiency occurs when the infant's body growth outstrips his iron stores. This takes place when he is approximately 2.5 times his birth weight, usually at 6–9 months of age in the term infant and as early as 2–3 months in the premature. Throughout childhood, however, iron deficiency is very common, especially in lower socioeconomic groups. A second peak of iron-deficiency anemia occurs in adolescence as the iron requirements of the rapid body growth exceed the teenager's intake. The situation is compounded in the menstruating or pregnant female.

Other causes of underproduction include chronic disease, chronic inflammation, plumbism, vitamin B_{12} or folate deficiency, and bone marrow infiltration or suppression.

The major causes of hemolysis are corpuscular defects, including hemoglobinopathies (e.g., sickle cell disease, thalassemia); enzyme deficiencies (e.g., G-6-PD), and membrane defects (e.g., hereditary spherocytosis). Extracorpuscular etiologies include autoimmune (Coombs-positive) hemolytic anemia secondary to collagen vascular diseases and drug-induced hemolytic anemia. Other causes include DIC, hemolytic-uremic syndrome, and infections (viral and bacterial).

Finally, ongoing blood loss is not a common pediatric problem, except for children with chronic gastrointestinal loss secondary to cow's milk intolerance and intestinal hookworms. In these situations, however, one must rule out a bleeding diathesis secondary to platelet abnormalities (e.g., idiopathic thrombocytopenic purpura, leukemia) or clotting factor disturbances (e.g., hemophilia, liver disease, Von Willebrand's disease).

Differential Diagnosis
History.

Underproduction. The course in a nursery of an anemic infant should be evaluated carefully. What was the length of gestation and birth weight? Was the infant sick as a newborn, suggesting multiple blood tests that might have depleted his iron stores? Was transfusion required?

What has been the baby's diet since discharge from the nursery? The bioavailability of breast milk iron obviates the need for supplementation for the first 6 months of life. Similarly, a diet of iron-fortified cow's milk formula does not require additional iron for 12 months. If, however, noniron-fortified cereals or foods high in plant fiber are added to the diet, the net amount of iron absorbed will decrease and might be insufficient. The use of nonfortified cow's milk in the first year will lead to iron-deficiency anemia unless supplementation is given. Goat's milk can lead to folate deficiency.

Does the nursing mother eat a complete diet, or is she a food faddist or vegetarian,

---

TABLE 5. ETIOLOGY OF ANEMIA IN INFANTS AND CHILDREN

Underproduction

Nutritional deficiency—common causes
  Iron
  Vitamin B_{12} (malabsorption syndromes)
  Folic acid (goat's milk diet)
  Protein (kwashiorkor)
  Ascorbic acid (scurvy)

Bone marrow depression
  Marrow-toxic drugs and chemicals (cancer chemotherapy, chloramphenicol)
  Infection
  Primary malignancy (leukemia)
  Metastatic malignancy (lymphoma, neuroblastoma)
  Chronic inflammation and chronic disease (liver disease, renal disease)
  Fanconi's anemia

Hemolysis

Congenital red blood cell defects
  Hemoglobinopathy (e.g., sickle cell, thalassemia, hemoglobin C)
  Enzyme deficiency (e.g., glucose-6-phosphate dehydrogenase, pyruvate kinase)
  Membrane abnormality (e.g., hereditary spherocytosis, elliptocytosis)

Acquired red blood cell defects
  Drug
  Toxin (oxidants, heavy metals)
  Infection
  Disseminated intravascular coagulation
  Microangiopathic hemolytic anemia
  Collagen vascular disease (systemic lupus erythematosus)
  Hemolytic-uremic syndrome

Blood Loss

Acute
Chronic (milk intolerance, hookworm infestation)

---

causing her milk to be deficient in vitamin B_{12} or iron?

Has the patient been ill? Chronic illness and inflammation are a common cause of anemia unresponsive to iron.

Is the child taking any drugs or medicines that might cause marrow suppression?

Does the child have a malignancy that can metastasize to the bone marrow, or is he receiving marrow-suppressive chemotherapy?

Is there a history of pica or peeling paint in the home, suggesting lead intoxication?

Blood Loss. Is the infant receiving cow's milk? Where is the child from? Intestinal hookworm with subsequent GI blood loss is a disease of the Southeastern states. Does the child have a liver disease that could cause a coagulopathy or a disease that can infiltrate the bone marrow, leading to thrombocytopenia?

Physical Examination. A healthy, vigorous infant or child usually is not suffering from a malignancy, severe malnutrition, severe liver or kidney disease, or bone marrow infiltration.

Skin. Jaundice can be caused by liver disease or hemolysis. With chronic hemolysis, patients may have a bronze skin color, especially if multiple transfusions have been given. Petechiae, purpura, multiple ecchymoses, and excessive bleeding from puncture sites are hallmarks of bleeding diathesis.

Lymph Nodes. Generalized lymphadenopathy suggests myeloproliferative disorders with marrow replacement.

HEENT. Frontal bossing, malar prominence, and malocclusion are seen classically in thalassemia major. They also occur in severe chronic hemolytic anemias. Anemia of any etiology causes pallor of the mucous membranes, especially the conjunctiva. Scleral icterus can be secondary to liver disease or a hemolytic process. A funduscopic examination may reveal the tortuous vessels and microaneurysms of sickle cell disease. Subconjunctival hemorrhages are seen in disorders of hemostasis.

Chest. An apical systolic murmur is a common finding in anemia of any etiology. A gallop rhythm and signs of congestive heart failure indicate a severe degree of tissue hypoxia.

Abdomen. Hepatomegaly is found in patients with hemolysis, liver disease, and malignancy and is seen also in a rapidly evolving anemia. In sickle cell disease, the spleen is not palpated after the first 3–5 years of life. Splenomegaly can also be seen in malignancies.

Extremities. A hypoplastic thumb can be seen in congenital hypoplastic anemia while koilonychosis (concave nails) occurs in severe iron-deficiency anemia. Leg ulcers suggest sickle cell disease.

Neurology. Paresthesias of the hands and feet can occur in association with vitamin B_{12} deficiency and megaloblastic anemia. These patients may lose vibration and position sense as well as deep tendon reflexes. Sickle cell patients are prone to cerebrovascular accidents resulting in fixed neurologic deficits.

Laboratory Examination. The anemia is discovered most commonly during routine screening or as an incidental finding during the work-up of another problem. Laboratory tests should be ordered selectively. An approach to the work-up is diagrammed in Figures 2 and 3. Since the most common cause is iron deficiency, it is appropriate to start iron supplementation without performing other tests, unless another etiology appears likely. Following initiation of treatment, a peak reticulocytosis should be seen in about 1 week,

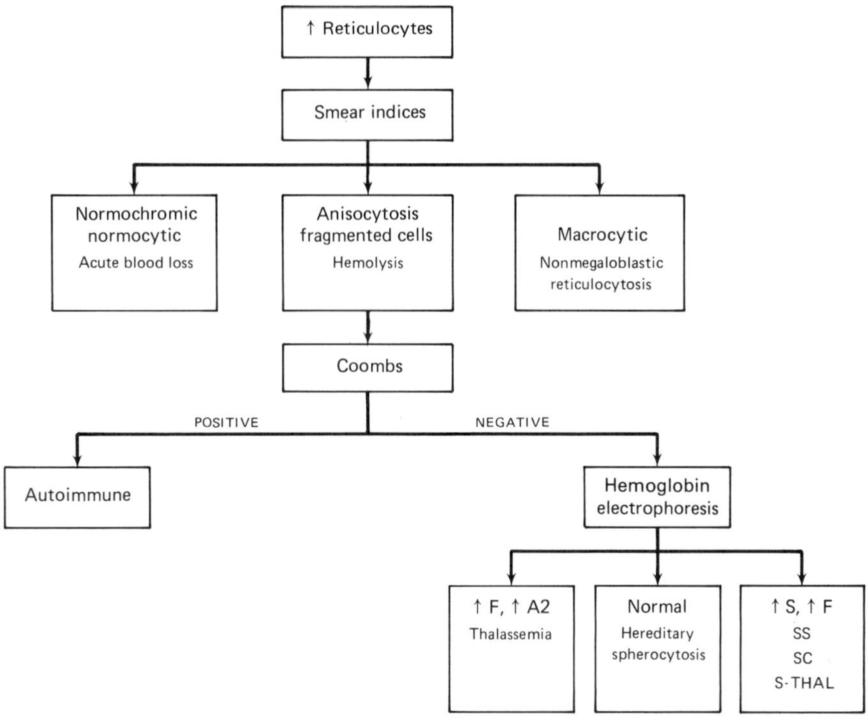

Figure 2. Work-up of anemia in infants and children.

but it is sufficient for diagnosis to demonstrate an increase in either the hemoglobin or the hematocrit after 1 or 2 weeks of therapy. A failure in the therapeutic response suggests another etiology or noncompliance, in which case a complete CBC should be performed, with white blood cell, differential, platelet, and reticulocyte counts, as well as red blood cell indices and morphology. As seen in Figure 2, the RBC smear is the first result to be considered; further diagnostic testing depends on the smear and reticulocyte count.

Underproduction. The hallmark of underproduction is a depressed reticulocyte count. Iron deficiency is the most common cause of a microcytic, hypochromic anemia— low mean corpuscular volume (mcv) and mean corpuscular hemoglobin concentration (mchc). (See Table 1.) However, if a therapeutic trial of iron fails, consideration must be given to lead intoxication, thalassemia minor, and chronic inflammatory or other diseases, in addition to noncompliance. The necessary tests are free erythrocyte protoporphyrin (FEP), ferritin, serum iron, and total iron-binding capacity (TIBC). The differential diagnosis is summarized in Table 6.

Iron deficiency leads to decreased serum ferritin and iron, along with an elevated-TIBC. Therefore, the percent saturation is greatly depressed.

Lead intoxication is usually manifested by a normocytic anemia with a markedly elevated FEP (> 160). Coexistent iron deficiency will lead to microcytosis. Basophilic stippling

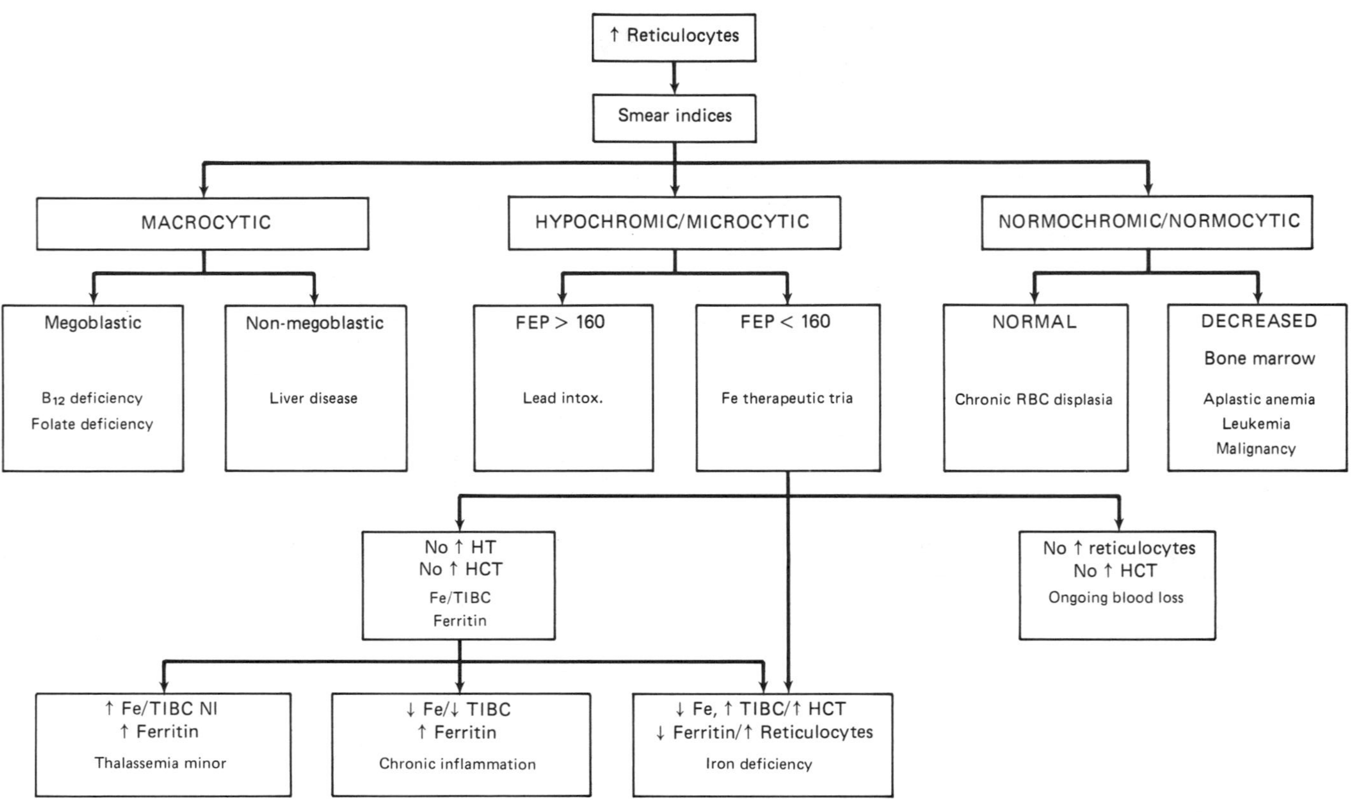

Figure 3. Work-up of anemia in infants and children.

TABLE 6. LABORATORY FINDINGS IN ANEMIA OF INFANTS AND CHILDREN 6 MONTHS TO 3 YEARS

Diagnosis	FEP	Ferritin	Fe	TIBC	% Saturation (Fe/TIBC)	MCV/RBC
Iron deficiency	50–160	<10	<40	>400	<10%	>14
Lead intoxication	>160	30–100	>50	200–350	20–35%	>14
Thalassemia minor	<30	30–100	>50	200–350	20–35%	<12
Chronic disease	40–100	>100	<40	100–200	>10%	>14

Fe, iron; FEP, free erythrocytic protoporphyrin; MCV, mean corpuscular hemoglobin; RBC, number of red blood cells; TIBC, total iron-binding capacity.

is nonspecific. In addition to plumbism, it is seen in iron deficiency and chronic illness.

In thalassemia minor, the serum ferritin and iron saturation are normal, while the MCV is low (Table 1). The discriminate index, or MCV/RBC, is under 12 in thalassemia minor, while MCV/RBC over 14 occurs in iron deficiency or lead poisoning.

Chronic disease and inflammation cause a microcytic or normocytic anemia with decreased serum iron and TIBC, so that the saturation remains normal. The ferritin is within the normal range.

If macrocytosis (mean corpuscular volume elevated, see Table 1) is noted, liver disease and megaloblastic anemia (vitamin B_{12} or and folate deficiency) should be considered.

If abnormality is noted in the white cell, differential, or platelet counts, either marrow suppression or replacement is occurring. Hematologic consultation is urgent so that the marrow can be examined.

Hemolysis. The hallmark of a hemolytic disorder is a reticulocytosis without an increase in hematocrit. As with underproduction, the initial step is the examination of the peripheral smear. A specific cell morphology, such as sickle cells (S-S, S-thalassemia, S-C) spherocytes (hereditary spherocytosis, autoimmune hemolytic anemias), or elliptocytes might be seen. In other cases target cells (thalassemia, hemoglobin C) or schistocytes

(intravascular hemolysis) might aid in securing the diagnosis. Polychromasia indicates the marrow's attempt at compensation.

If a hemoglobinopathy is suspected, a hemoglobin electrophoresis should be done. Children with sickle trait are not anemic, and, hence, this diagnosis should not be considered in a truly anemic child.

Screening tests for G-6-PD are readily available. It must be remembered that during an acute hemolytic episode in a black child, a quantitative assay is necessary since the younger RBCs have a higher level of the enzyme.

A Coombs test is necessary in the workup of an acute hemolytic episode in a patient without a prior history of a hemolytic disorder. A positive result is seen in collagen diseases and drug-induced hemolysis, while a negative Coombs test suggests infection or the hemolytic-uremic syndrome.

If an RBC enzyme defect or membrane defect is suspected, the patient should be referred to a hematologist for evaluation.

Blood Loss. Chronic blood loss is manifested either as a microcytic, hypochromic, iron-deficiency anemia or as a normochromic, normocytic anemia with a reticulocytosis. Usually, the source of the blood loss is the GI tract, and the stool guaiac is positive.

Acute blood loss causes a normochromic, normocytic anemia with reticulocytosis. If thrombocytopenia is the cause, abnormalities in the other cell lines suggest diseases of the marrow; ITP is manifested by thrombocytopenia only. In either case, a bone marrow aspiration is indicated.

If a coagulopathy secondary to liver disease is suspected, liver function tests (SGOT, SGPT, bilirubin) should be performed as well as a prothrombin time and partial thromboplastin time.

Management

Underproduction. The dose of iron for iron deficiency is 6 mg/kg/day of elemental iron as ferrous sulfate (20% elemental iron) in three equal doses until the hemoglobin is normal and then for 3 months more. Afterward, a maintenance dose of 2 mg/kg/day is prescribed. Oral iron may cause constipation, diarrhea, epigastric pain, and darkening of the stools. Proper compliance is proven by a peak reticulocytosis in 1 week as well as an increase in hematocrit of up to 1% each day. Failure of iron therapy implies an incorrect diagnosis, noncompliance, an ineffective iron preparation, improper administration, impaired absorption, ongoing blood losses, associated lead poisoning, or coexistent chronic disease.

If the infant is being fed unmodified cow's milk or a nonfortified formula, the diet should be changed to a formula containing 12 mg/liter of elemental iron. In addition to providing inadequate iron, unmodified cow's milk has been implicated as a cause of GI blood loss, so infants under 6 months of age should receive a modified cow's milk formula. In the second half of the first year of life, solid foods provide a good source of iron, especially iron-fortified cereals, which should be encouraged.

Replacement therapy with folic acid or vitamin B_{12} should be given as soon as the type of deficiency is diagnosed. Oral folate results in a reticulocytosis in 48 hours. For B_{12} deficiency, 50–100 mcg of B_{12} three times a day, or 1,000 mcg intramusculary

once a month, should lead to a reticulocytosis within 1 week.

The treatment of lead poisoning involves chelation therapy with calcium EDTA, 50 mg/kg/day IM, in three or four divided doses. The calcium EDTA should be mixed with procaine to ease the pain of the injections. Any child receiving this drug should be well hydrated. In severe poisoning (symptomatic or lead > 90 mg/dL), BAL 4 mg/kg/dose q4h is given IM alone for the first dose and then with calcium EDTA on the following doses. The total course is usually 5–7 days.

The anemia of chronic illness and inflammation will respond only to the treatment of the primary illness. The care of a child with a primary bone marrow illness is beyond the scope of this chapter. Such patients should be referred to a hematologist/oncologist.

Hemolysis. The family of a child with G-6-PD deficiency should be aware of potential oxidants (Table 4). Screening should be performed on other family members.

Children with other congenital red cell enzyme deficiencies and membrane defects should be referred to a hematologist. In the case of hereditary spherocytosis, splenectomy should be planned as a curative procedure.

In general, other than awareness of the diagnosis, no treatment is required in cases of thalassemia minor. However, hematologic consultation should be obtained for a child with thalassemia major. Hypertransfusion with or without deferoxamine chelation is the treatment for these patients. The course of sickle cell anemia is variable, with some children having such frequent, severe, painful crises or cerebrovascular accidents that a hypertransfusion regimen is indicated. Other patients will be relatively healthy, and the only concern is infection prophylaxis, either with Pneumovax, 0.5 ml at 2 years of age, or daily PO penicillin. The families of all children with hemoglobinopathies should undergo hemoglobin electrophoresis so that genetic counseling can be offered.

Any child with chronic hemolysis who develops gallstones and cholecystitis should be referred to a pediatric surgeon so that cholecystectomy can be arranged.

Blood Loss. The treatment of thrombocytopenia secondary to marrow invasion or coagulopathy secondary to malignancy should be performed in the hospital under supervision of a hematologist-oncologist. If liver disease is the etiology, vitamin K, 3–5 mg IM, should help restore the levels of the vitamin K-dependent factors.

As previously mentioned, an infant who is being fed cow's milk and presents with anemia and guaiac-positive stools should have his formula changed.

If hookworms are diagnosed, mebendazole 1 tablet twice a day for 3 days, is effective treatment.

Despite the variety and range of possible etiologies of anemia in infants and children, in most cases management consists solely of a therapeutic trial of iron, with appropriate follow-up. Unless acutely ill, most anemic patients can be treated in the practitioner's office without consultation with a hematologist-oncologist. In addition, in most cases when the cause is not iron deficiency, the management does not require a multitude of blood tests or subspecialist assistance. The child with lead intoxication, thalassemia minor, the anemia of chronic disease, hookworms, or mild intolerance should be followed by the practitioner. No hematology referral is necessary.

It must be remembered, however, that anemia can be the subtle presentation or feature of a much more complex, severe illness. Especially in the case of chronic or severe diseases, such as leukemia, renal failure, systemic lupus erythematosus, or chronic liver disease, a subspecialist's involvement is mandatory. No general practitioner can expect to care for such patients without adequate consultation and assistance. Instead, there is a need for coordination of services and support to the family.

BIBLIOGRAPHY

Dallman PR, Siimes MA: Percentile curves for hemoglobin and red cell volume in infancy and childhood. J Pediatr 94: 26, 1979

Duffy TP: Anemia in adolescence. Med Clin North Am 59:1481, 1975

Fuerth JS: Incidence of anemia in full-term infants seen in private practice. J Pediatr 79:560, 1971

Lubin B, Vichinsky E: Anemia in the newborn period. Pediatr Ann 8:416, 1979

Martinez-Torres C, Layrisse M: Nutritional factors in iron deficiency: Food iron absorption. Clin Hematol 2:339, 1973

Nutrition surveillance, United States, 1980. MMWR 30:521, 1981

Oski FA: Anemia in children. Hosp Practice Dec. 1976, p 63

Oski FA, Stockman JA: Anemia due to inadequate iron stores or poor iron utilization. Pediatr Clin North Am 27:237, 1980

Sullivan DW, Glader BE: Erythrocytic enzyme disorders in children. Pediatr Clin North Am 27:449, 1980

Wolfe LC, Lux S: Nutritional anemias of childhood. Pediatr Ann 8:435, 1979

Cross-Reference to *Pediatrics,* 17th ed.

SIX

Cough, Wheezing, and Stridor

Andrew P. Mezey

Cough is a common complaint in children; most often it is self-limited in duration and requires little or no therapy. Though at best it is an annoying symptom, at worst it may be a very frightening one, especially when associated with difficulty in breathing, such as when accompanied by wheezing and stridor. An appreciation of the causes, natural history, and treatment of cough, wheezing, and stridor is essential for those involved in the health care of children.

DEFINITIONS AND PATHOGENESIS

Cough

Cough is produced by a reflex response to stimulation of afferent end organs in the pharynx, larynx, trachea, and bronchi (but not the distal airways or alveoli). The sound occurs on expiration, due to the forceful movement of air against a closed glottis. Its characteristics are modified by the area responsible for the cough. Therefore, an experienced listener often is able to differentiate lower airway from upper airway disease based on the sound of the cough. Since force is required to produce the cough, variations in sound may be related also to the strength

or weakness of the individual. Decreasing cough associated with increasing difficulty in breathing suggests a worsening rather than an improvement in a patient's condition.

Wheezing

Wheezing is a sound most often heard only on expiration, due to active forceful expulsion of air through narrowed airways below the level of their exit from the pleural cavity (i.e., below the trachea). Airways inside the pleural cavity normally decrease in diameter during expiration due to increased intrathoracic pressure. When narrowing of these airways takes place during the course of disease, obstruction to flow results, expiration becomes active rather than passive, and wheezing occurs. Depending on the severity and location of the obstruction, the sound may be high or low pitched, localized or generalized, of long or short duration, and it may be present on inspiration as well as expiration.

Stridor

Stridor is a sound heard on inspiration due to an obstruction to flow in the airways above the pleural reflection (i.e., larynx and trachea). These airways decrease in size during normal inspiration. When a disease process narrows them further, requiring a more forceful entry of air on inspiration, stridor is produced. The quality of this sound varies with the location of the obstruction, the degree of narrowing, and the force used on inspiration.

ETIOLOGY

For the purposes of this discussion the various etiologies will be grouped by the symptom most often associated with that process, as shown in Table 1. Where it is felt that a process can cause cough with or without wheezing or stridor, it is placed in more than one category but is discussed under cough whenever possible.

Cough

An inflammation of the respiratory tract is the most common cause of cough. A wide variety of agents, including viruses, allergens, bacteria, fungi, mycoplasmas, and foreign bodies, may be at fault. The following discussion focuses on the most common causes, with an emphasis on acute rather than chronic cough (Table 1).

Upper Respiratory Infection (Common Cold). The common cold, or URI, can be caused by a number of viruses, though it is most commonly associated with rhinoviruses and coronaviruses. Coryza and sneezing are the cardinal features. Fever is not common, though malaise, fatigue, and myalgia may occur. Coughing is due to irritation of the posterior pharynx by secretions. Because of this, the cough is much more prominent during sleep, due to pooling in the recumbent position. Sore throat, when present, occurs upon arising and clears as the day progresses. The illness lasts only a few days. When it seems to persist, bacterial superinfection of the sinuses, middle ear, or lungs should be considered.

TABLE 1. CAUSES OF COUGH, WHEEZING, AND STRIDOR

Cough	Wheezing	Stridor
Acute	Acute	Acute
Upper respiratory infection	Allergy (asthma)	Laryngotracheitis (croup)
Allergic rhinitis	Foreign body aspiration	Epiglottitis
Lower respiratory infections	Lower respiratory infection	Retropharyngeal abscess
Croup	Chronic or recurrent	Foreign body aspiration
Bronchitis	Allergy (asthma)	Allergy (acute laryngeal edema
Bronchiolitis	Foreign body aspiration	or laryngospasm)
Pneumonia		Chronic or recurrent
Whooping cough		Congenital conditions
Chronic or recurrent		Intrinsic tracheal
Allergic rhinitis		Laryngomalacia
Asthma		Tracheal cartilage malfor-
Habit		mation
Lower respiratory disease		Laryngeal or tracheal web
Tuberculosis		Extrinsic tracheal
Bronchiectasis		Vascular rings
Cystic fibrosis		Retropharyngeal masses
Foreign body aspiration		Neck masses
Gastroesophageal reflux		Allergy (tracheitis, laryngitis)
with recurrent aspiration		

Allergic Rhinitis. The nature of cough due to allergic rhinitis is very similar to that of the common cold, since the irritation occurs also in the pharynx.

Lower Respiratory Infections. For purposes of discussion this section will be divided into five categories as seen in Table 1, under acute cough.

Croup. The term "croup" is used to describe a broad category of conditions associated with a barky cough and with varying degrees of inspiratory stridor. Pathologically, it is associated with disease in the subglottic area. Only the larynx and trachea are involved in most instances; extension to the bronchi is infrequent and is associated with more severe disease. Severity of illness is also determined by the degree of narrowing of the airway by either inflammation or edema. The etiology of croup is almost always viral; parainfluenza virus types 1 and 2 are the most common agents. However, croup may be caused by a variety of other viruses associated with respiratory infections, including respiratory syncytial virus, adenovirus, influenza A virus, and measles virus. For purposes of description and therapy, the clinical entity croup should be further subdivided into spasmodic croup, acute laryngotracheitis, and acute laryngotracheobronchitis.

Spasmodic croup is by far the most common form of croup. The typical history is that of an infant, usually 6 months to 2½ years, who develops a URI, goes to sleep for the night, and awakens within 2 or more hours with difficulty in breathing, associated with inspiratory stridor and a barky, seallike cough. This episode is frightening to both the parents and the child, and medical help is usually sought.

Acute laryngotracheitis is much less common than spasmodic croup, though it is difficult to assess accurately the comparative incidence. The usual age is 6 months to 2½ years, though children to age 8 years can be af-

fected. It is characterized by the development of a URI followed by the gradual development of a hoarse voice and barky cough, progressing to inspiratory stridor of varying degree, with or without fever. Occasionally, acute laryngotracheitis follows an episode of spasmodic croup that does not clear in the usual fashion. The stridor in laryngotracheitis is present all day, though it is worse at night. It may be present only with crying, or it may be audible with each breath, in which case it is usually associated with an increased respiratory effort. In young infants, the difficulty in breathing may interfere with feeding and sleeping, leading to starvation, metabolic acidosis, fatigue, and respiratory failure. These children require early evaluation and often hospitalization for proper treatment.

Acute laryngotracheobronchitis is the term used when there is evidence of bronchitis (rhonchi and coarse rales) as well as inspiratory stridor. It occurs either as a primary viral bronchitis (e.g., influenza A, measles) or a bacterial superinfection usually due to staphylococci. It tends to cause prolonged, severe disease, with fever and a toxic appearance as more prominent features. This illness is seen in the midst of outbreaks of influenza A and, in past years, with measles.

Bronchitis. In children, acute bronchitis is almost always due to a viral infection (influenza A or B, measles, adenovirus). The symptoms associated with it are those of the familiar flu syndrome: fever, loose cough, malaise, and myalgia. Acute bronchitis is more common in school-age children, with the acute symptoms lasting 3–4 days, and the cough persisting for 7–10 days. Diffuse ronchi and bibasilar rales are heard on auscultation of the chest.

Bronchiolitis. This is a disease of young infants from 2 to 18 months, usually less than 6 months, and is almost exclusively associated with a viral infection. The respiratory syncytial virus is by far the most common agent, though parainfluenza and adenoviruses may also cause this illness. The diagnosis is made when an infant develops a tight cough, associated with wheezing, after 3 or 4 days of an upper respiratory infection. Fever is usually absent, but tachypnea and difficulty with feeding are prominent features. As a general rule, the younger the infant, the more serious the disease, with almost all hospitalizations for bronchiolitis occurring in children under 6 months. On physical examination, bilateral expiratory wheezes, inspiratory rales, intercostal and subcostal retractions, and nasal flaring are noted. The severity of the disease generally peaks at 48–72 hours, with rapid resolution of the respiratory distress, though wheezing on auscultation may persist. In the rare case, respiratory failure may occur, necessitating supportive measures (mechanical ventilation). Acute bronchiolitis due to respiratory syncytial virus occurs in yearly epidemic form, usually in January and February, though April and May outbreaks are also seen. It is an interesting and important disease since maternal antibody does not provide significant protection, therefore placing the young infant at risk. It has been noted that after respiratory syncytial virus infection associated with wheezing, subsequent episodes of wheezing occur in up to 50% of these children, while asthma (recurrent episodes of reversible airway disease) is seen in 10–25%.

Pneumonia. Pneumonia can be defined as an infection of the lung that involves the alveoli or the interstitial supporting tissue. Though cough reflex receptors are not present in the alveoli or distal airways, cough is a prominent symptom in most patients with pneumonia, probably because of involvement of bronchioles and bronchi. However, cough may not be present early in the course of the disease.

The etiology of pneumonia varies according to age (Table 2). In the first 2 months, organisms associated with the mother's genital tract are most common, e.g.,

group B *Streptococcus pyogenes, Chlamydia trachomatis,* and cytomegalovirus. Viral infections are the major cause of pneumonia from 2 months to 5 years, with the respiratory syncytial virus being the most common etiology. *Streptococcus pneumoniae* and *Haemophilus influenzae* type b are the major bacterial causes of either primary or secondary pneumonias after 2 months of age, although as indicated in Table 2, they can also cause disease in the first 2 months. Primary bacterial pneumonia presents as fever without a source, with symptoms and signs subsequently localizing to the chest. If a blood count and blood culture are performed early in the course of the illness before respiratory symptoms emerge, the white blood count will usually be elevated above $15,000/mm^3$ and the blood culture may be positive. If a chest x-ray is taken, it may show pneumonia prior to the manifestation of respiratory symptoms. Most commonly, pneumonias, caused by *S. pneumoniae* and *H. influenzae* type b, are secondary pneumonias, i.e., a superinfection during the course of a viral respiratory illness, especially those due to influenza A and B or measles virus. This is recognized by the onset of fever over 39C., with or without respiratory distress, at a time when the patient should have begun to improve.

Mycoplasma pneumoniae as a cause of pneumonia is most common after 5 years of age. It frequently begins with a sore throat or cold symptoms and progresses to a cough, with or without fever. Physical findings may be minimal, while the chest x-ray usually shows areas of infiltration in the lower lobes. If wheezing is present on auscultation, or if a rash, especially erythema multiforme, is present, *M. pneumoniae* should be strongly considered. Just as respiratory syncytial virus is the most common infectious cause of wheezing in the infant, *M. pneumoniae* is the most common infectious cause of wheezing in the child over 5 years of age. This is usually a mild illness, often the cause of "walking pneumonia" in adults, clearing within 10 days even

TABLE 2. MAJOR ETIOLOGIES OF PNEUMONIA BY AGE GROUP

Newborn to 2 Months	2 Months to 5 Years	5 Years and Older
Febrile	Respiratory syncytial virus	*Mycoplasma pneumoniae*
Group B *Streptococcus (pyogenes)*	Adenovirus	Influenza A and B viruses
Staphylococcus aureus	Parainfluenza virus	Adenovirus
Streptococcus pneumoniae	Influenza A and B viruses	Parainfluenza virus
Haemophilus influenzae, type b	*S. pneumoniae*	*S. pneumoniae*
Klebsiella pneumoniae	*Haemophilus influenzae,* type b	
Gram-negative enteric bacteria		
Afebrile		
Chlamydia trachomatis		
Cytomegalovirus		
Respiratory syncytial virus		
Parainfluenza virus		
Adenovirus		
Pneumocystis carinii		

without treatment. However, children with sickle cell disease who develop *Mycoplasma* pneumonia seem not to fare well. They may develop severe systemic signs, including prolonged high fever and pleuritic pain, with pleural effusion on x-ray.

Whooping Cough (Pertussis). Whooping cough is an infection caused by the bacterium *Bordetella pertussis.* It produces a disease characterized by the development of a paroxysmal cough following an upper respiratory infection of about 2 weeks duration. The coughing paroxysms are often associated with cyanosis, vomiting, and the characteristic whoop. In between episodes of coughing, the child appears perfectly fine, without fever or respiratory distress, and the chest is clear to auscultation. Despite compulsory immunization, whooping cough is still seen. All four injections of killed pertussis vaccine are necessary for optimum protection, and the series is not completed until 18 months of age.

Pertussis is a disease whose management has provoked much controversy, since both the illness and the vaccine have associated neurologic morbidity. The present recommendations in the United States, however, are for continued vaccine usage.

The diagnosis of whooping cough can be made on clinical grounds only, i.e., without bacterial confirmation. Any infant or child presenting with a paroxysmal cough associated with cyanosis or vomiting, with or without a whoop, and who is without systemic signs (fever) and without adventitious sounds on auscultation of the chest should be considered to have pertussis. The presence of a marked lymphocytosis and a normal chest x-ray are helpful laboratory tests. The isolation of *B. pertussis* either by a fluorescent antibody technique or by growth on Bordet-Gengou medium is the definitive test but is not essential for the diagnosis.

Asthma. Asthma can be defined as an obstructive disease of the lower airways that is reversible, intermittent, and secondary to a variety of stimuli. The key features are that it is reversible and intermittent. The areas of the lung affected are the bronchi and bronchioles, and the stimuli producing the bronchoconstriction are many, including infectious agents (viruses and bacteria), noxious substances (tobacco smoke), cold air, exercise, emotional upsets, and a variety of allergens that release histamine (IgE mediated). The incidence is high, with a conservative estimate of occurrence of 1 in 30 individuals. It may be associated with a family history of allergy, such as hay fever, atopic eczema, or allergic rhinitis, or these conditions may be present along with the asthma in the patient. However, in some individuals with asthma, the family history is negative, and there are no symptoms of allergy. The natural history of asthma is that it becomes less severe with age and may remit entirely or produce only minor symptoms. However, a small minority of individuals develop progressive symptomatology, which interferes with their daily lives and may cause death during an acute attack.

When acute attacks occur the patient begins to cough with exertion or on taking deep breaths and progresses to difficulty in breathing. Because the airways affected are intrathoracic, they decrease in diameter on expiration, producing an obstruction to airflow. The expiratory component of breathing becomes active rather than passive, increasing the work involved. Physical examination reveals expiratory wheezes, with prolongation of expiration, intercostal and subcostal retractions, nasal flaring, and tensing of the sternomastoid muscles of the neck. If the obstruction is very severe, wheezing may not be heard since there will not be very much movement of air. If the attack is not treated, it may subside on its own after a few days, or it may progress to respiratory failure. The longer the disease goes on, the less reversible the airway disease becomes, since mucous plugging and atelectasis may occur. Status asthmaticus in children is usually defined as a failure to respond to subcutaneous injections of aqueous epinephrine and is life threatening. While many individuals with asthma never or rarely have an episode of status asthmaticus, other individuals have repeated, severe attacks.

Habitual or Psychogenic Cough. Every once in a while, a child presents with a persistent cough with no clear etiology. Sometimes the cough is so annoying that family life is greatly disrupted. Most often the symptoms begin following a routine illness and then persist and worsen. One should consider the possibility of the cough being related to emotional factors. Fortunately this condition is rarely seen in the pediatric population, but when it is encountered it sorely stresses the diagnostic abilities of the pediatric practitioner.

Foreign Body Aspiration. Aspiration of a foreign body is most often seen in children between 6 months and 2½ years and is associated with the ingestion of hard, round objects, such as peanuts, uncooked peas, and beads. Cough, stridor, or wheezing may be produced depending on the area in which the foreign body lodges. Cough alone is produced when there is irritation of cough receptors without airway obstruction. When narrowing of the tracheal airway occurs, stridor is produced, which varies from mild to severe depending on the extent of the obstruction. Wheezing is the most common manifestation of foreign body aspiration in children, since the objects generally are small and, therefore, can traverse the airways to the bronchi. Though one would expect localized wheezing to occur, this is not necessarily the case. Generalized wheezing is often heard after aspiration of a foreign body, although the wheezing is most pronounced in the area where the obstruction has occurred.

The diagnosis is based on a history of the acute onset of symptoms, appropriate physical examination, and help from the radiologist. The acute onset of stridor, especially in an awake child, should always make one think of foreign body aspiration. Over the past several years, we have seen two children die secondary to acute airway obstruction, one from a small checker, the other from an aspirated balloon. Both presented with the acute onset of respiratory collapse. More often the outcome is not tragic, for the objects do not occlude the airway completely. The sudden onset of wheezing and coughing, especially when it is associated with eating, should help one think of aspiration. Nuts are often put into a cake, which is fed to an infant, who then may aspirate a piece. The diagnosis can be made on physical examination if there are localized findings, but in our experience these are not always present. Consultation with a radiologist, who will help in obtaining special x-ray views of the chest, is most helpful. Most glass is radiopaque, even when it contains no lead, so it should be looked for carefully if it is suspected as the offending agent. Occasionally, the diagnosis of foreign body aspiration is not made, and the patient develops chronic cough or wheezing, the end result of which may be chronic or recurrent infection and bronchiectasis. We have seen one patient in whom aspiration was suspected, and where the diagnosis could not be made. The child persisted with intermittent wheezing and cough for a number of months until one day, during a paroxysm of coughing, an object was expelled, with relief of all symptoms.

Laryngomalacia. Laryngomalacia, tracheomalacia, and laryngotracheomalacia describe a benign, self-limited condition caused by abnormally soft and flaccid cartilages. While some authorities have tried to differentiate the above three terms, we believe that they are all the same condition. Infants present with an inspiratory cough (stridor) associated with crying, sometimes heard within the first few days of life. The noise produced can be very loud, especially when the child is on its back. There is no difficulty with feeding, and the infant grows well. Intercurrent respiratory infections cause an increase in noise but generally are no more severe than in children without laryngomalacia. Sometimes the

obstruction due to the soft cartilage is severe enough to produce costal and subcostal retractions or a mild pectus excavatum. In any case, after other etiologies are ruled out by x-ray and laryngoscopic examinations, parents can be assured that the symptoms will disappear by 1–1½ years of age.

Miscellaneous. Other causes of cough, stridor, and wheezing have either been covered in other chapters (epiglottitis, retropharyngeal abscess) or will not be dealt with in this book. The reader is referred to *Pediatrics,* 17th ed., for a detailed description.

DIFFERENTIAL DIAGNOSIS

History

Since cough is the underlying complaint, this aspect of the history will be stressed. The answers to certain key questions often provide the information necessary for accurate diagnosis and treatment.

- How long has the cough been present? Since cough is usually secondary to either upper or lower acute respiratory infection, the duration of symptoms generally is short. A cough of longer duration (2 weeks or more) expands the diagnostic possibilities greatly.
- Is there a history of recurrent cough in a child in whom the onset is acute? Recurrent cough should suggest the possibility of the presence of allergy involving either the upper or lower respiratory tract. A less likely cause is recurrent aspiration secondary to incoordination in swallowing or to gastroesophageal reflux. Even less likely are recurrent infections secondary to immune deficiency.
- Is the cough associated with any other symptoms, such as fever, rhinorrhea, wheezing, or inspiratory stridor? Cough with low-grade or moderate fever [39C

(102.2F) or less] is less likely to be associated with bacterial pneumonia than is a cough accompanied by a fever of 40C (104F). Rhinorrhea and low-grade fever are typical of an upper respiratory tract infection. The acute onset of inspiratory stridor is a symptom of croup (laryngotracheitis), whereas wheezing may be associated with either allergy or infection.

- Is the cough getting worse, or have any new symptoms appeared? Most acute respiratory infections in children have a characteristic natural history. They begin rather suddenly, plateau, and then begin to resolve after 1–3 days, the total duration of the disease usually lasting no longer than 4–5 days. Persistence of or increase in the severity of the cough or the addition of new symptoms, such as purulent rhinitis, fever, or respiratory distress, may signify a complication of the initial illness. This sequence is seen most commonly in children under 5 years and is usually due to a bacterial complication of a viral illness. Suppurative otitis media is the most common complication; sinusitis and pneumonia are less frequent.

- How would you describe the cough? Is it brassy, croupy, loose, dry, worse at night, worse in the morning? A brassy cough is associated with tracheitis or tracheobronchitis. Croupy or barky cough is typical of laryngitis or laryngotracheitis. A loose cough, usually worse in the morning, is often seen with bronchitis. A dry cough, which may be described as an unsuccessful attempt to cough something out, is heard in the early stages of pneumonia. Pooled pharyngeal secretions cause an irritative cough that is worse at night in a child with URI. A chronic cough that is worse at night is most likely associated with asthma, even when no wheezing is heard during the daytime. A cough productive of sputum in a young child is unusual, making this valuable piece of historical data in adult patients less helpful in pediatric practice.

- If the cough has been present for more than 2 weeks, a search must be made for the causes of its persistence. Persistent nighttime cough is most often associated with asthma, even without evidence of wheezing or allergy. A family history of allergies with or without asthma, previous episodes of wheezing with or without URIs, cough associated with exertion or cold temperatures, recurrent episodes of croup in the past or present are all helpful in making this diagnosis. Other features of the allergic child include a history of bluish discoloration under the eyes (allergic shiners), itchy nose, runny eyes, and persistent, clear nasal discharge.

 A history of weight loss or poor growth in a child with a chronic cough is important and generally signifies serious illness. Most children with asthma, even when severe, continue to grow normally over a long period of time. If there is true growth failure, cystic fibrosis should be suspected, especially in white children. Pertussis syndrome should be considered in any child with persistent cough, typically paroxysmal, and associated with vomiting, tearing of the eyes, and cyanosis during the cough. Tuberculosis, much less common now in the United States than previously, should also be considered in a child with chronic cough, as should foreign body aspiration, hypersensitivity pneumonitis, and neoplastic disease. Recurrent aspiration, either as a result of incoordinated swallowing or gastroesophageal reflux, and cow's milk allergy with or without pulmonary hemosiderosis can present with persistent wheezing. However, in a general pediatric practice, allergic asthma is by far the most common cause of chronic, persistent cough in an otherwise healthy child.

- Is there a history of possible foreign body aspiration? Aspiration can cause both acute and chronic cough depending upon the position of the foreign body. If an object lodges in the upper respiratory tract, inspiratory stridor occurs acutely, with the amount of respiratory distress related to the degree of obstruction of the airway. Chronic cough and wheeze can also occur following foreign body aspiration when the object is lodged in one of the smaller, more peripheral airways. In patients with either acute or chronic symptoms due to aspiration, a history is most often lacking, the diagnosis being established by clinical suspicion and appropriate diagnostic procedures.

Physical Examination

While the history is most important in establishing a diagnosis, the physical examination is most useful in determining the severity of the illness.

- Is the work of breathing increased? Is the work greater on inspiration or expiration? Normally expiration is a passive event; when lower airway obstruction occurs, it becomes active. Breathing is normally quiet; when severe obstruction occurs, either on inspiration or expiration, breathing becomes noisy. If very severe obstruction occurs, breathing becomes less noisy again, since less air is being moved. Observations on the work involved with breathing can be refined by looking for the presence of nasal flaring, supraclavicular, intercostal, and subcostal retractions, and contraction of the sternocleidomastoid muscle. Infants under 1 year of age tire more quickly, so it is especially important to gauge accurately the degree of respiratory difficulty. A good guide for this is observation of the ability to take a bottle. Difficulty in drinking is associated with significant distress, necessitating hospitalization.
- Is there any asymmetry in the movement of the chest or in breath sounds? Pain with breathing, due to pleural or abdominal disease, may cause splinting of one side of the chest. Differences in breath sounds heard on auscultation may be due to pneumothorax, pleural effusion, or pulmonary consolidation.
- Are there any adventitious breath sounds? The presence of expiratory wheezing, inspiratory stridor or wheezing, or inspiratory coarse or fine rales or rhonchi are helpful clues in diagnosis. Because of pressure differentials, the intrathoracic airways are narrower on expiration. Therefore, bronchospasm of mild or moderate degree will cause only expiratory wheezing. As the bronchial obstruction increases, wheezing will be heard on both inspiration and expiration. With further compromise of airways, air flow may be so diminished that wheezing will not be heard. The extrathoracic airway, however, is smaller during inspiration. Disease of the larynx and trachea, therefore, is associated with more difficulty on inspiration than on expiration (inspiratory stridor). Fixed inspiratory rales, especially toward the end of inspiration, are typical of pneumonia. When they are heard, the diagnosis of pneumonia can be made even without a radiograph.

Coarse bilateral diffuse rales or rhonchi present throughout inspiration or expiration are typical of bronchitis (disease of the larger airways). In these instances, it may be difficult to rule out pneumonia, since disease of both the large and small airways may be present, and the louder adventitious sounds may obscure the finer and less obvious inspiratory rales. Many practitioners treat these children with antibiotics, feeling that it is almost impossible to distinguish the two diseases.

Bronchiolitis, the most common infectious cause of wheezing in children under 2 years, is usually a mild disease of short duration, though in its severe form (infants below 6 months) it may cause respiratory failure. Wheezing associated with respiratory infection in the older child is most likely to be due to *Mycoplasma*. As mentioned above, aspiration of a foreign body can cause either acute or chronic symptoms with inspiratory stridor, expiratory wheezes, or evidence of pulmonary consolidation. It is noteworthy that the presence of bilateral, diffuse wheezing does not rule out foreign body aspiration.

- Is there any evidence of chronic pulmonary disease? Increased anterior-posterior diameter of the chest and clubbing of the fingers are both signs of longstanding pulmonary problems. Clubbing is unusual in children with asthma; when present it is more likely due to cystic fibrosis. Increased anterior-posterior diameter of the chest can be seen in older children with longstanding severe asthma as well as in those with other chronic respiratory problems, such as cystic fibrosis, emphysema due to alpha-1-antitrypsin inhibitor deficiency, and other rarer diseases.

Laboratory Diagnosis

Elevation of the white blood count with an increase in segmented and band forms in the child with evidence of lower respiratory disease may be helpful in differentiating bacterial from viral disease, especially if the elevated blood count is associated with fever (> 39.5C). Elevation of the white count with a marked predominance of lymphocytes is associated with pertussis syndrome. In the first 2–3 months of life, an afebrile infant with pneumonia and conjunctivitis who has an increased eosinophil count is likely to have a *Chlamydia* infection. Eosinophilia is also seen in children who wheeze secondary to allergies. However, marked eosinophilia (> 20% of white count) in a patient with wheezing is more likely associated with pneumonic phase of intestinal parasites or with allergic aspergillosis.

Radiography. A radiograph of the chest is helpful in differentiating acute and chronic causes of wheezing, stridor, and cough. However, it does have limitations. Most causes of both acute and chronic cough are associated with normal chest films. Pneumonia in children, but especially in infants, the most susceptible age group, may not be associated with a lobar infiltrate. If the film is taken early in the course of the illness, the radiograph usually is normal. Use of chest radiographs should be reserved for the diagnostic problems shown in Table 3.

A radiograph in a child in the midst of an acute attack of asthma is seldom helpful. Even if areas of pulmonary density are seen, they are most likely secondary to atelectasis and clear rapidly as the disease is treated with bronchodilators. In the child with the first episode of wheezing, a radiograph may be helpful in defining the etiology. Pneumonia may sometimes be the cause, but other diagnostic possibilities include compression of a bronchus by a node or obstruction by a foreign body.

Lateral radiographs of the neck are helpful in differentiating acute epiglottitis from croup. (See Chapter 18.) However, the diagnosis can usually be made on clinical grounds alone. Other diagnostic tests, such as lung scans, ultrasound, computerized tomography, special radiographic views, fluoroscopy,

TABLE 3. INDICATIONS FOR CHEST X-RAY IN THE CHILD WITH PULMONARY DISEASE

Lack of response to usual antibiotics
Positive tuberculin test
Toxic child with pulmonary symptoms (rule out pleural effusion, neoplasia, necrotizing pneumonia)
Infants below 3 months of age
Immunocompromised host
Chronic cough when cause not apparent
Chronic illness complicated by pulmonary symptoms
Suspicion of foreign body aspiration
Persistent fever without a source

and barium studies, are best obtained in consultation with a radiologist or pulmonary specialist.

MANAGEMENT OF ACUTE ILLNESS

The general management of upper respiratory illness depends on the particular diagnosis, while the specific management depends upon the severity of the illness. This section will deal with specific management with an emphasis on the severely ill infant or child.

Upper Respiratory Infection

Uncomplicated upper respiratory infection requires little or no specific management. In the first few months, infants may have greater difficulty with stuffed noses due to a decreased ability to switch to mouth breathing. In these instances, normal saline nose drops are very effective and safe. (A solution of the appropriate strength can be made by adding ¼ teaspoon salt to 6–8 ounces of water.) Sympathomimetics given either locally or systemically are not necessary and are potentially harmful in the young infant. In the older child, antihistamines, with or without sympathomimetics, may be helpful in relieving symptoms, especially at night. They have the disadvantage of changing the child's behavior (irritability), due either to sedation or stimulation. There is an occasional child with a URI whose cough at night is so severe that he keeps himself or the family up all night. In these cases, when a trial of an antihistamine/sympathomimetic agent has been unsuccessful, cough suppressants (dextromethorphan, codeine) may be used. It is unusual for the above symptoms to be due solely to a URI, and they may signify some other condition (e.g., asthma, otitis media). We believe, therefore, that the frequent use of cough suppressants by practitioners is an abuse of medication.

Allergic Rhinitis

When this diagnosis is made, antihistamines are used when the severity of symptoms indicates. If the condition is persistent or bothersome despite symptomatic treatment, referral to an allergist may be helpful. Allergists tend to be much more forceful than pediatric practitioners in cleaning houses to protect the allergic child. Occasionally, skin testing and hyposensitization is recommended for the treatment of allergic rhinitis or rhinoconjunctivitis, especially when symptoms persist despite good cooperation in environmental control. This is especially true when the rhinitis is associated with recurrent or persistent otitis media.

Croup

The management of croup depends greatly upon whether the child is at home or in the hospital. The decision to hospitalize the patient is dependent upon the judgment of the individual practitioner, but croup scores have been devised to help assess the degree of severity of illness (Table 4). They take into account the amount of respiratory distress, as judged by the presence or absence of cyanosis, nasal flaring, and supracostal or suprasternal retractions, and by the degree of elevation of respiratory rate and pulse. Scoring the degree of severity is useful for following a child's progress, but absolute numerical scores should not be used in making a judgment about hospitalization. The infant or child with stridor who feeds and sleeps well and who is playful and active need only be followed daily. As the disease continues, the stridor may become more severe, feeding may become more difficult, and the child's mood may worsen. This sequence occurs more frequently in infants under 1 year who are febrile ($\geq$ 39.5C). When this progression

TABLE 4. CROUP SCORE AS A GUIDE TO SEVERITY OF ILLNESS*

	Stridor	Cyanosis	Chest Retractions	Nasal Flaring	Elevated Pulse/ Respiration
None	0	0	0	0	0
With crying	1	1	1	1	1
At rest	2	2	2	2	2

*Degree of severity: 0–3, mild; 4–7, moderate; 8–10, severe.

is noted or the features are present from the outset, hospitalization is advisable. More rapid respiratory failure tends to intervene in younger infants due to increasing airway compromise and increasing fatigue.

Spasmodic Croup

In children who have typical spasmodic croup, improvement with treatment is almost always prompt, usually within 15–30 minutes. This is accomplished by the use of a number of tried and true remedies: hot, moist air generated by running the shower in the bathroom, cold moist air created by a fog generator, cold night air generated by a car ride, and time alone generated by patience. Previously, the induction of vomiting by the use of emetics such as ipecac was also used. We no longer recommend this therapy, believing that the four methods listed above are as effective and safer.

After the acute episode of difficulty in breathing subsides, the child is left with a barky cough and hoarse voice. The parents are left with palpitations and a rapid pulse, and the pediatric practitioner is left with interrupted sleep. This episode may recur that night or the next night; it is usually less severe than the first one. The child remains afebrile during the course of the illness, which usually lasts 3–4 days. If the child does become febrile, another source of infection, such as an ear infection or pneumonia, should be suspected.

Spasmodic croup tends to be recurrent, in association with URIs, and it may occur in other siblings, especially where there is a family history of allergy. No treatment other than humidification of the child's room for the duration of the illness is required. Elevation of the child's head may be helpful. Anecdotal evidence suggests that holding the child upright in front of the television set may also be effective in preventing a second episode. Antihistamines, cough remedies, antibiotics, and steroids are neither recommended nor indicated. Very rarely the degree of upper airway obstruction is so severe that the child may become cyanotic, have a seizure or a respiratory arrest, and become comatose. If these unusual events occur, establishment of an airway, oxygen therapy, and hospitalization are urgently required. In the private practice of the author, no such instance occurred during a period of 13 years. However, in a large hospital pediatric service, one or two such episodes associated with spasmodic croup may be seen in the course of a year.

Acute Laryngotracheitis/ Laryngotracheobronchitis

The treatment of acute laryngotracheitis is controversial (Fig. 1). Most authors agree that humidification of air is beneficial and that oxygen therapy should be used if indicated by arterial blood gas evaluation. However, nebulization of alpha-adrenergic agents, such as racemic epinephrine or phenylephrine, and the use of adrenocorticosteroids are controversial. We have used nebulized 2.25% racemic epinephrine in a 1:5 to 1:10 dilution, depending on severity and tolerance, as frequently as every 2 hours and on rare occasions hourly; the effect lasts 2–3 hours on the average. We strongly recommend that patients in whom racemic epinephrine has been used to improve inspiratory stridor be hospitalized, since the effect is only transitory. Antibiotics are not indicated when there is no evidence of bacterial superinfection. If the child is feeding poorly or tires after feeding, intravenous fluids are indicated. If oxygen requirements increase as evidenced by decreased PaO_2 levels in association with evidence of CO_2 retention (increased $PaCO_2$ levels), endotracheal intubation with ventilatory assistance may be required. We have not routinely used steroids in children with acute laryngotracheitis. A recent study has shown some effect on the rapidity of improvement, though the number of patients studied was small. It is our impression that in the very ill child with acute

laryngotracheitis, early use of steroids has not eliminated the need for endotracheal intubation.

The most important factor in the care of a child with acute laryngotracheitis is diligent observation, proper assessment of hydration and respiratory effort, and patience. The more severe the disease, the longer it tends to last, especially when associated with influenza A or measles. Inspiratory stridor of 2 weeks duration may occur. If the child is not tiring and if the arterial blood gases are stable, most children will improve with only supportive therapy and intermittent administration of nebulized racemic epinephrine.

Children who have acute laryngotracheobronchitis usually do not respond to the above measures. These infants get worse, develop high fever, tend to become more toxic with time, and require more oxygen. Treatment with antibiotics is indicated when mate-

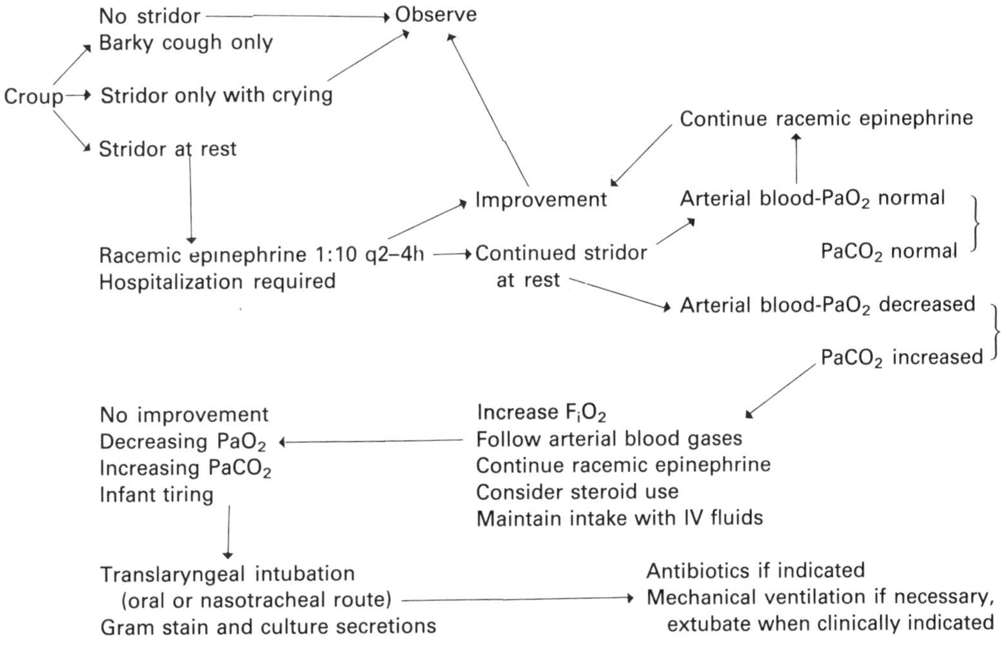

Figure 1. Management of Croup

rial aspirated following laryngoscopy and intubation is purulent and grows bacteria on culture. A recent report suggests that staphylococci may play a role in acute laryngotracheobronchitis. We use a combination of antibiotics active against *H. influenzae* type b, *S. pneumoniae,* and staphylococci while awaiting the results of culture. (Nafcillin or oxacillin 100 mg/kg/24 hr and chloramphenicol 100 mg/kg/24 hr in divided doses.)

Figure 1 is an algorithm for the management of the child with croup. It should be noted that hospitalization is required once the choice is made to use racemic epinephrine. Though not everyone agrees with this action, we believe that since the relief of stridor is only transient, observation in a setting where alpha-adrenergic agents can be repeated is indicated. It should also be noted that the use of adrenocorticosteroids is left to the individual practitioner's preference. In our experience, early use of steroids has not seemed to change the course of the illness in the patients with severe disease. Translaryngeal intubation, either oral or nasotracheal, is indicated when the patient begins to hypoventilate, as judged by a rising $PaCO_2$. The size of the endotracheal tube used should be at least 0.5 mm smaller than usual for the age; it is left in place for 3–7 days. As the subglottic swelling subsides, an air leak will become evident, and the child may vocalize; both of these events predict the likelihood of successful extubation. Occasionally, a child will develop subglottic stenosis as a result of the disease process or the intubation or both. In these instances a tracheostomy will have to be performed, as well as tracheal endoscopy to delineate the cause. When subglottic stenosis occurs, an otolaryngologist who is familiar with its management should be consulted.

Bronchitis

Since bronchitis is most often of viral etiology, no specific therapy is indicated. Cough suppressants should not be used routinely since the cough can be controlled for the most part by warm liquids and hard candies. It is not easy to prevent people from buying over-the-counter remedies, but one should try. In those rare instances when the cough is very bothersome and asthma and pneumonia have been ruled out, codeine 15–30 mg per dose is effective.

Bronchiolitis

This is most frequently a benign, self-limited illness, which requires only patience on the part of the parent and practitioner. Change of feedings to clear liquids may be necessary if the cough or rapid respiration interferes with eating, while humidification of the room may also help. In infants under 6 months of age, the respiratory distress occasionally is severe enough to require hospitalization and use of oxygen and intravenous fluids. Rarely, bronchiolitis may lead to respiratory failure, as evidenced by a rising $PaCO_2$ in the face of tachypnea. The standard therapy at this point has been to intubate the trachea and to use mechanical ventilation until the process subsides. We have had success with the use of intravenous aminophylline, as in the patient with asthma. In a number of infants between 2 and 5 months of age, hypercapnea has been reversed and tracheal intubation averted. Careful monitoring of theophylline levels is essential, for its pharmacokinetics in infants are less predictable than in the older child.

Pneumonia

Appropriate treatment of pneumonia is dependent upon an understanding of the changing etiologies with age, as can be seen in Table 2.

Newborn to Two Months. In this age group, fever or lack of it is helpful in predicting etiology. In the febrile, severely ill infant with pneumonia, antibiotic coverage must be adequate to treat a number of organisms (Table 2) and can be accomplished by the use of nafcillin or oxacillin 100 mg/kg/24 hr., gentamycin 7.5 mg/kg/24 hr., and chloramphenicol 100 mg/kg/24 hr. Aminoglycoside and chloramphenicol serum levels should be obtained to adjust the dosage. Culture results from the blood or pleural fluid (if present) will be helpful in selecting the most appropriate combination of antibiotics. Consultation with an infectious disease specialist may also be helpful.

Pneumonia in the afebrile infant is either viral or caused by *C. trachomatis*, with a rare case being caused by *Pneumocystis carinii*. The infant who presents with a staccato cough, tachypnea, bilateral, diffuse, fine inspiratory rales, bilateral infiltrates on chest x-ray, increased eosinophils on a peripheral blood smear, and a previous history of conjunctivitis should be considered to have pneumonia due to *Chlamydia*. Treatment with erythromycin 30–50 mg/kg/24 hr for 14 days is recommended. Our practice with infants has been to culture for *C. trachomatis* and to begin erythromycin. If the culture results are negative but the symptoms and signs very typical, we continue therapy anyway. If the symptoms and signs are not typical and the culture is negative, we discontinue therapy. If the infant is wheezing, has pneumonia on x-ray, the rest of the picture is not typical for *Chlamydia*, and we are facing an epidemic of bronchiolitis, we will neither culture nor treat but assume that the disease is secondary to respiratory syncytial virus. If the pneumonia is progressive despite antibiotic or symptomatic therapy, we consider doing an open lung biopsy with frozen and paraffin sections as well as viral and bacterial cultures. These procedures should be carried out in conjunction with pulmonary and infectious disease consultants.

Two Months to Five Years. In this age group, viruses are the most common etiology (Table 2). *S. pneumoniae* is the most common bacterial agent, with an occasional case due to *H. influenzae* type b. The usual management is to use either penicillin 100,000–150,000 U/kg/24 hr or ampicillin 100 mg/kg/24 hr for 10 days. If the child is very ill, the addition of chloramphenicol should be considered to cover for the possibility of ampicillin-resistant *H. influenzae*. In any case, the febrile child with pneumonia who is hospitalized should have blood cultures performed. Children treated as outpatients presumably are less ill and can be successfully treated using either ampicillin or penicillin in almost all cases. Chest x-rays are not usually indicated, especially in the older infant or child where a thorough and reliable physical examination can be done. Every so often, the etiology will prove to be tuberculosis, and it is worthwhile placing a tuberculin test on all patients who are treated for pneumonia.

Five Years and Older. In this age group, *M. pneumoniae* must be considered as a cause of pneumonia. Erythromycin is the treatment of choice in a dose of 30–50 mg/kg/24 hr., not to exceed 1 g. Children receiving over 1 g are likely to develop severe gastritis and vomiting. *S. pneumoniae* and *M. pneumoniae* are both sensitive to erythromycin, and since *H. influenzae* type b is an unlikely cause of pneumonia in this age group, this choice of antibiotic is a convenient and effective one.

Whooping Cough (Pertussis)

Fortunately, whooping cough is not a common disease any longer, for it is uncomfortable at best and potentially dangerous at worst. It is worthwhile to admit to the hospital infants under 6 months with pertussis and to consider for admission infants between 6 and 12 months, since it is the young infant who has the most difficulty with this disease. The treatment is supportive during paroxysms—suctioning and oxygen as required. Erythromycin is given 30–50 mg/kg/day for 10 days to eradicate the carrier state. It probably does not decrease the severity of symptoms or shorten the duration of the illness. If the infant is hospitalized and cannot be isolated, it is worthwhile giving erythromycin for 5 days to all susceptible children (those who have received less than four injections of pertussis vaccine) in the same room to prevent spread of the disease. The 5-day period is selected because it takes about that long to eradicate pertussis from the nasopharynx of the index case. Symptomatic treatment in the hospital is continued until cyanosis with paroxysms stops. For the older individual with pertussis, hospitalization is not required, only patience, for the disease persists for many weeks. Cough suppressants are not particularly helpful but may be tried. Old remedies, such as warm, moist air and honey are as effective as any others.

Asthma

It is impossible to fully describe the management of asthma in this chapter, but some basic areas will be covered.

Acute Management. In the child who develops an acute asthmatic attack, the treatment of choice is to use subcutaneous aqueous epinephrine 1:1000 at a dose of 0.01 ml/kg/dose to a maximum of 0.3 ml. This may be repeated twice (a total of three times), at intervals of 20–30 minutes. Most children will improve markedly within 10–15 minutes after receiving the first injection and may be begun on oral theophylline. Some physicians give a second injection simultaneously with the oral theophylline in order to prevent relapse. Others have stopped using epinephrine as a first-line treatment and have begun to use the newer beta-2-adrenergic medications by aerosol. In a hospital setting, this is possible to do, but in an office setting, subcutaneous epinephrine is more convenient. In either case, most individuals respond to the acute treatment as judged clinically or by measurement of the peak expiratory flow rate. The child with asthma who fails to respond should be hospitalized and treated with a combination of aminophylline, beta-2-adrenergic agents, and possibly adrenocorticosteroids. Aminophylline is given intravenously, 6–9 mg/kg initial dose, followed by 6 mg/kg every 6 hours. Theophylline levels should be measured to judge the appropriateness of the dose. The concentration should be maintained between 10 and 20 mg/L in order to be effective without producing toxicity (Fig. 2). Aerosolized beta-2-adrenergic agents are given every 4–6 hours. Arterial blood gases should be monitored as indicated by the clinical condition. Chest percussion and postural drainage are helpful adjuncts to the pharmocologic therapy.

Management of Chronic Illness. In children with only occasional episodes of wheezing, intermittent therapy is acceptable. However, for the child who has continuous symptoms, as judged by persistent cough or wheezing, especially at night with disturbance of sleep, chronic treatment with theophylline is recommended. The goal of treatment is to improve the quality of life by decreasing cough and wheezing. Maintenance of theophylline levels between 10 and 15 mg/L has been shown to be effective. When breakthrough symptoms occur, adjunctive therapy can be used, e.g., beta-2-adrenergic nebulizers or oral preparations. Slow-release forms of theophylline with predictable pharmacokinetics are now available and make this form of therapy reasonably simple to manage. This is especially true since theophylline serum levels are easily obtained through commercial laboratories. However, since the etiology of asthma is often related to allergy, it is worthwhile to refer patients with persistent symptoms to an allergist experienced in the treatment of children.

Foreign Body Aspiration

When this diagnosis is considered, consultation with a radiologist and an endoscopist comfortable with children is indicated. The pediatric practitioner's role in the manage-

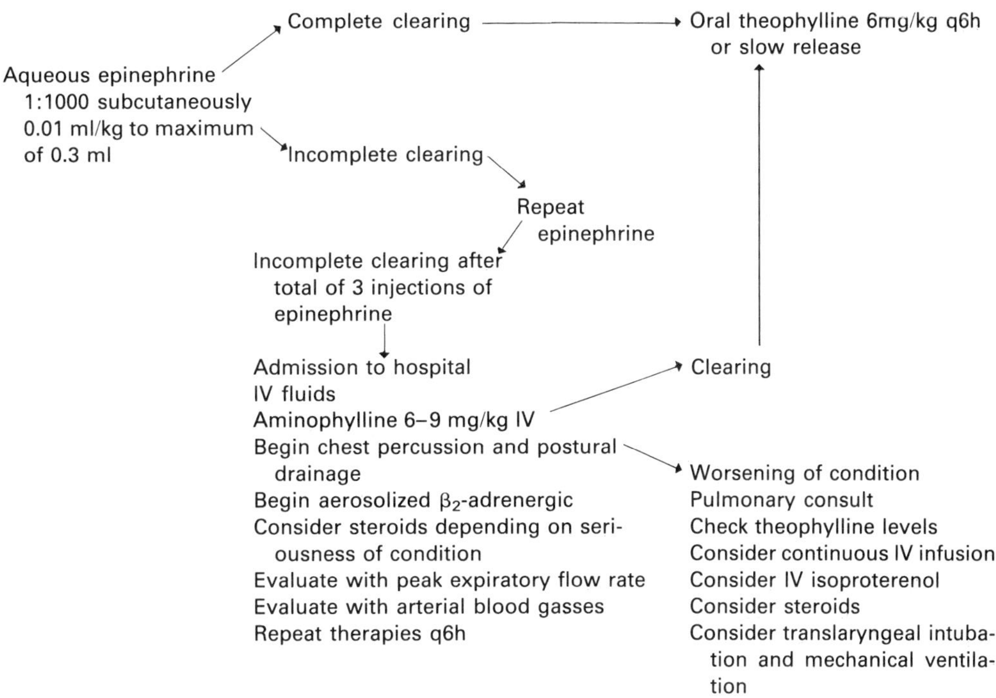

Figure 2. Management of the Acute Asthmatic Attack

ment is to make the diagnosis quickly in order to avoid either acute or chronic irreversible damage.

BIBLIOGRAPHY

Cherry J: The Treatment of Croup. J Pediatr 94:352, 1979

Ellis EF: Relationship between the allergic state and susceptibility to infectious airway disease. Pediatr Res 11:227, 1977

Hammerschlag M: Chlamydial Infections. Pediatrics in Review. 3:77, 1981

Leffert F: The management of acute severe asthma. J Pediatr 96:1, 1980

Ribble JG, Reed SE: Pneumonia caused by bacteria, mycoplasmata, viruses, and pneumocystis In Scarpelli EM, Auld PAM, et al. (eds.): Pulmonary Disease of the Fetus, Newborn, and Child. Lea & Febiger, 1978, p 355

Schley WS, Krauss, AM: Bronchitis and bronchiolitis. In Scarpelli EM, Auld PAM, et al. (eds.): Pulmonary Disease of the Fetus, Newborn, and Child. Lea & Febiger, 1978, p 274

Schley WS, Krauss, AM: Diseases of the Upper Airways. In Scarpelli EM, Auld PAM, et al. (eds.): Pulmonary Disease of the Fetus, Newborn, and Child. Lea & Febiger, 1978, p 254

Webb-Johnson DC, Andrews JL Jr: Bronchodilator therapy. N Engl J Med 297:477, 1977

Cross-Reference to Pediatrics, 17th ed.

SEVEN

Diarrhea and Vomiting

Andrew P. Mezey

The complaints of diarrhea and vomiting are not only among the most common in pediatric practice but are also among the most distressing to both the child and the parents. The anxiety of the parents may be so great that it will interfere with their ability to care for the child. The following discussion should provide an understanding of the problems and their management so that the principles of therapy may be more clearly conveyed to the family. Successful therapy of the diarrhea and vomiting will then be more likely.

For the purposes of this chapter, it is convenient to divide the subject of diarrhea and vomiting into three categories: (1) acute diarrhea (with or without vomiting), (2) chronic diarrhea, and (3) acute or chronic vomiting without diarrhea.

DEFINITIONS

Though diarrhea is usually thought of in terms of frequent, loose stools, it probably is defined more accurately as excessive losses of fluids and electrolytes in the stool. Generally, these losses are also accompanied by excessive losses of fat, carbohydrate (to a moderate extent), and protein (to a much lesser extent). The stools may be accompanied by abdominal cramping or distention or both, although these symptoms are not constant. The stools may be watery and clear, mucusy, or bloody; they may be semiformed or loose. The implications of the different characteristics are discussed below.

Acute diarrhea refers to diarrhea that has a relatively abrupt onset and usually lasts less than 2 weeks. Chronic diarrhea is considered to exist when it has been present for several weeks duration. It may have begun abruptly or have had an insidious or not clearly identifiable onset.

Vomiting is an obvious event, although in the young infant, drooling, "cheesing," or spitting-up may be confused with vomiting. Vomiting is generally a forceful rather than a passive act. The vomitus may be clear, greenish, bright green, bloody, or blood tinged. It may or may not be accompanied by nausea, a symptom that is difficult to assess in infants.

ACUTE DIARRHEA

Etiology

In the past several years there has been a clarification of the etiology of acute childhood diarrhea. The most important discoveries were identification of the rotavirus (duovirus, orbivirus, reovirus-like agents) and the Norwalk virus, which have been shown to be the most common of the identifiable infectious causes of diarrhea among children. In addition, newer bacterial identification tech-

TABLE 1. DISTINGUISHING CHARACTERISTICS OF THE COMMON ETIOLOGIC AGENTS ASSOCIATED WITH ACUTE DIARRHEA IN INFANTS AND CHILDREN

	Season	Transmission	Fever	Diarrhea Type
Viruses (major causes)				
Rotavirus	Cooler	Fecal-oral	Common, high in infants	Watery
Norwalk	Epidemic cooler	Fecal-oral	When present, low grade	Watery
Bacteria				
Shigella	Warm	Fecal-oral	Common	Watery or pus and blood
Salmonella	Warm	Fecal-oral	Common	Watery or pus and blood
Campylobacter	All year	Food, water, fecal-oral	Common	Watery or pus and blood
Yersinia	All year	Food, water, fecal-oral	Common	Watery or pus and blood
Escherichia coli				
Toxigenic (travelers')	Warm	Food, water	Low grade if present	Watery only
Invasive	Undefined	Undefined	Common	Watery—pus, rarely blood
Pathogenic (nursery)	Warm	Food, fecal-oral	Low grade if present	Watery only
Parasitic				
Giardia lambia	Warm	Water	Variable	Watery

niques have demonstrated *Campylobacter* species to be a frequent cause of bacterial diarrheas. *Yersinia* species to be an infrequent but possible cause, and *Escherichia coli* to cause three distinct diarrheal syndromes: enteropathogenic (EPEC), enterotoxigenic (ETEC), and enteroinvasive (EIEC). Table 1 is a summary of the discussion to follow.

Minor viral agents include adenovirus, astrovirus, calicivirus, coronavirus, and enterovirus. These viruses will not be discussed further.

Rotavirus. Infections with rotavirus are the most frequent cause of infantile diarrhea throughout the year, although a peak is seen in the winter months. Vomiting and fever frequently accompany and often precede the diarrhea, which is watery and without mucus. Upper respiratory symptoms are common. The syndrome of fever, vomiting, and watery diarrhea occurring in a young infant from November through May is most typical of rotavirus-induced disease. It is a self-limited illness, with the diarrhea lasting 3–5 days. However, because vomiting is a frequent symptom, dehydration may occur. Rotavirus is the cause in three fourths of infants between 7 and 24 months hospitalized for diarrhea.

Norwalk Virus. Infection with Norwalk virus occurs typically in epidemics among school-aged children and adults, the virus getting its

Diarrhea Duration	Vomiting	Ages Affected	Antibiotic Treatment
3–5 days	Common as presenting sign	Infants most common Older ages, less common	None
1–3 days	Common as presenting sign	Older chldren, adults	None
Variable	Uncommon	All	Often needed TMP-SMX
Variable	Common though not as presenting sign	All	Rarely indicated
Variable	Variable	All, more common in infants, young children	Unknown ? erythromycin
7–20 days	Common	All, more common in young children	Unknown, ? TMP-SMX
3–7 days	Variable	All	Not indicated
5–8 days	Uncommon	All	Unknown, possibly indicated
Variable	Common	Newborn nurseries	Often indicated (colistin)
Variable, can be chronic	Uncommon	All	Metronidazole, quinacrine

name from an epidemic that occurred in Norwalk, Ohio, in 1968. An abrupt onset, usually with nausea and abdominal cramps, followed by vomiting and diarrhea, is most common. The nausea, vomiting, and cramps usually subside within a few hours, while the diarrhea lasts from 1 to 3 days. Fever, when it is present, is low grade. Relapses are rare.

Bacteria. Bacterial causes of diarrhea tend to peak in the summer months. Their frequency varies from place to place. For example, *Shigella* is the most frequently identified cause of diarrhea in children in Houston, Texas, outranking rotavirus, but an infrequent cause of diarrhea in the New York City area. In New York, *Salmonella* species are more commonly encountered than *Shigella*, especially among hospitalized children.

Other. *Giardia lamblia* causes both acute and chronic diarrhea in children. It is often missed when only the stools are examined; duodenal intubation or use of a swallowed gelatin capsule (Enterotest) may be necessary to visualize the organism. Parasites and amebae are infrequent causes of diarrhea in children in most parts of the United States. Antibiotic-induced diarrhea also occurs, most commonly with ampicillin and clindamycin. This syndrome, when severe, is diagnosed as pseudomembranous colitis from its appearance on proctosigmoidoscopy. A bacterium, *Clostridium difficile*, has been implicated as the prime etiologic agent. When this diagnosis is made, treatment with vancomycin is indicated.

Pathogenesis.

The pathogenesis of infectious diarrhea depends upon the type of organism involved. Some elaborate exotoxins (ETEC) without invading epithelial cells, others release enterotoxins after invading cells (*Salmonella, Shigella*), and in others the mechanism is unknown (EPEC, rotavirus, *Yersinia, Campylobacter*). Organisms that invade the epithelium of the terminal ileum and colon produce diarrhea that typically contains mucus (pus cells or polymorphonuclear leukocytes) and are likely to be associated with severe systemic signs, including high fever, severe abdominal cramping, and a toxic-appearing patient.

Differential Diagnosis

History. The abrupt onset of diarrhea with or without vomiting is usually indicative of an acute intestinal infection, often referred to as "acute gastroenteritis." However, the stomach is involved much less than the intestines, so that this vomiting, when it is present, is generally much less severe than the diarrhea. Although all age groups suffer with diarrhea and vomiting, infants below 2 years of age are most vulnerable, due to their relatively higher fluid requirements and their more intense response to gastrointestinal infections. The major concern, of course, is that diarrhea or vomiting will lead to severe dehydration and vascular collapse.

Most often in a pediatric practice setting, the practitioner's first knowledge that a patient has diarrhea is from a telephone conversation; some simple questions permit assessment of the severity of the complaint. This is important in determining whether the child needs to be seen or if the problem can be managed over the phone.

- How old is the child? The child over 2 to 2½ years is relatively easy to manage, and rapid development of dehydration is uncommon.

The infant below 2 months is particularly at risk and should always be seen whether or not the child appears ill to the parents.

- When did the symptoms start, and are they getting better or worse? If vomiting and diarrhea began a few hours ago and the vomiting now has subsided, temporary procedures with a follow-up telephone call a few hours later are appropriate (if the child is not in the critical first few months of life). If on the other hand, the symptoms have persisted, the parents having taken some steps on their own, and there is no improvement, the child should be seen and evaluated.

- Is the child with diarrhea also vomiting, and are the symptoms associated only with feedings? Vomiting may occur with or without feeding. The latter situation is much more difficult to manage, generally requiring that nothing be given by mouth until the vomiting subsides. Antiemetics are not helpful and should not be used. When the vomiting occurs only with feedings, it can be managed easily by giving small amounts of clear liquids at frequent intervals.

- Diarrhea also generally is of two types. It may occur only after feedings, or it may occur independent of feedings. Diarrhea that is associated only with feeding is managed by decreasing the number of feedings. Diarrhea that is so severe that it occurs with and without feedings is best managed by not feeding until the symptoms subside or improve.

- Is the child febrile? If so, for how long, and how high is the temperature? Does the child have cramps? When did the vomiting start in relation to the diarrhea? These questions help differentiate bacterial from viral illnesses. The infant who has a temperature of 105F or greater, where the fever has lasted for 48 or more hours and is associated with severe cramping, is more likely to have a bacterial infection as a cause of gastroenteritis than the child without cramping and with a lower fever that disappeared within 24 to 36 hours. Vomiting preceding the onset of diarrhea is more likely to be of viral etiology.

- What is the nature of the stools? Are they watery and clear (yellow or green) or are they filled with mucus, with or without blood? The child with mucus in the stool is more likely to have an infection with an invasive bacterium. If the previous questions have revealed that the child is febrile, with severe cramps, and also has mucus in the stool, further diagnostic efforts are indicated. These include culture and examination of the stool for polymorphonuclear white blood cells. If the stool is watery, the child afebrile and without severe cramps, it is most likely a self-limited viral or bacterial infection.

- Has anyone to whom the child recently has been exposed been sick with a similar disease? Have any new foods been given? For example, has a breastfed infant been given a formula of cow's milk for the first time? Vomiting or diarrhea as a manifestation of cow's milk allergy is not unusual, but this bit of information may not be reported by the parent. If there has been no change in diet, and if the child has been exposed to someone with similar symptoms, an infectious etiology is more likely.

- Does the child appear sick? This is perhaps the most crucial question, although not necessarily the one to ask first. Gathering objective data first and then asking a subjective question (such as "How sick does the child appear to be?") may give the practitioner a more objective answer than would be obtained by asking the last question earlier.

- The time of the last urination may be difficult to determine, especially in infants with watery stools, the most common form of diarrhea in the young child. In addition, the parent is not used to paying much attention to urination since infants are always wet. However, it is worthwhile attempting to find out if the child has voided recently.

- Accurate answers to questions concerning doughy skin, sunken eyes, and decreased activity usually cannot be provided in the course of a telephone history. If it is thought necessary to ask these questions, it is necessary to see the infant.

Physical Examination. All patients with a history of diarrhea or vomiting who are sick enough to be seen in the office or clinic must be weighed (without clothes). It is helpful to know a recent weight when available. The sudden loss of weight is assumed to be due to loss of fluid only. When it is 7% or more of body weight, it indicates a serious problem. A weight loss of 10% or more means that the child requires hospitalization and treatment with intravenous fluids.

One should seek clinical evidence of dehydration. Sunken eyes, dry mucous membranes, poor skin turgor, sunken anterior fontanelle, and a decrease in tears with crying are all signs of dehydration. A scaphoid abdomen is sometimes seen, although often the abdomen is distended, tympanitic to percussion, with hyperactive bowel sounds on auscultation. A rapid pulse, with or without decreased blood pressure, is seen with severe vascular contraction, corresponding to a weight loss of 15% of more. Rapid deep respirations are associated with fever and acidosis. Decreased activity and lack of interest in the immediate environment are other important signs of severe illness.

A search for a source of infection outside the gastrointestinal tract is very important. Diarrhea or vomiting in response to otitis media, pharyngitis, pneumonia, or acute urinary tract infection is very common in young infants. Appropriate treatment of these conditions usually results in prompt cessation of symptoms of gastroenteritis.

Laboratory Diagnosis. The definitive laboratory diagnosis of infectious diarrhea must be made by microbiology laboratories using relatively sophisticated techniques for some organisms and very sophisticated techniques for others. However, information on the likelihood of a bacterial, invasive agent can be obtained by examining the stool under a microscope. The presence of neutrophils, with or without blood, is seen mostly with invasive organisms, such as invasive *E. coli* (EIEC), *Salmonella, Shigella, Yersinia,* and *Campylobacter.* Examination of the stool for pH and the presence of reducing substances may be helpful when looking for a secondary disaccharidase deficiency (pH less than 5.0). If a sugar cannot be metabolized, it passes into the large intestine, and fermentation takes place with production of acids and reducing substances, which in turn cause an osmotic diarrhea. Reducing substances can be tested for by using Clinitest tablets (but not glucose oxidase methods, such as Labstix or Testape) when liquid stools are present. A result of 2% or greater is considered positive.

Although the presence of a low pH or reducing substance in the stool is not helpful in making an etiologic diagnosis, these findings may help in directing treatment or may guide one to perform more specific tests.

Treatment

Regardless of etiology, the therapy of acute diarrhea or vomiting is similar. Although some infections require antibiotic therapy, the great majority occurring in the United States require only strict attention to fluid and electrolyte balance.

Most children can be managed with oral hydration if (1) the onset is not so severe that acute dehydration occurs before oral hydration can be begun or (2) vomiting, if present, relents and allows for replacement of losses with oral fluids. In other words, intake must keep up with, and preferably stay ahead of, output. Evidence that intake has been adequate is easily obtained by accurate measurements of weight and observation of urine output. The basis of therapy is the use of clear fluids that contain sugar and electrolytes, the most important of which is sodium. The

World Health Organization has developed an oral electrolyte solution for the management of acute gastroenteritis (Table 2). It is specifically designed to be used for secretory diarrhea, e.g., cholera, one of the major causes of diarrheal disease in underdeveloped countries. The electrolyte content of diarrheal water in cholera is high in sodium (90–100 mEq/L) and is the reason for the high content of sodium in the repair solution. In developed countries, however, most diarrheal disease is not secretory, and the sodium content of the stool tends to be much lower. Repair solutions for the viral type diarrheas seen in the United States and Western Europe can, therefore, contain less sodium, although recent experience suggests that the WHO oral rehydrating solution can be used safely for all forms of diarrhea, even in young infants. The induction of hypernatremia by the use of solutions containing as much as 90 mEq of sodium per liter appears to have been due to the osmotic effect of an excessively high concentration of carbohydrate in the solution, exacerbating the diarrhea, rather than the high intake of sodium per se. Commercial preparations for oral rehydration are available, such as Lytren and Pedialyte (Table 2). For short-term use, plain sugar water can be used (2 tablespoons of table sugar in 1 quart of water is approximately a 3% solution). Carbonated sodas (Coke, Pepsi, 7-Up, ginger ale) are also acceptable. We have a

TABLE 2. ORAL REHYDRATION FLUIDS

	Na	K	Cl	HCO$_3$/ citrate	Glucose G%
			mEq/L		
WHO oral	90	20	80	30	2
Lytren	30	25	25	36	4.5
Pedialyte	30	20	30	28	5
Pedialyrers	60	20	50	30	2.5
Infalyte	50	20	40	30	2.0

prejudice against the use of apple juice, feeling that diarrhea is sometimes exacerbated when large quantities are given to young infants. We have preferred not to allow parents to make up their own electrolyte solution (e.g., by adding salt to sucrose water) because of the possibility that a mistake will lead to salt poisoning. If prolonged therapy with clear liquids (greater than 24–36 hours) is required, the commercially available electrolyte solutions may be used. In general, most acute diarrhea responds quickly to oral clear liquids of any type. Our experience has been that the feedings can almost always be advanced after a short time. If they cannot, it often indicates severe underlying disease.

If the illness begins with vomiting not associated with food intake, the parent is asked not to feed the child until there has been no vomiting for about an hour. At that time small, frequent feedings with clear liquids are begun, with a gradual increase in the volume and the length of time between feedings. A typical regimen is shown in Table 3. If the

TABLE 3. SUGGESTED REFEEDING REGIMEN AFTER VOMITING

1. Wait 1 hour after last episode of vomiting*
2. Give 10 ml clear liquid every 10 minutes × 4
3. Wait 15 minutes
4. Give 15 ml clear liquid every 10 minutes × 4
5. If no vomiting has occurred, infant may leave clinic or office
6. At home begin 1 ounce (30 ml) every 15 minutes × 4
7. If no vomiting, begin clear fluids as tolerated every 3–4 hours
8. Review progress with parent after initial 24 hours or sooner if vomiting occurs or if diarrhea excessive
9. If infant is doing well, continue refeeding as per text

*Initial instructions (1–4) may be given to patient over telephone. If vomiting persists, the infant must be seen.

child is seen in the office, clinic, or emergency room with the complaint of diarrhea and vomiting, the infant is fed and observed. If vomiting does not take place, instructions are given for infrequent feedings (every 4 or more hours) of up to 8 to 10 ounces of clear liquids, and the parent is asked to call or come in the next day. It is made clear that milk cannot be given without the advice of the pediatric practitioner.

The decision whether to return or whether the patient can be managed on the telephone is based on the type of practice. In private offices, most patients with diarrhea are treated very effectively with telephone consultations. In inner city emergency room populations, diarrhea is managed by repeated visits, initially daily, when careful weights are obtained. If the vomiting and the diarrhea have stopped, the diet is advanced. Ideally, the child will have had a bowel movement that has form and consistency. Most times, however, the child will not have had a bowel movement at all once clear liquids have been started or will have had one or two watery movements and then nothing more through the night.

If the infant is old enough to be taking fruits and cereals, the diet should be advanced to rice cereal made with water, apple sauce (but not apple juice), and bananas, given in three meals. The next day, if the diarrhea is improving (loose, semiformed, or formed stools, as opposed to watery), vegetables and meat are added if they have previously been a part of the child's diet. Milk is the last food to be resumed and is begun by giving only 2 ounces twice the first day and then 4 ounces twice the second day. If there has been no exacerbation of the diarrhea, milk in its usual quantities is given on the third day.

In the case of the infant over 2 months of age who has been on cow's milk only, milk is reintroduced slowly, as described above. If there is exacerbation of the diarrhea, a soy milk preparation is started. In the infant under 2 months of age who has had a bout of diarrhea, soy milk is introduced after clear liquids.

These regimens, while empirical, have worked very well over many years. Their success is based on several possible mechanisms. There may be some degree of fat intolerance following diarrhea. Though skim milk is low in fat, it is not recommended for use in refeeding children with diarrhea because of a higher electrolyte and osmotic concentration, possibly leading to hypernatremia. Since fat intake should be decreased immediately after acute diarrhea, refeeding with cereals and fruits, which are low in fat, is preferred. The observation has been made by generations of grandmothers that rice, banana, and apple sauce are "binding." In any case, they seem to be helpful in not making diarrhea worse and by adding bulk and calories to the diet of a hungry child.

Some degree of secondary lactose intolerance is likely following diarrhea severe enough to be brought to the attention of the pediatric practitioner, especially when rotavirus is the etiology. We reintroduce milk last and slowly to circumvent this problem. In the infant who has not been fed anything but cow's milk but is over 2 months of age, we watch to see what happens when milk is given. Under 2 months, soy milk does not contain lactose and is given instead of cow's milk because of a greater concern for the nutritional status of the younger infant and its lesser ability to cope with stressful situations.

Fortunately, in the last few years the incidence of breastfeeding has increased in many population groups. Diarrheal disease occurs less frequently in totally breastfed infants, and when it does occur, it resolves much faster. We have found that when the child is not vomiting, having the mother continue to nurse has been the best therapy for infantile diarrhea. If the infant has vomited, the mother is asked to give one or two sugar-water feedings and then to resume nursing. Both diarrhea and vomiting subside quickly.

Antiemetics and antidiarrheal medications are not helpful in infants and may be hazardous. Promethazine, chlorpromazine, prochlorperazine, and trimethobenzamide all have been used for their antiemetic properties. If and when they do work, it is generally for centrally induced nausea and vomiting (e.g., associated with chemotherapy or radiotherapy) rather than for vomiting associated with acute gastroenteritis. Phosphorylated carbohydrate preparations (such as Emetrol) have been suggested as being useful antiemetics, perhaps by reducing smooth muscle contraction on contact with the wall of a hyperactive intestine. Coke syrup has been recommended for the control of vomiting, the mechanism of action allegedly being similar to that of phosphorylated carbohydrates.

It is not clear whether any of these medications are helpful in the vomiting of acute gastroenteritis. In any event, this type of vomiting is self-limited and responds very well to small, frequent, clear liquid feedings. Because of this and because in children extrapyramidal tract symptoms and signs (oculogyric crises, torticollis) are common toxic effects of phenothiazines, especially prochlorperazine, the use of specific antiemetic medications is contraindicated. Our experience has been that vomiting so severe that it does not respond to dietary measures is very unusual; a more serious condition should be considered.

Antidiarrheal medications are unnecessary and contraindicated for acute diarrhea of infancy and childhood. Narcotic preparations, such as tincture of opium or diphenoxylate with atropine, have been used. If the diarrhea is associated with an exotoxin, medications that decrease intestinal motility may be dangerous and may in fact prolong the disease state. In addition, the diarrhea in infants tends to be watery rather than loose, as is the diarrhea of adults. In such cases, medication sufficient to improve the consistency and decrease the frequency of stools may be associated with narcotization of the infant.

Kaolin-pectin preparations may be effective in very large doses in improving stool appearance. Some preparations have been flavored to make them more attractive to children. However, there is no evidence that the duration of disease is shortened with their use. Recently, bismuth subsalicylate (Pepto-Bismol) has been recommended for use in traveler's diarrhea (usually associated with toxigenic *E. coli*). This is an unusual cause of diarrhea in children, and treatment with bismuth is not recommended.

We prefer the therapy outlined above, i.e., in frequent feedings with large amounts of clear liquids once the child has stopped vomiting.

The use of infrequent feedings causes less stimulation of the gastrocolic reflex. Since in infants this reflex is maximal or near maximal in acute diarrhea, a small feeding does not cause any less of a bowel movement than a large one. The combination of infrequent large feedings, therefore, allows for the greatest oral intake with the least stimulation of the gastrointestinal tract.

Antibiotic therapy is seldom necessary and usually used only in the treatment of *Shigella* infection. Trimethoprim-sulfamethoxazole (TMP-SMX) is the medication of choice, with the following dosage schedule: TMP 8–10 mg/kg/day, SMX 40–60 mg/kg/day for 5 days. For the occasional child with EPEC or ETEC, oral neomycin 100 mg/kg/day in four doses for 3–5 days or colistin 15–20 mg/kg/day in four doses for 3–5 days is suggested. For EIEC (enterinvasive *E. coli*), when symptoms and signs warrant, ampicillin 100 mg/kg/day in four doses for 7–10 days is effective for sensitive strains. This regimen can also be used for *Salmonella* enteritis when indicated (in immunodeficient individuals or neonates). TMP-SMX, in the same dose as for *Shigella* enteritis, is effective therapy for *Salmonella* resistant to ampicillin. Treatment of uncomplicated *Salmonella* enteritis in infants or individuals other than those who are immunocompromised is not generally recommended, since treatment may not be effective, may prolong the carrier state, and may be associated with a higher clinical relapse rate. Hospitalized infants with *Salmonella* enteritis often have positive blood cultures (up to 30% in infants under 1 year of age in one study), leading to the recommendation that this group be treated with antibiotics for 14 days. We also recommend treatment of the rare older child with a severe form of *Salmonella* enteritis.

Numerous regimens have been suggested for intravenous resuscitation of infants who require hospitalization for dehydration secondary to diarrhea or vomiting. The child who requires hospitalization will appear sick, be apathetic, and have obvious evidence of dehydration. Sometimes hospitalization is required for instances in which the parent can no longer cope with a less severe illness. This is usually seen when diarrhea has been present for several days, has gotten better, and then has exacerbated. When this point has been reached, and when the parents feel they have done everything correctly, it is often wiser to admit the child to a hospital to allow some of the responsibility for care to be shouldered by others.

If accurate weights are not available, an estimation of the degree of dehydration is made. Seven to ten percent dehydration causes sunken eyes, decreased activity, decreased urinary output, diminished tears, dry mucous membranes, decreased skin turgor, but no evidence of shock. Twelve to fifteen percent dehydration is associated with a rapid weak pulse, evidence of peripheral vasoconstriction, and, at times, hypotension. The child with greater than 15% dehydration is close to moribund and requires rapid institution of fluid therapy.

The use of estimates of dehydration is helpful in planning therapy, but regardless of the estimated or actually known amount of fluid loss, therapy always begins with rapid reexpansion of the extracellular fluid volume. Either isotonic saline (0.9%) or Ringer's lactate, 20 ml/kg given intravenously over 30–60 minutes, is acceptable. The amount may need to be given once or twice again in the more severe case. It is rarely necessary to use colloid (5% albumin, plasmanate, or blood) although some clinicians recommend such treatment of patients in hypovolemic shock.

Prior to beginning IV fluids, blood should be obtained for performance of a CBC and measurement of sodium, potassium, chloride, bicarbonate, urea nitrogen, and glucose concentrations. By the time the initial hydrating solution has been given, the results of these laboratory tests should be known. Depending on the type of dehydration, a specific plan for fluid replacement is formulated. Generally speaking, fluid and electrolyte losses are replaced during the first 24 hours in the child with hypotonic or isotonic dehydration but over a 48–72-hour period in hypernatremic dehydration. This difference is related to the observation that rapid correction of hypernatremia may be associated with seizures. If electrolyte values are not known after the initial reexpansion, 90 mEq/L NaCl in 5% dextrose water is a good all-purpose fluid and is given at a rate allowing for one-half the fluid losses to be replaced in the first 8 hours. A complete description of the management of dehydration can be found in *Pediatrics,* 17th ed.

CHRONIC DIARRHEA

Etiology

Chronic Nonspecific Diarrhea. By far the most common cause of chronic diarrhea in children is termed "chronic nonspecific diarrhea (CNSD)." It originally was thought to be a part of the celiac syndrome and has also been called the "irritable bowel" or "irritable colon" syndrome. It typically occurs in children between 6 months and 2½ years of age and is never associated with malabsorption. The children grow normally but have loose movements (which may contain mucus) several times per day. There may be a family history of bowel problems. Generally, there is no abdominal pain or tenesmus associated with the passage of stool. Occasionally, there is a history of low-grade fever, but it is difficult to document. Sometimes these children are put on elimination diets high in carbohydrate and low in fat. However, addition of fat to the diet may result in resolution of the diarrhea. Gluten-free diets have been prescribed without appropriate laboratory studies and, if followed without supervision, may cause nutritional damage. Since malabsorption does not occur in these children, they should receive a normal diet.

Cystic Fibrosis. Cystic fibrosis (CF) should be considered in all children with chronic diarrhea, especially white children in whom it is associated with failure to thrive; other symptoms may or may not be present. The diagnosis is made by measuring the level of sodium or chloride in the sweat. The reliability of the sweat test is greater if it is done at a facility skilled in its performance. CF is the most common lethal genetic disease among white children; the frequency ranges from 1:2,000 to 1:3,500 live white births. Early recognition and aggressive therapy improve the prognosis. All these children should be referred to CF centers for the highly specialized care that is required.

Inflammatory Bowel Disease. Inflammatory bowel disease, which includes both ulcerative and granulomatous colitis, is uncommon before the age of 10 years, although it can be seen even in younger children. The diagnostic work-up, initial prescription for management, and help in follow-up should be done in consultation with a gastroenterologist. A complete description of inflammatory bowel disease, with therapy, can be found in *Pediatrics,* 17th ed.

Diarrhea with Failure to Thrive. The young infant with diarrhea associated with failure to thrive usually poses a very difficult diagnostic problem. Referral to a pediatric center is recommended, since this is a potentially life-threatening situation. The differential diagnosis ranges from A (aminoacidemia) to Z (zinc deficiency), as shown in Table 4. More detailed descriptions can be found in *Pediatrics*, 17th ed.

***Celiac Disease* (Gluten Enteropathy).** Celiac disease, once a common diagnosis, is rarely seen in the United States today, though it is still common in some other countries, notably Ireland and Poland. It is defined as an intolerance to wheat and rye gluten associated with malabsorption and with a characteristic flattening of intestinal villi on jejunal biopsy. Typically, it occurs after 6 months of age, probably because most pediatric practitioners do not introduce wheat or rye prior to that time. The diagnosis should not be made on the basis of a therapeutic trial of a gluten-free diet; it is established with a jejunal biopsy. The diagnosis of celiac disease requires life-long abstinence. This recommendation should not be made, therefore, without careful documentation of the diagnosis.

Chronic Diarrhea Due to Infection. Chronic infectious diarrhea, though uncommon in the United States, is most likely to be caused by *G. lamblia*, a motile protozoan. The diagnosis is made by finding the organism in the stool or, failing that, in duodenal secretions obtained by direct aspiration or by use of a swallowed gelatin capsule (Enterotest). Efforts are being made to develop serologic tests, which, if successful, may replace the other methods. Treatment is with quinacrine 2 mg/kg orally 3 times a day after meals for 5 days, up to a maximum dose of 300 mg. Its use should be avoided in individuals who have had psychiatric disturbances, as it may precipitate an acute psychosis. Metronidazole has also been used, but it has been reported to be possibly carcinogenic in animals. When metronidazole is used, it is given for 7–10 days, in two or three divided doses, after meals, in daily dosages as follows: under 2 years 125 mg, 2–4 years 250 mg, 5–8 years 375 mg, 9–12 years 500 mg, over 12 years 750 mg.

Amebiasis caused by *Entamoeba histolytica* is another infectious cause of diarrhea. It is less common in the United States than giardiasis and is usually treated with metronidazole in the dosages recommended above for giardiasis.

Other. A number of tumors secrete substances that can cause chronic diarrhea, including ganglioneuromas and pancreatic islet cell tumors. Immunodeficiency disorders, either congenital or acquired, may be associated with chronic diarrhea. Certain endocrinopathies, such as hyperthyroidism, hypoadrenalism, hypoparathyroidism, and hypopituitarism, also may be associated with chronic diarrhea.

A complete discussion of the differential diagnostic possibilities is not possible here, and more specific sources should be consulted. Table 4 provides a partial list of the most common causes of chronic diarrhea in children.

Differential Diagnosis

History. Persistently loose stools are a common complaint in pediatric practice. The major problem is to determine whether or not the bowel pattern is a normal variant, which is usually the case, or part of a chronic disease. Bowel patterns in children tend to be less regular than in adults. A child who has had formed bowel movements may begin to have looser, more frequent ones due to a change in eating habits. This may be interpreted by the parents as the onset of diarrhea, when in fact it is related only to a change in diet. The following questions help determine whether a problem truly exists.

• How long have the symptoms been present? Can you describe how it began? Did it begin with an acute episode associated with fever? If the diarrhea began acutely and has persisted, an infectious etiology is like-

TABLE 4. SOME CAUSES OF CHRONIC DIARRHEA

Giardia Lamblia	Cystic Fibrosis
Entamoeba Histolytica	Schwachman Syndrome
Fecal Impaction	Hyper and Hypothyroidism
Blind Loop Syndrome	Hypoparathyroidism
Intestinal Duplications	Congenital Adrenal Hyperplasia
Malrotation	Adrenal Insufficiency
Inflammatory Bowel Disease	Vasoactive Polypeptide Producing Tumors
Chronic Nonspecific Diarrhea	Neuroblastoma, Pheochromocytoma
Immune Deficiency Diseases	Acrodermatitis Enteropathica
Disaccharidase Deficiencies	Hartnup Disease
	Gluten Enteropathy (Celiac Disease)

ly. Giardiasis, though usually a self-limited illness, can become chronic. Mild secondary lactose intolerance may be a sequela of viral enteritis; diarrhea and cramping occur within several hours after milk intake. The insidious onset of diarrhea usually is associated with a chronic condition, such as nonspecific diarrhea in young infants or inflammatory bowel disease in older children.

- How old is the child? The frequency of the different conditions varies with age. Has there been weight loss or a decrease in the rate of growth? If growth has continued normally, serious causes of diarrhea are unlikely.
- Has the child's development been normal? Hypoparathyroidism, as well as a number of inborn errors of metabolism, such as Hartnup disease, congenital adrenogenital hyperplasia, and acrodermatitis enteropathica, may be associated with diarrhea.
- Does the child appear sick? Fever (intermittent or steady), lethargy, and poor appetite may all be associated with chronic systemic illness.
- Is there pain, blood, or mucus with bowel movements? Is the child awakened at night with diarrhea? These symptoms typically are associated with inflammatory bowel disease.
- Is there an urge to defecate, or does the stool leak out? Continuous soiling may not be diarrhea but represent fecal impaction secondary to constipation and stool withholding. Liquid stool from the right side of the large bowel may leak around a large retained mass of stool in the rectum.

Physical Examination. Evidence of chronic disease may be found on physical examination, including signs of weight loss, decreased subcutaneous tissue, wasted buttocks, protuberant abdomen, or decreased muscle tone. Hepatosplenomegaly as well as other abdominal masses should be sought. Skin rashes should be noted. Blood pressure should be taken, as some causes of chronic diarrhea are associated with increased catecholamines (ganglioneuroma, neuroblastoma, pheochromocytoma). Evidence of hypothyroidism or hyperthyroidism should be looked for. The physical examination must be very complete, since the list of diseases that can cause chronic diarrhea includes virtually all systems.

Laboratory Diagnosis. The search for the etiology of chronic diarrhea includes laboratory tests from the simple to the most sophisticated. A list of causes of chronic diarrhea is shown in Table 4. It is obvious from the diagnoses listed that a large number of laboratory tests may be appropriate depending on what illness is being considered.

Treatment

Treatment, if any exists, depends upon the etiology. For detailed descriptions of specific therapy, the reader is referred to *Pediatrics*, 17th ed. It must be emphasized that chronic diarrhea, when associated with poor growth and development in children, is a very serious problem. A diagnosis must be carefully sought and optimal therapy started promptly, usually in consultation with a pediatric gastroenterologist.

ACUTE AND CHRONIC VOMITING

Etiology of Vomiting

The abrupt onset of vomiting in children occurs commonly. Usually it is secondary to an acute illness, which may be either enteral or parenteral; it usually subsides quickly. Persistent vomiting, on the contrary, is uncommon and potentially serious, and its cause must be determined promptly.

Pyloric Stenosis. Pyloric stenosis is the most common cause of persistent vomiting associated with poor growth in the young infant. Though symptoms may begin in the first few days of life, vomiting usually is noted after the first week. The vomiting increases in severity, occurring with each feeding and becoming projectile by the third or fourth week of life. Decreasing weight gain or actual weight loss is common, although occasionally an infant with a persistent parent may continue to gain weight at near normal rates.

Pyloric stenosis is a familial disease that occurs much more frequently in males than females, with reported ratios varying from 5:1 to 8:1. The diagnosis is made by palpating a firm, olive-sized mass in the right upper quadrant of the abdomen. A peristaltic wave,

due to gastric outlet obstruction, is sometimes noted after a feeding; when present it is very suggestive of pyloric stenosis. Experienced pediatricians and surgeons usually have little trouble in making the diagnosis, but if there is a question, a barium swallow can be done. The characteristic findings are elongation of the pyloric channel (string sign) and retention of barium in an enlarged stomach.

Pyloric stenosis is treated in the United States by pyloromyotomy, a relatively simple and usually uncomplicated surgical procedure, which effects an immediate cure and after which recurrences are very unusual. In countries where reliable anesthesia and experienced surgeons are not readily available, medical management with anticholinergic drugs has been used. This is an acceptable and effective method but involves patient refeeding, a longer course of treatment, and a higher rate of relapse.

Gastroesophageal Reflux. Gastroesophageal reflux (chalasia) is due to incompetence of the cardioesophageal junction, with regurgitation of stomach contents. A minor degree of this condition is very common and is known as "cheesing" by parents. This type of regurgitation, associated with normal growth and development, disappears between 9 and 12 months, coincident with the time infants assume the standing position. In its severest form, which is unusual, symptoms begin within the first few days of life, and the vomiting leads to poor weight gain. The vomiting is not forceful although it is copious. The infant appears vigorous and healthy and feeds eagerly.

The best diagnostic test is a therapeutic trial of thickened feedings followed by placing the infant in a head-up prone position by use of a board. If successful, after 2 weeks or so the regimen can be modified by reinstituting regular feedings but continuing the prone, head-up position. Although the infant may continue to "cheese," normal weight gain should be maintained. If the diagnosis cannot be made with certainty by this therapeutic trial, a barium swallow with fluoroscopy should be performed.

In recent years the subject of gastroesophageal reflux has become quite confused, since the syndrome has been linked with recurrent or persistent wheezing and sudden infant death syndrome. Sophisticated tests, utilizing continuous lower esophageal recording of pH and pressure and endoscopy with and without biopsy, have been used to help confirm the diagnosis.

This discussion concerns itself only with the symptom of vomiting secondary to gastroesophageal reflux and its management. In the child in whom positional therapy coupled with thickened feedings fails, additional therapy using anticholinergics and antacids is used. In our experience, severe gastroesophageal reflux unresponsive to medical therapy occurs mainly in children with serious neurologic problems. In these instances, surgery, using a technique known as a Nissen fundoplication, is necessary. Sandifer's syndrome is an interesting condition in which there is torticollis associated with gastroesophageal reflux. The etiology is not known, but the torticollis is relieved as the esophagitis due to gastroesophageal reflux is resolved.

Achalasia. Achalasia is the end stage of gastroesophageal reflux and is rarely seen in children. Only a few cases have been reported. It is considered to be secondary to reflux esophagitis, with secondary stricture of the distal end of the esophagus. Treatment consists of dilating the stenotic segment, and it requires the help of an experienced gastroenterologist or surgeon.

Increased Intracranial Pressure. Increased intracranial pressure in an infant may be associated with hydrocephalus or an intracranial mass, usually a brain tumor in the posterior fossa. Vomiting may be present in a child with a chronic subdural hematoma, although it is less prominent than symptoms or signs of irritability, increasing head size, and seizures. Pseudotumor cerebri, a condition seen most commonly in adolescents (especially obese adolescent girls), may cause vomiting. Other symptoms include papilledema, headache, and diplopia associated with a sixth nerve palsy. Postconcussion syndrome also can be associated with vomiting and headache.

Nonspecific Persistent Vomiting of Childhood. Nonspecific persistent vomiting of childhood is only a descriptive term and includes all those children who vomit without apparent cause. It includes children who vomit with stress, in much the same way that others have stress-induced diarrhea, abdominal pain, or headache. However, vomiting occurring with stress is likely to cause concern about systemic disease on the part of the parents and physician. Our experience has been that it is not an unusual psychosomatic symptom, often associated with school problems or an unstable family situation. The diagnosis can be made in most instances on the basis of the history and physical examination without resorting to extensive invasive procedures. Treatment is aimed at helping the child and parents to understand the nature of the problem and working to alleviate it by marshalling the resources of the persons involved.

Anorexia Nervosa and Bulimia. Both these conditions are seen mainly in adolescent and young adult females. The vomiting is done in secret and often is associated with binge eating. The distinction between anorexia and bulimia may be artificial but is based on the presence of severe weight loss in anorexia and relatively normal weight with bulimia. These diagnoses are often difficult to make early on, help often coming from friends or school authorities. When an early diagnosis is made, psychiatric consultation is mandatory.

Late diagnosis (after severe weight loss has occurred) may require hospitalization and re-establishment of adequate nutrition.

Miscellaneous Causes of Vomiting in Infants. Poor feeding technique is said to be the most common cause of vomiting, though our experience in both private practice and clinic settings does not support this statement. When it is suspected, a disturbed parent-child relationship should be considered. Whatever the reason, when the diagnosis of poor feeding technique is made as a cause of vomiting, counseling and support for the parent is mandatory. It cannot be treated simply by giving instructions in proper feeding and burping techniques.

Differential Diagnosis

Pathogenesis. According to Davidson, vomiting due to causes other than gastric obstruction is associated with an atonic, distended stomach. Food is usually held up in the duodenum, which contracts during episodes of nausea and vomiting. The afferent stimuli for vomiting arise in the duodenum, the force for vomiting being supplied by abdominal muscle contractions.

History. It is worthwhile to consider the causes of vomiting in relation to the age of the child. Congenital lesions, as important causes of vomiting in the newborn, are much less likely to cause vomiting in infancy, the majority of cases being due to infections and, thus, self-limited. Recognizing that almost any systemic disease can cause vomiting, the following questions are designed to help recognize chronic disease. Diseases associated with abdominal pain, which have vomiting as a concomitant symptom, will be considered elsewhere.

- Is headache associated with vomiting? Increased intracranial pressure is associated with vomiting, even in the absence of specific neurologic findings, especially with a posterior fossa brain tumor in a young infant. Migraine, both typical and abdominal, and abdominal epilepsy are other causes of vomiting that may be associated with headache.
- Has the child been losing weight? Diabetic ketoacidosis, while generally a very acute disease, may sometimes present with a history of intermittent vomiting associated with the typical symptoms of polyphagia, polydipsia, and polyuria. Vomiting is a prominent symptom in adrenal insufficiency, especially in cases secondary to congenital adrenal hyperplasia. Urinary tract infection, especially in the young infant, sometimes presents with chronic vomiting or chronic diarrhea.
- Is there a recurrent pattern to the vomiting? Various forms of cyclic vomiting have been described. Some are associated with emotional disturbances; others are thought to be a form of autonomic epilepsy.
- Is the child taking any medications? This question is always worth asking, since the patient may have received the medication from someone else, or the practitioner may have forgotten which medications the patient is taking. Theophylline, nitrofurantoin, aspirin, digitalis, and erythromycin may all cause vomiting. Hepatotoxic medications may cause vomiting secondary to liver damage.

Physical Examination. The physical examination can be very helpful in making a specific diagnosis. Generalized abdominal distention with hypoactive or absent bowel sounds and bilious vomiting is indicative of paralytic ileus. The palpation of an olivelike mass in the right upper quadrant is the well-known sign of pyloric stenosis. Virilization of either a male or female infant who is vomiting suggests congenital adrenal hyperplasia. Congenital glaucoma, diagnosed by finding a large cornea or a large globe (buphthalmos or

TABLE 5. CONDITIONS IN WHICH VOMITING IS THE MAJOR SYMPTOM

Pyloric stenosis

Congenital malformations
- Annular pancreas
- Intestinal atresia
- Intestinal stenosis

Gastroesophageal reflux

Achalasia

Feeding technique

Congenital adrenal hyperplasia

Inborn errors of metabolism

Increased intracranial pressure
- Hydrocephalus
- Chronic subdural hematoma
- Posterior fossa brain tumor
- Pseudotumor cerebri

Emotional disturbances
- Ruminators
- School phobia
- Anorexia nervosa
- Bulimia nervosa

ox eye), sometimes is associated with vomiting. Increased intracranial pressure may be diagnosed by the presence of papilledema (which, however, does not uniformly occur in young infants). A child who appears chronically ill and who has lost considerable weight obviously needs to have a prompt, accurate diagnosis made. On the other hand, the investigation into the cause of persistent vomiting in a child who appears to be well is less urgent.

Laboratory Diagnosis. The laboratory procedures necessary to make a diagnosis depend upon the causes suggested by the history and physical examination. *Pediatrics,* 17th ed, should be consulted for the diagnostic aids for specific diagnoses. A list of the causes of vomiting as the primary symptom is shown in Table 5.

Treatment.

As in the discussion of chronic diarrhea, the therapy of acute or chronic vomiting varies with the cause. For detailed descriptions of specific therapy, the reader is referred to *Pediatrics,* 17th ed. Selection of the appropriate consultant will depend on the diagnosis.

BIBLIOGRAPHY

Black RE, Dykes AC, Sinclair SP, Wells JG: Giardiasis in day-care centers: Evidence of person-to-person transmission. Pediatrics 60:486, 1977

Blacklow NR, Cukor G: Viral gastroenteritis. N Engl J Med 304:397, 1981

Carpenter CJ: Mechanisms of bacterial diarrheas. Am J Med 68:313, 1980

Cohen SA, Hendricks KM, Mathis RK, Laramee S, Walker WA: Chronic nonspecific diarrhea: Dietary relationships. Pediatrics 64:402, 1979

Davidson M: Abdominal pain. In Rudolph A (ed), Pediatrics; 17th ed. New York, Appleton-Century-Crofts, 1982

Diagnosis and Management of Acute Diarrhea. Report of the Thirteenth Ross Roundtable on Critical Approaches to Common Pediatric Problems in Collaboration with the Ambulatory Pediatric Association and the University of Texas Health Science Center at Baltimore, Maryland. Brunell PA (chairperson), October 4 and 5, 1981

Finberg L: The role of oral electrolyte-glucose solutions in hydration for children—international and domestic aspects. Editorial. J Pediatr 96:51, 1980

Harland EG, Cox DL, Lyew M, Lindo F: Composition of oral solutions prepared by Jamaican mothers for treatment of diarrhoea. Lancet 1:600, 1981

Levine MM, Edelman R: Acute diarrheal infections in infants. I. Epidemiology, treatment, and prospects for immunoprophylaxis. Hosp Pract Dec 1979, p 89

Levine MM, Edelman, R: Acute diarrheal infections in infants. II. Bacterial and viral causes. Hosp Pract Jan 1980, p 97

Lloyd-Still JD: Where have all the celiacs gone? Pediatrics 61:929, 1978

Pickering LK, Evans DJ Jr, Munoz O, et al.: Prospective study of enteropathogens in children with diarrhea in Houston and Mexico. J Pediatr 93:383, 1978

Pickering LK, Woodward WE: Diarrhea in day care centers. Pediatr Infect Dis 1:47, 1982

Santosham M, Daum RS, Dillman L, et al.: Oral rehydration therapy of infantile diarrhea. A controlled study of well-nourished children hospitalized in the United States and Panama. N Engl J Med 306:1070, 1982

Tedesco F, Gurwith M, Markham R, Christie D, Bartlett JD: Oral vancomycin for antibiotic-associated pseudomembranous colitis. Lancet 2:226, 1978

Cross-Reference to *Pediatrics,* 17th ed.

EIGHT

Earache

Steven P. Shelov

A complaint of earache may be due to a variety of different causes, including trauma, infection of the middle ear or external canal, or foreign body in the external auditory canal. Although earache is not the only presenting complaint in a child with these conditions, it is the predominant one and, therefore, the most logical heading under which to discuss them.

DEFINITION

Earache is defined simply as pain localized to the area of the ear. In children over the age of 2 this is a useful complaint, as there is a high correlation with an actual, treatable problem. Below the age of 2, the infant and child may not be able to localize the pain, and thus the practitioner cannot rely on the complaint to point toward the ear as the source of the problem.

CAUSES OF EARACHE

Middle Ear Effusion
Purulent Otitis Media (POM). POM is most frequent in children under 2 years of age. Howie found that 66% of children seen in his practice had at least one episode of otitis by the time of their second birthday and 1 in 7 children had more than six episodes. Klein

found similar frequencies and reported, in addition, that more episodes of POM were observed in the first year of life than in any other one year. These very high frequencies would not have been revealed if the diagnosis had been made only in children complaining of earache or in those presenting with fever, the latter reported to be present in only 40 to 70% of children with POM.

The presenting complaint may be that the baby is pulling at his ear or repeatedly sticking his finger in his ear, or the first manifestation may be drainage from the ear. Occasionally, there is an association between pain when the baby is sucking on a bottle and swallowing, due to opening and closing of the eustachian tube, producing pressure changes in the middle ear that impact against an inflamed tympanic membrane (TM). Other suggestions of the presence of POM in a young infant include an acute onset of fever, presence of an upper respiratory illness for the 2 or 3 days preceding the complaints, or previous episodes of diagnosed POM presenting in a similar fashion. Mothers are often aware of subtle behavioral changes that indicate the onset of POM in their young child. A verbal child complaint of pain in the ear should be taken very seriously by the parent and practitioner; it requires immediate attention.

In most children with POM, the TM has not perforated at the time of diagnosis, and, hence, there is no visible discharge from the ear. If rupture of the TM has occurred, there may be purulent, foul-smelling material coming from one or both ears. More often, rupture occurs later and is accompanied by improvement in the ear pain.

Pathogenesis. The eustachian tube is an anatomic canal normally sterile and air-filled in nondiseased states. It has three physiologic functions: (1) protection of the middle ear from nasopharyngeal secretions, (2) drainage of the secretions from the middle ear into the posterior nasopharynx, and (3) ventilation of the normally air-filled middle ear to equilibrate air pressures inside of the TM with outside air pressure and allow for free mobility of the TM. Many conditions interfere with these functions and allow fluid to collect in the middle ear:

1. Children with cleft palate may have defects in their ability to open and close the nasopharyngeal part of the eustachian tube.
2. Adenoidal hypertrophy may block the nasopharynx and result in poor ventilation and increased negative pressure within the middle ear, creating two problems: (a) the increased negative pressure forces transudate into the middle ear; and (b) the increased pressure gradient between the posterior nasopharynx (positive) and the middle ear (negative) predisposes to introduction of posterior nasopharyngeal contents into the middle ear.
3. In allergic children, the mucosa of the eustachian tube is often swollen, producing a functional obstruction that prevents drainage from the middle ear. In addition, by interfering with ventilation of the middle ear, negative pressure is generated within it, and the same vicious cycle of negative pressure, transudate, poor drainage, and secondary infection ensues.

Once fluid has been introduced into the middle ear due to any cause, an ideal condition exists for bacterial overgrowth. There are several routes through which bacteria reach the middle ear:

1. Direct entrance through the eustachian tube from the posterior nasopharynx.
2. Hematogenous.
3. Through a perforation in the TM from the external auditory canal (much less common in infants, more common in older children).

Etiology. Numerous studies, using a variety of intricate techniques for middle ear aspiration, have documented bacteria in only about 75% of clinically diagnosed cases of POM. However, investigators generally agree that a child with POM, diagnosed on the criteria outlined below, should be assumed to have bacterial infection and considered to be a candidate for antibiotic therapy.

The most common bacteria causing otitis media in the older infant (older than 6 weeks) are *Streptococcus pneumoniae* and *Haemophilus influenzae.* Table 1 indicates the percent of infections due to different organisms in children 3 months to 6 years of age as reported by various investigators. The predominance of

TABLE 1. BACTERIAL PATHOGENS ISOLATED FROM MIDDLE EAR FLUID IN 3,583 CHILDREN AGED 3 MONTHS TO 6 YEARS WITH PURULENT OTITIS MEDIA

Microorganism	% of Children with Pathogen
Streptococcus pneumoniae	35
Haemophilus influenzae	20
Streptococcus, group A	8
Staphylococcus aureus	2
Neisseria catarrhalis	3
Gram-negative bacteria	1
Mixed culture	2
Nonpathogens	29

Summary of 11 reports from US, Finland, and Sweden, 1953–1975.

S. pneumoniae and *H. influenzae* appears to be present even in children in the older age groups.

The diagnosis of POM in the neonate has been a focus of attention, as its prevalence appears to be greater than once appreciated. Gram-negative organisms were reported to be the predominant cause of otitis media in neonates in the ICU setting. However, tympanocentesis done on a more representative population of neonates with POM seen as outpatients revealed the same organisms as seen in older infants and children, predominantly *S. pneumoniae* and *H. influenzae*.

Though POM is the major disease of the ear that causes ear pain in infants and children, it is important to give the pediatric practitioner a complete differential diagnosis prior to a description of optimum therapy and appropriate use of a consultant.

Serous Otitis Media and Secretory Otitis Media.

There are two forms of nonbacterial or nonsuppurative otitis media accompanied by a sterile effusion: (1) serous otitis media (SOM) and (2) secretory otitis media or mucoid otitis media (MOM). Serous otitis media is simply a collection of sterile, nonviscid fluid within the middle ear that obscures normal tympanic mobility. The consistency of the sterile effusion in secretory otitis media is much more mucinous or tenacious. This latter type of effusion impairs TM mobility and is much more difficult to treat.

Recurrent Otitis Media (ROM) of Infectious Etiology.

ROM is defined as repeated bouts of POM with apparently normal intervals between episodes. It is relatively uncommon, and little is known about its epidemiologic characteristics. The frequency of bouts of ROM is so great that the child is viewed by practitioner and parent alike almost never to be without an ear infection. The common causes of ROM are respiratory infection, genetics, mastoiditis, allergy, and environmental conditions.

Respiratory Infection.

Chronically diseased adenoidal tissue may persistently block the nasopharyngeal end of the eustachian tube and interfere with proper drainage of middle ear fluid, predisposing the child to persistent superinfection and POM. Infected adenoids are often associated with persistent sinusitis. These sites of persistent infection prevent full response of the POM to antimicrobial therapy, requiring further measures to completely eradicate the infection and prevent recurrence.

Genetics.

Certain tribes of American Indians, Alaskan Eskimos, and Guamanians have a much greater incidence and prevalence of ROM.

Mastoiditis or Persistent Perforation of the TM.

Latent infections in sites with direct communication to the middle ear are occasionally found as causes of ROM.

Allergy.

Controversy exists concerning allergy as a cause of ROM. However, there are considerable data to suggest an increased prevalence of ROM in allergic children.

Adverse Environmental Conditions.

In situations where there is greater crowding, poorer hygiene, and deteriorated living conditions, infectious diseases are seen more commonly. ROM is one of the diseases seen more frequently, probably due to a greater prevalence of respiratory infections and their complications.

External Auditory Canal

Otitis Externa.

The child with otitis externa usually presents during the summer often following swimming. The initial complaint is usually itching in one ear or both, followed by a discharge, and finally pain in the involved ear. Physical examination reveals a red, inflamed external canal with evidence of exudate that is sometimes foul smelling but usually more serious in nature. Culture of this exudate is usually not of value because of the presence of nonpathogenic organisms.

Foreign Body in the External Ear. Foreign bodies in the ear are seen most commonly in children between 1½ and 4 years. It should be suspected in children complaining of earache who have been playing with small toys or objects or with tissue paper. The identification of the foreign body is determined through a careful physical examination. Care should be taken not to push the foreign body further into the canal.

Pinna and Periauricular

Anaphylactic Insult. Allergic reactions of the ear due to bee sting or other bites cause a large, red, swollen ear that is pushed out from the head. The parents of the patient should be reassured that the symptoms will resolve with appropriate management (Table 2).

Trauma. Trauma represents a significant problem with respect to the ear because of the lack of subcutaneous tissue and the susceptibility of the underlying cartilage to infection, which may occur with minimal trauma and little abrasion of the skin.

DIFFERENTIAL DIAGNOSIS

The diagnosis usually can be accurate by taking a careful history and performing a careful physical examination. Though the laboratory may offer some confirmatory aid, it is rarely crucial to the diagnosis.

History

- Has the child had an upper respiratory infection? Most episodes of POM are concurrent with or follow a URI.
- Has the child had an ear infection before, and if so did the child behave similarly to the present? Often parents will note characteristic behaviors, fussiness, ear pulling, or other actions during episodes of otitis media. These observations are important for the practitioner to be aware of.
- Is there a discharge from the ear? Either a purulent otitis media with perforation would be suspected or, if it is the season, an otitis externa.
- Does the child appear to be hearing less? This suggests an effusion either suppurative or serous. After clinical assessment, verification with tympanometry and audiometry is imperative.
- In an older child, it is important to ask if the ear hurts. If so, did the pain come on abruptly, or was it a dull, aching fullness feeling? This will help distinguish a secretory effusion from a purulent one.
- Does the ear hurt when you touch it or move it? This suggests an otitis externa.
- Did the ear suddenly become bright red, and does it seem to stand out more prominently from the head (like a flag)? This suggests an anaphylactic response to an insect bite.
- Did you observe the child playing with small objects? Has the child ever put anything in his ear? It is important to always remember about foreign bodies.
- Was there any trauma to the ear? A traumatic perichondritis is extremely painful and can show little evidence on physical examination except pain.

Physical Examination

The examination should proceed in the following manner:

- The pinna and external meatus should be examined for erythema, induration, or any evidence of crusting from recent discharge from the external auditory meatus. Crusting around the meatus usually indicates either an otitis externa with a serous discharge or otitis media with perforation of the tympanic membrane.
- After careful examination of the external ear, careful traction on the pinna and pres-

TABLE 2. MANAGEMENT OF EARACHE

Diagnostic Consideration	Therapy	Indication for Consultation
Purulent otitis media (POM)	1. Penicillin V 50,000 U/kg/day × 4, 7–10 days Sulfisoxasole 150 mg/kg/day × 3–4 2. Ampicillin 75 mg/kg/day qid dosage, 7–10 days or Amoxacillin 25 mg/kg/day tid dosage, 7–10 days 3. Erythromycin 40 mg/kg/day × 4, 7–10 days Sulfisoxazole 150 mg/kg/day × 3–4, 7–10 days Fixed combination now exists which is acceptable Drugs or drug combination 1–3 have reasonably equal efficacy Second line medications when above regimens have failed are 4. Trimethropim-sulfamethoxazole 10 mg/kg/–200 mg/kg/day bid × 7 days 5. Cefaclor 20 mg/kg/day tid × 10 days (Current evidence suggests simultaneous use of decongestants is of no value and should not be used)	None
Serous otitis media (SOM)	Conservative use of eustachian opening exercises, consider use of one course of antibiotics	Persistence for more than 3 months with hearing loss
Recurrent otitis media (ROM)	Sulfisoxazole 500 mg bid during high incidence periods as prophylaxis	None
Secretory (mucoid) otitis media (MOM)	Conservative use of eustachian tube opening exercises, one course of antibiotics	Persistence for more than 3 months with hearing loss
Otitis externa	Local application of Lidosporin drops with placement of wick (if perforated TM, use solution; if nonperforated TM, use suspension)	None
Foreign body	Attempt to remove it within 3–4 mm of the external meatus	If greater distance from external meatus
Anaphylactic reaction	Cold compress, systemic antihistamine diphenhydramine 5 mg/kg/day or cyproheptadine 2 mg/kg/day	None
Trauma	Local cleansing, bacitracin, early use of systemic antibiotics	Significant laceration
Localized infection	Antistaphylococcal penicillin	None

sure at the tragus area should be exerted. This procedure is exquisitely painful in children with otitis externa but should not cause pain in children with uncomplicated POM. If a foreign body is suspected, careful inspection with light and no speculum should be performed first. This will prevent pushing a foreign body further into the canal.

- Once no foreign body is detected, careful insertion of a proper size speculum should follow. Some practitioners find holding the handle of the otoscope upward at 45 degrees and bracing the hand against the infant's head gives the most stable position. The more the otoscope can be stabilized, the less danger there is of injuring the canal should the child move.

Prior to examination of the TM, the canal should be sufficiently free of cerumen to permit clear visualization of the TM. Various techniques are available to clean cerumen from the canal, the choice of which depends on the skill and experience of the examiner.

1. If the cerumen is soft, several drops of 3% H_2O_2 followed in 20 minutes by cleansing with a Water-Pik at low velocity usually gives good results. This is the safest procedure.
2. If the pieces of cerumen are hard but discrete and are within easy reach by a curette, a No. 1 straight curette or fine bayonet forceps can be used through the surgical otoscope head.
3. If the canal has large amounts of impacted cerumen, application of 3% H_2O_2 followed by careful curetting may be needed.

Procedures 2 and 3 require considerable experience and skill.

Examination of the tympanic membrane (TM) is the most difficult and, in most instances, the most important part of the examination of an infant or child suspected of having POM. The normal tympanic membrane with identification of landmarks is shown diagrammatically in Figures 1, 2, and 3. The upper part of the drum, the pars flaccida or Shrapnell's membrane, should be examined first, since it is usually the first portion to become erythematous and to bulge outward. The remainder of the TM should then be examined for distortion of landmarks, especially failure to visualize the short process of the malleus and umbo and loss of the light reflex.

Finally, the TM should be examined for decreased mobility, evaluated best with the use of the rubber air insufflator attached to a pneumatic otoscope. In this examination, the largest speculum that can be inserted into the canal should be used to obtain the best seal, ensuring reproducible responses of the TM to changes in external canal pressure.

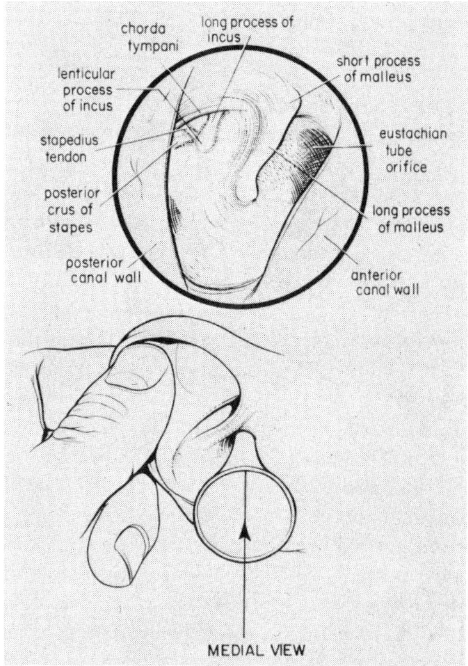

Figure 1. Normal tympanic membrane, medial view. (*Courtesy of Dr. R. Ruben.*)

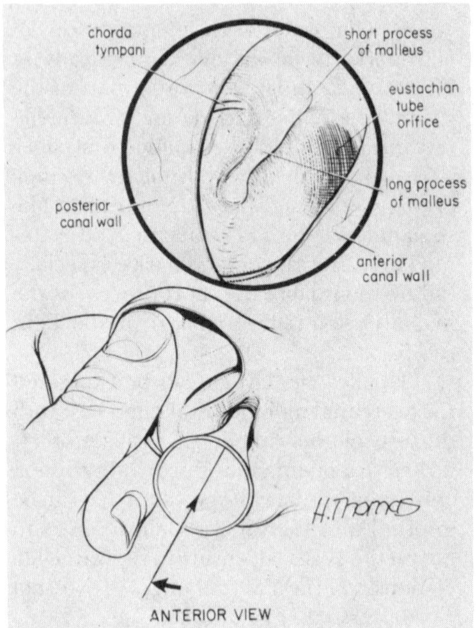

Figure 2. Normal tympanic membrane, anterior view. (*Courtesy of Dr. R. Ruben.*)

Laboratory Investigations

It is usually not necessary to perform extensive laboratory work-up or diagnostic procedures to confirm the diagnosis of the cause of a child's ear pain. However, several aids to diagnosis are available and may be useful in some patients.

Tympanometry. A more objective adjunct to assessing tympanic mobility, easily available for office use, is the tympanometer (Fig. 4). By inserting the probe of the tympanometer into the ear of a quiet, resting child, induced pressure changes alter the mobility of the drum and indicate whether or not there is fluid behind the drum. By altering the pressure in the external canal, either positively or negatively, the drum will be increasingly pushed or pulled, respectively. In a normal drum, with pressures equal on both sides, the TM is maximally mobile and will reflect the 600 Hz sound back to the microphone at minimum amplitude, indicating greatest compliance. As the pressure is changed, this mobility decreases to a minimum at extremes of negative and positive pressures. In a child with POM, the TM has decreased mobility due to fluid pressing against it. The tympanogram shown as type b in Figure 5 reflects this type of decreased mobility in contrast to a normal tympanogram (type a).

The diagnosis of POM is made by a combination of confirmatory history and the physical examination, including specifically a bulging drum, distorted landmarks, and abnormal tympanic mobility.

Sweep Audiometry. This test, easily used in the pediatric office, gives an estimate of hearing at several fixed amplitudes (25, 40db) covering a range of frequencies (500–

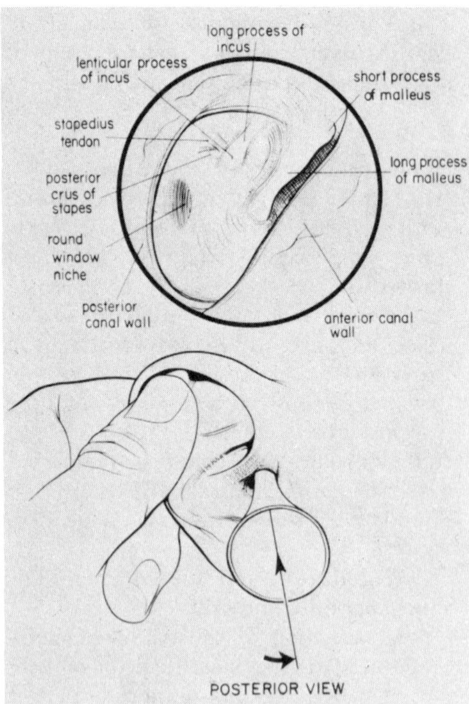

Figure 3. Normal tympanic membrane, posterior view. (*Courtesy of Dr. R. Ruben.*)

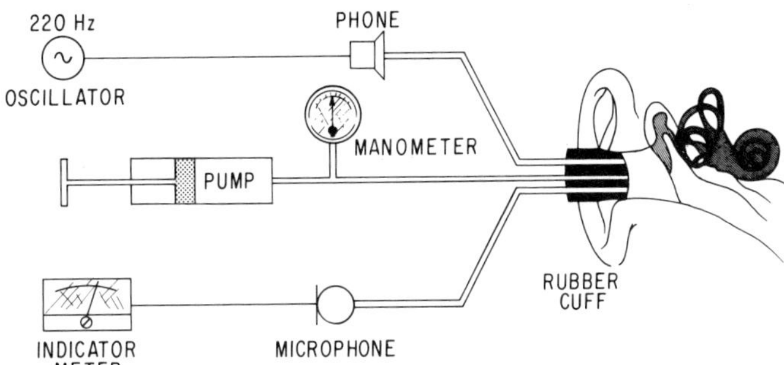

Figure 4. Simplified schematic diagram of the electro-acoustic impedance bridge. (*From Paradise J et al.: Pediatrics 65:17, 1980. Copyright American Academy of Pediatrics 1980.*)

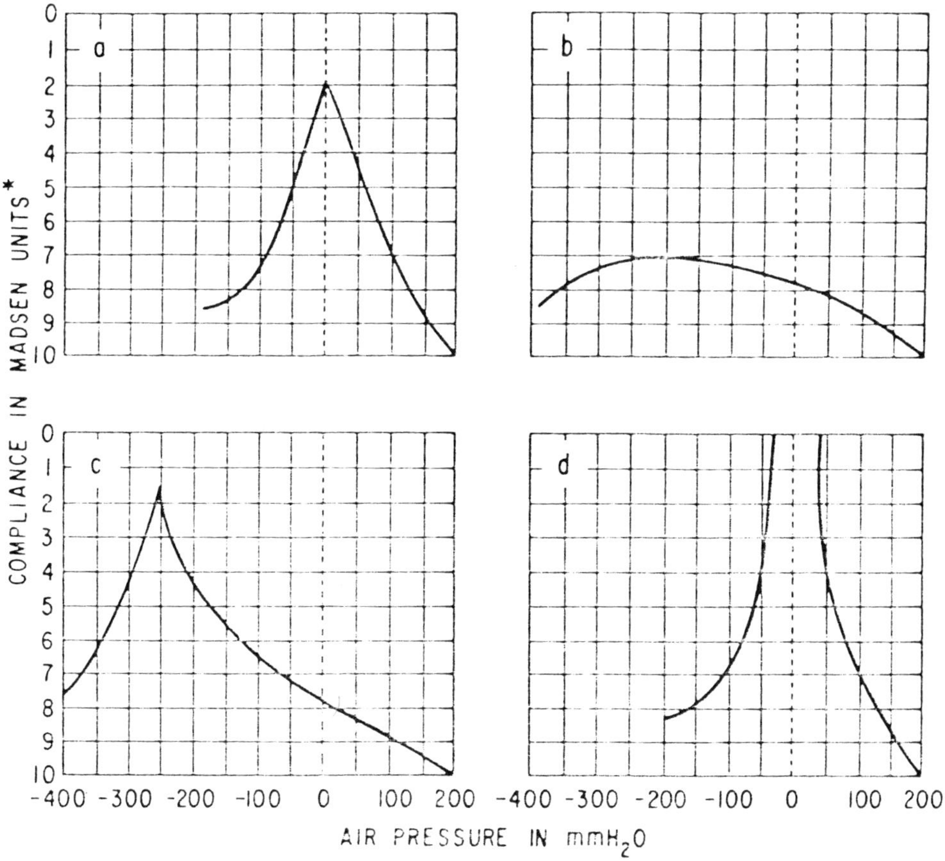

Figure 5. Tympanogram (b) reflects decreased mobility in contrast to a normal tympanogram (a). (*From Paradise J et al.: Pediatrics 65:931, 1980. Copyright American Academy of Pediatrics 1980.*)

2000Hz). Abnormalities in this test would alert the practitioner to the severity of the problem and to the realization that hearing loss, a frequent complication of POM and SOM, has occurred. Referral to a consultant would be indicated if this hearing loss persists for greater than 1 month.

Cultures. Cultures of ear discharge are usually not helpful, since contamination by flora from the external canal occurs so frequently that the practitioner cannot interpret with any validity the significance of the results of a positive ear culture.

Radiographs. These are indicated only when the diagnosis of mastoiditis is being considered as a complication of POM or ROM. Cloudiness or haziness of the normally pneumaticized cells in the mastoid area of an older child (older than 3 years) or in the mastoid antrum of a younger child would confirm the diagnosis of mastoiditis.

Myringoctomy. Myringotomies were performed commonly in patients with POM in the past. However, at present this procedure is done much less frequently in office practice. The indications for myringotomy are few. If adequate drainage of the middle ear is thought to require myringotomy, consultation should be sought.

Tympanocentesis. This is being used increasingly because of numerous reports of otitis media refractory to therapy. Tympanocentesis permits identification and determination of antibiotic sensitivities of the bacterial organism causing the otitis media. Indications for tympanocentesis in children with POM include:

1. Continuing fever after 6–7 days of antibiotic therapy
2. Very severe systemic manifestations
3. Failure to respond to a second course of an appropriate antibiotic when compliance has been good

Tympanocentesis can be performed as an office procedure for the above indication. However the pediatric practitioner who elects to do this should have been carefully instructed and supervised by a pediatric otolaryngologist or another pediatrician skilled in the technique. The proper technique should include:

1. Proper sedation of the child and secure immobilization
2. Cleansing of the external canal
3. Use of a specifically designed needle for middle ear aspiration. This needle is bent at an angle to pass easily through the external canal through the tympanic membrane.
4. Careful insertion of the needle using the operating otoscope
5. Aspiration should take place at the posterior-superior aspect of the TM

Sterile handling of the fluid is of utmost importance. Placement of aspirate on sheep blood agar plates, medium for *H. influenzae*, anaerobic medium, and blood culture bottles would be optimum.

MANAGEMENT

Diagnosis and treatment of a child with an earache must be prompt in order to prevent potential serious complications. Table 2 summarizes the diagnostic possibilities, the therapy indicated, and the suggested indications for consultation. Treatment of the major causes of earache are discussed here in more detail.

POM

It is generally believed that antibiotics should be given to patients with POM, although no properly controlled studies have demonstrated their value. In fact, one uncontrolled study of 2,000 patients in Sweden reported improvement in a large number of children who were not given antibiotics. At present, however, antibiotic treatment is recommended.

The choice of antibiotic is also somewhat controversial in that the number of instances of resistance of *H. influenzae* to commonly used first-line antibiotics (ampicillin, amoxacillin) is increasing. Should this increase continue as projected by some investigators, perhaps Cefaclor or trimethoprim-sulfomethoxazole will be indicated for initial treatment. The practitioner must stay current with recommendations from reliable, well-documented sources to assure appropriate treatment of patients with POM.

The ear pain of POM in a young infant or child often is quite severe and unrelenting. The irritability that often results is very upsetting to parents. Thus, often the parent would like to do something to relieve this pain. Once the practitioner is convinced that a perforated tympanic membrane is not present, instillation of several drops of hyperosmotic glycerol solution (Auralgan, Lidosporin) will result often in instantaneous relief for the infant (and parent).

SOM and MOM

At this time there is no proven, recommended medical therapy for serous otitis media. Numerous studies with various combinations of antihistamines and decongestants, decongestants alone, and even oral steroids have proven contradictory. Thus, until such an acceptable, proven regimen is available, a conservative approach is best. This approach should consist of:

1. Simple exercises, such as chewing sugarless gum or using other means to open the eustachian tube
2. Antihistaminic medications in children who are clearly allergic

3. Continued assessment of hearing; if hearing loss persists for over 3 months, consider intervention with myringotomy and tympanostomy tubes.

Tympanocentesis in children with these conditions usually reveal no bacterial growth. Recently, however, positive bacterial cultures have been reported, which has led some investigators to use an initial course of antibiotics in children with the diagnosis of SOM or MOM. Though several investigators are studying this question, no controlled trial results are available as yet.

ROM

Prevention of ROM is very important, since ROM may lead to chronic otitis media (COM) and permanent hearing impairment. However, two studies, one using ampicillin, and one using sulfisoxazole, Perrin et al Rochester 1974 have suggested the effectiveness of prophylactic antibiotics in preventing ROM. Further prospective controlled trials are required. In a child who has four to six bouts of POM in the course of one respiratory season and in whom resolution of each bout is documented, prophylactic sulfisoxazole might be tried as an adjunct to therapy of individual attacks. The presence of an unresolved mastoiditis, adenoiditis, or sinusitis must be ruled out in these cases.

In all of the situations described above, SOM, MOM, POM, and ROM, investigators are actively evaluating different methods of treatment. The pediatric practitioner must remain current with the results of well-controlled studies and alter the approach to intervention as some of the existing areas of controversy begin to be resolved.

CONSULTANT

The areas of greatest need for a consultant for a child with earache are the following:

Significant Ear Trauma

A surgeon should be consulted for any injury where laceration or avulsion requires placement of sutures.

Foreign Body

An otolaryngologist should be consulted to remove a foreign body that is deeper in the ear canal than 3–4 mm from the meatus.

Cholesteatoma

These are epithelial sacks filled with debris which cause resorption of adjacent middle ear bone and permanent middle ear changes. They appear as white, pearly excrescences on the TM. When they are diagnosed, consultation with an otolaryngologist should be done.

Persistent ROM

An otolaryngologist should be consulted to discuss adenoidectomy or mastoidectomy if there are persistent sites of infection in these areas.

Singificant SOM or MOM with Hearing Loss

The practitioner should consult with an otolaryngologist in caring for patients with a hearing loss or impaired language development due to ROM, SOM, or MOM.

The use of antihistamines or nose sprays in these patients has been very ineffective. The major alternative to be considered is placement of tympanostomy tubes after myringotomy and drainage. Although the long-term results of this procedure are not known,

TABLE 3. SUGGESTED GUIDE FOR TREATMENT OF MIDDLE EAR EFFUSION BY MYRINGOTOMY WITH OR WITHOUT TYMPANOSTOMY TUBE PLACEMENT*

Duration of Current Effusion†	History of Myringotomy during Preceding 12 Mo	Duration of Previous Effusion-Free Period‡		Recommended Treatment for Current Effusion§
		After Myringotomy	After Tube Extrusion	
<2 or 3 mo ‖	Irrelevant	...	...	No surgery
≥2 or 3 mo ‖	None	...	...	Myringotomy without tube placement
	Myringotomy without tube placement	≥6 mo	...	Myringotomy without tube placement
		<6 mo	...	Myringotomy with tube placement
	Myringotomy with tube placement	...	≥6 mo	Myringotomy without tube placement
		...	<6 mo	Myringotomy with tube placement

*See text for qualifications.

†If date of onset is uncertain, history and appearance of eardrum may permit reasonable estimate of duration. If in doubt, as to changing status, an observation period of 4–6 weeks—to include serial tympanometric testing, if available—may help clarify course direction.

‡If uncertain and cannot be reasonably estimated, assume <6 months.

§The treatment of each ear is to be considered individually.

‖ Use 3 months if there has been little or no ear disease in the past or prompt recovery from previous episodes. Use 2 months if previous episodes have been frequent or unduly protracted or have failed to resolve completely. (*From Paradise J, et al.: Pediatrics 60:86, 1980. Copyright American Academy of Pediatrics 1980.*)

the guidelines given in Table 3 have been drawn up by Paradise and co-workers and appear reasonable. Further data on the long-term consequences of tympanostomy are awaited to better evaluate their appropriate use. One recent study indicates that tube insertion appears preferable to myringotomy alone for prevention of persistent effusion. However, longer-term, larger studies are awaited before definitive recommendations can be made.

SUMMARY

The pediatric practitioner should be able to diagnose accurately and to treat 98% of the causes of earache in children. However, continuing proper care of these children will require the pediatric practitioner to remain current with the advances being made in the understanding of the etiology of these diseases and in diagnostic aids and treatment modalities currently under investigation. Given the frequency of this complaint, the ease of diagnosis and availability of appropriate interventions should allow for resolution of the problem and a satisfying result for practitioner, child, and parent.

REFERENCES

Cantekin EI, et al.: Lack of efficacy of a decongestant-antihistamine combination for otitis media with effusion (secretory otitis media) in children. N Engl J Med 308:6 297, 1983

Klein J, et al.: Increased resistance of *H. influenzae* to ampicillin. J Pediatr 92, 1978

Medical Letter, July 30, 1978: Recommendations for use of trimethoprim-sulfamethoxazole.

Northern J: Advanced techniques for measuring middle ear function. Pediatrics 61:761, 1978

Olsen AL, et al.: Use of decongestants and treatment of acute and serous otitis media. Pediatrics 61:679, 1978

Paradise J: Otitis media in infants and children. Pediatrics 65:917, 1980

Paradise J, et al.: Use of tympanostomy tubes. Pediatrics 60:86, 1977

Perrin J et al.: Use of antibiotics in recurrent otitis media. N Engl J Med 291:667, 1977

Rowe D: Acute suppurative otitis media. Pediatrics 56:285, 1975

Schwartz R, et al.: Acute purulent otitis media in children older than 5 years. JAMA 238:1032, 1977

Schwartz R et al.: Bacterial etiology of otitis 5–9 years of age. JAMA 238:1032, 1977

Schenberg B, et al.: Comparison of cephalexin and ampicillin. Pediatrics 58:532, 1976

Shurin PA, et al.: Bacterial etiology of acute otitis in infants 6 weeks old. J Pediatr 92:893, 1978

Cross-Reference to *Pediatrics*, 17th ed.

NINE

Fever, Meningitis, and Bacteremia

Joy Glaser

The thermometer invented in the 1600s by Sanctorus was over a foot in length, cumbersome to use, and employed only once if at all during an illness.[1] Today the thermometer is so readily available that it is usually nonprofessionals who quickly determine alteration in body temperature and present the physician with this objective measure of the presence of disease.

An elevated temperature accompanies many conditions, and in children the etiology of most of these febrile episodes is readily diagnosed. In some instances, a careful clinical approach combined with thoughtfully selected laboratory tests and the expertise of a consulting specialist are necessary before the cause is understood.

DEFINITION

Fever is defined as an elevation in body core temperature above normal. Generally, this normal temperature varies from 36.2C to 37.8C, but for any child the normal temperature may be slightly outside of this range. The rectal temperature is often higher than the oral temperature, but it is not more accurate, as some think, in reflecting core temperature.

An exaggeration of the normal late afternoon peak in body temperature in an active, healthy child is not unusual. Nevertheless, at most other times, an elevated body temperature is usually a sign of illness. Although the most common cause of fever in childhood is an infectious disease, at times malignancy and antigen-antibody reactions must also be considered.

Thermoregulation

The hypothalamus maintains thermal homeostasis by sending signals to a number of effector organs when core temperature is either above or below the hypothalamic set point. For example, during strenuous exercise, heat production initially exceeds heat loss, resulting in an elevated core temperature. Equilibrium is quickly restored by peripheral vasodilation, sweating, and panting, mechanisms initiated by stimuli from the thermoregulatory center to the autonomic nervous system. Fever secondary to most diseases is the result of disordered thermoregulation. The interaction of abnormal substances, such as bacteria, viruses, or immune complexes, with phagocytic cells initiates the production and release by the host

110

cells of endogenous pyrogen, a substance which resets the hypothalamic thermostat to an elevated set point.[2] To maintain homeostasis, increased muscular activity (in the form of chills) and peripheral vasoconstriction occur to raise body temperature. No matter what the stimulus, the pyrogen released by phagocytic cells (monocyte, neutrophil, eosinophil) is chemically the same. Although lymphocytes are not capable of producing pyrogen, they are able to produce soluble substances that promote production of pyrogen in phagocytic cells. Fever, then, which is so notable in calling attention to the existence of a disease, is nonspecific in defining either the etiology or pathogenesis of the disease process.

Fever Unassociated with Pyrogen Release

Most fevers in children are caused by a disease that initiates endogenous pyrogen release. However, there are some conditions associated with an elevated temperature that are the result of other processes.

1. In the late afternoon, peak body temperature may be as high as 38.5C in an active, healthy child. The child looks well, and the temperature declines without intervention as the child's activities diminish.
2. Elevated external temperatures, especially accompanied by overdressing in young infants, can produce a nonpathologic fever. This process is due to the decreased ability to sweat in this age group and is quickly reversed once the environment is altered or the excessive clothing is removed.
3. Exercise may result in a temporarily elevated temperature as heat loss fails to keep up with heat production.
4. In thyrotoxicosis, hypermetabolism results in an elevated body temperature.
5. Congenital or acquired central nervous system disease may affect temperature regulation.
6. The elevated temperature may be factitious.

ANTIPYRETICS AND FEVER

Fever which is not markedly elevated (< 40.0C–104F) or prolonged does not have a deleterious effect on the child. There is experimental evidence to show that fever may be beneficial to the infected host by increasing immunologic defenses. Maximum phagocytic activity for human leukocytes has been shown to occur between 38 and 40C, while human lymphocytes have increased activity at 39C. In addition, some bacteria are more susceptible to antibiotics at higher temperature, and the ability of viruses to replicate may be inhibited by elevated temperatures. There is recent epidemiologic evidence suggesting that salicylates may actually be harmful, since Reye's syndrome has been associated with the use of salicylates during a preceding episode of varicella or influenza.[3] The reflex use of antipyretics, therefore, for every febrile illness is neither advisable nor therapeutic. These drugs should be used mainly when the child is very uncomfortable, when the child is at risk of convulsions, or when the temperature is greater than 39.5C (103F).

Both acetaminophen and salicylates are effective antipyretics.[4] However, during certain viral illnesses as described above, acetaminophen is the antipyretic of choice.

DISEASES ASSOCIATED WITH FEVER

Infection is the most common cause of acute or prolonged fever in childhood.[5] A broad list of diseases associated with fever in children is presented in Table 1. A discussion of

TABLE 1. DISEASES ASSOCIATED WITH FEVER IN CHILDREN

Infectious Diseases*	Fungal infections
Bacterial infections	Rickettsial infection
Bacteremic infections	Parasitic infections
Associated with a septic focus	Unknown, presumed infectious diseases—
Unassociated with a focus	Reye's syndrome, Kawasaki's disease
Nonbacteremic infections	**Allergic Diseases**
Viral infections	
Mycobacterial infections	**Collagen Vascular Diseases**
Mycoplasma infections	**Neoplastic Diseases**

*For an in-depth presentation of the vast array of infectious diseases manifested by fever, the reader is referred to Feigin RD. Cherry JD (eds), Textbook of Pediatric Infectious Diseases, Philadelphia, Saunders, 1981.

each and its relation to fever is beyond the scope of this chapter. The subsequent sections, therefore, discuss evaluation, management, and therapy of selected bacteremic, febrile, infectious diseases.

Febrile Bacteremias

Pediatricians may encounter bacteremia in three clinical situations: (1) secondary to focal suppurative infections, (2) in 5% of previously healthy febrile children less than 2 years of age, many of whom have no identifiable source of the bacteremia, and (3) in febrile, immunosuppressed patients, in whom bacteremia often occurs with no primary focus.

Bacteremia Associated with an Infected Focus.

Some focal infections are frequently associated with bacteremia; these include epiglottitis, meningitis, osteomyelitis, septic arthritis, pyelonephritis, and suppurative thrombophlebitis. In addition, positive blood cultures are obtained in approximately 5–10% of children with bacterial pneumonia. Some focal infections not usually associated with bacteremia in older patients may be accompanied by bacteremia in the young child. These include staphylococcal infections of the skin, salmonella gastroenteritis, and *Haemophilus influenzae* type b cellulitis (Table 2).

Evaluation and Treatment of Focal Suppurative Disease.

For bacteriologic diagnosis, smears and cultures of the infected site should always be obtained, as well as two blood cultures. Even appropriately handled material taken from the infected site will not always yield the organism. A list of the commonly encountered organisms in various age groups with focal bacteremic disease is presented in Table 2 as a guide to antibiotic therapy before culture results are obtained because unusual organisms or organisms with altered antibiotic sensitivities will sometimes be encountered, making recovery of the etiologic agent vital for proper antibiotic therapy.

For many of the focal infections listed, antibiotic therapy should be coupled with adequate drainage. Consultation with other specialists, such as orthopedists, surgeons, and the infectious disease team, is, therefore, often required.

Bacterial Meningitis

Children less than 5 years of age are unusually susceptible to bacterial meningitis. Indeed, about 60% of all cases of purulent meningitis occur in this age group.[6] The organism most commonly encountered is *H. influenzae* type b. However, *Neisseria meningitidis* and *Streptococcus pneumoniae* remain important etiologic agents. In infants less than 2 months, it is the group B streptococcus, *Escherichia coli*, other enteric gram-negative organisms, and *Listeria Monocytogenes* that are responsible for most central nervous system disease.

Clinical Findings. Clinical manifestations of meningitis include *fever,* which is present in over 95% of patients. A temperature $\geq 41.1C$ (106F)is associated with a 10% incidence of meningitis; therefore, a spinal tap is recommended in any child with this degree of fever.

Altered mental status manifested by irritability, confusion, or coma is seen in 90% of children. Twenty percent have a seizure prior to admission to the hospital, and 14% have focal neurologic findings on admission, indicating a poor prognosis. We have encountered a rapidly progressive form of meningitis in a few children who suddenly became obtunded or went into coma during a benign febrile illness. In these children, in whom encephalitic symptoms predominated, the spinal fluid showed only a mildly elevated cell count, but myriads of organisms were easily visible in the sediment of a centrifuged sample of spinal fluid. Because the differential diagnosis in these patients includes subdural empyema, brain abscess, and viral or

TABLE 2. ORGANISMS MOST OFTEN ENCOUNTERED IN FOCAL BACTEREMIC DISEASE OF CHILDHOOD

Focus of Infection	Age		
	2 wk–2 mo	2 mo–2 yr	>2 yr
Bone	*Staphylococcus aureus* *Escherichia coli* Group B streptococci	*S. aureus* Group A streptococci *Haemophilus influenzae* type b	*S. aureus* Group A streptococci
Joint	*S. aureus* Group B streptococci *E. coli*	*S. aureus* *H. influenzae* type b Group A streptococci	*S. aureus* Group A streptococci
Skin:			
Cellulitis	Group A or Group B streptococci *S. aureus*	*H. influenzae* type b Group A streptococci *S. aureus*	Group A streptococci *S. aureus*
Abscess*	*S. aureus*	*S. aureus* Group A streptococci	*S. aureus*†
Meningitis	Group B streptococci *E. coli* *Listeria monocytogenes*	*H. influenzae* type b Pneumococcus Meningococcus	Pneumococcus *H. influenzae* type b Meningococcus
Pyelonephritis	Enteric gram-negative	Enteric gram-negative	Enteric gram-negative
Lung	Pneumococcus *S. aureus*	Pneumococcus *H. influenzae* type b *S. aureus*	Pneumococcus
Gastroenteritis	Salmonella	Salmonella	

*Although *S. aureus* is the most common cause of skin abscess in certain clinical situations, other etiologies must be considered: (1) anaerobic and aerobic mouth flora are commonly cultured from submandibular abscess in children older than 3 yr of age; (2) an abscess on the lower abdomen or groin area may be caused by anaerobic and aerobic gram-negative bacteria.
†Bacteremia mainly occurs in children less than 2 yr of age.

toxic encephalopathy, it is advisable to perform a CT scan before the lumbar puncture. If the scan cannot be done immediately to rule out brain a consultation with the pediatric neurologist should be obtained to consider the advisability of slowly withdrawing a small amount of spinal fluid for examination.

Meningeal signs, such as neck stiffness, positive Brudzinski sign, or positive Kernig sign, are rarely seen in neonates or infants but are usually present in older children. Some young infants develop a bulging fontanel as evidence of meningeal infection.

Headache alone or with photophobia occurs in most older children. It tends to be unresponsive to mild analgesics.

Anorexia and *vomiting* are frequent symptoms in children with meningitis.

The decision to perform a spinal tap on a febrile child is based on the presence of suggestive clinical manifestations, as discussed.

Laboratory Diagnosis of Purulent Meningitis.

The CSF should be collected in four sterile tubes, the first used for microbiology, the second for chemistry, the third for cell count, and the fourth placed in the refrigerator for additional studies, such as counterimmune electrophoresis.

Examination of the CSF should always include the following:

Appearance.

The number of cellular elements determines if the CSF is clear (< 200 cells per cu mm), hazy (200–500) or turbid (> 500). Counts ranging from less than 100 cells per ml of CSF to 87,000 per ml have been recorded in patients with acute purulent meningitis.

Measurement of Pressure.

The pressure is usually elevated (> 200 mm water), and only a small amount of fluid should be removed if the pressure is very high.

Cell Count.

Cell count is elevated, due to a predominance of polymorphonuclear leukocytes. The total cell count is determined on the uncentrifuged CSF in a hemocytometer counting chamber. The white blood cell count is determined by lysing the red cells and recounting the cells. The differential cell count is done using a Wright stain preparation of the CSF sediment. The presence of any polymorphonuclear leukocytes in the spinal fluid is abnormal in children and may be indicative of a purulent meningitis.

Measurement of Protein and Sugar.

The concentration of protein in the CSF is elevated, while the concentration of sugar is decreased. A blood sugar must be obtained to determine the CSF:blood sugar ratio. The normal CSF glucose is greater than or equal to 50% of a simultaneously obtained blood sugar.

Gram Stain of Sediment.

This examination will usually reveal organisms when there are 10^5 or more per ml. In some instances, an organism seen on the gram stain does not grow on culture. The gram stain may then help guide subsequent antibiotic therapy and should be saved to be reviewed if necessary.

Culture.

Culture of the CSF and determination of antibiotic sensitivity of bacterial isolates are crucial for appropriate antibiotic therapy and eradication of disease. The CSF culture is positive in 90% of children with untreated purulent meningitis, while in partially treated meningitis, CSF culture is positive in only 70%.[8]

The cell count, gram stain, and wright stain must always be done by the physician caring for the child.

Management.

The complications of acute purulent meningitis include:

1. Focal neurologic disease
2. Seizures
3. Acute hydrocephalus
4. Syndrome of inappropriate release of ADH
5. Disseminated intravascular coagulation

6. Shock
7. Focal suppurative disease in other organs, e.g., pneumonia, purulent pericarditis, septic arthritis

The child with meningitis is critically ill and must be admitted to an intensive care unit for frequent monitoring of neurologic and vasomotor status. It is often necessary to include the infectious disease team and the neurologists in the care of these patients.

The initial choice of antibiotics depends on the organisms most commonly encountered in each age group, the findings on the Gram stain, and, if available, results of counterimmune electrophoresis.

For early therapy in suspected neonatal meningitis, we are presently using a combination of ampicillin, an aminoglycoside antibiotic, and a third-generation cephalosporin (moxalactam, cefotaxime) known to give high CSF levels. No one drug is adequate for the major organisms often encountered in this age group (group B streptococci, *Escherichia coli, Listeria*).[9] Until more data are available on the efficacy of the newest cephalosporins for the organisms causing neonatal meningitis, we feel more comfortable using a combination of the three antibiotics. It is already known that neither moxalactam nor cefotaxime is effective against *L. monocytogenes,* nor is moxalactam effective against group B streptococci.

Children over 2 months of age are generally treated with ampicillin and chloramphenicol until the organism and its antimicrobial sensitivity are known.

We perform only the initial diagnostic spinal tap in the child over 2 months of age with an *uncomplicated* purulent meningitis caused by the meningococcus, *H. influenzae,* or the pneumococcus. We have not found repeated examinations of the spinal fluid helpful. In addition, because some CSF abnormalities (elevated cell count, decreased sugar) may persist even after successful therapy, a spinal tap after the course of antibiotics is not helpful and may be confusing.

Prophylaxis for Diseases Caused by Meningococcus and Haemophilus Influenzae Type b.

Meningococcus. Close family contacts, both children and adults, and contacts in day care centers should receive a 2-day course of rifampin (children 20 mg/kg/day divided bid, adults 600 mg/day divided bid). This eliminates nasopharyngeal organisms and helps to prevent secondary cases. Vaccines against type A and type C organisms are available and are useful along with rifampin when these serotypes are encountered. The patient should also receive rifampin, since organisms in the nasopharynx may not be eradicated during therapy for the disease.

Haemophilus influenzae Type b. Four days of rifampin therapy is recommended for those who have been in close contact with the patient. The dose is as recommended for the meningococcus but is continued for a longer period. The patient should also receive rifampin.

Nonfocal Bacteremia in Febrile Children Less Than Two Years of Age

For a number of years, pediatricians have been aware that fever in infants less than 2 months of age may be due to nonfocal bacteremia. A recent study demonstrated that this occurs in approximately 5% of febrile young infants.[10] However, in the past 5 to 7 years, we have learned that bacteria can be identified in the blood of a significant number of febrile children who are older than 2 months but less than 2 years of age, with diagnoses such as "febrile URI" or "fever with no source."[11]

To put this phenomenon into perspective, most febrile children below age 2 years with no source for the fever are not bacteremic and have only a self-limited viral or bacterial disease. However, the children whose febrile illness is accompanied by bacteremia should be identified, since serious complications may develop.

Certain aspects of the clinical presentation and physical assessment help in predicting nonfocal bacteremia in the child less than 2.

Fever. There is a direct correlation between the height of the fever and incidence of bacteremia

Temperature (C)	Incidence of Bacteremia (%)
38.9–40.4	4.5
40.5–41.0	13.0
>41.1	23.0

Symptoms. A decreased appetite, decreased activity, increased sleep, and increased irritability are subtle symptoms of more serious illness.

Physician's Examination. A number of investigators have reported that the *clinical judgment* of an experienced observer (practicing physician, house officer, nurse) can be used to predict those febrile children in need of blood cultures. In most of the reported studies, each participant developed his own criteria to determine the degree of illness. Most important was that the observer had to take time to assess the functional capacity of the child before doing the physical examination. Clinical assessment was found to be valuable, along with a CBC and ESR, even in very young infants 2 weeks to 2 months of age.[10]

Laboratory Evaluation. Predicting bacteremia by various objective tests has been explored by a number of investigators. An ESR $\geq$ 30, WBC $\geq$ 15,000, neutrophil count $\geq$ 10,000, and band count $\geq$ 500 have been used alone or in combination as guides in deciding whether or not to obtain a blood culture. Each test has its proponents and opponents, and further investigations seem necessary to determine which are most useful.

Etiology. The organisms responsible for bacteremic disease without a focus depend mainly on the age of the child (Table 3). Choice of the appropriate antibiotics before culture reports are available is based on this knowledge. From age 2 weeks to 2 months the organisms include those which colonize newborns, such as group B streptococci, *E. coli*, other enteric gram-negative organisms, and *Listeria*. In children older than 2 months, the pneumococcus is responsible for the majority of nonfocal bacteremias. However, *H. Influenzae* type b has also been cultured from a significant number of febrile children with no recognizable source.

Management. The febrile child over age 2 months with otitis media or no focus for the fever and who may be bacteremic (criteria above) should be further evaluated as an outpatient with a chest x-ray, urinalysis, urine culture, CBC, and blood culture. An unsuspected focus may be revealed on the basis of these tests. The child who appears ill enough to require a lumbar puncture should be admitted to the hospital for closer follow-up.

Therapy for a suspected occult bacteremia is advisable, since it can be prolonged and lead to metastatic infection. However,

TABLE 3. ORGANISMS ENCOUNTERED IN NONFOCAL BACTEREMIA

Patient's Age	Organism
2 wk–2 mo	Group B streptococcus *Escherichia coli* *Listeria* Other enteric gram-negative
2 mo–2 yr	Pneumococcus *Haemophilus influenzae* type b

one must be aware that some instances of occult bacteremia clear without therapy and that in one retrospective study oral antibiotics did not alter the incidence of meningitis occurring during this process. Nevertheless, children who receive antibiotics early in the course of their bacteremia did clinically better than those who were not started on medication.[11] Ampicillin (amoxacillin) is considered the drug of choice. In geographic areas where a significant number of strains of *H. influenzae* type b are resistant to ampicillin, erythromycin and a sulfa drug would be appropriate. Close follow-up for the next 48 hours of those children suspected of being bacteremic is mandatory, whether or not antibiotics are started, since some children will not recover with oral antibiotics alone. If very close follow-up with the family is not possible, admission to the hospital is advised. In no case should antibiotics be given to a child suspected of being bacteremic without first obtaining blood cultures and performing the other diagnostic tests outlined above.

When a pathogenic organism is recovered from the blood and *the child is already taking antibiotics:*

1. Continue outpatient treatment for 10 days if the child is improved and afebrile
2. Admit for further evaluation and parenteral therapy if the child is still febrile

If the child is not taking antibiotics:

1. Begin outpatient therapy and continue for 10 days if the child is afebrile
2. Admit for further work-up and parenteral antibiotics if the child is still febrile

The above recommendations have been made for febrile children who may be bacteremic but do not appear ill enough to require hospitalization. Certain febrile children must be admitted for evaluation, therapy, and close observation. These include:

1. Febrile children who appear very ill
2. Children who require a spinal tap
3. Febrile children with temperature ≥ 41.1 C because of the high risk of bacteremia (23%) and meningitis (10%) in this group
4. Immunosuppressed febrile children in whom overwhelming sepsis may develop
5. Febrile children less than 2 months of age. Data are presently being collected which may allow us to distinguish the young infants with serious illness who are in need of hospitalization from the majority of febrile babies with benign disease who can be managed safely at home.

FEVER IN THE IMMUNOCOMPROMISED HOST

Fever in the immunosuppressed child or the child with an implanted foreign body (e.g., ventriculoperitoneal shunt) is often a sign of very serious disease. The immunosuppressed child should be seen as soon as possible when febrile, and cultures of any possibly infected site, no matter how small, should be taken. Blood cultures should also be obtained, since nonfocal bacteremia occurs frequently in this group, and hospital admission for antibiotic therapy and close observation is usually necessary. A lung biopsy in those patients with interstitial pneumonia who do not respond to initial therapy can be very helpful in guiding subsequent therapy. Because these patients are prone to a number of very serious viral infections as well, it is helpful to obtain viral cultures early and to obtain serum for acute and convalescent viral titers. Although children with sickle cell disease are prone to pneumococcal, *H. influenzae* type b, and salmonella infections, other immunosuppressed children, such as children with nephrotic syndrome, and neutropenic children and those on cancer chemotherapy or transplant immunotherapy, may also be bacteremic with these organisms. However, enteric gram-negative organisms, *Staphylococcus aureus,* protozoa, and fungi must also be considered in this latter group. Initial antibiotic therapy will depend on results of the clinical evaluation, laboratory tests, and host factors that make certain infectious diseases most likely.

The child who is febrile and has a synthetic device implanted, such as a ventriculoperitoneal or ventriculoatrial shunt, should have appropriate cultures taken (shunt and blood) before antibiotics are begun for treatment of an infection elsewhere (such as otitis media). It often takes many weeks while the child remains febrile before the correct diagnosis is made because of the difficulty growing the organisms from the CSF once antibiotics are begun.

SUMMARY

Fever is an important mechanism for calling attention to disease and probably helps shorten the course of many infectious diseases by increasing host defenses. As Thomas Sydenham said in the seventeenth century, "Fever is Nature's engine which she brings into the field to remove her enemy." It is more important to evaluate the cause of the fever than to lower it with various antipyretics. Focal or nonfocal bacteremias associated with fever are not rare in young children and those who are immunosuppressed. Initial antibiotic therapy for suspected bacteremic disease depends on the age of the child and the underlying process, while subsequent therapy depends on the organism recovered from cultures obtained before antibiotics are begun.

REFERENCES

1. Clendening L: The history of certain medical instruments. Ann Intern Med 4:176, 1930

2. Bernheim HA, Block LH, Atkins E: Fever: pathogenesis, pathophysiology and purpose. Ann Intern Med 91:261, 1979

3. Committee on Infectious Diseases: Aspirin and Reye's syndrome. Pediatrics 69:810, 1982

4. Eden AN, Kaufman A: Clinical comparison of three antipyretic agents. Am J Dis Child 114:284, 1967

5. Pizzo PA, Lovejoy FH, Smith DS: Prolonged fever in children: review of 100 cases. J Pediatr 55:468, 1975

6. Gerseler PJ, Selson KE, Levin S, Reddi KT, Moses VK: Community acquired purulent meningitis: A review of 1,316 cases during the antibiotic era, 1954–1976. Rev Infect Dis 2:725, 1980

7. McCarthy PL: Controversies in pediatrics: what tests are indicated for the child under 2 with fever? Pediatr Rev 1:51, 1979

8. Feigin RD: Bacterial meningitis beyond the neonatal period. In Feigin RD, Cherry JD (eds): Textbook of Pediatric Infectious Diseases. Philadelphia, Saunders, 1981

9. Schaad UB, McCracken GH, Threlkeld N, Thomas ML: Clinical evaluation of a new broad-spectrum oxa-beta-lactam antibiotic, moxalactam, in neonates and infants. J Pediatr 98:129, 1981

10. Crain EF, Shelov SP: Febrile infants: predictors of bacteremia. J Pediatr 101:686, 1982

11. Teele DW, Marshall R, Klein JO: Unsuspected bacteremia in young children. Pediatr Clin North Am 26:773, 1979

12. McCarthy PL, Jekel F, Stashwick CA, et al.: Further definition of history and observation variables in assessing febrile children. Pediatrics 67:687, 1981

Cross-Reference to *Pediatrics,* 17th ed.

TEN

Gastrointestinal Bleeding

Ellen F. Crain

Gastrointestinal (GI) bleeding occurs commonly during childhood. The task confronting the pediatric practitioner is to determine when this complaint is secondary to a relatively minor cause and when it heralds a serious and potentially life-threatening condition, such as massive hemorrhage or necrosis of part of the gastrointestinal tract.

Most causes of gastrointestinal bleeding in children are unique to the pediatric age group, and within this group they vary markedly with age. Thus, a consideration of the child's age, combined with a thorough history and careful physical examination, should allow the practitioner to narrow down the differential diagnosis, decide whether or not the bleeding is serious, and help determine which diagnostic tests are required to pinpoint the diagnosis.

DEFINITION

GI bleeding is defined as the microscopic or macroscopic passage of blood originating anywhere along the GI tract from the esophagus to the anus; it may occur as hematemesis, melena, or hematochezia. *Hematemesis* is defined as the vomiting of blood that has been swallowed or comes from the esophagus, stomach, or duodenum proximal to the ligament of Treitz. It can be bright or dark red or take on the appearance of coffee grounds when the blood is exposed for a time to the hydrochloric acid in gastric juice. If the blood is not vomited but passes into or is produced by the small bowel anywhere above the ileocecal valve, it takes on a tarry black appearance because of alteration by digestive enzymes. Passage of this tarry black material per rectum is called *melena*. Finally, bright or dark red blood passed per rectum is termed *hematochezia;* it suggests bleeding from the colon or rectum.

The character of the blood can help to localize the site of bleeding: a dark brown or black color suggesting upper GI bleeding and a bright red color lower GI bleeding. However, blood in the gastrointestinal tract stimulates peristalsis, and, therefore, with massive hemorrhage from the upper gastrointestinal tract, bright red blood may be passed per rectum.

ETIOLOGY OF GI BLEEDING IN INFANTS AND CHILDREN

Many causes of GI bleeding in children can be handled by the pediatric practitioner alone, although most require hospitalization at least for observation. The most common causes of bleeding by age and the site from which blood is recovered are listed in Table 1.

GI Bleeding in the Newborn

Typically, the pediatric practitioner will be called to see an apparently healthy newborn who has had an episode of GI bleeding within 48 hours of birth. Unless the infant is bleeding profusely and shows signs of inadequate circulating blood volume, there is ample time to make a careful assessment.

Conditions That Can Be Handled by the Pediatrician Alone. Bleeding in newborns is unexplained in over 50% of cases, but swallowed maternal blood and anorectal trauma account for nearly 90% of the known causes of GI bleeding in newborns and often can be handled by the pediatric practitioner alone.

Swallowed Maternal Blood. One of the most common causes of hematemesis, hematochezia, or melena is swallowed maternal blood, occurring either during the birth process or during nursing on a bleeding nipple.

TABLE 1. COMMON CAUSES OF GASTROINTESTINAL BLEEDING

	Blood Recovered from	
Age/Conditions to be Considered	**Upper GI Tract**	**Lower GI Tract**
Newborn period		
Conditions that can be handled by the pediatrician alone		
Swallowed maternal blood	+	+
Local anorectal trauma	0	+
Conditions that may require consultation		
Hemorrhagic disease of the newborn	0	+
Infectious diarrhea	0	+
Stress ulcers	+	+
Conditions that require immediate consultation		
Necrotizing enterocolitis	0	+
Volvulus	0	+
Older infants		
Conditions that can be handled by the pediatrician alone		
Anal fissure	0	+
Conditions that require consultation		
Ulcer disease	+	+
Meckel's diverticulum	0	+
Intussusception	0	+
Volvulus	0	+
Children older than 1 year		
All the lesions in older infants plus conditions that require consultation		
Colonic polyps	0	+
Esophageal varices	+	+
Peptic ulcer disease	+	+
Inflammatory bowel disease	0	+

Typically the infant looks well, has stable vital signs, and no other evidence of bleeding; he may be spitting up some of his feedings. The diagnosis is confirmed by passing a nasogastric tube and performing the Apt-Downey test on the return or on the infant's stool.

Anorectal Trauma. Anal fissures, secondary to passage of a large stool or to an overly vigorous digital examination, account for approximately 10% of cases. These infants, who look well, have passed a small amount of bright red blood per rectum or have blood-streaked stools. They do not have melena or hematemesis. The tear is seen on careful spreading of the perianal skin.

Conditions That May Require Consultation.

Hemorrhagic Disease of the Newborn. Hemorrhagic disease of the newborn was the second most common cause of neonatal GI bleeding before the administration of vitamin K to newborns became standard practice. It is now extremely uncommon but may occur, for example, in sick newborns or premature infants who are most likely to leave the delivery room without receiving vitamin K and are likely to develop this syndrome because of hepatic dysmaturity. It occurs typically between the second and fourth days of life when low stores of vitamin K result in a deficiency of coagulation factors II, VII, IX, and X. Symptoms include hematochezia or melena (or both) and, less commonly, hematemesis. There may also be evidence of cutaneous bleeding, which suggests that the bleeding is not secondary to swallowed maternal blood. Nevertheless, an Apt test should be performed because ecchymoses and petechiae may be secondary to birth trauma. Unless blood loss has been massive, which is unusual, these infants look well. Specific inquiry should be made about maternal intake of Coumadin and Dilantin.

Colitis. Infections with *Escherichia coli* and other bacterial agents can cause bloody diarrhea in the newborn, either sporadically or as part of a nursery epidemic. The onset of illness is often insidious. The infant may be listless or irritable and may have frequent watery stools followed by bloody, mucoid stools. The nasogastric aspirate should be negative for blood, and the abdominal x-ray reveals a normal gas pattern. Complications include otitis media, pneumonia, bacteremia, peritonitis, pyelonephritis, and, with extreme dehydration, renal venous thrombosis. Any infant with bloody diarrhea should be isolated from other infants and have a work-up for infection. The stool should be cultured and examined for white blood cells.

Stress Ulcers. Documented stress ulcers account for a small percentage of cases of GI bleeding, although they may be an unrecognized cause of bleeding in many infants in the idiopathic group. They occur more commonly in premature infants, and there is often an associated history of a difficult delivery or hypoxic episode. These infants usually look sick, so that the possibility of hypoglycemia or sepsis must be considered. Although bleeding may be massive, it is usually short-lived.

Conditions That Require Immediate Consultation.

Occasionally, GI bleeding is the presenting sign in infants with ischemia of the bowel. These patients require immediate consultation with a neonatologist and a pediatric surgeon.

Necrotizing Enterocolitis. Necrotizing enterocolitis (NEC) usually occurs in premature infants after they have begun to feed, but any newborn who has undergone significant stress is susceptible. Rectal bleeding, which usually is not massive, is a late sign, though the development of occult bleeding may be the earliest indication. Several factors distinguish the rectal bleeding of NEC from that of a gastric ulcer, including (1) the lack of blood in the stomach, (2) the development of abdominal distention and crepitance, and (3) a typical appearance of the intestines on x-ray, ranging from edema of the wall to free air in the peritoneum or the portal vein.

Volvulus. Gangrenous bowel with signs of obstruction is caused most commonly by small bowel volvulus. These newborns present with lethargy, poor feeding, and irritability, accompanied by bilious vomiting and hematochezia. In addition, there is usually abdominal distention and a palpable abdominal mass. The x-ray shows air-fluid levels in the small bowel and often no air beyond the duodenum. Any delay in operating on these infants may permit bowel ischemia to proceed to necrosis, with diastrous consequences. The differential diagnosis includes intussusception, but this entity is uncommon in the newborn period. The triad of obstruction, abdominal mass, and rectal bleeding in the newborn signifies volvulus. Barium enema is not indicated because the volvulus is nearly always of the small bowel. If barium enema is done, however, it will show the cecum to be in an abnormal position.

Common Causes of Bleeding in Infants after the Newborn Period

Causes That Can Be Managed by the Pediatrician Alone.
Anal Fissure. By far the most common cause of GI bleeding in older infants is anal fissure. The infant presents with a history of either bright red blood passed with or after the stool or a stool streaked with blood. He looks alert and vigorous. He may recently have had an episode of diarrhea or constipation, but the stools may have returned to normal by the time the bleeding is first noticed. The sequence often is that diarrhea resulted in anal irritation and pain on defecation, which in turn led to voluntary fecal retention. When the child cannot withhold any longer, a large

hard stool is passed that tears the anal mucosa, opening a fissure and leading to more pain as well as bleeding. The diagnosis is made on the basis of this typical history in a healthy looking child. It is confirmed by spreading the buttocks, everting the anus, and visualizing the fissure or its sentinel skin tag.

Causes that Require Consultation.
Ulcer Disease. Most ulcers in infants are acute stress ulcers secondary to severe injury, such as CNS trauma (Cushing ulcer), burns (Curling ulcer), ulcerogenic drugs (such as steroids and aspirins), and malignancies. Children with stress ulcers usually develop GI bleeding while being treated for a serious illness. Although hematemesis is present at some time in nearly 100% of patients and vomiting may be a presenting sign in young infants, signs of obstruction are absent. Many of these children have coagulation problems, such as thrombocytopenia and disseminated intravascular coagulation, which can aggravate the amount of hemorrhage. These children require intensive observation.

Meckel's Diverticulum. Meckel's diverticulum accounts for approximately 5% of cases of GI bleeding in infants. However, it is the most common cause of significant lower GI hemorrhage in previously well youngsters without evidence of obstruction.[1] The bleeding may be massive. Typically, it is either painless or accompanied by mild midabdominal tenderness secondary to diverticulitis. After age 3 or so, children may have a history of repeated episodes of bleeding. The physical examination is usually not helpful. Hematemesis rarely if ever occurs in this entity, and a gastric aspirate should be negative for blood. Rectal examination may reveal a melanotic stool or frank blood. The abdominal x-ray is not revealing. The most consistent finding, present in about 80% of children with proven Meckel's diverticulum, is a low hemoglobin, usually below 8 g/dl.[2] The most specific diagnostic test is a technetium pertechnetate abdominal scan, often called a Meckel's scan.

Causes for Which Immediate Consultation Is Required.

Intussusception. The second most common cause of GI bleeding in infants beyond the neonatal period is intussusception. The triad of colicky abdominal pain, vomiting, and bloody stools should make one think of intussusception and mandates immediate consultation with a pediatric surgeon and radiologist.

Most cases of intussusception occur during the second half of the first year of life. The diagnosis is rare in infants under 3 months and in children over 3 years of age. The history, signs, and symptoms are fairly typical. Except perhaps for a cold or diarrheal illness shortly before the onset of acute symptoms, a thriving infant suddenly cries out in pain, which then subsides, allowing him to return to play or to sleep. These cycles of crampy pain and relief recur at varied intervals. Vomiting may accompany the pain and eventually becomes bilious. A normal stool may be passed at the start of the episode, but some time later, a dark red, bloody mucoid stool, described as currant jelly, is passed as edema and ischemia of the bowel develop. Usually only a minimal to moderate amount of blood is lost, but significant blood loss may be masked by dehydration. Hematemesis and a positive gastric aspirate are not part of the picture of intussusception.

On physical examination, the abdomen is soft, with tenderness noted over a sausage-shaped mass, which is almost always palpable in the upper abdomen. In the most common type of intussusception, in which an ileocecal segment intussuscepts into the ascending or transverse colon, the right lower quadrant may seem empty (Dance's sign). Rectal examination may produce bloody mucus, and occasionally the intussusception can be palpated. Dilated loops of small bowel and a soft

tissue mass in the upper abdomen can be seen on x-ray.

Volvulus. Volvulus is far less common in older infants than in those under 3 months of age. About one third of patients present with hematochezia. A history of pain and bilious vomiting is common, and occasionally there is a history of similar pain in the past. Vomiting may decompress the upper segment (hematochezia reflects the fact that the distal limb of the twisted bowel segment is not completely obstructed), so that the abdomen is not always distended.

Common Causes of GI Bleeding in Older Children

The causes of GI bleeding in children beyond infancy include those discussed above. However, other causes become more common. Consultation for these patients is helpful but usually not urgent.

Colonic Polyps. Nearly half of the cases of GI bleeding in children older than 1 year are due to colonic polyps, although they are extremely rare below that age. Polyps occur more commonly in males between the ages of 2 and 6, who typically present with an episode of painless bright red or maroon rectal bleeding. The blood is frequently clotted or appears as several small streaks, but bleeding is not significant enough to lower the hematocrit. Twenty percent of patients may complain of some mild lower abdominal pain.

The physical examination is unrevealing, except that the polyp may often be palpated on digital rectal examination and occasionally prolapses out of the rectum on its long stalk. If the rectal examination does not reveal a polyp, proctoscopy should be done by a pediatric gastroenterologist, since 75% of these polyps are in the rectum and 80% are within the reach of the sigmoidoscope.

Juvenile polyps are always benign and in most cases are solitary. However, in the syndrome of juvenile polyposis coli, there are large numbers of juvenile polyps in the colon. Children with this syndrome may be thought at first to have familial multiple adenomatous polyposis of the colon, an autosomal dominant disease in which the mucosa of the entire colon is pebbled with premalignant adenomatous polyps.

Two other syndromes involve juvenile polyps. These are generalized gastrointestinal juvenile polyposis, in which juvenile polyps are found throughout the gastrointestinal tract, and the Cronkhite-Canada syndrome, in which generalized juvenile polyposis is associated with alopecia, hyperpigmentation, and dystrophic nails. Children with these syndromes may suffer from repeated episodes of intussusception and obstruction.

Polyps associated with the Peutz-Jeghers syndrome can also present with relatively painless passage of small amounts of blood, but these children can be identified by the characteristic pigmentation of the lips noted on physical examination long before they develop intestinal symptoms. This syndrome is inherited through an autosomal dominant gene. The polyps are primarily in the small bowel, and patients may present with small bowel obstruction, including intussusception as well as hematemesis if the lesions are proximal to the ligament of Treitz. Although the polyps in Peutz-Jeghers syndrome are hamartomatous and not malignant, there is a 3–5% incidence of gastrointestinal malignancies in patients with this syndrome.

Like Peutz-Jeghers syndrome, Gardner's syndrome should be identifiable before its associated polyps cause problems. Patients with this syndrome first develop soft tissue tumors, then bone tumors, and finally adenomatous polyps, usually, but not solely, in the colon. Fifty percent of these patients will develop colorectal cancer.

Esophageal Varices. Esophageal varices account for 5–10% of cases of GI bleeding in children older than 2 years and are the most common cause of massive upper GI bleeding in that group. In 75% of cases the cause is extrahepatic portal hypertension. Children who develop varices secondary to the portal hypertension that accompanies cirrhosis also have bleeding episodes. However, hematemesis is unlikely to be the first presenting sign, since the diagnosis is usually made long before any bleeding episodes occur. Children with extrahepatic portal hypertension typically appear well, with no evidence of failure to thrive or stigmata of chronic liver disease. Often the only abnormal finding on physical examination is an enlarged spleen. If splenomegaly is not appreciated, the diagnosis may not be made until the child presents with an episode of hematemesis. The child suddenly looks pale, complains of epigastric pain, and vomits a large amount of fresh blood. Passage of a melanotic stool may follow this episode. On physical examination, the child is pale, perhaps diaphoretic, and often tachycardic and hypotensive. The clue to the diagnosis is finding a palpable spleen, but it may not be easily felt immediately after the bleeding episode because of decompression. Dilated veins may be present on the abdomen, but there should be no other physical evidence compatible with liver disease. A history of sepsis, omphalitis, dehydration, or umbilical vein catheterization during the newborn period in a child who presents with this picture strengthens the likelihood of the diagnosis. The bleeding may be massive, but it usually stops spontaneously with only supportive care.

Splenomegaly and esophageal varices can also be caused by diseases associated with intrahepatic portal hypertension. Most of these, however, should be fairly easily distinguished from extrahepatic portal hypertension, since they are usually associated with the development of cirrhosis. In these patients, it is important to try to make a specific diagnosis, since therapy is sometimes available (galactosemia, chronic active hepatitis, and Wilson's disease, for example). Thus, an alpha-1-antitrypsin, a serum ceruloplasm, and a sweat test should be part of the screening tests on any patient with upper GI bleeding or portal hypertension of unknown origin.[3] Unlike patients with extrahepatic portal hypertension, these patients do not tolerate variceal bleeding well.

Peptic Ulcer Disease. Ulcers in older children are generally of the adult or chronic type and are found primarily in the duodenum. Melena and hematemesis occur in nearly 100% of children with peptic ulcer, but it is usually not until late childhood that a typical ulcer history can be elicited. In young children there may be a history of periumbilical pain and vomiting with meals but no consistent relationship of the pain to eating. Equally often, however, there is no history of pain but simply anemia and a history of melanotic stools. In older children, the pain is more reliably epigastric, burning in nature, and relieved by eating. The physical examination may elicit some epigastric tenderness but is otherwise unremarkable except for pallor and tachycardia if anemia is present. A family history of ulcers can often be elicited in cases of duodenal ulcer. A nasogastric tube should be passed; if the return is positive for blood, endoscopy or an upper GI series should be performed, when the child is stable, to identify the source of the bleeding and confirm the diagnosis.

Inflammatory Bowel Disease. Inflammatory bowel disease, especially ulcerative colitis, may present with bloody diarrhea or with blood mixed with normal stool. Nearly 15% of cases occur before the age of 16. Usually, the child has been well until the onset of frequent, loose, watery stools with blood, passed during the night and early morning. Bowel movements during the night are a sign of severe illness. Pain develops typically in the lower abdomen and is accompanied by tenesmus. Weight loss is a constant feature. Lower GI bleeding is usual as a presenting sign in ulcerative colitis, and severe hemorrhage can occur during an exacerbation in a child whose disease was previously diagnosed. The sedimentation rate is a useful test to do, in addition to stool cultures, in a middle-aged child or adolescent who presents with bloody diarrhea. A gastroenterologist should be consulted.

DIFFERENTIAL DIAGNOSIS

Many causes of GI bleeding in children can be handled by the pediatric practitioner alone, although most require hospitalization, at least for observation. Even for those entities that require consultation, much of the preliminary work-up in attempting to narrow down the differential diagnosis should be done by the pediatric practitioner. Therefore, the approach here will be to outline the most important conditions that cause GI bleeding at various ages and indicate how to recognize and to treat them.

History

Certain questions in the history may help to narrow down the diagnostic considerations.

- How old is the patient? Surgical causes of GI bleeding are quite uncommon in the newborn, but their incidence increases with age.
- Does the patient show signs of chronic illness? If so, the character of that illness may suggest the etiology of the bleeding. For example, in an adolescent with a history of inflammatory bowel disease, who presents with bloody diarrhea and pain, one would think first of a flare-up of the underlying disease.
- What is the character of the bleeding? Although the type of bleeding cannot be relied on exclusively, whether the child presents with hematemesis alone, hematochezia alone, melena and hematochezia, or some

other combination is very helpful in localizing the site of the bleeding. For example, melanotic stools may be secondary to either a bleeding ulcer or a Meckel's diverticulum. However, the former is nearly always accompanied by hematemesis, while the latter may practically be ruled out by such a finding.

- What is the quantity of the blood? Although frightened caretakers have difficulty estimating the amount of bleeding that has occurred, this assessment can be helpful. Polyps are a common cause of rectal bleeding in children older than 1 year, but the bleeding is usually limited to streaks or small clots of blood. Bleeding from a Meckel's diverticulum, on the other hand, frequently is massive.
- Is this the first episode of bleeding? If not, how many have there been, and when was the first episode? Repeated episodes of massive bleeding widely separated in time are common with esophageal varices, ulcers, and a Meckel's diverticulum but unlikely with polyps, volvulus, and intussusception.
- Is the blood mixed with or on the surface of the stool, or is it passed independently of the stool? Conditions associated with hematemesis may produce stools mixed with blood. Intussusception and, occasionally, midgut volvulus are associated with bloody stools. In acute colitis and enteritis, bloody diarrhea is a common finding. In an infant with an anal fissure, the stools are typically streaked with blood or followed immediately by a few drops of bright red blood. Polyps and such conditions as Meckel's diverticulum or intestinal telangiectasia, which may lead to significant hemmorrhage, may cause blood to be passed independently of the stool.
- If hematemesis is present, was blood noticed from the onset or after several episodes of vomiting? Blood noted from the onset suggests swallowed blood or a sub-stantial upper GI bleed. Blood noticed only after several episodes of vomiting is a sign of gastritis, reflux esophagitis, or a Mallory-Weiss tear of the esophageal mucosa.
- Has the patient been taking aspirin or other substances, such as acid, alkali, or iron, which could cause bleeding from erosive gastritis?
- Is the bleeding associated with pain? A short history of cramping abdominal pain in a healthy infant who passes dark red mucoid stools is characteristic of intussusception.
- Painless bleeding without hematemesis suggests a Meckel's diverticulum or a bleeding hemangioma. Pain before or a few hours after meals in an older child or adolescent followed days to weeks later by bleeding suggests an ulcer.
- Is there any family history of ulcers, polyps, hemangiomas, or a bleeding tendency? A positive response to any of these questions suggests the possible cause and may guide further investigation.
- Finally, is the material really blood? It should be remembered that beets, clingstone peaches, red gelatin and food coloring, and red crayons, and certain medications, such as ampicillin and iron, can turn the stool red or black, and inquiries about their ingestion should be made

Physical Examination

Together with history, the physical examination will enable the pediatric practitioner to decide if and how rapidly consultation is needed in the evaluation of a child with GI bleeding. Table 2 presents the major physical findings that might aid in the differential diagnosis.

Laboratory Examination

In most cases, it is only lesions that produce lower GI hemorrhage that require immediate surgical intervention, because these are

TABLE 2. DIAGNOSTIC CONSIDERATIONS BASED ON PHYSICAL EXAMINATION IN THE DIFFERENTIAL DIAGNOSIS OF GI BLEEDING IN INFANTS AND CHILDREN

Physical Examination	Diagnostic Considerations
General appearance	Wasted appearance suggests long-standing disease; habitus compatible with Turner's syndrome may give a clue to intestinal telangiectasias; delayed growth or short stature may be the only sign of inflammatory bowel disease
Vital signs	Serious aberrations would suggest shock
Blood pressure	Orthostatic changes suggest signficant blood loss as in a Meckel's diverticulum or bleeding varices, or shock from infection or necrosis
Pulse	Tachycardia can reflect blood loss, shock or the increased metabolic demands of infection or inflammation
Fever	Suggests an infectious etiology, viral or bacterial, or, if prolonged, an inflammatory etiology, such as ulcerative colitis or regional enteritis
Skin	
Pallor	Anemia from blood loss
Presence of petechiae and/or ecchymoses	May reflect systemic infection, coagulopathy, or local trauma
Purpura	Hemolytic-uremic syndrome, Henoch-Schönlein purpura
Telangiectasia	Superficial sign of GI telangiectasia, as in Rendu-Osler-Weber syndrome
Spider angiomata	Suggests cirrhosis
Skin lesions, such as erythema nodosum, pyoderma gangrenosum, erythema multiforme	Inflammatory bowel disease
Head	
Subcutaneous nodules on the scalp or face; tenderness over the mandible	Gardner's syndrome
Eyes	
Visual abnormality, pain, redness, photophobia, cataracts	Consider uveitis which may suggest inflammatory bowel disease
Nose	
Signs of recent epistaxis	Swallowed blood may cause hematemesis and mimic upper GI hemorrhage
Mouth	
Melanotic pigmentation of the lips and buccal mucosa	Peutz-Jeghers syndrome
Stomatitis, gingivitis	Regional enteritis

(*continued*)

TABLE 2 (*Continued*)

Physical Examination	Diagnostic Considerations
Chest	
Bruits	Rendu-Osler-Weber syndrome
Abdomen	
Examination	
Fullness	Obstruction hepatomegaly
Ascites	Cirrhosis, extrahepatic portal hypertension
Caput medusae	Cirrhosis
Palpation	
Tenderness	
Epigastric	Ulcer, gastritis
Other areas	Peritoneal irritation from necrosis, perforation, or stretching of the bowel wall by intraluminal contents
Mass	Intussusception, duplication, volvulus
Hepatomegaly	Liver disease, liver congestion from congestive heart failure, portal hypertension
Splenomegaly	Extrahepatic portal hypertension, infection, parasites
Auscultation	Abnormality of bowel sounds may accompany impending or established obstruction, blood in GI tract may stimulate peristalsis
Percussion	
Tympanitic	Obstruction
Rectum	
Perirectal abscess	Infectious process, inflammatory bowel disease
Skin tag	Anal fissure
Fissure	Anal fissure
Hemorrhoids	Commonly follow period of constipation or diarrhea but can accompany Crohn's disease or portal hypertension with cirrhosis
Rectal examination	
Hard stool	Fissure
Polyp	Colonic polyps
Bloody mucus	Intussusception, ulcerative colitis

the lesions that can obstruct or cause ischemia. In addition, it has been found that lesions that primarily produce upper GI hemorrhage usually respond better to medical rather than surgical intervention during the acute phase. Thus, the first step, when the source of bleeding is not obvious, is to pass a nasogastric tube and test the return for blood. In addition, although hematologic disorders are uncommon causes of GI hemorrhage beyond the newborn period, they can certainly influence the course of the bleeding. Therefore, all patients admitted to hospital for GI bleeding should have a platelet count and a prothrombin time (PT)/partial thromboplastin time (PTT) to rule out a bleeding diathesis. With this information and with a general idea of the location of the source of bleeding, the pediatric practitioner can decide on the basis of the history and physical examination what additional studies or therapeutic measures should be performed.

In newborns, swallowed maternal blood is the most common cause of GI bleeding and can be diagnosed by performing the Apt-Downey test on the gastric aspirate or stool.[4] One part stool or gastric aspirate is mixed with 5 or 10 parts water and centrifuged for 1–2 minutes. One ml of 25N (1%) sodium hydroxide is added to 5 ml of the above mixture. Maternal hemoglobin turns brown-yellow, while fetal hemoglobin stays pink. A false negative result will occur if the test is done on tarry stool in which the oxyhemoglobin has already been converted to hematin.

Beyond nasogastric aspiration, coagulation studies, and, in newborns, the Apt-Downey test, further laboratory investigations are dictated by the type of bleeding encountered, as outlined in Figures 1 and 2.

When confronted by a patient with upper GI bleeding, it is important to remember that the upper GI series misses many lesions responsible for bleeding, particularly superficial lesions like those in gastritis and esophagitis. It is a very unreliable technique for determining the site of bleeding and so should not be used for children with active hemorrhage. The most sensitive technique for diagnosing upper GI bleeding is endoscopy, which should be performed as soon as the patient is stable and within 24 hours of the onset of the bleeding. In cases of massive bleeding, when blood flow is at least 0.5ml/min, angiography may be the procedure of choice.

In children over 1 year of age with lower GI bleeding, one should think first of a Meckel's scan, since it should be done prior to barium studies. Radioactive labeled technetium is concentrated by the gastric mucosa present in two thirds of all Meckel's diverticula and in more than 80% of those that

bleed. Sequential imaging will reveal an area of abnormal uptake, usually in the right lower quadrant. False positive scans can result from accumulation of the technetium in other structures, including the intestine if the stomach is emptied, a hydronephrotic kidney, hydroureter, or pelvic kidney, inflammatory lesions, an AV malformation, an obstructed loop of bowel, an intussusception, or a duplication.[5] Although false positive scans are uncommon, they do occur, so an experienced person must read the scan. The usefulness of a Meckel's scan has been well established, with positive scans occurring in as many as 90% of patients with proven Meckel's diverticulum. False negative results can occur if the diverticulum contains no gastric mucosa, which is unusual, or, more commonly, if it contains only a small amount.[5]

Following this test, one may elect to move on to endoscopy or contrast studies in an attempt to make a specific diagnosis.

MANAGEMENT

Most cases of GI bleeding in infancy and childhood require consultation, although some can be handled by the pediatric practitioner alone. However, even in cases where consultation is required, the pediatrician plays an important role in patient management.

Newborn Period
Conditions That Can Be Handled by the Pediatrician Alone.
Swallowed Maternal Blood. Swallowed maternal blood is the most common cause of GI bleeding in the newborn period and requires little treatment. It should resolve in 1–3 days as the blood is evacuated from the GI tract with the infant's stools. In some cases, it may be useful to empty the infant's stomach with a DeLee catheter, since blood is irritating to the gastric mucosa and may lead to vomiting.

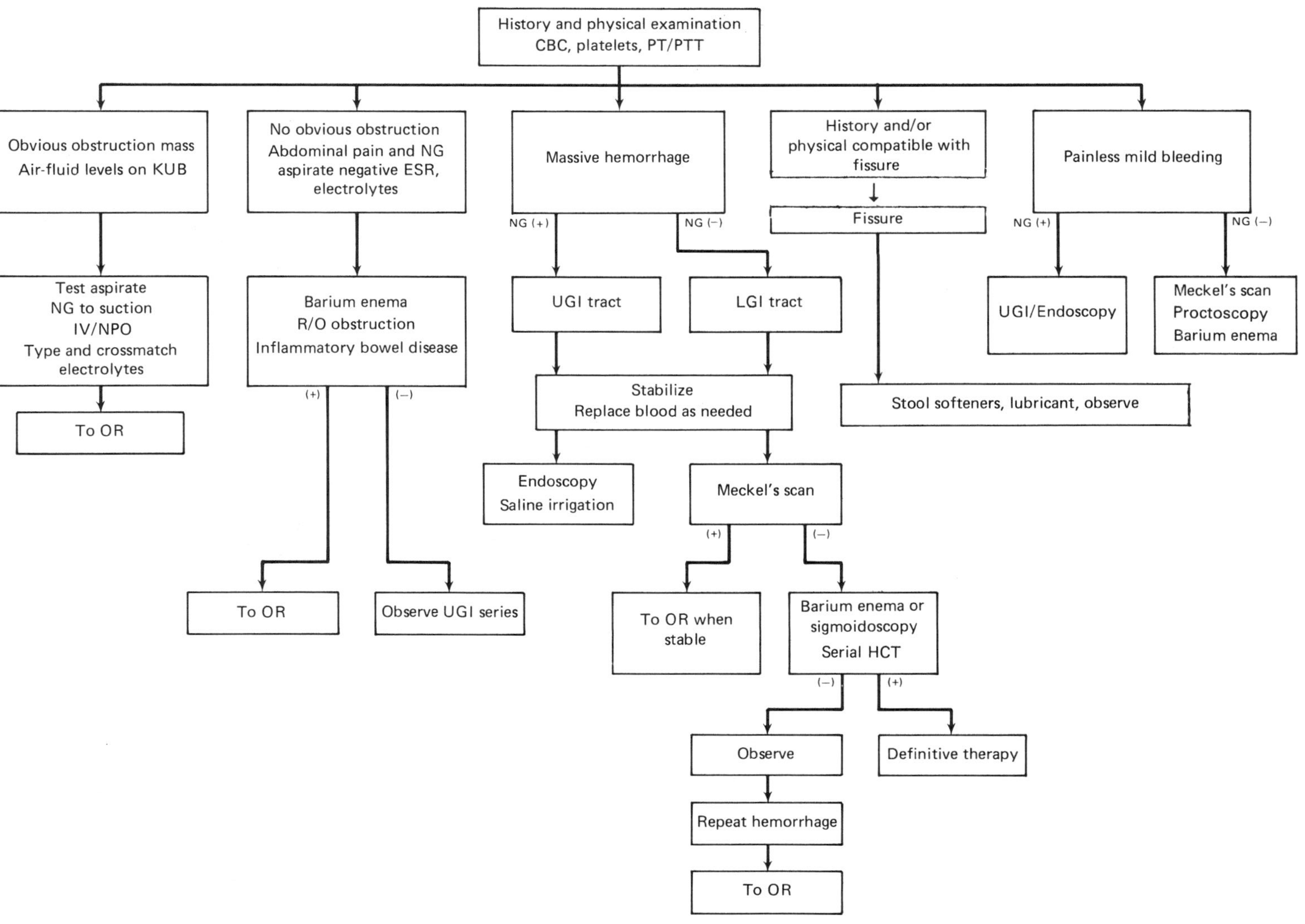

Figure 1. An approach to the work-up of GI bleeding in infants and children.

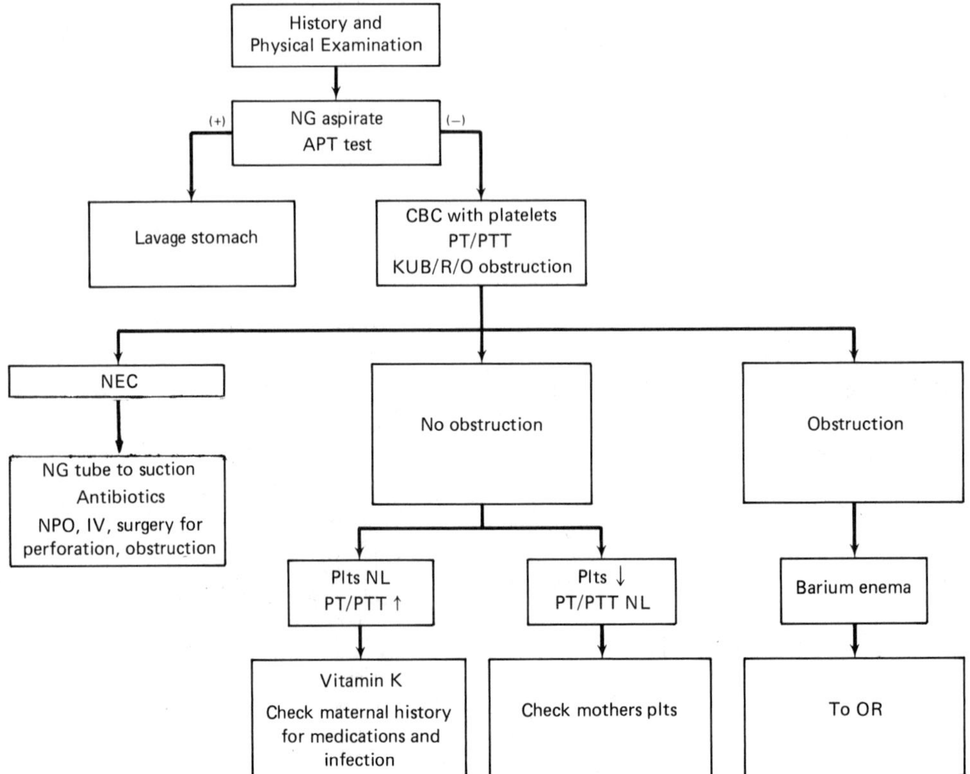

Figure 2. An approach to the work-up of GI bleeding in newborns.

Anorectal Trauma. The newborn with local anorectal trauma also looks well and usually has a fissure visible at 12 o'clock or 6 o'clock on careful examination of the anus. If the history and physical examination are compatible with this diagnosis, one need look no further for a cause of bleeding. The tear heals rapidly, and treatment consists only of the application of petroleum jelly to the anus.

Conditions That May Require Consultation.

Hemorrhagic Disease of the Newborn. All infants with the diagnosis of hemorrhagic disease should be transferred to a neonatal intensive care unit. In infants with bleeding secondary to vitamin K deficiency, the PT and PTT should be prolonged, but the platelet count and fibrinogen are normal. These infants should be given 1 mg of vitamin K (Aqua Mephyton) IM regardless of a history of having received it earlier. Hemorrhagic disease of the newborn responds to parenteral vitamin K with the cessation of bleeding within 4–5 hours and a return of the PT/PTT to normal within 24 hours. Premature infants and infants with liver disease may require an infusion of fresh frozen plasma

(10 ml/kg) if the PT is very prolonged and does not respond to vitamin K administration.

Colitis. Infectious diarrhea can be sporadic or the result of an epidemic. Stool cultures should be taken in all young infants with diarrhea. Blood cultures should be obtained and a full sepsis work-up performed in most cases, certainly if the infant appears ill or has fever. Most infants with diarrhea will be started on parenteral antibiotics pending the results of the culture.

One's concern increases as the amount of blood in the stool increases. Infants with grossly bloody stools are at risk for serious conditions, such as necrotizing enterocolitis, congenital lesions of the gastrointestinal tract, and Hirschsprung's disease with colitis. In the face of worsening diarrhea or signs of obstruction, consultation with a neonatologist is imperative. A stool smear for PMNs may suggest a bacterial process. Strict intake and output must be recorded for infants with gastroenteritis, along with daily weight and urine specific gravity. Infants with mild diarrhea may often be maintained on oral feedings of electrolyte solution. Fluids should be administered intravenously if the infant has worsening diarrhea or continues to lose weight, and daily electrolyte measurements must be obtained. In addition, infants with diarrhea must be isolated from others, and strict handwashing must be enforced.

Stress Ulcers. Stress ulcers occur frequently in seriously ill infants but can occur in infants who look well. Appropriate management for all of these infants includes transfer to a neonatal intensive care unit and consultation with a neonatologist. All infants should have an intravenous line placed, blood drawn for type and hold, and hematocrit and a nasogastric tube placed for suctioning and lavage. Serum electrolytes and an arterial blood gas should be measured to rule out acidosis secondary to hypovolemia or sepsis. Obstruction must be ruled out by history, physical examination, and an abdominal film. Serial hematocrits should be followed and blood replaced as needed. An upper GI series and barium enema examination are not helpful. A pediatric surgeon should be consulted if the hemorrhage is massive and does not abate or if peritoneal signs develop. The bleeding, although often massive, usually only lasts a short time.

Conditions That Require Consultation.
Necrotizing Enterocolitis. Treatment, pending surgical consultation, is to withhold feedings and decompress the abdomen with a nasogastric tube attached to continuous suction. An evaluation for sepsis should be performed if the baby is stable and should include blood and stool cultures. Antibiotic coverage should be started with ampicillin and an aminoglycoside parenterally, in addition to oral kanamycin. Fresh frozen plasma should be given if clotting studies are abnormal. These infants need close monitoring and should be transferred promptly to a neonatal intensive care unit. Hyperalimentation should be started under the supervision of a neonatologist.

Volvulus. Once the diagnosis of volvulus is made, the objective is rapid surgical intervention to prevent necrosis of the ischemic bowel segment. While awaiting the surgeon, the management should include the establishment of a secure intravenous line, and obtaining a blood type and crossmatch, arterial blood gases serial hematocrits, electrolytes, and a complete blood count.[6] A nasogastric tube will help to decompress the proximal segment and should be attached to suction. Strict intake and output records should be started and the infant transferred immediately to an intensive care unit. Shock may go unnoticed because of the high hematocrit in the newborn, so careful attention must be paid to serial vital signs and changes in the hematocrit.

Older Infants
Conditions That Can Be Handled by the Pediatrician Alone.
Anal Fissure. This condition can be managed in the same way as it is in the newborn. In addition, however, one should add a stool softener to the diet, such as malt extract, bran, or prune juice, since fissures are more likely to be secondary to an episode involving constipation.

Conditions That May Require Consultation.
Ulcer Disease. Acute ulcers in children are not thought to be related to an ulcer diathesis. Thus, surgery is usually not indicated, although consultation with a pediatric surgeon is indicated if the bleeding is massive. The treatment of acute ulcers in children should be discussed with the gastroenterologist who initially sees the child in consultation for the episode of hematemesis and/or melena. The pediatrician should be aware of the need to rule out the presence of shock and to obtain an abdominal film to look for perforation, which requires immediate surgery.

Meckel's Diverticulum. If the scan is positive, the diagnosis is made, and a surgeon should be consulted after the patient is stabilized. If the scan is negative, one may elect to discontinue oral intake, follow the hematocrit and transfuse if necessary, and observe whether or not the bleeding stops. It has been found that unless the hemorrhage is massive and the child is under 2 years of age, a Meckel's diverticulum is usually not found at laparotomy. If the child has repeated small episodes of bleeding or a second major hemorrhage, laparotomy is indicated, and in these cases, a Meckel's diverticulum is found in close to 50% of patients.

Conditions That Require Consultation.
Intussusception. When the diagnosis of intussusception is considered, a pediatric surgeon and radiologist must be consulted immediately.

The initial treatment is a hydrostatic barium enema unless symptoms have been present for more than 48 hours or there are signs of peritonitis or shock. Hydrostatic reduction is successful in about 75% of cases, particularly when there is a lead point, such as a polyp, lymphoma, Meckel's diverticulum, or hemangioma. The older the patient, the more likely there is to be a lead point. Recurrences can occur and are common in cystic fibrosis, Henoch-Schönlein purpura, and parasitic infestations. If the enema is not successful, i.e., if the radiologist is unable to see contrast material flow into the terminal ileum, the patient must be taken to the operating room for surgical reduction.

Volvulus. The treatment of volvulus is surgical and, as in younger infants, when the diagnosis is seriously entertained, a pediatric surgeon must be consulted. The pediatrician may stabilize the patient in preparation for the operating room by starting an intravenous line to insure adequate fluids and drawing the necessary bloods for a CBC, electrolytes, and a type and crossmatch. A nasogastric tube should be inserted and attached to continuous suction to decompress the proximal bowel.

Children Older than One Year
Conditions That Require Consultation.
Colonic Polyps. Children with the diagnosis of probable polyps should be managed in consultation with a pediatric gastroenterologist.

In any child with a history and examination consistent with the presence of a polyp, the pediatrician should take a careful family history for polyps and look for stigmata associated with Peutz-Jeghers or Gardner's syndromes. These patients may have one or more episodes of minimal to moderate bleeding, but they almost never present in shock. Accessible polyps should be removed by a gastroenterologist for biopsy and to prevent further episodes of bleeding or obstruction. If pathology confirms the diagnosis of juvenile polyp, one need do no more unless symptoms continue or recur. If no polyp is found on sigmoidoscopy, a barium enema with air contrast should be performed. Where biopsy proves or barium enema suggests adenomatous polyps associated with familial polyposis or Gardner's syndrome or the hamartomatous polyps of Peutz-Jeghers syndrome, close observation and early laparotomy may be indicated.

Esophageal Varices. Patients with GI bleeding secondary to esophageal varices should be admitted to a pediatric intensive care unit. Those whose varices are secondary to intrahepatic obstruction usually will tolerate the bleeding poorly. Those with extrahepatic causes usually will do well with medical management but will need close observation. In the latter group surgical intervention usually is not indicated, since the bleeding typically stops spontaneously. With time, bleeding episodes become less frequent and usually stop altogether by the late teens. Initial management includes keeping the patient in a semisitting position in a quiet environment, gastric lavage, and blood replacement. If the bleeding continues after consultation with a gastroenterologist, vasopressin can be given as a constant intravenous infusion.

Peptic Ulcer Disease. Children with GI bleeding secondary to peptic ulcer disease should be admitted to the hospital and managed in conjunction with a pediatric gastroenterologist. In the face of significant bleeding, vital signs and the hematocrit must be closely followed and blood replaced as necessary. As long as there is no perforation, these patients can usually be managed medically. These patients should be kept in a semisitting position with a nasogastric tube on intermittent suction. Antacids can be instilled into the stomach and left for some time between periods of suctioning. After the bleeding has subsided, the patient should be started on small frequent feedings every 2–3 hours interspersed with antacids and/or milk. This diet needs to be continued for only 4–6 weeks until the ulcer has healed.

Inflammatory Bowel Disease. Management of patients with inflammatory bowel disease should be determined after consultation with a gastroenterologist. The most likely diagnosis is ulcerative colitis, though Crohn's disease can present with rectal bleeding. bleeding.

Most patients in whom this diagnosis is made should be hospitalized for teaching and psychosocial intervention if not for aggressive medical treatment. Severely ill children may require steroids by enema, mouth, or IV and parenteral alimentation. For patients on oral feedings, one may want to withdraw milk from the diet, as there is a transient decrease in lactase activity. Many experts suggest the gradual introduction of salicylazosulfapyridine for the long-term management of these patients. More radical therapies involve immunosuppressive drugs or surgery.

SUMMARY

There are many causes of GI bleeding in the pediatric population. However, in each major age group (newborns, infants, and older children), relatively few lesions account for the majority of cases. This chapter has considered the most common causes of GI bleeding with the aim of enabling the pediatric practitioner to arrive at a diagnosis and decide quickly whether or not the bleeding represents a potentially life-threatening emergency for which immediate consultation is required.

REFERENCES

1. Spencer R: GI hemorrhage in infancy and childhood: 476 cases. Surgery 55:727, 1974

2. Shandling B: Laparotomy for rectal bleeding. Pediatrics 60:789, 1965

3. Roy C, Silverman A, Cozzetto F: Pediatric Clinical Gastroenterology, 2nd ed. St. Louis, Mosby, 1975, p 595

4. Apt L, Downey W: Melena neonatorum: the swallowed blood syndrome. J Pediatr 47:??, 1955

5. Case records of the Massachusetts General Hospital, N Engl J Med 302:959, 1980

6. Abrams R, Lynn F: Rectal bleeding in children. Am J Surg 104:831, 1962

BIBLIOGRAPHY

Berman W, Holtzapple P: Gastrointestinal hemorrhage. Pediatr Clin North Am 23:4, 1975

Cox K, Ament M: Upper gastrointestinal bleeding in children and adolescents. Pediatrics 63:??, 1979

Jaros R, Schuphein A, Levy M: Preoperative diagnosis of bleeding Meckel's diverticulum utilizing 99m technetium pertechnetate scinti-imaging. J Pediatr 82:45, 1973

Luk G, Bynum T, Hendrix T: Gastric aspiration in localization of gastrointestinal hemorrhage. JAMA 241, 1979

Shaw A: Guidelines for diagnosing children who bleed through the rectum. Hosp Phys ??:36, 1974

Cross-Reference—to *Pediatrics,* 17th ed.

ELEVEN

Headache

Steven P. Shelov

Headache is a common complaint in pediatric practice. The major problem is to decide when a headache is due to a relatively minor cause, as is usually the case, or when it is a presenting symptom of a serious condition that requires extensive and often traumatic investigation. In most instances, it is relatively easy to differentiate clinically between causes of headache that are serious and those that are not. The complaint of persistent or recurring headache requires a thorough and systematic history, physical examination, and sometimes selected laboratory examinations.

DEFINITION

Headache is defined as discomfort in any portion of the upper part of the head, extending from the orbit to the suboccipital area. Headaches are classified as shown in the following list, with important etiologies to be considered:

    I. Psychogenic
        A. Emotional–functional
        B. Muscle contraction (tension)
   II. Intracranial
        A. Meningitis, encephalitis
        B. Brain abscess
        C. Brain tumor
        D. Head trauma
        E. Pseudotumor cerebri
        F. Arteriovenous malformation
        G. Ruptured aneurysm
  III. Extracranial
        A. Sinusitis
        B. Ocular abnormalities
        C. Dental disorders
        D. Systemic infections
   IV. Vascular
        A. Classic migraine
        B. Common migraine
        C. Hemiplegic migraine
        D. Ophthalmoplegic migraine
        E. Basilar artery migraine
        F. Cluster headaches
        G. Epilepsy equivalent

The causes of headache will be discussed, first considering those where no consultation is required and then those conditions where consultation is recommended. Fortunately, the majority of children who present to the pediatrician will have conditions in the first category.

CAUSES OF HEADACHE IN CHILDREN FOR WHICH CONSULTATION IS NOT IMMEDIATELY NECESSARY

Psychogenic

Emotional–Functional. Headaches due to emotional disturbances are the most common type seen by the pediatrician; they occur usually in children from about 6 years old through adolescence. These headaches may be triggered by identifiable emotional or traumatic events, for which evidence should be sought. The psychopathology may be simple anxiety or tension or, less commonly, a severe depression. Such issues as school rivalry or disturbed family or peer relationships are often involved. The headache is often of prolonged duration, sometimes lasting for weeks or more. It is not accompanied by abnormal neurologic signs or symptoms, and its severity, frequency, and duration are not progressive. Associated behavioral changes, such as poor school performance, sleep disturbances, aggressive behavior, lack of energy, weight loss, and self-deprecatory behavior, are often seen.

The diagnosis of psychogenic headache can usually be made from a careful history and physical examination and usually does not require any laboratory investigation. Consultation with an appropriate mental health professional is often necessary for successful intervention.

Muscle Contraction (Tension). Chronic, recurrent headaches in childhood are frequently caused by tension. There are no prodromal signs. The discomfort is symmetrical and usually begins in the neck or in the muscles of the shoulder or upper back and often moves anteriorly to the forehead or top of the head. The headache is characterized by being dull, achy, or like "a tight band around my head." It is not described as pulsing or throbbing. The symptoms are often triggered by a strong emotional or stressful episode.

The diagnosis of headache due to muscle contraction can usually be made from a careful history with no additional laboratory or radiographic investigations.

Intracranial Lesions

It is understood that though the expectation is for the primary care pediatrician to diag-

nose and manage the following entities, there might be a need ultimately for a consultant.

Meningitis. Headache in meningitis is usually an early symptom. It is generally quite severe and is often accompanied by nuchal rigidity. The pain is generalized, constant, and often described as "throbbing all over." Headache with fever but with little nuchal rigidity is often the presenting symptom in viral (aseptic) meningitis, seen more often during the summer. Headache may or may not be present in the child with encephalitis, in whom change in level of consciousness is often a more prominent symptom.

Headache Associated with Mild Head Trauma. A history of mild head trauma is very frequent. Ninety percent of major head trauma in children is of the nonpenetrating, closed type, and in most patients there is only slight alteration of consciousness. Headache, often localized to the area of impact, is a frequent complaint. In older children who complain of headache following trauma but who have normal neurologic examinations and no progression, there is usually no underlying pathophysiologic abnormality. It is often an expression of a functional complaint, and, though it should be taken seriously, it rarely indicates a serious or progressive pathophysiologic problem. It usually resolves in short course.

Closed head injury may result in significant sequelae, with associated headache, but there are usually other, more diagnostic aspects of the history and physical examination. These are discussed in a later section.

Extracranial Causes
Sinusitis. Sinusitis is occasionally the cause of headache in children, the ethmoid sinuses being involved most commonly in young children and the maxillary sinuses in older children. Frontal sinusitis is not seen in children under the age of 7 years, at which time this

sinus becomes functionally present. Young children with ethmoid sinusitis usually do not present with the typical adult symptoms of fever, tenderness over the sinus, and headache. It is most often associated with a periorbital or orbital cellulitis.

The history and physical examination vary with the age of the child: the child of 3 to 6 years complains of pain referred to the teeth or to the cheek area, there is a persistent morning headache, with purulent unilateral nasal drainage, and persistent postnasal drip, and generalized fatigue and irritability are frequent.

In children age 7–14 years with frontal headache, there is throbbing above or behind the eye and pain in response to percussion over the center of the forehead. The symptoms and findings may be acute or subacute. The underlying problem is usually obstruction of the nasofrontal duct, in which case purulent discharge is often not found. If the maxillary sinus is involved, there is usually pain either over the cheek or referred to the dental area. Maxillary sinusitis may occasionally follow dental extractions. Ethmoiditis in this age group presents more commonly with headache. Careful history often elicits pain referred to the nasal area or behind the eyes.

Physical examination may reveal tenderness directly over the sinus. Transillumination may help in the diagnosis but is not totally reliable. Fever often accompanies sinusitis and correlates directly with the degree of obstruction and inflammation.

Ocular Abnormalities. Headaches due to ocular or visual abnormalities are often diagnosed but rarely established. Characteristically, the history is one of late afternoon or evening headaches after much visual activity. Occasionally, it can present as morning headache when there has been reading in poor light late at night. The headache due to eyestrain usually subsides after the visual strain is stopped.

True ocular problems as a cause of headache are usually heralded by visual fatigue, photophobia, and localized tenderness, swelling, and inflammation. The headache is usually generalized and may extend throughout the head and heck.

Dental Disorders. Headache secondary to dental decay, abscess, or secondarily infected gingiva is probably mediated through the fifth cranial nerve. The pain usually can be induced by stimulating the involved dental structure, thereby identifying its source. The history is also helpful in that minor dental manipulation, such as chewing in the involved area, can aggravate the pain and suggest the correct diagnosis.

Systemic Infections. Headache may be part of the clinical presentation in a child with a systemic infection. Children with streptococcal pharyngitis often present with headache, which may occur with many other bacterial and viral infections. Fever is characteristically present. When fever is present and concern about systemic infection arises, appropriate laboratory investigation should be performed, as detailed in Table 1. When the site of infection is identified, probable etiology discovered, and therapy instituted, the headache promptly resolves. If the headache does not resolve, which is unusual, further investigation for an undiscovered source must be initiated.

Headache of Vascular Origin—Migraine Syndrome

Definition. Migraine headaches are best defined as paroxysmal headaches that are often unilateral, accompanied by nausea, and begin with a prodromal or preheadache phase with visual aura. They are usually found in a child with a very strong family history. These headaches occur as frequently as once or twice a week or as infrequently as several

TABLE 1. DIAGNOSTIC CONSIDERATIONS MANAGED PRIMARILY BY THE PEDIATRICIAN

Category	Diagnostic Work-up and Anticipated Results
Psychogenic	Exploration of psychosocial environment
Intracranial	
Meningitis	Lumbar puncture
	Tests for:
	Opening pressure
	Gram stain and culture for microbial etiology
	Cells
	Glucose
	Protein
Bacterial	CSF pleocytosis with PMNs predominating, $\downarrow$ CSF glucose, $\uparrow$ protein
Aseptic (viral)	CSF pleocytosis with lymphocytes predominating, CSF $\uparrow$ protein, $\pm$ normal CSF glucose
Extracranial	
Acute	
Sinusitis	Culture smear of purulent nasal discharge
	Lateral film, Waters view (occipitomental), Caldwell (occipitofrontal)
	Sphenoid opacification, maxillary opacification, ethmoid and frontal opacification
Ocular abnormalities	Visual acuity near and far
	No abnormality usually found
Dental abnormality	After careful inspection results in suspected positive findings, referral should be accomplished
	None or per consultant if abscess suspected
Systemic infections	Lumbar puncture
	Blood culture
	ESR
	CBC with platelets
	Urine C and S
	None unless point tenderness or localized findings
Migraine syndromes	
Classic or common	None
Hemiplegic	EEG
	Normal CT scan
Ophthalmoplegic	Must rule out intracranial mass
	Normal CT scan
Basilar artery	EEG
	No radiographic study is indicated if all other etiologies are ruled out
Epilepsy equivalent	EEG
	No radiographic study is indicated if all other etiologies are ruled out

times a year. The child with migraine has been characterized as compulsive, tense, anxious, and ambitious. This generalization, however, has not been substantiated by well-conducted, systematic studies.

Age and Sex Distribution. The age of onset is usually greater than 5 years. In a study by Burke of 92 cases of migraine, the average age of onset was 7 years, and the presence of migraine increased from 2.5% in the 7–9-

year-old group to 4.6% in the 10–12-year-old group. The frequency of migraine in children, as in adults, appears to be higher in females.

Pathogenesis and Etiology. The etiology of migraine attacks is not clear, but it appears to be mediated by a vasoactive transmitter. Classically, two phases of migraine are described. Initially there is a vasoconstrictive phase lasting from 1 minute to 15 minutes that results in some transient cerebral ischemia, which may or may not be clinically manifested by a visual aura, paresthesias, or a numbing sensation. Following this phase, vasodilation takes place, and the true headache phase occurs, manifested clinically by pulsating and throbbing. It is often unilateral but may be bilateral and sustained.

Abnormal EEG patterns have been reported to occur more often in patients with migraine than in normal children, suggesting that migraine may be an epileptic equivalent. However, it is more likely that certain forms of seizures are manifest by headaches and that migraine headaches are a distinct entity not having a true epileptogenic focus. This question is considered further under Epileptic Equivalent Syndrome below.

Incidence. In a study of 8,993 school children in Uppsala, Bo Bille reported that 3.9% had migraine headaches; of the remainder, 41.4% had no history of headache, 48.0% had infrequent nonmigrainous headaches, and 6.8% had frequent nonmigrainous headaches.

Predisposing Factors. Heredity undoubtedly plays a large role in predisposing the individual to migraine. Although a compulsive personality type, seen often in adults, is not observed in children, migrainous children do seem to be more prone to temper tantrums, phobias, and nightmares. Stress and emotional factors play a large role in triggering migraine headaches.

Classification. Subtypes of the migraine syndrome are classified as listed below:

- Classic
- Common
- Hemiplegic
- Ophthalmoplegic
- Basilar artery
- Cluster
- Epilepsy equivalent

Classic Migraine. The classic type of migraine occurs in the two phases described above. Afterwards, the child often sleeps for 1–2 hours. Upon arising, the headache is gone. There are no postheadache sequelae.

Common Migraine. This form is more common in children than is classic migraine. It differs from classic migraine in that the symptoms are much more variable, the aura is usually absent, and the prodromal phase often consists only of personality changes and malaise. Also, the headache is less often unilateral. The fact that this is a migraine headache has been well established through the presence of other findings, the strong family history, the throbbing of the headache itself, and the need to sleep prior to remission of the symptom.

The following subtypes of migraine are included in this section, but often consultation with a pediatric neurologist is appropriate in diagnosing and managing these children.

Hemiplegic Migraine. This form is much less frequent in children. It is characterized by recurrent episodes of paralysis associated with migrainous or vascular headaches. Occasionally, the hemiplegias may be alternating. The etiology is believed to be a vasoconstrictive phenomenon in the vascular distribution of the internal carotid artery. The only important confusion in differential diagnosis is with an arteriovenous malformation. However, the latter condition is associated with repetitive pain on the same side, and other neurologic signs are present.

Ophthalmoplegic Migraine. The term "ophthalmoplegic migraine" is used to describe a condition in a child, occasionally even an infant, who has transient ptosis or complete third nerve palsy, manifested by outward movement of the eye, accompanied by eye pain. Initially, these symptoms last only several moments, but, with frequent recurrence of attacks, they can persist for days or even weeks. Very young children, who cannot complain of headache, often become very irritable at the time of appearance of the physical findings. The signs and symptoms in ophthalmoplegic migraine usually disappear after the age of 10 years.

Basilar Artery Migraine (BAM) and Acute Confusional State. These entities are described together because they appear to be related pathophysiologically. BAM usually occurs in children with a family history of headache. It is more common in girls than boys. There are intermittent neurologic findings, such as alternating hemiparesis and vertigo, which resolve quickly after the headache subsides. Signs and symptoms referable to the cerebellum or to the distribution of the basilar artery are characteristic. Occasionally, an acute confusional state is the only symptom, in which case, the name Alice in Wonderland syndrome has been used to describe the acute confusional migraine episode. The page from the book Alice in Wonderland shown in Figure 1 indicates why the name is applied.

These children often have episodes of delerium and seem not to be in touch with the world. They appear as if they are under the influence of hypnotic medication. There is a strong family history of migraine. Radiographic evaluation is negative. The entire episode resolves in the course of 4–6 hours, usually after a period of sleep. Once the previous good state of health and normal mental status are regained, questioning reveals there

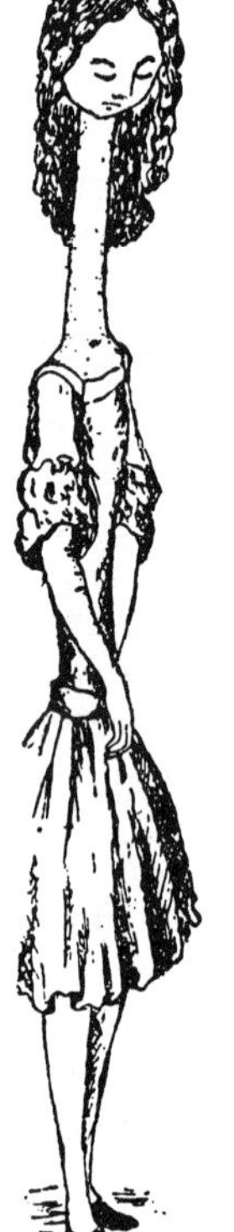

Figure 1. Alice in Wonderland. (*From A. P. Friedman, E. Harms, Ed., Headaches in Children, 1967. Courtesy of Charles C. Thomas, Publisher, Springfield, Illinois.*)

was evidence of a headache prior to this episode.

Cluster Headaches. These headaches occur rarely in children. The diagnosis can be made when a child presents with unilateral, severe periorbital pain, with tearing and occasionally facial flushing on the side involved. The symptoms often recur many times a day over a period of weeks and then subside for intervals of months between attacks. These attacks are often confused with a psychogenic type of headache but can be differentiated by the following characteristics: severity of pain, associated autonomic signs, short intervals of symptoms with long pain-free periods, and preponderance in males.

Epilepsy Equivalent Syndrome—Cyclic Vomiting. This particular syndrome has been poorly delineated, and until this time the nosology is still confused. The names *migraine variant, abdominal epilepsy, visual epilepsy, epileptic variant, convulsive variant,* and *abdominal migraine* have all been used to describe a syndrome consisting of headache, abdominal discomfort or vomiting, and an abnormal EEG.

Though many have found a strong association between epilepsy and migraine, most authors believe that the two conditions are separable through the following five guidelines developed by Friedman et al.

1. In epilepsy, the onset of headache is abrupt and of maximal severity. It is frequently accompanied by impairment of consciousness and followed by drowsiness, sleep, or stupor. In migraine, the onset of the full-blown headache is gradual and is not generally accompanied by impairment of consciousness, though it may be followed by drowsiness or sleep.
2. Epileptic headaches are occasionally associated with gastrointestinal disturbances, but these symptoms are much more frequent and severe in patients with migraine. In fact, cyclic vomiting in children is thought to be a precursor to migraine in later years.
3. A positive family history may be present in both conditions but is more frequent in migrainous disorders.
4. The electroencephalogram most frequently reveals specific abnormalities in epilepsy, whereas in migraine it is usually normal or shows nonspecific electrical irregularities.
5. Ergot preparations are of no value in controlling the acute headache of epilepsy,

whereas these drugs generally abort or attenuate the headache phase of migraine. A specific 14 and 6/sec positive spike pattern occurs in a large proportion of patients with the diagnosis of epilepsy. However, in one study of 24 patients with classic migraine, 42% were found to have this pattern. Because of this association, some investigators conclude that migraine is a form of epilepsy, although the relationship remains controversial and inconclusive.

CAUSES OF HEADACHE IN CHILDREN FOR WHICH PROMPT CONSULTATION IS RECOMMENDED

Intracranial Lesions

These causes of headache are the most immediately life threatening and require early consultation and intervention to prevent morbidity and mortality.

Brain Abscess. Headaches may be associated with an intracranial, subdural, or extradural abscess due to a variety of infectious agents, mainly staphylococci, respiratory flora, anaerobic organisms, and, occasionally, fungi. The initial stages are nonspecific and usually heralded by fever, generalized headache, vomiting, and sometimes convulsions. If the abscess has followed perforation of a frontal or maxillary sinus, there may be tenderness over these sinuses. If the abscess goes undiagnosed, symptoms will progress, and the neurologic sequelae of increased intracranial pressure will appear, including severe, intractable headache, focal neurologic signs, papilledema, and progressive deterioration in state of consciousness. The nature of the headache in this later stage of brain abscess is similar to that due to a brain tumor.

Brain Tumor. Intracranial tumor should be suspected in a child who presents with headache, vomiting, and diplopia. The headache in this case is rarely localized, but it has a characteristic pattern. Initially, it is usually intermittent, but it then recurs with increasing frequency and severity. The headache occurs often after sleep and may be most severe on early rising; it may even awaken the child. It is often accompanied by nausea and vomiting. Occasionally, the headaches are aggravated by coughing or straining at stool. Severe occipital headache may indicate that the tumor is in the occipital area, and frontal localization may reflect a supratentorial mass.

It is most important to identify the presence of localizing neurologic signs. Double vision may be the result of sixth nerve paralysis, secondary to increased intracranial pressure. A tendency for the child to tilt the head or to turn the head laterally or squint in order to see is reported more often than is true diplopia. This behavior indicates abducens paralysis and the attempt of the child to compensate to observe objects clearly. Other focal neurologic signs seen in children with brain tumors are impaired vision, nystagmus, personality changes, ataxia, focal pyramidal deficit, and seizures. Careful neurologic examination should include funduscopic examination. Evidence of a choked disc or papilledema confirms the diagnosis of increased intracranial pressure and further substantiates the suspicion of an intracranial mass.

Significant Head Trauma

Most cases of head trauma do not need consultation. Only two conditions for which consultation is indicated are discussed here. A more detailed discussion of additional traumatic causes of headache can be found in *Pediatrics,* 17th ed.

Epidural or Extradural Hematoma. An epidural hematoma is a localized accumulation of blood between the skull and the dura that occurs as the result of tearing of the dural veins or meningeal veins. It occurs in about 1% of children hospitalized for head trauma. In one study, half of the patients were less than 2 years of age.

The history usually includes a severe fall on the occiput, followed by persistent impairment of consciousness, headache, vomiting, and stiff neck. Unlike adults, children rarely have a lucid interval between the initial alteration of consciousness and subsequent deterioration. More commonly, the child is stunned or, at worst, has a brief period of unconsciousness. After a variable period, which may be minutes to a day, the onset of headache, vomiting, and progressive change in state of consciousness heralds the expanding epidural hematoma.

Subdural Hematoma. The clinical manifestations of a subdural collection of blood differ according to the age of the child. The condition occurs most commonly in infants with a history of either significant birth trauma or environmental trauma (child abuse).

In older children and adolescents, clinical manifestations of either an acute or chronic subdural hematoma are due to increased intracranial pressure. The acute subdural hematoma usually results from arterial bleeding following head trauma. The symptoms of change in consciousness and other signs of rapidly evolving increased intracranial pressure occur within 1 or 2 days following such an injury.

Chronic subdural hematomas are uncommon in young children. They are seen more often in adolescents, who present with headache, unilateral in 80% of the cases, and occurring often without a preceding history of head trauma. Over a short period of time, there is evidence of a personality change, changes in state of consciousness, and, without intervention, progressive and rapid deterioration. Headache combined with a personality change in an adolescent should suggest the possibility of chronic subdural hematoma.

Pseudotumor Cerebri. Pseudotumor cerebri is a condition in which there is increased intracranial pressure with no evidence of a space-occupying lesion. It has been associated with many primary disorders, a partial list of which is given in Table 2.

The cause of the increased intracranial pressure is not known, but there are probably multiple mechanisms involving the balance between CSF production and absorption.

Clinically, these children present with intermittent headaches, vomiting, blurred vision, and, occasionally, diplopia. Although physical examination reveals papilledema, there is no alteration in the level of consciousness or in intellectual functioning, in contrast to the findings in any of the space-occupying lesions discussed in the preceding section.

Diagnosis is made by finding markedly increased CSF pressure on lumbar puncture after excluding space-occupying lesions. The latter is accomplished with computerized tomography.

Intracranial Hemorrhage Secondary to an Arteriovenous Malformation or Ruptured Aneurysm. Arteriovenous malformations (AVM) are the most common vascular lesions in the CNS and may be located along any part of the neuraxis. The lesions occur more often in males than in females. Only about one half of AVMs are symptomatic during the lifetime. Of these, 20% become clinically manifest during the first decade, the remainder by the second or third decade.

The clinical course is characterized by the sudden onset of a severe headache. Following this, nuchal rigidity, irritability, and vomiting occur, followed by progressive hemiparesis, focal or generalized seizures, and progressive deterioration of consciousness. Depending on the site of the AVM, different neurologic syndromes are encountered.

Ruptured aneurysms occur less frequently than AVMs in children. The presentation of a ruptured aneurysm is similar to that seen in AVMs, but examination of the CSF reveals frank blood or significant xanthochromia more often in the latter condition.

Diagnosis. Diagnostic evaluation of a child who presents with the symptoms and signs noted above should involve (1) immediate hospitalization and neurologic consultation, (2) skull radiographs (PA and lateral), and (3) CT scan with and without contrast. For children with a suspected intracranial mass, prompt neurosurgical management of an expanding epidural or subdural collection of blood can be lifesaving. It must be emphasized that a lumbar puncture is contraindicated until it is certain that there is no intracranial mass. For management of these conditions, see *Pediatrics*, 17th ed.

TABLE 2. CONDITIONS ASSOCIATED WITH PSEUDOTUMOR CEREBRI

Middle ear infection	May account for as many as 25% of cases
Thrombosed lateral dural sinus 2° to mastoiditis	
Hypovitaminosis and hypervitaminosis A	
Withdrawal from adrenocortical steroid therapy	
Tetracycline and chlortetracycline therapy	
Profound Fe deficiency	Extremely rare
Hypoparathyroidism	
Addison's disease	
SLE	
Hypercarbia 2° to chronic lung disease	
Galactosemia	

DIFFERENTIAL DIAGNOSIS

In most cases, a careful history and physical examination will allow the pediatric practitioner to ascertain the correct etiology of the child's headache. Only in certain selective cases should laboratory tests be employed.

History

Certain questions in the history have special significance in evaluating a child complaining of headache and in determining the seriousness of the problem.

- When did the headache first begin? If the headache has begun within the past 1–2 weeks, a search should be made for events that may be causally related, such as an ingestion, physical trauma, or psychologic trauma.
- Is there anything that either relieves the headache or makes it worse? If the headache is persistent but relieved with analgesics, it is probably functional in origin. If position changes its severity, especially if lowering the head increases it, sinusitis should be considered a possible cause.
- Does it occur at special times of the day or night? Early morning headaches are typical of sinusitis and, less frequently, of intracranial mass lesions, which occasionally awaken children from sleep. Late afternoon or early evening headaches are more often functional, tension, or psychogenic.
- Were there any warning symptoms of the onset of the headache? Though not as reliable a sign in children as in adults, visual or auditory auras may precede the headache in classic migraine.
- Is the headache accompanied by any associated symptoms, such as photophobia, nausea, or vomiting? With migraine headache associated with prodromal nausea, vomiting may accompany the actual headache. Headaches due to increased intracranial pressure usually progress in severity over weeks or months and culminate in early morning, projectile vomiting.
- Does anyone else in the family have headaches? A strong family history of headaches suggests the diagnosis of migraine.
- What is the quality of the headache? Throbbing or pulsating types are seen more often in migraine headaches. Sharp, severe, excruciating, unilateral headaches occur in the cluster type of migraine headache. Dull, static headaches are more frequent in tension or psychogenic headache.
- Is the headache so severe that activity must stop? Migraine or the less common cluster type may be so severe that activity is interrupted at the vasodilatory stage when throbbing is most intense. Interruption of activity due to headache may also be due to an expanding intracranial lesion, especially following an interval of progressively increasing severity and persistence of the headache.
- How long does the headache last, and how frequently does it occur? Classic or common migraine headaches usually last ½–2 hours. They are followed by periods of somnolence or sleep lasting for 1–3 hours. They occur 1–2 times per week but may be as frequent as daily. Cluster type headaches are, as indicated by the name, severe debilitating headaches, localized to a specific location in the head and occurring in intense, multiple episodes over the course of days or weeks. After these intensely painful episodes, there may be intervals of months of freedom from headache.
- Are the symptoms increasing in severity, or have they remained the same since they began? If the headache has been intermittent but begins to occur at shorter intervals and with increasing intensity, there should be concern about an intracranial cause.
- Where is the pain felt? Unilateral or bilateral parietal or parietotemporal headaches are usual in migraine. Patients with a tension or psychogenic headache more often identify the occipital area as the site of their pain. However, the occipital region may be the site in some children with intracranial tumors and in the rare cases of migraine headaches of the basilar artery type. Frontal headaches accompanied by frontal tenderness are more often associated with sinusitis.

TABLE 3. DIAGNOSTIC CONSIDERATIONS ON THE BASIS OF PHYSICAL EXAMINATION

Physical Examination	Diagnostic Considerations
Vital signs	Serious aberrations suggest a major disease process
Blood pressure	Increased—consider headache secondary to hypertension (rare in childhood)
Fever	Infectious etiology—bacterial or aseptic meningitis, meningoencephalitis, sinusitis, systemic infection
Skin	
Presence of petecchia	Possible hematologic or infectious etiology, meningococcal meningitis, sepsis in older child
Stria and obesity	Cushing's disease
Head	
Acute enlargement	Obstructive hydrocephalus
Large head	Arrested hydrocephalus
Bruit	Arteriovenous malformation
Sinus tenderness or positive transillumination	Sinusitis
Eye	
Acute onset of strabismus	Ocular muscle paralysis secondary to increased intracranial pressure—may be a manifestation of tumor, ruptured arteriovenous malformation, gradually expanding subdural hematoma, or other type of expanding mass, or ophthalmoplegic migraine
Abnormal funduscopic examination	No venous pulsation suggests early increased intracranial pressure to expanding intracranial mass or pseudotumor cerebri Blurred disc margin suggests more serious stage of increased intracranial pressure due to above causes
Visual abnormality	
Refractive error	Headache as a result of eye strain
Hemianopsia	Possible intracranial mass
Ear	Either purulent otitis media or serous otitis media may give referred headache; mastoiditis is often accompanied by headache
Mouth	Peritonsillar, posterior pharyngeal, or dental abscess or infection
Nervous system	
Focal neurologic finding, fixed or progressive	Several considerations (in order of most life-threatening to least life-threatening)—intracranial lesion, arteriovenous malformation, tumor, ruptured aneurysm
Focal neurologic changes (transient)	Basilar artery type of migraine
Acute change in personality or affect	Intracranial mass, arteriovenous malformation, tumor, basilar artery or classic migraine

TABLE 4. DIAGNOSTIC CONSIDERATIONS FOR WHICH PROMPT CONSULTATION IS RECOMMENDED

Category	Diagnostic Work-up and Anticipated Results
Intracranial	
Brain abscess	CT scan with and without contrast to identify localized mass, non-vascular space-occupying lesion
Brain tumor	Do *not* do lumbar puncture (LP) CT scan with and without contrast to identify space-occupying lesion
Head trauma	
Significant, serious	Consider monitoring ICP CT scan to show cerebral edema, small ventricles, or evidence of accumulation of blood in subdural, subarachnoid, epidural, or intracerebral spaces
Simple, posttraumatic	Skull x-ray—concerned only if diastatic fracture noted
Pseudotumor cerebri	Do *not* do LP until after CT scan confirms absence of a space-occupying lesion; CT scan shows cerebral edema—no localized collection or space-occupying lesion
AVM, ruptured aneurysm	If signs of herniation impending, do *not* do LP CT scan with and without contrast Angiogram to show vascular mass intracerebral, Dx-confirmed bag of worms seen on angiogram.

Physical Examination

Table 3 presents the essential components of the physical examination and indicates diagnostic implications of certain physical findings.

Laboratory Investigations

Only rarely will specific laboratory tests be helpful in establishing the accurate diagnosis. Tables 1 and 4 summarize these diagnostic situations in which a laboratory test would be

TABLE 5. DIAGNOSTIC CONSIDERATIONS FOR MENTAL HEALTH CONSULTANT

Consultation Probably Not Necessary	Situations Where Outside Consultant Is Recommended
Headache intermittent with identifiable, triggering tension or situation	Emotion or tension creating the situation not identifiable
Headache present <2 months	Headache persistent for >2 months and occurs more than once/week
Family/child willing and eager to talk about situation that might be contributing to the headache in open way	Family and child reluctant to discuss the possible environmental settings in which the headache occurs
No prolonged school absences	School absence significant
No bizarre behavior	Evidence of other abnormal behavioral problems
Developmental milestones intact	Delayed or abnormal developmental milestones
Family is not being disrupted by these symptoms	Family becoming significantly disrupted either as a possible contributing factor to or result of these persistent headaches

TABLE 6. DIAGNOSTIC CONSIDERATIONS MANAGED PRIMARILY BY PEDIATRICIAN

Category	Therapeutic Intervention	Consultant Called
Intracranial		
Meningitis	Suspected bacterial, initiate antibiotics: ampicillin 300 mg/kg/day IV, chloramphenicol 100 mg/kg/day IV, await culture and sensitivity results from microbiology laboratory	None
Extracranial, acute		
Sinusitis	Ampicillin, decongestant, inhaled warm moist air	If chronic, otolaryngologist
Systemic infections	Appropriate antibiotics	None
Vascular migraine	Cafergot ½ tab and then 1 tab q30/ minutes, total 3 tabs/attack/day Prophylaxis—propranolol 10–20 mg tid	Only occasionally, a neurologist

useful and what the anticipated results might be.

MANAGEMENT

Psychogenic and Tension-induced Headache

The pediatrician usually plays the central role in diagnosing the etiology of headaches in children. As noted in the beginning of this chapter, headaches in children are, for the most part, functional. Management in this case should consider first an in-depth exploration of the environment of the child, over the course of discussions with child and family, and an understanding of tensions that play a part in the child's headaches. Often there is an improvement in the symptomatology. The pediatric practitioner will often find that skills of listening, understanding, and some appropriate reassurance and intervention are all that is required. However, the pediatric practitioner should be alert to the significant hallmarks of such functional headaches where the situation should not be managed in his own practice and may require outside mental health consultation and possible intervention (Table 5).

The other diagnostic considerations that can be managed by the pediatrician alone are summarized in Table 6.

Migraine Headache

Table 7 lists other categories of migraine with therapeutic intervention and the consultant to be called. Table 8 presents management steps in those patients requiring consultation. More detail can be found in *Pediatrics*, 17th ed.

SUMMARY

The pediatric practitioner must be aware that the major cause of headache in children is

TABLE 7. MIGRAINE, OTHER SUBTYPES

Category	Therapeutic Intervention	Consultant
Hemiplegic	None specific	Neurologist
Ophthalmoplegic	None specific	Neurologist
Basilar artery	None	Neurologist
Epilepsy equivalent	Consider anti-convulsant medication	Neurologist

TABLE 8. DIAGNOSTIC CONSIDERATIONS FOR WHICH PROMPT CONSULTATION IS RECOMMENDED

Category	Therapeutic Intervention	Consultant
Intracranial		
Brain abscess	Immediate: Surgical exploration and drainage Antibiotics—chloramphenicol, penicillin	Neurologist Neurosurgeon
Brain tumor	Surgical exploration, chemotherapy dependent upon type of tumor	Neurologist Neurosurgeon
Head trauma	If significant: Mannitol 1.5 g/kg IV Dexamethosone 0.3 mg/kg IV q6h Hyperventilation Surgical drainage if displacing subdural or epidural	Neurologist Neurosurgeon
Pseudotumor cerebri	If not severe, no therapy If severe, repeated LP to decrease pressure which will relieve symptoms Rx specific cause found (Table 4)	Neurologist
AVM, ruptured aneurysm	Surgical intervention if herniating If no herniation, stabilize and consider intravenous embolization If embolization not effective, as revealed by angiogram, must surgically intervene Anticonvulsant Rx Physical rehabilitation if hemiparesis has resulted	Neurologist Neurosurgeon

functional. Given the systematic approach to a child with a headache outlined in this chapter, it is hoped that a rational approach to diagnosis and intervention can be accomplished and alleviation of this often debilitating symptom will be the result.

BIBLIOGRAPHY

Caviness VS et al: Headache. N Engl J Med 302: 446, 1980

Day WH: Diseases of Children. Philadelphia, 1881

Elkind AM, Friedman AP: Review of headache, part I. N Y State J Med, 255, 1967

Friedman AP: Recurring headache. Primary Care, 1: 275, 1974

Friedman AP, Harms E:Headaches in Children. Springfield, Ill, Charles C Thomas, 1967

Golden GS, French JH: Badilar artery migraine in young children. Pediatrics 56:722, 1975

Rothner A David: Headaches in children: A review. Consultant, 159–161, 1979

Cross-Reference to *Pediatrics,* 17th ed.

TWELVE

Hemoptysis and Epistaxis

Jeffrey Gershel

HEMOPTYSIS

Hemoptysis is the expectoration of blood or blood-tinged sputum deriving from the respiratory tract. In children, it is most often a complication of severe pneumonia. True hemoptysis is infrequent in children. Most suspected cases are actually instances of blood from the esophagus or oropharynx being mixed with sputum and then expectorated.

Etiology

The causes of hemoptysis can be considered in two categories, infectious and noninfectious diseases (Table 1).

Infectious Etiology. The vast majority of cases of hemoptysis are secondary to infection, with the most frequent etiology being bacterial pneumonia leading to bronchiectasis or airway erosion. This can be from either acute or recurrent infection. Bronchiectasis is a well-known complication of cystic fibrosis. It occurs also in association with the chronic lung changes seen in low-birth-weight infants with bronchopulmonary dysplasia.

Uncommon infections that cause hemoptysis include tuberculosis and coccidioidomycosis. Rarely, recurrent bacterial infections occur in association with pulmonary sequestration.

Noninfectious Etiology. The most common noninfectious etiologies are foreign bodies and fractured ribs. Foreign body in the airway is a disease peculiar to toddlers, who present with hemoptysis in conjunction with an asthmalike illness, pneumonia, or acute upper airway obstruction. In some patients, a period of months or years separates the aspiration and the presentation of the illness. Trauma to the chest wall can cause a rib fracture, and the sharp end of the rib can then lacerate the pleura or parenchyma, with subsequent hemoptysis.

Although uncommon, pulmonary and mediastinal masses can cause extrinsic airway and blood vessel compression and erosion. Examples include bronchogenic cyst, lymphoma, and teratoma. A pulmonary arteriovenous malformation and pulmonary hemosiderosis are rare diseases that can present with massive hemoptysis.

A bleeding diathesis secondary to thrombocytopenia (idiopathic thrombocytopenic purpura), platelet dysfunction (von Willebrand's disease) or a coagulopathy (liver disease, Coumadin ingestion) can be the cause of hemoptysis.

TABLE 1. CAUSES OF HEMOPTYSIS AND CLINICAL AND LABORATORY FEATURES

Diagnosis	Nature of Hemoptysis	Chest Roentgenogram	History and Clinical Findings
Infectious			
Acute bacterial pneumonia	T	Infiltrate	Fever, cough, rales, chest pain Previously well
Bronchiectasis	T/BR	Normal or infiltrate	Recurrent infections, chronic cough History of BPD or cystic fibrosis
Tuberculosis	T/BR	Infiltrate, calcified node	Cough, weight loss, fatigue Contact with known case
Coccidioidomycosis	T/BR	Localized density	Cough
Noninfectious			
Foreign body aspiration	T/BR	Unilateral hyperlucency	Acute: respiratory distress Chronic: cough, asthma
Fractured rib	T/BR	Fracture	History of trauma to chest Point tenderness over fracture
Arteriovenous fistula	BR	Localized density	Massive acute bleeding Heart murmur and chest wall thrill
Mediastinal tumor	T/BR	Mediastinal widening	Can be asymptomatic Fatigue and weight loss
Bronchogenic cyst	T/BR	Localized density	Recurrent infections Substernal discomfort
Pulmonary sequestration	T/BR	Infiltrate	Recurrent infections
Hemosiderosis	BR	Infiltrate	Iron deficiency anemia

T, tinged; BR, bright red.

Differential Diagnosis

History. Useful information can be obtained by asking the following pertinent questions.

- Is the child ill with fever, cough, rapid breathing, or chest pain? The major cause of hemoptysis is severe respiratory infection.
- Have there been past episodes of hemoptysis? If so, what have been the frequency and severity? Recurrent hemoptysis suggests a chronic disease, such as cystic fibrosis, pulmonary sequestration, or hemosiderosis.
- Has there been an episode of cyanosis? This is seen in massive pneumonia and pulmonary arteriovenous malformation.

- Has there been trauma to the chest wall that might suggest a fractured rib?
- Are there any signs of a bleeding diathesis, such as bloody urine or stools, excessive tendency to bruise, or petechial or purpuric rash? Is the patient taking any drugs that might interfere with hemostasis, such as Coumadin, heparin, or aspirin? Are there signs of liver disease, such as jaundice, light-colored stools, or dark urine? Liver disease might result in a bleeding diathesis or esophageal varicosities.
- Was the child noted to be gagging or choking, especially after eating or playing with a small object? Foreign body aspiration is a major cause of hemoptysis between 18 months and 4 years of age.

- Has there been a nosebleed, hematemesis, or blood in the mouth? As previously mentioned, the bleeding source in many cases of suspected hemoptysis is not in the respiratory tract.
- Has the child been chronically ill, with recurrent respiratory infection, failure to thrive, and diarrhea? This clinical picture raises the possibility of cystic fibrosis.
- Has the child had contact with a known case of active tuberculosis?

Physical Examination. Most children with acute hemoptysis are quite sick, with marked findings on physical examination. The extent of acute blood loss can be assessed by the presence of tachycardia, hypotension, pallor, weakness, and cardiac gallop. It must be remembered that anemia may also be present in cases of chronic, recurrent hemoptysis. A bleeding diathesis is suggested by petechiae, purpura, subconjunctival hemorrhages, oozing from puncture sites, hepatomegaly, or lymphadenopathy. Fingernail clubbing suggests long-standing hypoxemia, as in arteriovenous fistula.

The chest should be carefully examined for signs of external trauma or point tenderness secondary to a broken rib. Auscultation might reveal rales of acute infection, wheezing of airway obstruction (i.e., foreign body), or decreased breath sounds. The diagnosis of an AV fistula may be suggested by palpation of a thrill.

Careful inspection of the oropharynx and nasopharynx might reveal the true origin of the bleeding.

Laboratory Examination. In general, the only laboratory examinations required are anteroposterior and lateral chest roentgenograms. The common findings are lobar infiltrate, mediastinal widening, and peripheral density. Infiltrates suggest acute pneumonia, tuberculosis, or hemosiderosis. Mediastinal widening is seen with mediastinal tumors and lymphadenopathy. Localized, peripheral densities include AV fistula, pulmonary sequestration, bronchogenic cyst, and mediastinal tumor. Foreign body aspiration is suggested by unilateral hyperlucency, especially when the affected side is dependent. Inspiratory-expiratory films and fluoroscopy reveal expiratory mediastinal shifting away from the affected side. On occasion, the foreign body is opaque. Evidence of chronic lung disease with blebs and fibrosis suggests bronchopulmonary dysplasia or cystic fibrosis. The latter possibly indicates the need for a sweat test.

A chronic iron deficiency anemia occurs in hemosiderosis. Conversely, polycythemia is seen with an AV fistula.

Work-up of a possible bleeding diathesis includes a CBC, reticulocyte count, prothrombin time, partial thromboplastin time, and fibrinogen level.

If tuberculosis, coccidioidomycosis, or histoplasmosis is being considered, appropriate skin tests should be performed.

Treatment

The underlying cause of the hemoptysis will determine specific treatment. Severe hemoptysis mandates hospitalization. The management of acute blood loss and anemia are considered in Chapter 5. Regardless of the etiology, packed red blood cell transfusions are given as required to maintain an adequate hematocrit.

A foreign body is removed by bronchoscopy. A fractured rib requires no special treatment if the bleeding is controlled and there is no respiratory embarrassment.

Consultation

Except for the child with blood-tinged sputum caused by an acute pneumonia, a consultant's assistance will usually be needed. A thoracic surgeon should be consulted if there is a mass lesion (bronchogenic cyst, mediastinal tumor, AV fistula), foreign body, or uncontrolled bleeding. A hematologist is required to facilitate work-up and management of a bleeding diathesis. The care of a child with hemoptysis secondary to cystic fibrosis is best managed by a pediatric pulmonologist.

EPISTAXIS

Epistaxis is bleeding from the nose, usually from the anterior nasal septum (Little's area). The vessels involved are part of Kisselbach's plexus supplied by the external carotid. Much less commonly, the source is the posterior part of the inferior turbinate, in which case the bleeding usually is more severe. On occasion, the blood may cross behind the nasal septum so that the bleeding appears to be bilateral. True bilateral bleeding, however, occurs only with a nasal septal fracture. Sometimes, if the site is posterior or if the child is sleeping, the blood is swallowed, and the child presents with hematemesis.

The incidence of epistaxis is impossible to determine, as in most cases medical help is not sought. Nosebleeds are most common between the ages of 3 and 10 years. They are rare in infancy and infrequent in adolescence, although occasional episodes occur at menarche. There is a marked male predominance in the preschool and school-age years secondary to an increased incidence of blunt external trauma due to falls or punches and nose-picking. Usually, such children require treatment only, as the etiology is evident.

Etiology
Anatomic Causes. As mentioned above, the majority of nosebleeds are secondary to trauma and arise from an anterior nasal site. Blunt external trauma and nose-picking are frequently found circumstances. In addition, excessive use of nasal sprays and excessively dry, overheated environments have all been implicated without any specific anatomic abnormality. In these cases, the only pathology seen is the bleeding vessel. Occasionally, a toddler will present with a nasal foreign body that has caused mucosal ulceration and bleeding.

The presence of an anatomic lesion as the cause of a nosebleed is much less common. Hemangiomas, telangiectasias, and polyps are seen both anteriorly and posteriorly and, occasionally, are the cause of massive bleeding. Very rarely, epistaxis occurs after tonsillectomy and adenoidectomy.

Hematologic and Systemic Disorders. Any child with either massive, prolonged, or recurrent epistaxis, with or without other signs of a bleeding diathesis, should be evaluated for a platelet disorder. Most commonly, the problem is thrombocytopenia, secondary to idiopathic thrombocytopenic purpura or bone marrow invasion, as in leukemia or lymphoma. Other causes are disseminated intravascular coagulation (many etiologies, including sepsis), hypersplenism secondary to liver disease and cirrhosis, and drug-induced thrombocytopenia (cancer chemotherapy, diuretics, sulfonamides, penicillins). The most common cause of platelet dysfunction is von Willebrand's disease. Children with this disorder have a normal platelet count and a prolonged bleeding time; epistaxis is a common manifestation.

Clotting factor deficiencies less frequently result in epistaxis. Hemophilia (factor VIII deficiency), Christmas disease (factor IX deficiency), and liver disease (factors I, II, V, VII, IX, X deficiencies) are all possible etiologies. Hypertension can cause spontaneous epistaxis, although central nervous system symptoms (headache, blurred vision, seizures) are much more common. Rarely, a child will be taking Coumadin, heparin, or aspirin to prevent thrombolic or embolic disease. These drugs predispose to abnormal bleeding episodes.

Differential Diagnosis
History. Usually, taking a thorough history will obviate the need for any further work-up of a child with epistaxis.

Anatomic Causes.

- Is there a history of blunt nasal trauma, insertion of a foreign body, or nose-picking? These are the most common causes of epistaxis, the latter being the most frequent etiologic factor.
- Has the patient had a cold or rhinitis of any cause, including allergic? The nasal mucosa is more readily traumatized with resultant bleeding.
- Does the patient complain of drying or cracking of the nasal mucosa? These are associated with overheated homes in winter and excessive use of antihistamines and nasal sprays, both of which predispose to mucosal ulceration.
- Has the patient undergone tonsillectomy or adenoidectomy in the past day or two? Postsurgical epistaxis is an infrequent but difficult problem to handle.

Hematologic and Systemic Causes.

- Has there been bleeding from other sites, including urine or stools, or after toothbrushing or other minor trauma. These suggest a bleeding diathesis. Similarly, is there excessive bruisability or a petechial or purpuric rash? Is the patient taking drugs that might interfere with hemostasis, such as heparin, Coumadin, or aspirin?
- Does the child have signs of liver disease (jaundice, dark urine, light stools) with resultant clotting factor deficiency or hypersplenism?
- Has the child had chronic nosebleeds? Although this history usually indicates the less serious etiologies, a bleeding diathesis must be considered.
- Does the child have a history of hypertension or renal disease that could lead to high blood pressure?
- Is there a family history of epistaxis or other bleeding diathesis? Hemophilia and Christmas disease (X-linked recessive) occur in other males of the family, while von Willebrand's disease (autosomal dominant) can affect either sex.

Physical Examination.

Anatomic Disorders. The most pertinent part of the physical examination is evaluation of the head and neck, to localize the site of bleeding and to confirm the diagnosis. However, a general examination should always be performed.

GENERAL. Weakness, lassitude, and pallor should be noted as an indication of severe blood loss.

SKIN. The presence of cutaneous hemangiomas or telangiectasias raises the possibility of similar lesions of the nasal mucosa.

HEENT. The nasal septum and cavities are examined to localize the bleeding site and to note the presence of a hemangioma, telangiectasia, polyp, or foreign body. Preferably, this is performed with the patient in a sitting position, using a bright light, such as an otoscope. If a source of bleeding is found, the search is ended, as multiple bleeding sites are distinctly unusual except in the case of a nasal fracture. In such instances, the septum is deviated and irregular. A septal hematoma (extreme bluish swelling) should be sought, as it must be evacuated as soon as possible to prevent septal infection or necrosis.

If no source is found anteriorly and the blood is seen trickling down the back of the throat, it can be assumed that the bleeding is from a posterior site in the nasal cavity.

Attention should be paid to signs of an upper respiratory infection (drainage of mucus) or allergic rhinitis (watery drainage, transverse crease of the nasal bridge). Conjunctival pallor suggests a significant amount of blood loss.

HEART AND LUNGS. Auscultation can confirm the presence of a respiratory infection, while tachycardia or gallop suggest significant amounts of blood loss.

Hematologic and Systemic Disorders.

GENERAL. A debilitated appearance

might indicate a severe illness, such as malignancy, liver disease, or renal disease. The blood pressure should be recorded to rule out hypertension.

SKIN. Multiple bruises and petechiae or excessive bleeding from puncture sites suggest a bleeding diathesis. Jaundice secondary to liver disease can be associated with clotting factor deficiency.

LYMPH NODES. Generalized lymphadenopathy suggests leukemia or other malignancy.

HEENT. In addition to the thorough examination described previously, the conjunctivae are examined for hemorrhages (suggesting a bleeding diathesis) and icterus (suggesting liver disease).

ABDOMEN. Hepatosplenomegaly is seen in leukemia and other malignancies. An enlarged liver could be associated with a clotting factor deficiency. Splenomegaly can lead to thrombocytopenia.

Laboratory Examination.
Hematologic and Systemic Diseases. In general, laboratory tests are not necessary, although in some cases certain specific examinations are indicated. If the patient appears ill, one should investigate for anemia secondary to excessive blood loss, a bleeding diathesis, liver disease, and malignancy.

Appropriate studies are done to evaluate hypertension, bone marrow or platelet disease, renal disease, or disseminated intravascular coagulation.

Figure 1 summarizes the overall approach to the evaluation of a child with epistaxis.

Management
Anatomic Disorders.
Most nosebleeds from Kisselbach's plexus respond to 5 minutes of firm, continuous local pressure. The child should be kept upright, with his head tilted forward, to prevent swallowing of blood trickling down the throat. If this maneuver is unsuccessful, cotton soaked in 1:1000 aqueous epinephrine solution should be placed in the anterior nasal cavity. Alternatively, the nasal cavity can be packed with ½ inch diameter Vaseline gauze or Gelfoam (oxidized cellulose). After hemostasis is obtained, the site can be cauterized for three seconds with a silver nitrate stick. Appropriate measures should be taken to prevent recurrence. For example, Vaseline and humidification prevent drying of the nasal mucosa, while the chronic nose-picker might have to wear mittens while asleep.

Foreign body removal can be attempted with forceps or suction. In some instances, the object can be removed by passing an uninflated Foley catheter beyond the object, then inflating the balloon and withdrawing the catheter and the object. Occasionally, the child must be admitted to the hospital for removal of the foreign body under general anesthesia.

An otolaryngologist should be called for both posterior and postsurgical (tonsillectomy, adenoidectomy) bleeding, as well as when routine measures are ineffective in achieving hemostasis. In these cases, the proper (posterior) packing is placed, and the child is admitted for observation.

If a hemangioma, telangiectasia, or polyp is found, an otolaryngologic consultation is obtained in order to plan elective excision. In general, these lesions respond to pressure or anterior packing. Cautery should not be used.

Hematologic and Systemic Diseases.
If the cause of the epistaxis is a bleeding diathesis, local pressure and anterior packing can be used, but cautery is contraindicated, as the tissue might slough. The specific treatment of these illnesses is beyond the scope of this chapter. However, such children should always be admitted to the hospital to facilitate the work-up and management. Hematology-oncology consultation is necessary for cases of suspected malignancy, thrombocytopenia, or thrombocytopathia.

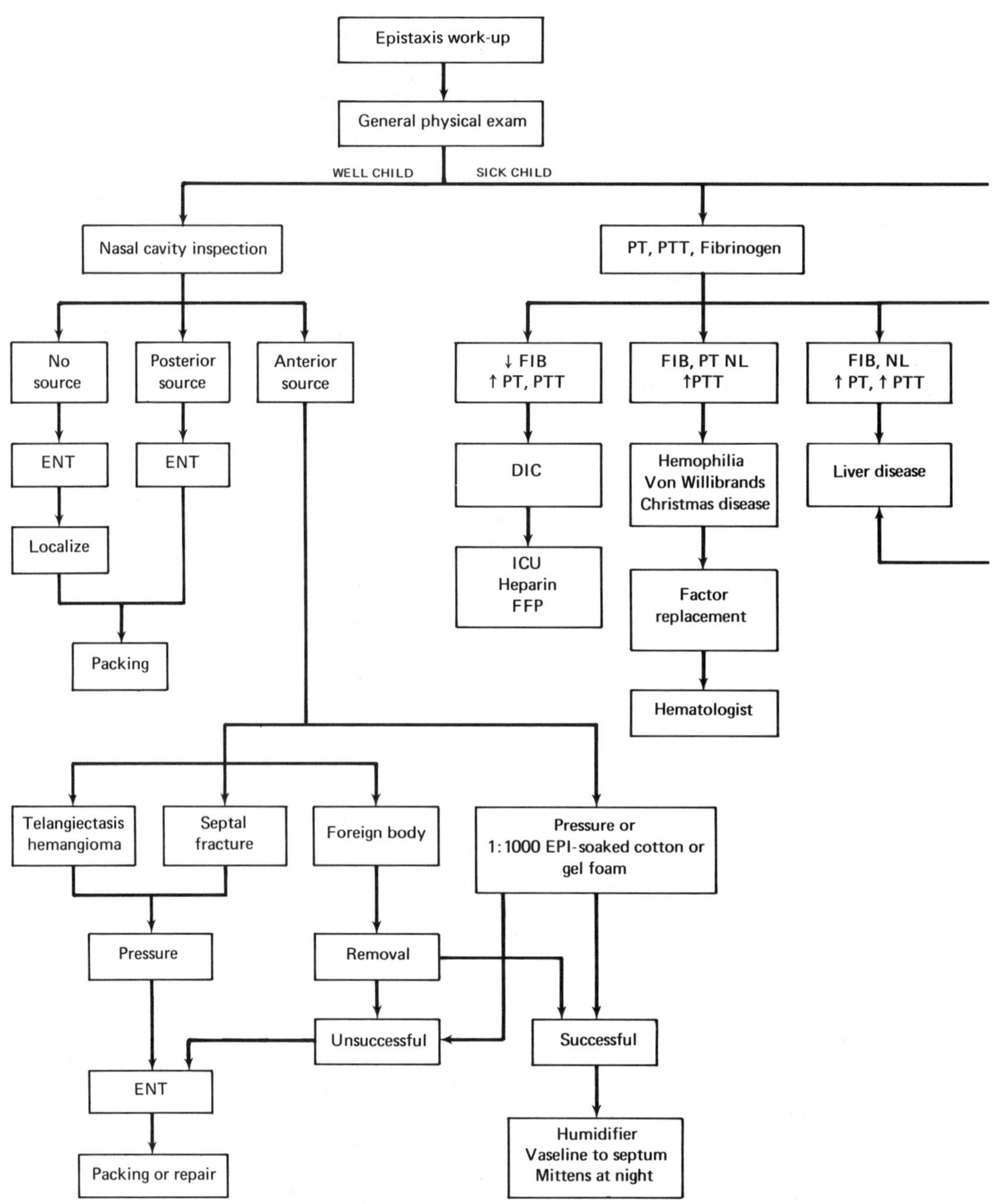

Figure 1. Overall approach to the evaluation of a child with epistaxis.

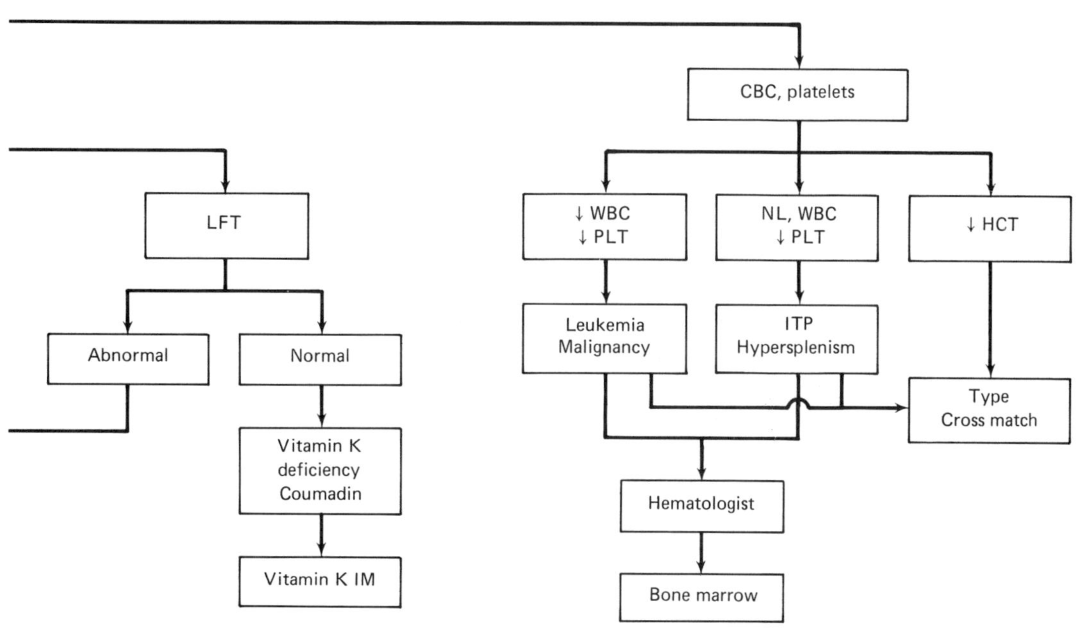

CBC, platelets
LFT
↓ WBC
↓ PLT
NL, WBC
↓ PLT
↓ HCT
Abnormal
Normal
Leukemia
Malignancy
ITP
Hypersplenism
Vitamin K
deficiency
Coumadin
Type
Cross match
Vitamin K IM
Hematologist
Bone marrow

BIBLIOGRAPHY

Hemoptysis

Green M: Pediatric Diagnosis. Philadelphia, Saunders, 1980, pp 511–512

Holsclaw DS, Grand RJ, Shwachman H: Massive hemoptysis in cystic fibrosis. J Pediatr 76:829, 1970

Tom LW, Wersman RA, Handler SD: Hemoptysis in children. Ann Otol Rhinol Laryngol 89:419, 1980

Epistaxis

Barelli PA: The management of epistaxis in children. Otolaryngol Clin North Am 10:91, 1977

El Bitar H: The etiology and management of epistaxis: a review of 300 cases. Practitioner 207:800, 1971

Juselius H: Epistaxis, a clinical study of 1724 cases. J Laryngol Otol 88:317, 1974

Lingeman RE: Epistaxis. Am Fam Physician 14:78, 1976

Cross-Reference—to *Pediatrics*, 17th ed.

Hypotonia

Jeffrey Gershel

Hypotonia is defined as diminished resistance to passive movement. Clinically, the condition is manifested by excessive joint motion, decreased spontaneous movement, or unusual body postures. Weakness is defined as diminished muscular strength and, therefore, is not synonymous with hypotonia. The floppy infant syndrome includes any combination of hypotonia and weakness.

Although the primary disorder in a weak or hypotonic patient may lie outside the neuromuscular system, most often the pathology is within one particular part of the system, especially the central nervous system, but also the peripheral nerves, muscles, myoneural junction, or spinal cord.

Because of the wide variability in the degree of hypotonia and weakness, their incidence is impossible to determine. The underlying causes can be considered in three major categories: the floppy infant syndrome, acute diseases of childhood, and chronic diseases of childhood.

THE FLOPPY INFANT SYNDROME

Etiology

The etiology of the floppy infant syndrome can be considered in two major categories, acquired (most common) and congenital diseases (Table 1).

Perinatal Causes. The increasing rate of survival of low-birth-weight and very-low-birth-weight infants has resulted in a corresponding increase in the occurrence of anoxic injury or cerebral palsy. Although a newborn who is immediately postasphyxic may be hypotonic, in general the condition at that time has no prognostic significance. An asphyxiated newborn should not be considered floppy until he no longer is receiving life-support measures, antibiotics, or intravenous fluids. Conversely, hypotonia may not be appreciated until several months of age. Often, spastic cerebral palsy will develop after a variable period of hypotonia.

Intracranial Bleeding. In addition to hypoxia, prematures and especially newborns who are small for gestational age are at risk of developing intracranial bleeding. This most commonly is an intraventricular bleed in a newborn whose birth weight is under 1,500 g. Hypoxia, acidosis, hypernatremia, and birth trauma increase the risk of bleeding. The signs and symptoms are variable and nonspecific, although hypotonia is often seen. The ultimate prognosis for these infants is controversial, but most authorities feel that permanent neurologic disability is the rule.

Birth Trauma. Birth trauma can cause spinal cord injury, especially if the delivery was difficult with the baby in a breech presentation.

TABLE 1. ETIOLOGIES OF THE FLOPPY INFANT SYNDROME

Congenital	Acquired

Chromosomal syndromes (Down's, some cases of Prader-Willi)	Perinatal
	  Anoxia (cerebral palsy)
	  Intracranial bleed

Neuromuscular diseases
  Spinal cord (spina bifida)
  Anterior horn cell (Werdnig-Hoffmann)
  Peripheral nerve (polyneuropathy)
  Neuromuscular junction (myasthenia gravis, neonatal and congenital)
  Muscle (muscular dystrophies, congenital myopathies, myotonic dystrophy)
	Spinal cord trauma
	Polyneuropathy (hereditary)
	Neuromuscular blockade (botulism)
	Renal (renal tubular acidosis)
	Endocrine (hypothyroidism)
	Collagen vascular disease (dermatomyositis)

Endocrine (congenital hypothyroidism)	

Metabolic
  Aminoacidopathy (hyperlysinemia, hyperglycinemia)
  Lipidoses (Tay-Sachs, Nieman-Pick)
  Glycogen storage disease (Pompes)	

Collagen (Marfan's, Ehlers-Danlos)	

The newborn is floppy, but usually, after a variable period of floppiness, hypertonia develops below the level of the lesion.

Congenital Causes. In contrast to the acquired lesions, most congenital causes of the floppy infant syndrome are rare. There may be an evident dysmorphologic picture, as in Down's syndrome, Prader-Willi syndrome, and spina bifida. In such patients, the diagnosis is usually apparent early in infancy.

Neuromuscular diseases of the newborn and infant can affect any level of the system and cause hypotonia and weakness. Spinal muscular atrophy, or Werdnig-Hoffmann disease, affects the anterior horn cells. Although the severity is variable, symptomatic newborns and young infants have a grave prognosis. Proximal muscle weakness, diminished deep tendon reflexes, tongue fasiculations, and difficulty in swallowing are features of the disease.

Myasthenia gravis, a disease of the myoneural junction, can present as respiratory and feeding difficulties in an offspring of a mother with myasthenia gravis. If a newborn's respiratory distress cannot adequately be explained by pulmonary or cardiac disease, a trial of neostigmine can be lifesaving. This condition is a transient one which usually resolves within the first week of life. Congenital myasthenia presents later in infancy with weakness and the classic ocular findings (ptosis, external ophthalmoplegia) that are not seen in the neonatal variety.

Myotonic dystrophy can present either in a newborn of an affected mother, with respiratory and feeding difficulties (neonatal myotonia), or later in life in the infant of either affected parent (congenital myotonia). Distal muscle weakness with preservation of the deep tendon reflexes and sustained muscle contractions (myotonia) are seen. The diagnosis is confirmed by eliciting myotonia in one of the parents.

Inborn errors of metabolism can involve glycogen storage disease (Pompe's), lipid disorders (Tay-Sachs, Niemann-Pick), and aminoacidopathies (hyperlysinemia, hyperglycinemia). In general, these present after the infant has started taking formula containing fats or protein. Hypotonia out of proportion to weakness, metabolic acidosis, vomiting, failure to thrive, and seizures are the common signs and symptoms. Dietary manipulation is curative in some of these disorders.

Differential Diagnosis

History. A careful, complete history often enables the practitioner to identify the correct diagnosis. The character of the initial abnormality and the age at which it was noted are of particular importance. Questions pertinent to the floppy neonate will be considered first.

- Was the newborn noted to have a weak grasp, poor suck, or weak cry? Were there any respiratory difficulties in the nursery? Were decreased spontaneous movements or floppiness evident? These are the earliest presentations of a floppy infant. If present, the disease is either congenital (Down's, Prader-Willi, myasthenia, Werdnig-Hoffmann, myotonic dystrophy, some myopathies) or acquired in the perinatal period (cerebral palsy, intraventricular hemorrhage).
- What was the child's neonatal course? The nature of the delivery and the level of the Apgar score may suggest the possibility of perinatal anoxic insult (cerebral palsy). Was the child on a respirator? If so, for how long? This suggests possible anoxia or motor unit pathology (congenital myasthenia, Werdnig-Hoffmann, or myopathy). Were there seizures or a cardiopulmonary arrest, suggesting the possibility of brain damage?
- Was the baby a breech presentation and a difficult delivery, which could lead to damage of the spinal cord?
- Did the child's mother note a lessening of fetal activity during the third trimester?

This is occasionally seen with Werdnig-Hoffmann disease.

- Beyond the neonatal period, the rate of progression is most important. Is the infant achieving his gross motor milestones appropriately? Since this age group attains new skills rapidly, an infant who remains at a certain level may in reality have a progressive condition (lipid or glycogen storage disease, Werdnig-Hoffmann, aminoacidopathy) rather than a static lesion (cerebral palsy).
- In which muscle(s) was the weakness first noted? Onset in proximal muscles occurs with muscular dystrophies and Werdnig-Hoffmann disease, while distal pathology suggests a neuropathy or myotonic dystrophy.
- Does the patient have feeding difficulties? This can be a feature of infant botulism, myasthenia gravis, myotonic dystrophy, Werdnig-Hoffmann disease, Prader-Willi syndrome, some congenital myopathies, and postasphyxia.
- Has the infant been fed honey, which has been implicated as a source of botulism toxin?
- Is the child mentally retarded (i.e., delayed language and social-adaptive behavior)? This is a feature of Down's syndrome, Prader-Willi syndrome, congenital hypothyroidism, aminoacidopathies, Pompe's disease, and myotonic dystrophy.
- Are there any family members who are similarly affected? Some disorders are autosomal dominant (myotonic dystrophy, Marfan's syndrome, Ehlers-Danlos syndrome), autosomal recessive (Werdnig-Hoffmann, limb-girdle muscular dystrophy, Tay-Sachs), or X-linked (Duchenne's).

Physical Examination. Although the neurologic examination is of paramount importance, the remainder of the physical must not be neglected. Findings pertinent to securing an etiology for the floppy infant syndrome are summarized in Table 2.

TABLE 2. PHYSICAL FINDINGS IN THE FLOPPY INFANT

System	Findings	Possible Diagnosis
General	Low-birth-weight or small for gestational age	Cerebral palsy or intracranial bleed
Skin	Loose, elastic skin	Ehlers-Danlos
	Erythematous rash	Dermatomyositis
HEENT	Micro- or macrocephalic	CNS lesion
	Patent posterior fontanel	Hypothyroidism
	Cherry red macula	Tay-Sachs disease
	Large tongue	Hypothyroidism
Neck	Palpable thyroid	Hypothyroidism
Lungs	Newborn respiratory distress	Werdnig-Hoffmann, congenital myopathy, neonatal myasthenia
	Acute respiratory distress	Infant botulism
Heart	Cardiomegaly, murmur	Pompe's, Down's syndrome
Abdomen	Umbilical hernia	Hypothyroidism
Genitalia	Hypogonadism	Prader-Willi
Rectal	Decreased sphincter tone	Spinal dysrhaphia or trauma
Back	Scoliosis	Muscular dystrophy, Werdnig-Hoffmann, myotonia
	Sacral dimple or hair tuft	Spinal dysrhaphia
Extremities	Arthrogryposis, club feet	Werdnig-Hoffmann, congenital myopathy, myotonic dystrophy

Neurologic Examination of the Floppy Infant. The neurologic examination of the newborn and infant is particularly challenging. However, the practitioner should be able to gather enough information so that a differential diagnosis can be made.

MENTAL STATUS. A complete Denver Developmental Screening Test is most useful, as the results will define either a central nervous system etiology (global failure, including language and social-adaptive) or a neuromuscular disorder (gross and fine motor delays only).

REFLEXES. The newborn should have symmetrical Moro, palmar and plantar grasp, and placing reflexes, in addition to rooting and a strong suck. Although the deep tendon reflexes are intact, usually the triceps reflex cannot be elicited. Up to 10–12 beats of ankle clonus is considered normal. Any abnormalities suggest either a congenital disease or perinatal insult. The deep tendon reflexes are usually normal but sometimes decreased later in the course of Prader-Willi syndrome, Tay-Sachs disease, dermatomyositis, and the aminoacidopathies.

From 2 to 5 months of age, the tonic neck reflex should be present. This should never be obligate (persistent beyond 30 seconds) and should not be present after 6 months of age. At 8–9 months, the parachute reflex occurs.

MUSCULAR ACTIVITY AND STRENGTH. The baby should be observed in the prone and supine positions for spontaneous movements of all four extremities. Symmetry is tested by withdrawal from pain, the face-cover test (removal of a blanket from his face, 4–5 months), lateral propping (extension of the arm as the sitting infant is tipped sideways, 6 months), and parachute reflex (extension of both arms as the suspended prone infant is thrust toward the examining table, 8–9 months).

At 3–5 months, head lag should be absent, and the baby should sit at 6 months. At 8–9 months the infant can stand holding on by himself. The average child begins to take steps alone at 12 months. The most common cause of motor delay is cerebral palsy, although young infants can be suffering from Pompe's disease, an aminoacidopathy, or Werdnig-Hoffmann disease.

The ability to turn over from supine to prone before 6 weeks of age suggests hypertonia, while a hand preference that develops before 2 years of age implies contralateral weakness. In both cases, a central nervous system etiology should be suspected.

TONE. The baby is held in ventral suspension to gauge his tone. The ability to bring the foot to the chin or adduct the elbow past the midline is a sign of hypotonia or excessive joint laxity.

SENSORY. As mentioned, the baby's withdrawal from a noxious stimulus will assess his sensation.

CRANIAL NERVES. The examination of the cranial nerves of an infant is very difficult, but with patience much useful information can be obtained.

III, IV, VI. Ptosis and external ophthalmoplegia occur in congenital myasthenia, while ptosis is almost universally present in myotonic dystrophy.

VII. Facial weakness is seen in myotonia and some congenital myopathies.

IX, X. Drooling and difficulty in swallowing occur in myasthenia gravis and infant botulism.

XII. Tongue fasiculations occur in Werdnig-Hoffmann disease.

Laboratory Examinations. A detailed consideration is given only to examinations that a generalist might request.

Serum Enzymes. The creatine phosphokinase (CPK) is elevated in muscular dystrophies, Werfnig-Hoffmann disease, and myotonic dystrophy. The CPK is normal in neuropathies and sometimes in myotonic dystrophy. Other assays, such as aldolase, SGOT, LDH, and SGPT, are also elevated in myopathic conditions, but there is no definitive pattern to discriminate one disease from another.

Urine Amino Acid Screen. This is mandatory in the work-up of any floppy infant who has not suffered a hypoxic event.

Tensilon Test. This is indicated in any newborn with respiratory distress along with ptosis and swallowing difficulties, suggesting neonatal myasthenia gravis.

Other Tests. If a central nervous system lesion is suspected, a CT scan can confirm the diagnosis in cases with hydrocephalus, porencephalic cysts, intracranial bleed, or cortical atrophy. Unfortunately, there are no pathognomonic findings for cerebral palsy.

Specific tests should be performed to rule out suspected systemic diseases (e.g., thyroid functions, blood urea nitrogen and creatinine, complete blood count).

Schema for Evaluation

Neonate. Since the vast majority of floppy newborns are suffering from acquired central nervous system lesions, secondary either to anoxia or intracranial bleeding, all such infants require a CT scan. Some centers, however, advocate ultrasonography to diagnose intracranial bleeding. Either of the radiographic studies will establish the diagnosis, or no abnormality will be found, suggesting anoxia as the etiology.

Vomiting, seizures, or an unexplained metabolic acidosis, especially if the onset coincided with the institution of formula feeding, suggests an inborn error of metabolism. Blood gas and pH, urine and blood for quantitative amino acids, blood ammonia, and urine ferric chloride tests should be performed and appropriate consultation obtained.

If a neuromuscular disorder is suspected, a neurologist must be consulted immediately. Neonatal myasthenia must be ruled out with a trial of neostigmine, and the mother should be examined for myotonia. Sophisticated testing (electromyogram, nerve conduction, muscle biopsy) should be performed at the neurologist's discretion.

Infancy. As in the case of the neonate, if a central nervous system lesion is suspected, a CT scan is indicated. Vomiting, seizures, or failure to thrive demands a metabolic work-up and consultation.

Similarly, the work-up of a neuromuscular disorder is identical to the schema for the newborn.

Management

Unfortunately, most of the diseases considered here have no specific treatment. Many etiologies, such as Down's syndrome, cerebral palsy, Prader-Willi syndrome, spinal cord transection and dysrhaphia, involve static lesions without any expected progression of the hypotonia. For such patients, management includes physical therapy and range of motion exercises, splints to prevent flexion contractures, and attention to other involved organ systems.

The patient with myasthenia is treated with an anticholinesterase, such as neostigmine bromide. If unsuccessful, thymectomy and corticosteroids are other options.

Infant botulism is a medical emergency. The child is admitted to an intensive care unit where assisted ventilation is readily available. Type-specific antitoxin is given for 5 days.

Specific treatment for any nonneuromuscular disease is mandatory. This may involve thyroid replacement, corticosteroids (dermatomyositis and polymyositis), bicarbonate therapy (renal tubular acidosis), and so on.

No matter what the diagnosis, if the genetics of inheritance is known, genetic counseling is mandatory so that decisions can be made by the parents regarding additional children.

HYPOTONIA AND WEAKNESS IN CHILDHOOD

Etiology

After infancy, hypotonia and weakness can result either in an acute or chronic process. The most significant causes to be considered in these two major categories are listed in Table 3.

Acute Conditions. Acute hypotonia and weakness usually are secondary to an insult to the neuromuscular system, either traumatic, infectious, or toxic. The injury can be at the level of the spinal cord, as in the case of a cord transection or compression. Usually, there is a variable period of hypotonia (spinal shock) below the level of the lesion, after which spasticity evolves. Bladder and bowel dysfunction commonly are seen. Depending on the level of the lesion, the upper extremities may be completely unaffected.

The anterior horn cells are acutely affected by poliomyelitis. A history of incomplete immunizations, along with fever, rash, nuchal rigidity, and asymmetrical findings are hallmarks of this disease. Lower motor neuron signs are present, including muscle atrophy, decreased deep tendon reflexes, and downgoing toes. On occasion, respiratory difficulties and difficulties in swallowing are seen. A cerebrospinal pleocytosis is a consistent finding.

Guillain-Barré syndrome, or polyneuritis, is an ascending paralysis that occurs in response to some offending agent. This most commonly occurs 1–3 weeks after a viral infection (Ebstein-Barr virus, herpes zoster, mumps, measles, Coxsackie, echo, or influenza) or an immunization (live virus of diphtheria-pertussis-tetanus). The onset can

TABLE 3. ETIOLOGIES OF HYPOTONIA AND WEAKNESS IN CHILDHOOD

Acute Neuromuscular Disorders	Chronic Neuromuscular Disorders

Spinal cord trauma or compression
Anterior horn cell (poliomyelitis)
Peripheral nerve
  Guillain-Barré syndrome (immunization, viral infection)
  Peripheral neuropathy (heavy metal, vincristine, isoniazid)
Myoneural junction (aminoglycoside antibiotics)
Myositis (dermatomyositis, systemic lupus erythematosus)
Nonnervous system
  Electrolyte imbalance (hyper- and hypokalemia)
	Central nervous system (Down's syndrome, Prader-Willi syndrome, hypotonic cerebral palsy)
	Spinal cord (dysrhaphia)
	Neuromuscular system
	  Anterior horn cell (Werdnig-Hoffmann disease)
	  Peripheral nerves (hereditary polyneuropathy)
	  Myoneural junction (myasthenia gravis)
	  Muscle
	    Muscular dystrophy (Duchenne's, Becker)
	    Myotonic dystrophy
	    Myopathy (limb-girdle, fascioscapulohumeral)
	Nonnervous system
	  Renal (renal tubular acidosis)
	  Endocrine (hypothyroidism, hyperthyroidism)

be abrupt (over several days to weeks) or more insidious, with only paresthesias seen initially. Bilateral facial involvement is characteristic, and the bulbar and respiratory muscles often are involved as well. The deep tendon reflexes are lost, while the sensory deficit, if any, is variable. The laboratory hallmark is an elevated cerebrospinal fluid protein without a pleocytosis (so-called cytoalbuminogenic dissociation).

An acute peripheral neuropathy can be caused by infection (diphtheria), toxins (heavy metals), drugs (vincristine, isoniazid), or metabolic disturbances (uremia and diabetes). Lower motor neuron signs and distal muscle weakness are found. In addition, impairment of sensation, especially vibration and light touch, in the region served by the affected nerve is a pathognomonic finding in a peripheral neuropathy.

Finally, acute hypotonia and weakness can be secondary to a primary muscular disorder, as with polymyositis or dermatomyositis. In general, proximal muscles are affected in a subacute manner, with muscle pain and tenderness being the most common complaints. A faint erythematous rash is sometimes noted. In general, the erythrocyte sedimentation rate and muscle enzymes are elevated, while the cerebrospinal fluid is normal.

Chronic Conditions. In contrast to acute diseases, chronic hypotonia and weakness in childhood usually are caused by diseases intrinsic to the neuromuscular system. Werdnig-Hoffmann disease, a disorder of the anterior horn cell, causes proximal weakness and hypotonia of variable progression. Atrophy of the tongue and fasiculations and absent deep tendon reflexes are usual features, while sensation and intelligence are normal. These patients commonly succumb to respiratory failure in the first or second decade of life.

Juvenile myasthenia gravis is a disease of the postsynaptic myoneural junction that occurs primarily in females over 10 years of age. Fatigability and generalized weakness are seen. Ptosis and external ophthalmoplegia causing double vision are almost universal findings. The diagnosis is confirmed by a reversal of symptoms after a test dose of Tensilon. Treatment consists of administration of a long-acting anticholinesterase, such as neostigmine.

A number of different diseases can affect the muscles, causing gradual weakness, with intact sensation, no muscle atrophy, and intact bladder and bowel control. Duchenne's muscular dystrophy is an X-linked recessive disorder with a significant rate of spontaneous mutation. There is proximal weakness and the loss of the deep tendon reflexes, with the exception of the ankle-jerk response. Frequently, the problem is first noticed when the child is late in walking unassisted. Marked elevation of the creatine phosphokinase is characteristic, as in the progressive course, culminating in death secondary to respiratory infection or failure. In myotonic dystrophy, the weakness is distal, with myotonia (sustained muscular contractions) being the distinguishing feature. Ptosis is seen, as well.

Differential Diagnosis

History. Once again, attention to taking a complete history is essential, as the several most likely diagnoses should be made evident.

- How rapid was the onset of the disorder? If the hypotonia and weakness developed over a period of minutes or hours, trauma is usually the etiology. Development over several days suggests infections or toxins (Guillain-Barré, peripheral neuropathy, or poliomyelitis) or electrolyte abnormalities (hypokalemia or hyperkalemia). A more insidious onset suggests one of the chronic, primary, neuromuscular etiologies.
- What was the rate of progression of the hypotonia and weakness? Rapid progression occurs in an acute infection or toxin exposure, while a subacute course is seen in the muscle disorders and anterior horn cell diseases. No change suggests a static lesion, as seen in spinal cord trauma.
- At what age did the patient achieve gross motor milestones? This will provide an in-

dication of age of onset as well as severity. Progression implies a period of normal development followed by the loss of previously acquired skills. It must be remembered, however, that since young children develop quickly, a patient who remains at a given developmental level might in fact have a progressive lesion. In general, more acute diseases (toxins, infections, acute trauma) are ruled out if the motor history is abnormal, while a delay is common in Werdnig-Hoffmann disease and the myopathies.

- In which muscle(s) was the weakness first noted? Onset in proximal muscles occurs with muscular dystrophies and Werdnig-Hoffmann disease, whereas distal pathology suggests a neuropathy, myotonic dystrophy, or Guillain-Barré syndrome. Generalized weakness is seen in myasthenia gravis, and intact upper extremity functioning despite leg weakness occurs in spinal cord pathology.
- Does the child have difficulty climbing stairs? This suggests a proximal muscle weakness instead of a distal problem.
- Are there difficulties with bladder and bowel control, as seen in spinal cord pathology?
- Does the patient have difficulty swallowing? This can be a feature of poliomyelitis, myasthenia gravis, myotonic dystrophy, and Werdnig-Hoffmann disease.
- Has there been a recent febrile illness, rash, headache, tick bite, or immunization, which suggest the possibility of the Guillain-Barré syndrome?
- Has there been vomiting and diarrhea or intravenous hydration, which might lead to an abnormal serum potassium?
- Is the child receiving drugs (vincristine, isoniazid) or been exposed to any toxins (lead, hydrocarbons, heavy metals) that could cause a peripheral neuropathy or block the myoneural junction (aminoglycosides)?
- Has there been trauma to the neck or back that could result in damage to the spinal cord?

- Is the child mentally retarded (delayed language or abnormal social-adaptive behavior), suggesting Down's syndrome, Duchenne's syndrome, muscular dystrophy, Prader-Willi syndrome, or myotonic dystrophy?
- Does the child have a voracious appetite, as is seen in Prader-Willi syndrome?
- Are there any family members who are similarly affected? Some disorders are inherited as autosomal dominant (myotonic dystrophy, Ehlers-Danlos syndrome), autosomal recessive (Werdnig-Hoffmann syndrome, limb-girdle muscular dystrophy, Tay-Sachs disease), or X-linked (Duchenne's syndrome) disorders.

Physical Examination. The pertinent findings on physical examination are summarized in Table 4.

Neurologic Examination. The neurologic examination should enable the practitioner to assess the anatomic site of the pathology (Table 5) in addition to suggesting the most likely diagnosis. The findings on the neurologic examination of the child are summarized in Table 6.

CRANIAL NERVES.

III, IV, VI. Ptosis and external ophthalmoplegia occur in myasthenia, while ptosis is almost universal in myotonic dystrophy.

TABLE 4. PHYSICAL FINDINGS IN THE CHILD WITH HYPOTONIA AND WEAKNESS

System	Findings	Possible Diagnosis
General	Chronically ill	Renal tubular acidosis, acute lymphoblastic (anemia)
	Obese	Prader-Willi
	Tall, lanky	Marfan's, Ehlers-Danlos
	Fever	Poliomyelitis
Skin	Loose, elastic skin	Ehlers-Danlos
	Erythematous rash	Dermatomyositis
	Petechial rash	Enterovirus
HEENT	Large tongue	Hypothyroidism
Neck	Palpable thyroid	Hypothyroidism
	Nuchal rigidity	Poliomyelitis
Lungs	Acute respiratory distress	Werdnig-Hoffmann, poliomyelitis, Guillain-Barré, muscular dystrophy
Heart	Cardiomegaly, murmur	Down's syndrome, Duchenne's (late)
Abdomen	Umbilical hernia	Hypothyroidism
Genitalia	Hypogonadism	Prader-Willi
Rectal	Decreased sphincter tone	Spinal dysrhaphia or trauma
Back	Scoliosis	Muscular dystrophy, Werdnig-Hoffmann, myotonia
	Sacral dimple or hair tuft	Spinal dysrhaphia
	Lordosis when weight-bearing	Duchenne's, muscular dystrophy
Extremities	Arthrogryposis, club feet	Werdnig-Hoffmann, congenital myopathy, myotonic dystrophy
	Muscle atrophy	Werdnig-Hoffmann, poliomyelitis, peripheral neuropathy
	Muscle pain, tenderness	Myositis
	Calf pseudohypertrophy	Duchenne's

TABLE 5. LEVEL OF NEUROLOGIC PATHOLOGY

Level of Pathology	Diagnosis	Comment
Cerebrum Increased reflexes Upgoing toes Ankle clonus	Cerebral palsy or intracranial bleed	Positive neonatal history Variable retardation Birth trauma Premature, low-birth-weight
Spinal cord Increased reflexes Upgoing toes	Dysrhaphia or transection	Sensory level Bladder and bowel affected Strength intact above level
Anterior horn cell Muscle atrophy Diminished reflexes Downgoing toes	Werdnig-Hoffmann Poliomyelitis Pompe's	Progressive, normal intelligence Tongue fasciculations and atrophy Asymmetrical findings Fever, nuchal rigidity No polio immunizations Retardation and cardiomegaly
Peripheral nerves Absent reflexes Distal weakness Muscle atrophy Sensory defects	Polyneuropathy Guillain-Barré	Family history/offending agent Slowed nerve conduction Exposure to offending agent Ascending, symmetrical weakness Cytoalbuminogenic dissociation
Myoneural junction No muscle atrophy Respiratory distress	Myasthenia gravis Infant botulism	Ptosis, external ophthalmoplegia (+) Tensilon test History of honey ingestion Constipation, drooling

Muscle
Normal reflexes
No muscle atrophy
	Congenital myopathy
	Duchenne's muscular dystrophy
	
	Myotonic dystrophy
	
	Myositis
		Proximal weakness
		Ankle jerk preserved, waddling gait,
		  elevated CPK
		Distal weakness and ptosis, mother's
		  examination is positive
		Elevated sedimentation rate

VII. Facial weakness is seen in myotonia, some myopathies (fascioscapulohumeral), and some cases of the Guillain-Barré syndrome. A blank facial expression is a feature of myotonic dystrophy.

IX, X. Drooling and difficulty in swallowing occur in poliomyelitis, myasthenia gravis, and myotonic dystrophy.

XII. Tongue atrophy and fasciculations suggest anterior horn cell disease, such as Werdnig-Hoffmann and poliomyelitis.

DEEP TENDON REFLEXES. Abnormally increased or brisk deep tendon reflexes, along with positive Babinski signs and ankle clonus, are seen in upper motor neuron lesions that involve the central nervous system or the spinal cord. Examples include cerebral palsy, spinal cord transection, and spinal dysrhaphia. Absent or markedly diminished deep tendon reflexes are always seen in neuropathies (including Guillain-Barré) and anterior horn cell diseases, such as poliomyelitis and Werdnig-Hoffmann disease. The deep tendon reflexes are usually normal but sometimes decreased later in the course of the muscular dystrophies, Prader-Willi syndrome, and myositis. The reflexes are always preserved in myasthenia. However, in Du-

TABLE 6. NEUROLOGIC EXAMINATION FINDINGS

Examination	Finding	Diagnosis
Cranial nerves	Ptosis	Myasthenia gravis, myotonia
	External ophthalmoplegia	Myasthenia gravis
	Facial weakness	Myotonia, fascioscapulohumeral dystrophy, Guillain-Barré
	Drooling, difficulty swallowing	Poliomyelitis, botulism, myasthenia gravis, myotonia
	Tongue atrophy and fasciculations	Poliomyelitis, Werdnig-Hoffmann disease
Deep tendon reflexes and Babinski sign	Brisk with ankle clonus and upgoing toes	Cerebral palsy, intracranial bleed, spinal dysrhaphia, or cord transection
	Absent or diminished	Peripheral neuropathies, Guillain-Barré, poliomyelitis, Werdnig-Hoffmann, infant botulism, aminoglycosides
	No change	Prader-Willi, inborn errors of metabolism, muscular dystrophy, myositis, myasthenia gravis
	Ankle jerk preserved	Duchenne's muscular dystrophy
Sensation	Diminished	Peripheral neuropathies
Gait	Wide-based	Muscular dystrophies
	High-stepping	Peripheral neuropathies
	Toe-walking	Muscular dystrophies, Werdnig-Hoffmann disease
Muscle strength	Proximal weakness	Muscular dystrophies, myopathies
	Distal weakness	Peripheral neuropathies, myotonia
	Fatigability	Myasthenia gravis, hyperthyroidism

chenne's muscular dystrophy, all deep tendon reflexes are lost, with the exception of the ankle-jerk response. Hung-up reflexes (prolonged contraction phase) is a feature of hypothyroidism.

The diagnosis of myotonic dystrophy is aided by tapping the thenar eminence or tongue to see the myotonic response (sustained contraction). Often, the diagnosis can be confirmed by documenting myotonia in the patient's mother.

SENSORY. Any paresthesia or loss of sensation implies that the process primarily involves the peripheral nerves. Paresthesias are not seen in myopathies, central nervous system disease, or anterior horn cell disease. Pinprick, light touch, position, and vibratory sense should all be tested. Alterations in light touch and vibratory sense are seen in neuropathies, while decreased pain sensation is a feature of spinal cord transection and Werdnig-Hoffmann disease.

GAIT. The child must be observed walking, specifically to see if his gait is wide or narrow-based and to see if he is capable of heel-walking, toe-walking, and tandem gait. A child with a myopathy will have a wide-based waddling gait with toe-walking. Footdrop or a high-step gait is indicative of a peripheral neuropathy.

STRENGTH. It is often necessary to differentiate muscle weakness due to a myopathy from that caused by a peripheral neuropathy. Classically, the weakness of myopathy involves proximal muscle, i.e., shoulder and hip, so that the deltoid and iliopsoas muscles should be tested. In peripheral neuropathies and myotonic dystrophy, the weakness is distal, so that there is a footdrop while walking. The child should be asked to climb stairs and to get up from the floor. If he assists himself by placing his hands on his legs (Gower's sign), hip weakness (myopathy) is proven.

In general, good muscle strength despite significant hypotonia is seen in children suffering central nervous system disease, while a decrease in both strength and tone are seen in disorders of the neuromuscular system. Excessive fatigability, as seen in myasthenia, is elicited by asking the child to perform repetitive actions, such as climbing stairs or making fists. Fatigability is a feature of hyperthyroidism, also.

Children with myotonic dystrophy are unable to release the examiner's hand after shaking and have garbled speech after eating ices.

Laboratory Examinations. As for the floppy infant, consideration will be given only to the examinations that a generalist might request.

Serum Enzymes. Most useful is the creatine phosphokinase, which is markedly elevated in Duchenne's muscular dystrophy. High levels are seen also in other muscular dystrophies (limb-girdle, fascioscapulohumeral), Werdnig-Hoffmann, myotonic dystrophy, and muscle trauma. The CPK is normal in neuropathies and myotonic dystrophy. Other assays, such as aldolase, SGOT, LDH, and SGPT, are also elevated in myopathic conditions, but there is no definitive pattern to discriminate one disease from another.

Lumbar Puncture. An examination of the cerebrospinal fluid is indicated in any hypotonic patient who is febrile with meningeal signs or is suffering an acute change in the level of consciousness. In the Guillain-Barré syndrome of any etiology, the protein is elevated without a pleocytosis. In poliomyelitis an elevated protein can be seen along with a lymphocytosis. On occasion, the protein is elevated with peripheral neuropathies.

Tensilon Test. This is indicated in any patient with generalized weakness, ptosis, ophthalmoplegia, and dysphagia, suggesting myasthenia gravis. The dose is 0.2 mg/kg up to 10 mg maximum of Tensilon (edrophonium).

Serology. If Guillain-Barré is suspected, serologic testing for *Mycoplasma*, Ebstein-Barr virus (heterophil antibody), and herpes zoster is indicated.

Other Tests. Specific tests should be performed to rule out suspected systemic diseases (thyroid functions, blood urea nitrogen and creatinine, complete blood count). An ESR and collagen-vascular work-up (antinuclear antibody, lupus erythematosus preparation, VDRL) are indicated if a myositis is suspected.

If the suspected diagnosis is a primary neuromuscular disorder, a neurologist should be consulted to facilitate the further work-up with specialized examinations (e.g., electromyography, nerve conduction studies, muscle biopsy).

Schema for Evaluation

A careful history should enable the practitioner to decide whether the illness is acute or chronic in nature. The physical examination will add other clues, especially whether the weakness is primarily proximal or distal or if the illness is outside the neuromuscular system (central nervous system, endocrine, renal, collagen-vascular, and so on). A schema for the evaluation of neuromuscular diseases follows.

Acute proximal weakness is caused by myositis, acute myoneural blockade, and possibly myasthenia gravis. Removal of any offending agent, an erythrocyte sedimentation rate, and the Tensilon test should help to establish the diagnosis.

Acute distal weakness suggests the Guillain-Barré syndrome or a peripheral neuropathy. If there is any possible offending agent, it should be removed. A lumbar puncture is indicated to differentiate these two. If spinal cord pathology is the etiology, the CSF opening pressure will be elevated (compression) or the fluid will be xanthrochromic (trauma).

Chronic proximal weakness is caused by a primary muscle disorder or myasthenia gravis. If ptosis and double vision are findings, a Tensilon test is mandatory. If the neurologic examination reveals loss of all deep tendon reflexes except for the ankle-jerk, the diagnosis is Duchenne's muscular dystrophy. Otherwise, these are the patients who should be seen by a neurologist for a complete neuromuscular evaluation.

Finally, chronic distal weakness is seen in myotonic dystrophy and hereditary polyneuropathies. The patient's mother must be tested for a myotonic response, especially if ptosis is noticed. Otherwise, these patients also are referred to a neurologist for work-up.

Management

Unfortunately, most of the diseases considered here have no specific treatment. Many conditions, such as Down's syndrome, Prader-Willi syndrome, and spinal cord transection and dysrhaphia, involve static lesions without any expected progression of the hypotonia. For such patients, management consists of special education, physical therapy and range of motion exercises, splints to prevent flexion contractures, bladder and bowel hygiene programs, and attention to other involved organ systems. The management of these patients is usually shared with a neurologist and rehabilitation specialist.

Many of these children are confined to a wheelchair or bed and, therefore, are prone to decubitus ulcers. Frequent position changes, lamb's wool padding, and rigid skin care protocols can minimize the incidence of skin breakdown and subsequent bacterial infection. Once an ulcer has occurred, aggressive therapy is indicated, including wet-to-dry dressings, avoidance of sitting or supine postures, and antibiotics (dicloxacillin or cephalosporin). This should facilitate healing and prevent extension to an osteomyelitis.

Patients with myotonic dystrophy, myopathies, and Werdnig-Hoffmann disease all will suffer lifelong, progressive, incurable disabilities. Therefore, treatment is aimed at maximizing the quality of life, as described above, and maintaining mobility for as long as possible with the use of braces, night splints, and exercises. These patients eventually suffer pulmonary complications secondary to their muscle weakness, with aspiration pneumonias and eventually respiratory failure. Acute episodes are treated with vigorous pulmonary toilet and broad-spectrum antibiotics, with particular attention to anaerobic coverage (penicillin, clindamycin). In some centers, tracheostomies are performed to facilitate the removal of secretions.

In the cases of peripheral neuropathy or Guillain-Barré syndrome, the offending agent should be removed if possible. Once again, there is no specific treatment, only supportive measures to maximize function once the patient's strength returns (e.g., exercises, splints).

The patient with myasthenia is treated with an anticholinesterase, such as neostigmine bromide. If unsuccessful, thymectomy and corticosteroids may be of value.

Specific treatment for any non-neuromuscular disease is mandatory. This may involve thyroid replacement, corticosteroids (dermatomyositis and polymyositis), bicarbonate therapy (renal tubular acidosis), and so on.

No matter what the diagnosis, if the genetics of inheritance is known, genetic counseling is mandatory so that there will not be other affected siblings without the parents' knowledge of the chances of recurrence.

BIBLIOGRAPHY

Arnon SS, Midura TF, Clay SA, et al.: Infant botulism:Epidemiological, clinical, and laboratory aspects. JAMA 237:1946, 1977

Dubowitz V: Muscle Disorders in Childhood. Philadelphia, Saunders, 1978

Evans OB: Polyneuropathy in childhood. Pediatrics 64:96, 1979

Hanson PA: "Floppy baby" (Oppenheim's disease, amyotonia congenita). Pediatr Ann, 1977

Markland LD, Riley HD: The Guillain-Barré syndrome in childhood. Clin Pediatr 6:162, 1967

Rabe EF: The hypotonic infant, a review. J Pediatr 64:422, 1964

Rapin I: Progressive genetic-metabolic diseases of the central nervous system in children. Pediatr Ann, 1976

Spiro AJ: Approach to diagnosis in the child with muscle weakness. Pediatr Ann, 1977

Wright FS: An approach to hypotonia in children. Postgrad Med 50:116, 1971

Cross-Reference to *Pediatrics*, 17th ed.

FOURTEEN

Diagnosis and Management of Jaundice

Gabriel Dinari and Michael I. Cohen

DEFINITION

Clinical jaundice results from the staining of tissues with bilirubin. While this is a dramatic manifestation of hyperbilirubinemia, jaundice may not become obvious until the bilirubin concentration exceeds 6 mg/dl in the neonate or 2.5 mg/dl in the older infant and child.

A serum bilirubin concentration exceeding 1 to 1.5 mg/dl is considered to be physiologic in the first 1 or 2 weeks of life but is otherwise always abnormal and may suggest a variety of clinical situations, including hematologic, hepatobiliary, metabolic, and infectious disorders. Bilirubin is an innocuous metabolic compound except in the newborn, where it may cause brain injury. Thus, the etiology of neonatal jaundice should always be promptly investigated to avoid permanent damage.

Several approaches to the classification of jaundice exist, but one of the more useful is that which separates the causes of jaundice into those with unimpeded bile flow and those with reduced or obstructed bile flow. The first group is characterized by an increase of the unconjugated fraction of bilirubin. It is due to excessive pigment formation or a deficiency of the hepatic uptake of bilirubin from the plasma or of the bilirubin-conjugating mechanism within the hepatocyte. Unconjugated hyperbilirubinemia (UHB) is therefore generally defined as a state in which the conjugated fraction is 15% or less of the total bilirubin concentration. If it is greater than 30%, a conjugated hyperbilirubinemia (CHB) is said to exist.

Causes of jaundice associated with reduced or obstructed bile flow and defined as demonstrating a CHB are often referred to as "cholestatic" conditions. These are associated with the retention of substances normally excreted in bile, such as conjugated bilirubin, bile acids, and cholesterol. They may be due to hepatocellular damage, functional disturbances in bile excretion, or mechanical obstruction to the flow of bile. Morphologic hallmarks include cholestasis with plugs of bile in hepatic biliary canaliculi and degenerative changes in the hepatocytes. Rarely, in such entities as the Dubin-Johnson and Rotor syndromes, there is a presumed hereditary metabolic defect of bilirubin excretion but not of other biliary components, and a CHB is the principal finding.

Some clinical entities may present with unimpeded bile flow (UHB) or with reduced or obstructed bile flow (CHB). Severe hemolytic anemia may be associated with hepatocellular damage and a CHB, although hemolytic states usually demonstrate UHB. Similarly, sepsis, galactosemia, and Wilson's disease are usually characterized by a CHB but may sometimes initially present as a predominantly UHB.

ETIOLOGIC CLASSIFICATION OF JAUNDICE

Significant jaundice in the newborn and young infant is unique in that it may be the initial manifestation of a serious metabolic, infectious, or structural disease. The potential severity of the jaundice is clearly influenced by the state of maturity of the infant. Most importantly, the pigment alone may cause brain injury in this vulnerable population. The etiologic considerations are thus different from those at any other age and are noted separately (Tables 1, 2, 3, 4), although the definitional issues of conjugated versus unconjugated bilirubin cited above remain very useful in approaching the differential diagnosis of infants and children with jaundice.

Some Disorders Associated with Unconjugated Hyperbilirubinemia

Physiologic jaundice of the newborn. Over 90% of newborns have serum unconjugated bilirubin concentrations which exceed 1.5 mg/dl during the first week of life. Jaundice appears during the second or third day of life, rarely exceeds 12 mg/dl in the term neonate, and persists for about a week. These infants are clinically well and have no abnormalities on physical examination, and, except for the hyperbilirubinemia, laboratory studies are normal. In the premature infant, serum concentrations may reach 15 mg/dl, peak at 5–7 days of age and return to normal after 2 weeks.

TABLE 1. ETIOLOGIC FACTORS INVOLVED IN PREDOMINANTLY UNCONJUGATED HYPERBILIRUBINEMIA IN INFANCY

Physiologic jaundice	Crigler-Najjar syndrome
Hemolysis	Gilbert's syndrome
Rh, ABO, or minor group incompatibility	Galactosemia
G6PD deficiency	Intestinal obstruction
Pyruvate kinase deficiency	Pyloric stenosis
Hemoglobinopathies	Annular pancreas
Spherocytosis	Duodenal, jejunal, or ileal atresia
Nonspherocytic hemolytic anemia	Meconium plug or ileus
Polycythemia	Hirschsprung's disease
Maternofetal or fetofetal transfusion	Drugs
Delayed cord clamping	Vitamin K analogs
Placental insufficiency	Novobiocin, chloramphenicol
Maternal diabetes	Parenteral nutrition solutions, sulphonamides
Hematoma	Digoxin, gentamicin
Cephalhematoma	Hypoglycemia
Subdural hematoma	Hypothyroidism
Tissue bleeding	Generalized septicemia
Jaundice associated with breastfeeding	Hypoxia
Lucey-Driscoll syndrome	Acidosis

TABLE 2. ETIOLOGIC FACTORS INVOLVED IN PREDOMINANTLY CONJUGATED HYPERBILIRUBINEMIA IN INFANCY

Infections
  Toxoplasmosis
  Cytomegalovirus
  Rubella
  Hepatitis B
  Coxsackie virus
  Herpes simplex
  Varicella zoster
  Echovirus
  Adenovirus
  Listeriosis
  Syphilis
  Reovirus
  Bacterial infections
Specific metabolic and genetic disorders
  Hereditary fructose intolerance
  Galactosemia
  Tyrosinemia
  Cystic fibrosis
  Alpha-1-antitrypsin deficiency
  Niemann-Pick disease
  Gaucher's disease
  Wolman's disease
  Cholesterol ester storage disease
  Glycogen storage disease
  Chromosomal disorders
    Trisomy 17-18, 21, Turner syndrome
  Zellweger's syndrome
    (cerebrohepatorenal syndrome)
  Dubin-Johnson syndrome

Drugs, phenols, parenteral nutrition solutions
Severe hemolysis
Hypoxia
Congestive heart failure
Intrahepatic cholestatic syndromes
  Familial persistent or recurrent intrahepatic
      cholestasis
    Byler's disease
    Aagenes syndrome
    Arteriohepatic dysplasia
    Inherited defects in bile acid metabolism and
      secretion
    Idiopathic benign recurrent intrahepatic
      cholestasis
  Sporadic (nonfamilial) persistent or recurrent intra-
      hepatic cholestasis
  Paucity of intrahepatic bile ducts
Anatomic biliary tract disorders or obstruction
  Biliary atresia
  Biliary hypoplasia
  Choledochal cyst
  Caroli's disease
  Bile plug syndrome
  Spontaneous perforation of extrahepatic bile ducts
  Compression of bile ducts from enlarged lymph
      nodes, abdominal mass, duodenal atresia
  Duplication of bile ducts
  Hemangioma of bile ducts
Idiopathic neonatal hepatitis syndrome

At virtually every juncture along the normal pathway of bilirubin metabolism, one may invoke an etiologic basis for the formation of physiologic jaundice in the newborn. Bilirubin production is increased from non-heme sources and as a result of decreased erythrocyte life span. Defective hepatic uptake of unconjugated bilirubin circulating in the plasma, decreased activity of the hepatic conjugating enzyme, UDP-glucuronyl transferase, and the increased enterohepatic circulation of previously conjugated bilirubin are among the factors contributing to this neonatal hyperbilirubinemia. These normal metabolic pathways are even more compromised in the premature infant. Factors, such as fasting, hypoalbuminemia, acidosis, respiratory distress, and certain drugs, may increase circulating bilirubin levels while simultaneously increasing the unbound protein fraction and the risk of central nervous system tissue injury.

Hemolysis. This is one of the most frequent causes of neonatal jaundice. ABO or Rh blood group incompatibility may cause severe jaundice developing during the first 36 hours of life. Anemia, hepatosplenomegaly, and hydrops may develop. Hereditary spherocytosis and G6PD deficiency are relatively

TABLE 3. ETIOLOGIC FACTORS INVOLVED IN PREDOMINANTLY UNCONJUGATED HYPERBILIRUBINEMIA IN OLDER CHILDREN

Hemolysis
  Congenital hemolytic anemias
  Autoimmune hemolytic anemia
  Hemoglobinopathies
  Hemolytic-uremic syndrome
  Hypersplenism
  Generalized septicemia of bacterial or viral
    origin
  Wilson's disease
Gilbert's syndrome
Congestive heart failure
Hyperthyroidism
Type II Crigler-Najjar syndrome

common congenital causes of hemolysis and neonatal jaundice. A positive family history is often present. Because of genetic heterogeneity, an increased risk of neonatal jaundice exists in caucasians and orientals with G6PD deficiency but is less frequent in full-term black babies. Other congenital defects of the red cell membrane, enzymatic red cell pathways, or the hemoglobin structure are much rarer causes of neonatal jaundice. Hemolysis is also a common cause of UHB in the older child. Adverse drug reactions and autoimmune disorders are much more frequently found in this older group than in the neonate. Wilson's disease at times presents as an acute hemolytic episode and should always be excluded in unexplained hemolysis.

Hematomas. Rapid degradation of hemoglobin and absorption in the circulation of this large pool of bilirubin previously contained in a hematoma may produce bilirubin overload and jaundice. This is mainly a phenomenon of the newborn.

Hypothyroidism. Prolongation of physiologic jaundice may be the initial manifestation of neonatal hypothyroidism. Jaundice persists until appropriate therapy is initiated.

While the mechanism is not clear, it is thought to be due to the defective uptake and conjugation of bilirubin.

Intestinal Obstruction. An UHB occurs in approximately 10% of infants with pyloric stenosis and in a smaller percentage of patients with other causes of upper intestinal obstruction, such as atresia or annular pancreas. Jaundice may appear at any time during the first 2–3 weeks of life, is of variable intensity, and always clears after surgery. Decreased hepatic glucuronyl transferase activity, reduced portal blood flow, and an increased enterohepatic circulation of bilirubin due to hypomotility and fasting may all be responsible for the jaundice.

Jaundice Associated with Breastfeeding. Breastfed infants not infrequently develop a prolonged UHB. The jaundice does not usually become evident before the end of the first week of life. Bilirubin concentrations do not commonly exceed 20 mg/dl, and no case of kernicterus has as yet been described associated with this syndrome. Physical examination is completely normal, and the baby thrives and gains weight adequately. Jaundice may persist for as long as breastfeeding is continued and usually up to several months of age. It decreases within a few days after breastfeeding is stopped and, surprisingly, rarely rebounds if breastfeeding is resumed. Some clinicians use brief cessation of breastfeeding with an associated fall in serum bilirubin levels as a diagnostic test.

The pathophysiology of this syndrome is unclear. A factor inhibiting hepatic glucuronyl transferase activity was found in breast milk, but its specific identification is subject to continued controversy. A steroid, 3-alpha-20-beta-pregnanediol, was initially identified as the inhibitor compound, but evidence now suggests unesterified fatty acids (UFA) as the culprit. Inhibitory breast milks contain abnormal spontaneous lipase activity, and this is responsible for the increased concentrations of UFA. It is postulated that fatty

TABLE 4. ETIOLOGIC FACTORS INVOLVED IN PREDOMINANTLY CONJUGATED HYPERBILIRUBINEMIA IN OLDER CHILDREN

Acute*	Chronic or Recurrent
Infections	Chronic hepatitis (persistent, active)
Viral (hepatitis A, B, non A-non B, CMV, EB virus, herpes)	Cirrhosis
Bacterial	Biliary (cystic fibrosis, ascending cholangitis, biliary atresia, biliary hypoplasia, drugs, idiopathic)
Parasitic	Postnecrotic (hepatitis B, non A-non B, postneonatal hepatitis, inflammatory bowel disease)
Fungal	Metabolic-genetic (may be due to any of the entities detailed in the metabolic-genetic section in Table 2 plus Wilson's disease, Rotor syndrome, Dubin-Johnson syndrome)
Toxic	Congestive (constrictive pericarditis, Budd-Chiari syndrome, veno-occlusive disease)
Drug-induced	Indian childhood cirrhosis
Parenteral nutrition solutions	Idiopathic
Malnutrition	Intrahepatic cholestatic syndromes (detailed in the intrahepatic cholestatic syndrome section of Table 2)
Irradiation	Familial persistent or recurrent intrahepatic cholestasis
Vascular	Nonfamilial persistent or recurrent intrahepatic cholestasis
Congestive heart failure	Paucity of intrahepatic bile ducts
Hypoxia	Anatomic biliary tract disorders
Shock	Sclerosing cholangitis
Postoperative	Caroli's disease
Budd-Chiari syndrome	Choledochal cyst
Vasculitis	Biliary stricture
Disseminated intravascular coagulopathy	
Autoimmune disorders	
Indeterminate	
Reye's syndrome	
Histiocytosis	
Biliary tract disorders or obstruction	
Cholecystitis	
Cholelithiasis	
Choledochal cyst	
Caroli's disease	
Bile duct stricture	
Ascending cholangitis	
Hepatic neoplasms	
Hepatoma	
Lymphoma	
Leukemia	
Hemangioendothelioma	

*Although a distinction has been made between acute and chronic causes of CHB in older children, for purposes of tabulation it should be noted that, infrequently, chronic liver damage may follow an acute insult. Conversely, some chronic disorders may present acutely, so that the distinction made is not as sharp as it might appear.

acids may not be completely esterified in the immature neonatal gut and could then reach the liver and inhibit glucuronyl transferase. Inhibitory milks have recently been shown to facilitate absorption of bilirubin from the intestinal lumen of laboratory animals.

Crigler-Najjar Syndrome. Two variants of this syndrome of chronic congenital nonhemolytic UHB are now recognized. In type I, an inherited autosomal recessive disorder, severe jaundice occurs shortly after birth and persists indefinitely. Serum bilirubin levels range between 18 and 50 mg/dl, and kernicterus is an inevitable consequence if prompt treatment is not initiated. There is no hepatosplenomegaly or hemolysis, and severe neurologic defects are the usual causes of death in early childhood.

Type II Crigler-Najjar syndrome is a benign disorder which is inherited as an autosomal dominant with variable penetrance. Jaundice usually appears at birth but occasionally not until later in life. Serum bilirubin concentrations range between 6 and 25 mg/dl but are usually less than 20 mg/dl. Kernicterus is uncommon, and normal survival with no intellectual impairment is the expected clinical course of this disorder. In both types I and II of the syndrome, hepatic bilirubin glucuronyl transferase activity is undetectable. Type I is characterized by the absence of bilirubin and its conjugates in the bile, whereas these substances appear in bile in type II patients. Unlike type I, there is a dramatic response to phenobarbital therapy in type II. It has been suggested that type I results from the complete absence of bilirubin conjugation, while in type II, there is an inability to add a second glucuronic acid molecule to the bilirubin-monoglucuronide moiety. Phototherapy and/or exchange transfusion are the limited therapeutic options for the infant with the type I defect, and neither is very acceptable.

Gilbert's Syndrome. This syndrome is characterized by mild UHB in the 2–3 mg/dl range and rarely exceeding 6 mg/dl. Liver function tests are normal, and overt hemolysis is absent. Jaundice usually appears after 10 years of age or at the time of puberty, although neonatal cases have been reported. The level of the hyperbilirubinemia fluctuates and is exacerbated by infection or physical exertion. Occasionally, abdominal discomfort and malaise may accompany the jaundice. Familial transmission appears as an autosomal dominant with variable penetrance, and males are affected more often than females. The pathogenesis is not completely known. Decreased hepatic glucuronyl

transferase activity and impaired hepatic uptake of circulating bilirubin have been documented. Bilirubin overproduction and mildly reduced red cell survival are often associated findings. Fasting, especially lipid deprivation, increases the serum bilirubin level, and this may be used as a diagnostic aid. Administration of phenobarbital reduces the jaundice, but its use is not recommended for this benign albeit lifelong condition.

Disorders Associated with Conjugated Hyperbilirubinemia

Acute Viral Hepatitis. Infectious agents (bacterial and viral) may cause hepatic damage and jaundice at any age. In the neonate, extrahepatic manifestations, such as microcephaly, chorioretinitis, cataracts, or hepatosplenomegaly, often point to the correct diagnosis as well as the specific etiologic agent. In most instances, specific viral agents can be clearly identified. In other cases, especially in the newborn, the clinical picture may be indistinguishable from idiopathic neonatal hepatitis or biliary atresia. Generalized bacterial infections should always be considered in the differential diagnosis of jaundice at all ages even if other features of sepsis are absent. Urinary tract infection caused by *Escherichia coli* is the usual source of sepsis associated with jaundice in the older child. Hepatocellular and canalicular dysfunction, as well as hemolysis, are among the factors responsible for the production of jaundice in bacterial infections in these children. However, in most children, acute viral hepatitis resulting from one of three viral groupings is most frequently observed. The viruses causing hepatitis A (HAV) and hepatitis B (HBV) have recently been well characterized. HAV is a 27 nm RNA virus, while HBV is a 42 nm DNA virus. The entire HB virion, called the Dane particle, has an outer shell containing a surface antigen (HB_sAg) and an inner portion containing a core antigen (HB_cAg). A soluble antigen (HB_eAg) is associated with chronicity and infectivity. The distinction between HAV and HBV infections has allowed the further discovery that about 80% of postperfusion-associated hepatitis and 15 to 20% of non HAV clinical viral hepatitis are caused by one or more additional viruses, now termed non A-non B. The clinical manifestations associated with these various viruses are similar. There is usually a prodromal stage lasting about a week and characterized by anorexia, nausea, and vomiting. The latter symptoms clear rapidly with the onset of jaundice. The icteric phase lasts 1–4 weeks, with complete recovery in most cases.

Anicteric hepatitis occurs in over 90% of the patients who are infected and may be completely asymptomatic. Prolonged cholestasis, or relapsing hepatitis, may occur. Fulminant hepatitis, culminating in hepatic coma and death, has been described and occurs in less than 1% of all infected patients. Chronic hepatitis may follow HBV and non A-non B infections but is not thought to occur after HAV infections. Some differences in the clinical manifestations of the various infections exist. HA hepatitis has a shorter incubation period (15–50 days) than HB (50–180 days) and non A-non B infections (35–70 days). HAV is usually spread through the fecal-oral route from contaminated food and water, while the other viruses are more commonly spread through contact with blood or other body fluids of infected individuals. HBV infection is often associated with extrahepatic manifestations, such as arthritis, nephritis, or a serum sicknesslike disorder, while these associations are rare in the other types of acute viral hepatitis. In most cases of HA hepatitis, the virus is excreted from 2 weeks prior to onset of symptoms up to 1 week after jaundice disappears. The corresponding antibody is detectable 1–4 weeks after exposure, reaches a peak at 4–6 weeks, and may persist for years or become lifelong. The HB_sAg appears 2–5 weeks prior to the onset of symptoms. It is normally cleared from the plasma in 1–5 months but may persist for years in chronic HB infection. The corresponding surface antibody (HB_sAb) ap-

pears 5–6 months after exposure. The core antibody (HB_cAb) is detectable just prior to or at the onset of symptoms, and it falls gradually after recovery, remaining high only in chronic infection. HB hepatitis in the neonate may be acquired directly from the mother during the perinatal period. There is a greater chance of the infant acquiring the infection if the mother had acute HB hepatitis during the third trimester and if she is HB_eAg positive. A chronic carrier state in the mother and infection early during the pregnancy are less often associated with transmission to the baby. Although most infected infants are asymptomatic or become chronic carriers, acute hepatitis with jaundice is a well-documented phenomenon.

Chronic Hepatitis. This diagnosis is established when there is clinical or biochemical evidence of hepatic inflammation for more than 6 months. A history of a preceding acute episode is elicited in only a minority of cases. Two types of chronic hepatitis, persistent and active, can be distinguished on the basis of selective histologic criteria.

Chronic persistent hepatitis is a mild disease with an excellent prognosis. The child is often asymptomatic or may experience mild fatigue, malaise, and abdominal discomfort. Jaundice may be mild and is usually intermittent or absent. The liver is slightly enlarged, and serum transaminase values are only mildly elevated. Histologic review of biopsy material reveals inflammation that is usually confined to the portal spaces. No treatment is recommended for this illness.

Chronic active hepatitis is a serious disorder which may progress to cirrhosis, liver failure, and death. It is associated with HB hepatitis, non A-non B infections, and certain drugs, such as methyldopa or isoniazid, but in many instances the etiology is unknown. Wilson's disease may sometimes present as chronic active hepatitis. The clinical features are very variable. Childhood and adolescence rather than infancy are peak periods for this disorder, and there is a marked female preponderance. An acute hepatitis-like onset occurs in a third of the children, but an insidious expression is common, with malaise, abdominal pain, and intermittent jaundice. Extrahepatic manifestations are common and include arthropathy, rash, nephritis, thyroiditis, and hemolytic anemia. Laboratory studies reveal elevated serum transaminase levels of more than twice normal, hyperglobulinemia, and impairment of various tests of liver function. Antinuclear, antismooth muscle and antimitochondrial antibodies are often present in the serum of these patients. When chronic active hepatitis is associated with HB hepatitis, often high titers of HB_sAg and DNA polymerase, absent HB_sAb, and the presence of HB_eAg are characteristically found. Changes of acute hepatitis, bridging necrosis, and cirrhosis may be present on review of histopathologic biopsy material, but the most distinguishing feature is the presence of piecemeal necrosis of the portal area limiting plate. Treatment includes the use of steroids with or without azathioprine for those with moderate to severe disease but especially in children who are HB_sAg negative on serologic assessment.

Galactosemia, Hereditary Fructose Intolerance, Hereditary Tyrosinemia. These three entities have similar clinical presentations. Failure to thrive, vomiting, bleeding episodes, jaundice, and hepatomegaly present shortly after birth or when fructose-containing substances are added to the diet in the case of hereditary fructose intolerance. Renal involvement, with a Fanconi-like syndrome is often found. In galactosemia, cataracts may be present at birth or develop later. If the child is not treated, cirrhosis, liver failure, and death may occur.

Alpha-1-Antitrypsin Deficiency. Symptomatic liver disease occurs in 10–20% of patients with the homozygous form of alpha-1-antitrypsin deficiency, usually of the PiZZ phenotype. Prolonged neonatal jaundice with variable degrees of cholestasis is charac-

teristic. Jaundice appears during the first days of life and usually before 10 weeks of age. Many of these infants have a spontaneous remission of the cholestatic phase after a few months but may present later in life with cirrhosis or milder degrees of liver dysfunction. Some infants have a histologic pattern demonstrating a paucity of intrahepatic bile ducts, which is clinically associated with pruritus, hypercholesterolemia, and jaundice lasting for many years. In still others, only a variable degree of biochemical liver abnormalities may be found. Lung disease, especially emphysema, may be noted in the older patients.

Cystic Fibrosis. Jaundice appearing during the first 3 weeks of life is a rare manifestation of cystic fibrosis. Bile and mucous plugs with focal biliary cirrhosis are characteristic histologic findings. Cirrhosis with its various complications is not infrequent in older children and adolescents with this disease.

Wilson's Disease. Because of the accumulation of copper in various organs, especially the liver, jaundice is a potential early presenting finding. Asymptomatic hepatomegaly, progressive liver failure resembling chronic active hepatitis, an acute viral hepatitis-like syndrome, and acute hemolytic anemia are some of the common clinical features which usually occur in children over 6 years of age. Neurologic manifestations, such as speech or behavioral impairment, dystonic movements, and Kayser-Fleischer rings, are later manifestations. The diagnosis is confirmed by finding reduced serum ceruloplasmin and copper levels, increased hepatic copper concentrations, and increased urinary copper excretion in response to a penicillamine challenge. The latter drug is the mainstay of current therapy.

Dubin-Johnson Syndrome. This is a benign familial disorder that is transmitted in an autosomal recessive fashion. The onset may occasionally be abrupt and mimic viral hepatitis but is more usually insidious. It is characterized by a fluctuating and predominantly conjugated hyperbilirubinemia, which may be exacerbated by infection, exertion, emotional stress, or drugs. The disease may clinically manifest itself at any age but is often first recognized in the adolescent age group. While the more commonly used tests of liver function are normal, there is a defect in the excretion of a number of organic molecules in the bile. This is responsible for nonvisualization of the gallbladder on cholecystography. The centrilobular accumulation of pigment gives the liver a characteristic black appearance on biopsy or laparoscopy. An abnormality in urinary coproporphyrin excretion has been described. The prognosis in this disease is excellent, and no treatment is currently recommended.

Intrahepatic Cholestatic Syndromes. Children with cholestasis that is associated with functional abnormalities of bile secretion or nonspecific structural hepatic defects have been described. A few familial syndromes have been recognized, while numerous instances of sporadic cholestasis occur that may mimic the familial syndromes. Jaundice, although occasionally manifest during the neonatal period, often is delayed until later childhood.

Byler's disease is an autosomal recessive syndrome first described in an Amish kindred. Intrahepatic cholestasis occurs within the first half-year of life in 50% of the patients. Pruritus, jaundice, steatorrhea, progressive hepatocellular damage, cirrhosis, and death within the first decade are characteristic. A variant with mental retardation has also been described.

Aagenes syndrome has been reported in several sibships of common Norwegian ancestry. It consists of recurrent episodes of cholestatic jaundice with pruritus persisting throughout childhood. At the time of puberty, these patients develop lymphedema associated with hypoplasia of the lymphatic vessels of the lower extremities, while non-

specific hepatic abnormalities, giant cell transformation, and cirrhosis are also noted.

Arteriohepatic dysplasia is a form of intrahepatic cholestasis with jaundice and pruritus that may occur in the neonatal period and persist into adulthood but with a relatively good prognosis. Cardiac anomalies, especially peripheral pulmonic stenosis, and a characteristic facies of high forehead, deepset eyes, clubbed nose, and pointed chin are constantly noted. Anomalies of the vertebrae, hypogonadism, mild mental retardation, and growth failure coupled with a paucity of intrahepatic bile ducts are characteristic findings, as originally described by Alagille and co-workers.

Benign recurrent cholestasis is a syndrome characterized by episodes of pruritus and jaundice, with variable and often prolonged remissions. The initial episode occurs in about 20% of patients in the first year of life but rarely in the neonatal period. During these cholestatic episodes, serum bile acids and alkaline phosphatase concentrations are elevated. Hepatic histologic changes are nonspecific and nonprogressive. One variant of this syndrome may be the recurrent cholestasis noted during pregnancy.

"Paucity of intrahepatic bile ducts" is the term currently used to replace the syndrome of "intrahepatic atresia" and denotes a reduced number of bile ducts in the hepatic portal spaces. It is now recognized that this is a nonspecific finding and does not imply a primary structural defect as the cause of the jaundice. The paucity of these ducts may be associated with many of the familial or sporadic syndromes of intrahepatic cholestasis already described, with some cases of alpha-1-antitrypsin deficiency, the rubella syndrome, or inborn errors of bile acid metabolism. The extrahepatic bile duct system is usually patent, although secondary intrahepatic hypoplasia may occur in some children with extrahepatic biliary atresia.

Drug-induced Liver Injury. Drugs classified as hepatotoxins either predictably cause liver damage in exposed humans and animals, often in a dose-related mode, or unpredictably cause hepatic injury due to an idiosyncratic host response (Table 5). Sex, age, genetic factors, and nutrition may influence the hepatic response to drugs in either group. Drug-induced jaundice may be either cholestatic or hepatocellular in origin, although mixed types are frequently observed. Rash, arthritis, and eosinophilia are associated with some drug reactions. Androgens and oral contraceptives often cause granulomas, peliosis hepatitis, or adenomas.

Choledochal Cyst. This is believed to be a congenital malformation of the common bile duct. Dilatation may involve the entire common duct, present as a common duct diverticulum or as a choledochocoele of the intraduodenal part of the common duct. There may also be associated cystic dilatation of a variable number of intrahepatic bile ducts. The disease occurs more commonly in females in ratio of about 4:1. In older children, the classic triad is that of intermittent abdominal pain, an abdominal mass, and jaundice. In young infants, the clinical presentation usually consists of prolonged neonatal jaundice. Surgical intervention is clearly the only appropriate treatment.

Bile Plug Syndrome. Some infants with prolonged conjugated hyperbilirubinemia are found to have obstruction of the common bile duct by a bile and mucous plug. This should not be confused with the "inspissated bile syndrome," an obsolete term used to denote prolonged jaundice as a consequence of erythroblastosis fetalis.

Extrahepatic Biliary Atresia. This disorder is characterized by atresia of part or all of the extrahepatic bile ducts and is responsible for approximately one third of the cases of neonatal conjugated hyperbilirubinemia. Jaundice usually becomes manifest during the first 6 weeks of life and is progressive, nonfluctuating, and associated with a firm, enlarged liver and usually acholic stools. In most infants, no other associated anomalies are present. The natural course is that of progressive biliary cirrhosis, with almost certain death before 2 years of age, although a small percentage of untreated infants survive to midchildhood. Although the exact etiology remains unclear, an ongoing obstructive cholangiopathy leading to progressive obstruction of the bile ducts suggested that biliary atresia was one end of an inflammatory spectrum, the other end being idiopathic neonatal hepatitis. Recent data suggest this

TABLE 5. COMMON EXAMPLES OF DRUGS WHICH INDUCE LIVER INJURY

Cholestatic		Hepatocellular	
Predictable	Nonpredictable	Predictable	Nonpredictable
Anabolic steroids	C-17 alkylated steroids	Acetaminophen	Halothane
Azathioprine	Phenothiazines	CCl_4	Isoniazid
Chlorambucil	Chlorothiazide	Methotrexate	Methyldopa
	Diazepam		Rifampin
	Penicillin		Imipramine
	Erythromycin estolate		MAO inhibitors
	Phenytoin		Probenicid
			Sulphonamides

may be secondary to a perinatal reovirus infection. Early diagnosis has become mandatory with the advent of hepatic portoenterostomy, since successful bile drainage may be achieved in up to 80% of the infants operated upon prior to 2 months of age.

Idiopathic Neonatal Hepatitis. The term is reserved only for those infants in whom the etiology remains unknown after an exhaustive diagnostic effort and in whom hepatic histology shows characteristic features of giant cell transformation, bile stasis, and a variable degree of inflammatory cell infiltrates in the portal triad. Together with extrahepatic biliary atresia, it accounts for 70–80% of neonatal conjugated hyperbilirubinemia. The clinical picture is variable. Onset of symptoms may occur at any time after birth, but they appear in the first weeks of life in over 50% of the patients. The infant is most often clinically well but may fail to thrive and develop progressive liver failure. After a variable period of sustained jaundice, frequently lasting weeks to months, the majority of patients recover fully. Hepatic disease may persist in less than 10% of the infants, and a fatal outcome is rare. The prognosis is worse in familial cases.

Cholecystitis. While rare in childhood, acute cholecystitis has been amply documented. Acalculous cholecystitis may be associated with cystic duct malformations, acute systemic disorders, septicemia, or dehydration, but in most cases the etiology is obscure. Acute onset with abdominal pain, vomiting, fever, and jaundice is characteristic. An enlarged gallbladder is often palpable, and treatment is surgical.

Cholelithiasis and associated cholecystitis are probably more common in childhood than previously thought. Many reports of pediatric patients without underlying hemolytic disorders or biliary malformations have appeared, especially among adolescent females. The symptoms of acute calculous cholecystitis in children are similar to those in adults. Fever, right upper abdominal tenderness, and sometimes a mass are typical. Jaundice is often present. New radiologic imaging techniques allow for early diagnosis, and treatment is surgical.

APPROACHES TO THE DIAGNOSIS OF SPECIFIC CAUSES OF UNCONJUGATED HYPERBILIRUBINEMIA

History

A family history of jaundice or anemia suggests the possibility of a congenital hemolytic anemia, such as spherocytosis, G6PD deficiency, or a hemoglobinopathy. The diagnosis of a blood group incompatibility, the Lucey-Driscoll syndrome, and the Crigler-Najjar or Gilbert's syndrome are also aided by a careful family history. Some disorders, such as G6PD deficiency, are also more common in certain geographic regions and among specific racial groups. Consanguineous marriage should raise the possibility of congenital hemolytic anemia, the recessive type of Crigler-Najjar syndrome, and Wilson's disease.

Many perinatal events may initiate or aggravate neonatal jaundice, and such factors should be carefully sought. Congestive heart failure, sepsis, acidosis, hypoxia, prematurity, delayed clamping of the cord, and maternal diabetes are some examples of these perinatal risk factors. The dietary history must be noted, since prolonged unconjugated hyperbilirubinemia in a nursing infant suggests breast milk jaundice. Galactosemia is rarely manifested as an unconjugated hyperbilirubinemia in infants consuming lactose-containing diets.

Some disorders associated with jaundice have a sex predilection. G6PD deficiency is sex linked and appears mainly in males, while hypothyroidism is 3 times more common in girls. Certain drugs and foods specifically initiate hemolysis in G6PD-deficient subjects or cause an autoimmune hemolytic anemia. The specific age of onset of jaundice is among the most vital historical facts to be obtained, since it often excludes many possible entities.

Physical Examination

The child with physiologic jaundice, Gilbert's syndrome, breast milk jaundice, and an absorbing hematoma is usually well and thriving. Sepsis should be suspected in a lethargic and poorly feeding infant while acute hemolysis at any age may cause tachycardia, weakness, and congestive heart failure. Splenomegaly may accompany some congenital hemolytic anemias. Cephalohematomas, other enclosed hematomas, or signs of bleeding anywhere should be carefully noted.

The signs of syndromes associated with polycythemia should be sought. The features of the infant of a diabetic mother are well known. A pale twin suggests a fetofetal transfusion, and a small for gestational age infant may be a result of placental insufficiency. An increased incidence of polycythemia occurs in Down's and Beckwith's syndromes.

Are early signs of intestinal obstruction present with jaundice? Vomiting, dehydration, the presence of peristaltic waves, a pyloric tumor, and other signs of obstruction are obvious and often point to the correct diagnosis. Signs of neonatal hypothyroidism should be sought in the presence of jaundice, while cataracts, hypoglycemia, and hepatomegaly suggest galactosemia. The latter may rarely present as an unconjugated hyperbilirubinemia.

Laboratory Evaluation

Systematic laboratory evaluation is important for the diagnosis of the specific causes of unconjugated hyperbilirubinemia. Some pertinent studies are presented in Table 6. Serial determination of the serum concentration is the most critical diagnostic approach, as is the need for constant fractionation of the total bilirubin value.

APPROACHES TO THE DIAGNOSIS OF SPECIFIC CAUSES OF CONJUGATED HYPERBILIRUBINEMIA

History

A history of jaundice in the family suggests the possibility of any of the metabolic and genetic disorders or the recurrent cholestatic

TABLE 6. LABORATORY EVALUATION OF UNCONJUGATED HYPERBILIRUBINEMIA

Condition	Test
Hemolysis	Typing of maternal and infant blood groups; complete blood count, red cell morphology; reticulocyte count; peripheral normoblast count; Coombs test; G6PD and pyruvate kinase activity; hemoglobin electrophoresis; osmotic fragility of RBC; serum haptoglobin concentration
Metabolic disorders	Blood and/or serum concentration of glucose, electrolytes, ceruloplasmin, and copper; red cell UDP-galactose-transferase activity; urinary reducing substances
Infections	Urinalysis; bacterial and viral blood, urine, and CSF cultures; appropriate serologic studies for specific etiologic agents
Intestinal obstruction	Appropriate radiographic studies of the intestinal tract
Breast milk jaundice	Demonstration of an inhibitor in milk of glucuronyl transferase activity
Crigler-Najjar syndrome	Decreased or absent liver glucuronyl transferase activity
Gilbert's syndrome	An increased serum bilirubin concentration after fasting

syndromes outlined previously. A history of meconium ileus or chronic lung disease should suggest cystic fibrosis or alpha-1-antitrypsin deficiency. Consanguineous marriage may also point to the possibility of a genetic or metabolic disorder associated with jaundice even if none has been previously described in the family.

A history of repeated abortions may suggest a possible intrauterine infection. Perinatal transmission of HB infection may occur, especially if the mother had acute hepatitis during the third trimester, or if she is a chronic HB_sAg carrier and is HB_eAg positive. A history of maternal medication use or the administration of a blood transfusion should be sought.

A few relatively simple points concerning the dietary history are worthy of note. Symptoms of fructosemia develop only after the addition of fructose-containing foods, such as sucrose or fruits, and symptoms of galactosemia will not develop unless lactose is ingested. Aversion to fructose-containing foods is seen in older children. Ingestion of shellfish or other contaminated foods may transmit hepatitis A infection.

The age and sex of the child remain essential distinguishing factors in several conditions. Biliary atresia is usually manifest during the first 2–6 weeks of life, while the jaundice associated with idiopathic neonatal hepatitis is very variable as to time of clinical appearance. Biliary atresia is considered by some to be twice, and choledochal cyst four times, as common in females as in males while the reverse is found in neonatal hepatitis. In the older child, hepatitis B infection is more common during adolescence, and chronic active hepatitis, especially when HB_sAg negative, is much more common in females, as are cholecystitis and cholelithiasis.

Previous bouts of jaundice often suggest chronic liver disease. Pulmonary infections may signify cystic fibrosis or alpha-1-antitrypsin deficiency, and the presence of cardiac disease suggests congestive liver damage or arteriohepatic dysplasia. Decreased school performance may be a subtle sign of Wilson's disease. A history of prior contact with a jaundiced individual suggests the possibility of hepatitis, as does exposure to inoculations and blood transfusions. Drug abuse, travel to hepatitis endemic areas, or homosexual behavior are all important historical points to note.

Previous surgery may contribute to the development of jaundice. Biliary tract surgery raises the possibility of retained stones or choledochal stricture. Hepatic metastases may cause jaundice after resection of a tumor, while halothane administration will rarely cause hepatitis.

A careful history of the rapidity of the presentation of jaundice is also noteworthy. The onset is usually insidious with extrahepatic obstruction but acute and rapid in hepatocellular disease or with a hemolytic cause for the jaundice. A prodromal stage of anorexia, fatigue, and nausea before the appearance of jaundice suggests hepatitis. While a history of acholic stools implies complete biliary obstruction and is present in 80% of babies with biliary disease in the first 10 days of hospitalization, such stools are also seen in 25% of infants with hepatocellular disease and are, therefore, of interest but not of diagnostic value.

Physical Examination

The majority of infants with conjugated hyperbilirubinemia do not appear clinically well, although the rare infant with Dubin-Johnson syndrome is usually thriving and well. Surprisingly, so may be the child with the earliest symptoms of biliary atresia. A lethargic, jaundiced, and poorly feeding infant who looks ill should be evaluated promptly for a possible septic process. While infants in the initial phase of neonatal hepatitis may look clinically well, feeding difficulties and failure to gain weight are not uncommon soon after the onset of jaundice, and in many of the metabolic disorders associated with jaundice, irritability, diarrhea, and failure to thrive are prominent features.

The older child with acute viral hepatitis or with decompensated chronic liver disease is often severely ill and demonstrates vomiting, malaise, and anorexia. Fever and chills follow, and the patient may progress to symptoms of systemic portal encephalopathy. Many of these features also occur in acute cholecystitis, and thus infection of the gallbladder with or without cholelithiasis must always be considered in the older child and adolescent with presumed acute viral hepatitis. The child with compensated chronic liver disease may appear completely well except for mild jaundice for prolonged periods of time, but, more commonly, chronic liver disease severely affects normal growth and development.

In support of an intrauterine infection as the cause of jaundice, the presence of microcephaly, hepatosplenomegaly, petechiae, cataracts, and chorioretinitis are helpful adjunctive diagnostic features. These findings suggest the possibility of congenital rubella, *Toxoplasma,* or cytomegalovirus infections. Cutaneous vesicles may implicate herpes simplex and myocarditis or meningoencephalitis, Coxsackie B infections. Signs of congenital syphilis are easily recognizable if kept in mind by the astute clinician. The presence of cardiac anomalies strongly suggests the rubella syndrome or arteriohepatic dysplasia. Pulmonic stenosis and peculiar facies with a high forehead, deep and wideset eyes, a pointed chin, and a clubbed nose further point to the latter diagnosis.

Hepatosplenomegaly and a bleeding diathesis in a poorly feeding and vomiting infant should suggest the diagnosis of galactosemia, fructosemia, or tyrosinemia once the proper dietary setting has been established. The presence of early cataracts strengthens the suspicion of galactosemia. The lipidoses may also present with jaundice and hepatosplenomegaly. Biliary atresia has been associated with the asplenia syndrome, as suggested by a midline liver and situs inversus. The signs of Zellweger's syndrome are a high forehead, brachycephaly, hypotonia, hepatomegaly, and cerebral and renal involvement.

The presence of an abdominal mass in the young jaundiced infant should alert the examiner to a choledochal cyst or obstructed extrahepatic bile ducts by extrinsic pressure from enlarged kidneys or an intra-abdominal tumor. Acute hydrops of the gallbladder or cholecystitis in the older infant or child is also associated with jaundice and an abdominal mass.

The presence of jaundice in association with physical signs secondary to chronic liver disease is a critical diagnostic aid. Chronic disturbances of liver function may cause peripheral edema, ascites, distended abdominal veins, cutaneous spider hemangiomata, and signs of portal hypertension or hepatic failure. The presence of these features, however, is not helpful in the specific diagnosis of the chronic disease. Xanthomas tend to be present early in intrahepatic cholestasis or incomplete obstruction but are generally absent in extrahepatic biliary atresia. Pruritus as manifested by evidence of scratching or a rash is often a sign of intra- or extrahepatic cholestasis. Malnutrition and growth retardation are not infrequent in chronic liver disease, and changes in mental status may be due to portosystemic encephalopathy, Wilson's disease, or fulminant hepatic failure.

The consistency and degree of smoothness or nodularity of the liver and spleen may sometimes be of help in suggesting cirrhosis. A tender and slightly palpable liver suggests acute hepatitis, congestive heart failure, or bacterial cholangitis, while a tender gallbladder is often a sign of cholelithiasis with or without cholecystitis. A very large liver extending many centimeters below the costal margin suggests a storage disease, while a small, nonpalpable, and minimally percussable liver usually points to severe cirrhosis.

Laboratory Evaluation

The orderly, systematic, and rapid use of laboratory tests will exclude most diagnostic problems presenting as a conjugated hyper-bilirubinemia. Those that remain include the urgent need to differentiate extrahepatic biliary atresia from other causes of cholestasis in the neonate and young infant and the need to differentiate intrahepatic cholestasis, obstructive jaundice, and hepatocellular damage in the older child and adolescent.

Commonly used tests of liver function, such as serum bilirubin or serum transaminase and alkaline phosphatase activities, have not proved helpful in the differentiation between biliary atresia and neonatal hepatitis. Gamma glutamyl transpeptidase activity of over 300 IU and 5'-nucleotidase levels of over 30 units may have better discriminative value, with the above levels favoring the diagnosis of biliary atresia. Many other tests have been suggested as being helpful in differentiating biliary atresia from neonatal hepatitis, but further studies have shown that significant overlap exists. These less than satisfactory discriminating tests include elevated serum alpha-fetoprotein suggestive of neonatal hepatitis and elevated lipoprotein X, abnormal vitamin E absorption and peroxidase hemolysis, and a decreased ratio of trihydroxy to dihydroxy bile acids, all suggestive of biliary atresia. Among the older, yet more reliable tests used is the ^{131}I rose bengal excretion test. A 3-day stool collection, with careful avoidance of contamination by urine, is essential. Excretion into the stool of over 10% of the administered dose of rose bengal indicates patency of the bile ducts. Stool collection may be replaced or supplemented by serial abdominal x-ray scanning, and the appearance of the radioactive rose bengal in the intestinal lumen indicates patency of the bile ducts.

Recently, scanning by [99m]technetium IDA derivatives has shown promise as an aid in this differential diagnosis. Presence of radioactivity in the intestine within 24 hours of administration of the radioactive compound indicates patency of the bile ducts. However, its failure to appear in the intestinal lumen on scanning has been seen in severe intrahepatic cholestasis associated with neonatal hepatitis. In order to increase the sensitivity of some of these tests, repeat studies after 7–14 days of cholestyramine or phenobarbital treatment is suggested. Decreased lipoprotein X levels and the appearance of intestinal radioactivity after rose bengal or technetium administration indicate patency of the bile ducts. Passage of time and the choleretic effects of the drug explain the better diagnostic results achieved after treatment with either of these two agents.

A recent description of the presence or absence of visual bilirubin on a 24-hour collection of duodenal fluid has been suggested as a rapid and accurate test for differentiating neonatal hepatitis from biliary atresia. Percutaneous transhepatic cholangiography using a thin, flexible needle has been successful in demonstrating the bile ducts in 50% of the cases reported. Ultrasonic examination of the right upper abdominal region showing a gallbladder 1.5 cm or larger correctly excluded biliary atresia in one study. These are all recent advances and, while promising, require further confirmation. Sonography may also identify anomalies, such as a choledochal cyst, a polycystic liver, or the presence of an abdominal mass. If a definitive diagnosis has still not been reached by the use of many, if not most, of the previous tests, percutaneous needle liver biopsy is clearly indicated. An accurate differentiation can be made in over 95% of patients, but if the diagnosis remains in doubt, and patency of the bile ducts has not been established, exploratory laparotomy with intraoperative cholangiography is mandatory. The entire diagnostic work-up must be concluded prior to 2 months of age, as biliary drainage may not be achieved if portoenterostomy for biliary atresia is performed after this age.

The laboratory differentiation of extrahepatic obstruction, intrahepatic cholestasis, and hepatocellular jaundice in the older child and adolescents remains a relatively uncomplicated process. Common tests of liver function, while nondiagnostic, may be helpful in this differential diagnosis. Transaminase activities are more often elevated in hepatocellular disorders, while marked elevation of liver alkaline phosphatase, gamma glutamyl transpeptidase, and 5′-nucleotidase activities suggests a cholestatic syndrome. Improvement of prothrombin time after parenteral administration of vitamin K implies extrahepatic obstruction, and an absence of response is more compatible with hepatocellular disease. An absence of urinary urobilinogen suggests biliary obstruction. Liver biopsy is most often diagnostic in hepatocellular disorders.

Recent advances in abdominal imaging techniques are extremely helpful in the differential diagnosis of a conjugated hyperbilirubinemia. Hepatic scanning with ^{99m}technetium sulfur colloid may identify focal hepatic lesions or point to generalized liver disease, while ^{67}gallium citrate primarily is concentrated in neoplasms and inflammatory tissues, such as hepatic abscess. Technetium-labeled derivatives of hepatic iminodiacetic acid (HIDA) are excreted into the bile even in the presence of jaundice, giving a clear image of the gallbladder and biliary tract. Acute cholecystitis, biliary obstruction, choledochal cysts, and Caroli's disease are some of the conditions that have been easily diagnosed by using these new imaging agents.

Ultrasonography of the liver may also identify focal intrahepatic lesions. Dilated bile ducts suggesting extrahepatic obstruction secondary to an enlarged gallbladder, the presence of gallstones, or a congenital anomaly, such as a choledochal cyst, are all easily diagnosed. Computerized tomography has similar applications and is complementary to sonographic examination of the abdomen.

In rare instances, there may be a need to utilize two diagnostic procedures primarily used in adult patients for identification of le-sions in the biliary tract. They are percutaneous transhepatic cholangiography (PTC) and endoscopic retrograde pancreatocholangiography (ERCP). PTC is performed with a thin, flexible needle. It has a reported success rate in delineating the biliary tract of almost 100% when the bile ducts are dilated and 60 to 95% when they are not. The incidence of bile leakage following the procedure is low, but the complication rate approaches 5%. ERCP has a similar success rate in demonstrating the biliary system, especially when it is not dilated, but it requires very specialized technical expertise. Both procedures appear to have limited applicability among pediatric patients.

APPROACHES TO THE MANAGEMENT OF UNCONJUGATED HYPERBILIRUBINEMIA

Many of the disorders associated with this form of jaundice will be identified and must be treated regardless of the intensity of the jaundice. The major, if not only, objective of management from the perspective of jaundice is the prevention of central nervous system damage and, most specifically, kernicterus. This is an issue only in the newborn, since in older children danger from kernicterus is usually not a consideration. Three major treatment modalities are currently available.

Exchange Transfusion

Usually 2 times the circulating blood volume of the infant should undergo exchange transfusion if the serum bilirubin approaches 20 mg/dl in the full-term patient or 10–15 mg/dl in the premature infant. The presence of complicating factors, such as infection, hypoxia, acidosis, or severe hemolysis, may make exchange transfusion necessary at lower serum bilirubin levels. Specific lower levels have not been universally accepted, but a consulting neonatologist would prove helpful as a member of the team deciding upon the indications for the procedure. This technique allows for a rapid fall in serum bilirubin concentrations.

Phototherapy

Exposure of the affected infant to light at a wavelength of 450 μm reduces serum bilirubin levels through the formation of presumably nontoxic photoisomers. Some side effects have been described, including dehydration and ocular reactions, while other as yet unknown effects may exist. Cholestyramine at 1.5 gram kg/day has recently been shown to shorten the time necessary for phototherapy in term infants. It will also reduce the daily duration of chronic phototherapy in type I Crigler-Najjar syndrome. This technique permits a slow fall in serum bilirubin concentration, and so its use requires initiation at lower serum bilirubin levels than described with exchange transfusion.

Pharmacotherapy

Phenobarbital causes an induction of hepatic enzymes, including glucuronyl transferase, and may also increase the hepatic uptake and excretion of bilirubin. There is a lag period of about 48 hours before its effects are clinically apparent. It has no place in the management of established chronic jaundice, except in the type II Crigler-Najjar syndrome. In this disorder, chronic administration of 5 mg/kg/day causes a reduction of serum bilirubin level. Type I Crigler-Najjar syndrome does not respond to phenobarbital administration. administration.

In the clinically well full-term infant with a low or very slowly rising serum unconjugated bilirubin level and in the absence of any complicating factors, management is relatively simple. It consists of observation and/or a short course of phototherapy. Because of the potential for central nervous system injury when complicating factors, such as prematurity, hypoxia, and infection, are pre-sent, a neonatologist should be consulted early in the course of the disease. Consultation may similarly be required when faced with some of the more uncommon genetic and metabolic causes of neonatal unconjugated hyperbilirubinemia.

APPROACHES TO THE MANAGEMENT OF CONJUGATED HYPERBILIRUBINEMIA

In all instances, no specific therapy for conjugated hyperbilirubinemia is necessary, since an excessive serum concentration of this pigment has no serious consequences short of its cosmetic impact. Therapy is, therefore, directed at specific causes of the jaundiced state. Antibiotic treatment is obviously indicated for all bacterial infections, and diets free of galactose and fructose and low in phenylalanine are employed when the diagnosis of galactosemia, fructosemia, and tyrosinemia, respectively, have been made. Penicillamine is lifesaving in Wilson's disease, and steroid therapy is indicated in many children with chronic active hepatitis.

Nonspecific management is directed toward the maintenance of adequate nutrition and the treatment of general complications associated with acute or chronic liver disease. The diet should be balanced and nutritionally adequate. Medium-chain triglycerides are absorbed in the face of reduced intestinal bile acid concentrations and can beneficially replace long-chain fatty acids in the diet. Water-soluble preparations of vitamins A, D, K, and E should be used.

Cholestyramine binds bile acids in the intestinal lumen and increases hepatic bile acid secretion in those children where some bile flow into the intestine exists. This orally administered exchange resin is given in doses of 4 to 8 g/day to neonates and up to 16 g/day to older children, in divided doses and with meals. The drug should be given especially at breakfast, so that the resin may bind with the large amount of bile released from the gallbladder after an overnight accumulation. Cholestyramine therapy causes reduction in serum bilirubin and bile acid levels, alleviation of bile salt-induced pruritus, and the disappearance of skin xanthomas. Mild steatorrhea, metabolic acidosis, intestinal obstruction, and unpalatability are the major complications attendant on its use. Phenobarbital has also been shown to have a salutory effect on enhancing bile acid secretion and thus is helpful in some cases of intrahepatic cholestasis. Both drugs have been used in combination.

Hepatic portoenterostomy, as described by Kasai and others, has now been shown to result in successful bile drainage and a concomitant fall in serum bilirubin in up to 80% of infants with biliary atresia operated upon prior to 2 months of age. Unfortunately, the presence of bile drainage does not avoid repeated bouts of cholangitis. Portal hypertension and progressive liver disease with cirrhosis occur in a large number of these infants. Choledochal cyst, choledocholithiasis, cholecystitis, and other causes of extrahepatic obstruction may require surgical correction with a prompt fall in some bilirubin concentrations. All other medical and surgical treatment modalities are not primarily employed for the relief of jaundice. Improvement, as evidenced by a fall in serum bilirubin, is a minor secondary gain associated with a vigorous approach to the underlying hepatobiliary problem.

Most of the disorders causing a conjugated hyperbilirubinemia in the neonate have a prolonged or even lifelong effect on the child and his environment. A consultant should become involved early during the diagnostic and therapeutic efforts. If the possibility of a potentially operable disorder seems likely, a pediatric surgeon is needed promptly. In the older child, many of the acute causes of jaundice are self-limiting disorders and can be managed comfortably by a primary care physician. When, however, the etiology is unknown, the course is complicated, or the child's condition deteriorates, consultation should be sought immediately. Chronic liver disease at all ages continues to pose a major therapeutic dilemma.

BIBLIOGRAPHY

Abramson SJ, Treves S, Teele RL: The infant with possible biliary atresia: Evaluation by ultrasound and nuclear medicine. Pediatr. Radiol 12:1, 1982

Alagille D, Odievre M: Liver and Biliary Tract Disease in Children. New York, Wiley, 1979

Andres JM, Mathis RK, Walter WA: Liver disease in infants, parts I and II. J Pediatr 90:686, 864, 1977

Chandra RK (ed): The Liver and Biliary System in Infants and Children. Edinburgh, Churchill Livingstone, 1979

Javitt NB: Cholestasis in infancy. Status report and conceptual approach. Gastroenterology 70:1172, 1976

Morecki R, Glaser J, Cho S, Balistreri W, Horwitz M: Biliary atresia and reovirus type 3 infection. N Engl J Med 307:481, 1982

Ostrow JD: Jaundice in older children and adults. Algorithms for diagnosis. JAMA 234:522, 1975

Sass-Kortsak A: Management of young infants presenting with direct reacting hyperbilirubinemia. Pediatr Clin North Am 21:777, 1974

Sherlock S: Diseases of the Liver and Biliary Systems, 6th ed. Oxford, Blackwell, 1981

Thaler MM: Jaundice in the newborn. Algorithmic diagnosis of conjugated and unconjugated hyperbilirubinemia. JAMA 237:58, 1977

Watkins JB, Katz AJ, Grand RJ: Neonatal hepatitis: A diagnostic approach. Adv Pediatr 24:399, 1977

Cross-Reference to *Pediatrics*, 17th ed.

FIFTEEN

The Child with a Limp

Paul Harris

Limp is an extremely common complaint in pediatric practice. It may be subtle or quite obvious, of sudden onset or of long duration, intermittent or persistent, with or without pain. However, limp is never normal, and the symptom should never be considered unimportant or accepted without a thorough investigation to determine its cause.

Limp represents a disturbance of gait, a normal function that is usually taken for granted. Parents will usually not allow symptoms of limp to persist for more than a short time before seeking advice, and pediatricians must be prepared to evaluate the symptom skillfully and with an organized approach to determine its etiology. The causes of limp vary greatly in significance from conditions as trivial as a plantar wart, ingrown toenail, and foreign body to those as serious as septic arthritis and osteogenic sarcoma. Limp or pain in the lower extremities may represent the first manifestation of a systemic or chronic disease, or it may reflect a specific entity localized to the musculoskeletal system.

Although a history of trauma may be helpful in distinguishing between the two broad entities of traumatic vs nontraumatic limp, the presence or absence of such a history may be of no help at all, or it may even be misleading. Active children sustain multiple episodes of minor trauma daily and may be unable to recall a specific significant event even after sustaining serious injury. Conversely, parents or children frequently associate the onset of limp or pain with a specific traumatic event that may bear no causal relationship to it. Since the management and prognosis of traumatic limp differ in such important ways, the unreliability of a history of a very specific traumatic event must be understood.

Unlike disturbances involving the upper extremities, where localization of pain or dysfunction is likely to indicate the specific anatomic site of involvement, the symptom of limp or painful gait is a complex summation of functions of the entire lower extremity and even the lower abdomen. Conditions arising in toes, foot, ankle, leg, knee, thigh, hip, inguinal region, or abdomen may all be contributing factors resulting in limp. Furthermore, conditions affecting the nervous system, skeleton, muscles, joints, skin, soft tissues, and even the psyche may precipitate limping as the major or sole presenting symptom. With the most severe form of limp, the child may refuse to walk, making localization of the problem even more difficult.

DEFINITION

Orthopedic problems involving the lower extremities in children may be classified broadly into two major groups: (1) those that interfere with function, e.g., resulting in limp

TABLE 1. ORTHOPEDIC PROBLEMS OF LOWER EXTREMITIES

Types of Functional Derangements (Limp)

Trendelburg gait (gluteus medius limp)

Gluteus maximus limp

Quadriceps femoris limp

Steppage gait

Short swing gait

Unequal leg length limp

Mimetic limp

Enigmatic limp

Posttraumatic limp

Conditions That Result in Pain without Dysfunction

Trauma to soft tissue, bone

Infection of bone (osteomyelitis), soft tissue

Avascular necrosis, Legg-Calvé-Perthes disease

Vascular, e.g., hemangioma

Congenital

Developmental, e.g., pes planus, pes cavus

Tumor, e.g., osteoid osteoma, osteochondroma, osteogenic sarcoma, leukemia

Ewing's sarcoma, neuroblastoma, neurofibromatosis, benign exostosis and bone cysts

Collagen diseases

Growing pains

Conditions That Cause Pain Associated with Dysfunction

Trauma

Infection of joint

Avascular necrosis of bone, Legg-Calvé-Perthes disease

Vascular

Developmental, e.g., unequal leg lengths

Tumors, advanced

Collagen diseases, advanced involvement of joints

(which we will now define as any disturbance of normal gait), and (2) those that cause pain or leg aches (Table 1). As will be seen, there is a significant overlap of these two groups in that limp causing pain may secondarily interfere with function, even though there is no functional limitation of motion. However, at either end of the spectrum, there are purely functional conditions and purely painful conditions that must be considered.

ETIOLOGY

In general, conditions that combine derangement of function with both limp and pain require urgent and definitive diagnostic evaluation. They represent potentially dangerous situations with significant sequelae if there is a delay between onset of symptoms and intervention, whereas limp without pain usually indicates a less acute process. The dif-

ferential diagnosis of conditions causing both pain and alteration of function is also challenging and extremely important to resolve but here again is of different significance than the combination of alteration of function, limp, and pain.

ETIOLOGY AND CLINICAL FEATURES

Hip

There are four major diseases of the hip that may cause a limp in children: transient synovitis, Legg-Calvé-Perthes disease, slipped capital femoral epiphysis, and septic arthritis. In addition to trauma, a variety of systemic disorders may affect the hip joint and produce symptoms. These include juvenile rheumatoid arthritis, acute rheumatic fever, osteomyelitis, tuberculosis, postviral syndrome, neuroblastoma, collagen disease, and sickle cell disease. Other less common specific conditions that may involve the hip are avascular necrosis of adolescence, osteochondritis dissecans, idiopathic chondrolysis, and congenital hip dysplasia.

Transient Synovitis. Transient synovitis, also known as toxic synovitis, is the most common cause of nontraumatic limp in childhood. Although this condition is relatively benign, self-limited, and of short duration, it is very significant because of potential difficulties in distinguishing it from other more serious conditions.

Transient synovitis occurs in children of both sexes between the ages of 2 and 12 years, but it is most common in boys between the ages of 5 and 10. The etiology is unknown, but many children have an antecedent history of a mild viral illness, such as an upper respiratory infection, associated with intermittent fever.

The presenting complaint is usually the gradual onset of unilateral limp. The child may complain of knee or hip pain and often will bend forward at the hip on the affected side, since flexion of the joint relieves symptoms. The child either refuses to walk or manifests a mildly painful gait with only moderate discomfort and is usually afebrile but occasionally has a low-grade fever.

Examination of the hip reveals no tenderness, warmth, or swelling, but discomfort is elicited on extension, internal rotation, and abduction of the hip. The gait and natural resting position of the affected side reflect flexion, external rotation, and adduction of the hip joint.

Legg-Calvé-Perthes Disease. Legg-Calvé-Perthes disease is a potentially serious condition if not recognized early. Fortunately, it is not as common as generally thought. It has an estimated annual incidence of 1:18,000, occurs most often in Caucasian children between the ages of 4 and 9 years, and has a sex predominance for boys over girls of 5:1.

Legg-Calvé-Perthes disease is an aseptic or avascular necrosis of the femoral head and is usually considered to represent an osteochondrosis of the capital femoral epiphysis. The etiology is unknown. Low-birthweight children, children with constitutional delay of growth, and children with retarded bone age have a significantly higher incidence than the general population. Children with an antecedent history of transient synovitis are susceptible. The condition is bilateral in 10–18%, and there is an increased familial frequency.

Children with Legg-Calvé-Perthes disease most often present with an intermittent limp of insidious onset, associated with knee pain. The gait is antalgic, with pain in the groin, lateral hip, or inner aspect of the knee. However, there may be no pain at all, and often the history is so subtle that the diagnosis is delayed because the parents or the physician do not attribute sufficient significance to the symptoms.

On examination there is shortening of the stance phase in symptomatic children, and there is limitation of internal rotation and abduction on passive manipulation of the hip joint. In long-standing cases, there may also be some flexion contraction and mild atrophy of the leg muscles on the affected side. These children are afebrile.

Slipped Capital Femoral Epiphysis. Slipped capital femoral epiphysis is a serious, common condition of obese preadolescents or early adolescents. It occurs in males between 10 and 17 years of age and females between 8 and 15 and is bilateral in 20–30% of patients. Before fusion of the epiphyseal plate has taken place, males have the disorder 2–4 times more frequently than females; blacks are more predisposed than whites. About 80% of cases fall into this category, with a slowly progressive chronic slip of the femoral shaft off the capital head through the epiphysis. The remaining 20% have a more acute process, usually associated with significant trauma. This latter group is comprised of younger children, including newborns, who have sustained shearing trauma, especially from automobile accidents or abuse. Typical presentation of the former, larger group involves an antalgic gait with pain in the knee, groin, buttock, or lateral hip. Again, the limp may be subtle or intermittent and the pain not particularly severe. A chronic low-grade slip may be exacerbated by superimposed trauma. Symptoms may have been present for many months before being recognized, but the moment the diagnosis is suspected or confirmed, immediate hospitalization is indicated to prevent further slip.

The physical examination is performed classically by placing the child in the supine position and passively flexing the hip. In the patient with slipped capital femoral epiphysis, the hip will abduct and rotate externally instead of flexing in the same neutral plane as the knee. This maneuver should be made a part of the routine examination for adolescents, as the history of limp or pain may frequently appear later in the course of the disease.

Septic Arthritis of the Hip Joint. Septic arthritis is the most important diagnosis to make promptly in the differential diagnosis of hip joint disease. In its classic form, the findings are fairly straightforward, but atypical or early presentations may mimic other conditions. Subsequent morbidity due to destruction of the femoral head and neck is directly proportional to duration of delay in recognition and instituting treatment. This condition must be considered, therefore, whenever there is recent onset of limp associated with joint findings. The diagnosis must be made early and treatment instituted promptly.

Septic arthritis of the hip joint may arise at any age from the neonatal period through adolescence. It is usually bacterial in origin, with organisms entering the joint space via a hematogenous route from a distant site of infection or by direct skin portal of entry from recent trauma or puncture. Pneumonia, otitis media, pharyngitis, or skin infection have all been associated with subsequent septic arthritis. Organisms responsible for the infection include *Haemophilus influenzae* in neonates and young infants, and the pneumococcus, streptococci, the gonococcus, and salmonella, the latter occurring especially in children with sickle cell disease.

The history is that of a sudden onset of fever, hip pain, limp, or total failure to move the extremity, often associated with or following an infection.

On examination, the patient appears seriously ill. Pain is elicited by any movement of the affected joint, with swelling and erythema overlying the proximal thigh. The joint is splinted in flexion, external rotation, and abduction. Tenderness to palpation of the overlying soft tissues is often elicited.

Other Conditions.

Rubella Vaccination. Arthritis lasting for variable periods of time (sometimes as long as a year) has been reported following rubella vaccination. Myeloradiculitis involving the lumbosacral region may cause an aching in various locations of the lower extremity. The gait is described in typical cases as toe walking with both hips and knees flexed.

Sickle Cell Disease. Children with thromboembolic crisis may have pain in any extremity and may limp or refuse to walk. In addition, sickle cell disease may produce an aseptic necrosis of the femoral head indistinguishable from Legg-Calvé-Perthes disease.

Appendiceal Abscess. Occasionally, a child with a retroperitoneal abscess presents with a limp. The patient walks bent over from the waist because of hip flexion; a low-grade fever may be present.

Inguinal Adenitis. Adenitis causing tenderness or pain in the inguinal region may present as limp. This condition may be due to a variety of systemic or cutaneous causes, including cat scratch fever.

Posttraumatic Limp. Following injury, with or without casting, children may limp for prolonged periods of time after the original injury has healed. These patients are sometimes referred to as having the "stiff knee syndrome," which may be due to either voluntary limitation of motion or decreased range of motion about the knee joint from prolonged disuse.

Toddler's Fracture. Without the parents being aware of it, young children may sustain significant injury to the lower extremities while learning to walk and run or while in the playpen. These injuries include spiral fractures of the tibia and impacted (torus) fractures of the tibia resulting from compression injury.

Mimetic Limp. "Mimetic limp" is the term used to describe children who imitate an older person who limps and may thus be brought to the pediatrician. The child may be imitating a much admired person in the family, such as grandpa or an uncle, who receives much secondary gain and attention from a chronic condition resulting in limp or use of a cane. Children are great imitators and will unintentionally develop a mimetic limp that focuses the center of attention on them. At other times, anxiety over a close relative's serious or fatal illness may lead a child to subconsciously experience the same symptoms as the affected individual. Limp is one of the more commonly shared symptoms that may be an expression of anxiety. A careful family and social history will help to elucidate this symptom, which is suggestive of an emotional problem and should not be ridiculed as a form of malingering. Once the relationship of the child's limp to an affected family member, close friend, or TV personality is determined and the patient has an opportunity to verbalize his feelings, the symptom usually disappears. If, however, the symptom is of long standing or of great importance to the child's current mechanisms of coping, more aggressive psychosocial intervention may be required.

Disorders Involving the Knee

The knee is a common site of pathology that results in the symptom of limp. The knee is essential for normal gait, all ambulatory activity, and standing. One general rule is that conditions affecting the knee joint usually interfere with the joint function per se, i.e., flexion, and not with the stance phase of gait or locked position. More frequently, the knee buckles or causes pain when flexed but remains relatively asymptomatic and stable in full extension, even with a significantly weakened quadriceps femoris musculature.

The most common conditions affecting the knees include chondromalacia, osteochondritis dissecans, acute leukemia, sickle cell anemia, hemophilia, Osgood-Schlatter disease, subluxation or dislocation of the patella, and injuries of the menisci.

Nonspecific or systemic conditions that may affect the knee include juvenile rheumatoid arthritis, acute rheumatic fever, osteomyelitis, suppurative arthritis, neoplasms, and trauma, including fracture, periostitis, tendonitis.

Osgood-Schlatter Disease. Probably the most common condition involving the knee region is Osgood-Schlatter disease. This painful entity is most common in preadolescents and adolescent children who are actively engaged in contact sports; basketball seems to be a particularly common offender. In prior years, Osgood-Schlatter disease, which does not actually involve the joint itself, was most prevalent among males, but with the more recent increased participation of girls in competitive sports, the sex ratio has shifted toward equality.

The diagnosis of Osgood-Schlatter disease is made on clinical grounds alone and should be suspected whenever there is pain and swelling with tenderness over the anterior tibial tuberosity. X-rays are not helpful, since the tibial tubercle is usually irregular, and there are no radiographic criteria for the diagnosis. The condition, which represents a partial avulsion of the tibial tubercle at the insertion of the patellar tendon, is self-limited and responds to conservative management, namely, rest, diminution of precipitating sporting events, and analgesics. A discussion with the family and patient usually suffices to balance the degree of athletic activity against the degree of symptomatology. Recurrences are common until growth is completed in late adolescence, when the only residual is nontender "knobby knees."

Chondromalacia Patellae.

Chondromalacia patellae may be related to excessive athletic activities or trauma. It involves the knee joint itself and is not necessarily self-limited. Degenerative softening of cartilage results from repetitive mechanical stress from direct trauma or indirect forces sustained during strenuous physical activity, such as jogging, cycling, or calesthenics.

Another cause of this condition is excessive femoral anteversion, with compensatory external tibial torsion leading to patellofemoral malalignment syndrome. When the patella is pulled laterally out of its groove by the quadriceps tendon, undue stress leads to chondromalacia.

Osteochondritis Dissecans.

Osteochondritis dissecans is another condition of the knee joint (less frequently other joints) affecting predominantly adolescent males and resulting in intermittent painful limp following strenuous activity. It is often associated with stiffness, a clicking sensation, buckling, or locking phenomena. It is due to separation of a fragment of cartilage from its underlying subchondral bone, which subsequently undergoes vascular necrosis, becoming detached and floating free in the joint space. A

family history or history of trauma may be helpful.

Other Conditions.

A variety of other traumatic conditions of the knee, including subluxation, dislocation or fracture of the patella, meniscus injuries, and fracture of the anterior tibial spine, result in functional impairment of the knee joint with antalgic gait. Two painful conditions that do not usually limit function but result in chronic pain especially prominent at night are various tumors of bone and "growing pains." The most common tumor is the benign osteoid osteoma, which is diagnosed by x-ray. Growing pains, which occur in a significant percentage of 4–14 year olds, cannot be dismissed by even the most skeptical clinicians, even though their etiology and pathogenesis remain obscure. Perhaps the single most important aspect of this symptom is that it not be dismissed as an inconsequential condition without adequate history and physical examination to rule out underlying organic disease. At best, this is a diagnosis of exclusion, but since all diagnostic procedures are within normal limits, good judgment must be used to determine the extent of the work-up indicated.

Foot Pain

Limp in children can also be caused by pain in the foot. Table 2 lists the major etiologies that must be considered.

As may be seen from Table 2, the causes of foot pain are multiple but may be divided according to the frequency of this occurrence in various age groups. It is beyond the scope of the chapter to describe individually all the causes of foot pain. It may be noted, however, that developmental conditions, such as pes cavus and pes planus, stress fractures, and sprains, and certain tumors of bone are more likely to appear in older children, whereas infections, occult fractures, and inflammatory conditions are more prevalent in younger children. Conditions, such as ill-fitting shoes,

TABLE 2. PROBABLE CAUSES OF FOOT PAIN BY AGE

0–6 Years	6–12 Years	12–19 Years
Ill-fitting shoes	Ill-fitting shoes	Ill-fitting shoes
Foreign body	Foreign body	Foreign body
Occult fracture	Accessory navicular	Ingrown toenail
Osteomyelitis	Occult fracture	Pes cavus
Juvenile rheumatoid arthritis	Tarsal coalition (peroneal spastic flatfoot)	Hypermobile flatfoot with tight Achilles tendon
Rheumatic fever	Ingrown toenail	Ankle sprains
	Ewing sarcoma	Stress fractures
		Ewing sarcoma
		Synovial sarcoma

From: Gross R: Pediatr Clin North Am 24:815, 1977.

foreign body, plantar warts, and trauma, may occur at any age.

The major function of shoes at any age, including infancy, is to protect the feet from trauma, such as puncture wounds. Children and infants who go without shoes (especially in summertime) will be exposed to a greater variety of traumatic conditions than those wearing shoes or sneakers. A history of going barefoot is helpful in arriving at the diagnosis of local trauma.

DIFFERENTIAL DIAGNOSIS OF THE CHILD WITH A LIMP OR PAINFUL LOWER EXTREMITY

Since the majority of children with limp or lower extremity pain come first to the attention of the pediatric practitioner rather than a specialist (orthopedist, neurologist, rheumatologist), and since many of the conditions responsible for those symptoms can and should be managed principally or with subsequent consultation by primary practitioners, such practitioners must be thoroughly familiar and comfortable with the differential diagnosis of limp, as well as the diagnostic work-up and management. Even with a history of trauma, the limping child should not be immediately or automatically referred, since this common condition usually can be managed entirely by an experienced pediatric practitioner. On the other hand, there are many conditions that require surgical intervention or diagnostic procedures that involve surgical skills and expertise for which a consultant or specialist is required promptly in order to participate early in the course of events. The practitioner must, therefore, have a general familiarity with all of the most common causes of limp or pain and also know when and whom to call for consultation. Consultation with an orthopedist or other specialist does not mean automatically relinquishing clinical responsibility for the child but rather an ongoing presence and partnership with the consultant. Particularly since many of the conditions to be considered may or may not require surgery or other unusual procedures, the practitioner has an important role to play in participating with the consultant and family in decisions concerning whether a particular diagnostic or therapeutic plan is warranted or indicated.

In the following sections, we outline the various aspects of history, physical examination, and laboratory investigation helpful in the differential diagnosis. In each instance, however, the approach embodies the following principles:

1. The most common conditions causing limp or lower extremity pain usually involve trauma, which should be the first diagnosis considered.
2. Conditions that are most likely to result in progressive damage must be ruled out promptly.
3. Noninvasive techniques that may be applied simply by the pediatrician should be considered before more aggressive invasive procedures.
4. The necessity for consultation with an appropriate specialist (orthopedist, neurologist, physical therapist) should be considered at each step along the way.
5. Refinement of the diagnosis to include the less frequent causes of limp should be considered as additional clinical data are gathered.

It is imperative that communication with patients and their parents be maintained throughout the orderly process of arriving at a diagnosis. In addition to meeting their psychologic needs, their participation will enhance the physician's ability to arrive at an accurate assessment and to assure compliance with the therapy indicated. Just as it is nonproductive for the physician to consider either rare or the most serious causes of limp first in the differential diagnosis, it tends to be more helpful to parents to inform them about positive findings and pertinent negative findings and to discuss the most probable causes of the limp or pain that their child is experiencing, rather than to burden them with the entire gamut of less likely and more serious possibilities.

History

It is frequently stated that the history is the most important part of the physician-patient encounter, that up to 90% of diagnoses can be made on the basis of history alone, that the physical examination constitutes another 5% and that the remaining 5% is accomplished through diagnostic procedures. Assessment of a child with limp or lower extremity pain

conforms to this generalization. Although a greater proportion of information than usual is provided by further diagnostic procedures, mainly radiographs, 50% of diagnoses can be made from history alone. The most salient points in the history include the following.

- *Age.* Certain conditions occur more often at specific ages, e.g., slipped femoral capital epiphysis 10–17 years (adolescents), Legg-Calvé-Perthes disease 4–9 years, osteogenic sarcoma and Ewing sarcoma in the second decade of life.
- *Sex.* Congenital dislocation of the hip has a 6:1 preponderance in females vs males, and Legg-Calvé-Perthes is 5 to 6 times more common in boys than girls.
- *Race.* Although some conditions are rare in certain ethnic groups, e.g., Ewing sarcoma in blacks, too much significance cannot be placed on race as a differential point in the history.
- *Onset.* When was the limp or pain first noted? Was it sudden, gradual, or insidious? These questions will help to clarify the duration or chronicity of the condition. It is most important to determine whether or not it is a condition of recent onset or is long standing. Conditions with sudden or recent onset are more likely to be secondary to trauma or to require more aggressive, prompt intervention. The limp or pain associated with Legg-Calvé-Perthes disease, slipped capital femoral epiphysis, or juvenile rheumatoid arthritis may well be intermittent, whereas persisting pain of recent onset may be associated with toxic synovitis or septic arthritis.
- *Character of Pain.* Is the pain or limp intermittent or constant? Is it severe, mild, or only present at certain times? Is it worse during the day or night? Does the pain interfere with normal activities, such as running or walking? Symptoms in conditions involving bones, such as osteoid osteoma, are likely to be more severe at night, whereas conditions involving joints or weight-

bearing surfaces become more symptomatic with daytime activities.

- *Location of Pain.* Where is the pain experienced most acutely? It may be extremely helpful if the child or parent can localize the pain to a particular region of the lower extremity, such as the toes, foot, ankle, or knee. One significant exception to this rule involves knee pain. A history of pain in the knee may indicate a local problem, such as arthritis, osteomalacia of the patella, or a problem with ligaments or cartilage of the joint. Knee pain, however, is a frequent complaint in conditions affecting the hip joint, such as Legg-Calvé-Perthes disease or slipped capital femoral epiphysis. Children with either of these conditions may have no symptoms referable to the hip but present only with referred intermittent knee pain. Similarly, back pain in children may be a symptom of problems with the lower extremities, such as the fairly common condition of unequal lengths of the legs, which may produce an almost unrecognizable disturbance in gait. Even intra-abdominal conditions, such as acute appendicitis, may cause an abnormal gait and lower extremity pain on the affected side; inguinal adenitis may also produce a painful gait. Is there a history of trauma? What are the circumstances surrounding the incident? As previously mentioned, a history of trauma may be exceedingly helpful in elucidating the problem, but it may also be misleading. The absence of a definitive history of trauma does not rule it out as the precipitating event.

- *Systemic Symptoms.* Does the ill child have any more generalized symptoms or signs? Is there a history of fever or rash? Are joints other than the lower extremity involved? Is there weight loss, fatigue, or anorexia? A history of fever associated with joint pain should alert the clinician to such conditions as septic arthritis, toxic synovitis, juvenile rheumatoid arthritis, and acute rheumatic fever, whereas the absence of fever or other systemic symptoms is more likely to implicate trauma, developmental conditions, or tumor. Leg pain may be the presenting complaint of a child with acute leukemia who subsequently is noted to have other manifestations of systemic illness.

- *Function and Limitation of Motion or Activities.* Does the presenting pain or discomfort interfere with, alter, or curtail daily activities, such as school sports, climbing stairs, walking, running? Osgood-Schlatter disease may be exacerbated by and prevent active participation in contact sports but may cause relatively little discomfort while swimming or bicycling. Is there limitation of motion or pain involved in a particular joint? Where does the patient think the pain emanates from?

- *Relief of Symptoms.* What treatment or home remedy seems to relieve the pain? Does aspirin or rest help? Does using either exacerbate or relieve symptoms? Is the condition more noticeable at the beginning of the day or in the evening? Joint pain associated with juvenile rheumatoid arthritis is classically more prominent in the morning but becomes less noticeable as things loosen up during daytime activities.

- *Family History.* Do other family members have or have they had similar symptoms? Children are great imitators and may at times mimic a favorite relative or other household member for attention or other secondary gain. Some conditions, such as unequal leg lengths, have a familial pattern, which may be revealed by an accurate history. What do the family and the patient think is the cause of the pain or limp? This seemingly naive question will frequently bring out pertinent historical data that would not otherwise have been gleaned by routine questioning. In addition, it will inform the pediatric practitioner of what the family is most worried about and whether it is real or irrational. Of course, this question may also elicit a great deal of material that is or appears to be irrelevant, but the time it takes is usually well spent.

Physical Examination

A complete and thorough physical examination should always be done. Evaluation of the apparent site of pain or dysfunction must include examination of all adjacent structures, including abdomen, back, and inguinal region, before any further diagnostic procedures are considered. Since many of the specific entities being considered affect the function of walking, observation of the child's stance and gait, with and without shoes and with and without clothing, should be made. It is often helpful to ask the cooperative child to run back and forth, as this action may accentuate, unmask, or eliminate an otherwise subtle or exaggerated limp.

In order to analyze disturbances in a limping child, it is essential to understand the components of a normal gait. Gait is an effortless action of rapidly alternating movements of the lower extremities divided into a stance phase (weightbearing phase) and a swing phase (nonweightbearing, movement phase). In walking, as opposed to running, one lower extremity is always in the stance phase while the opposite is in the swing phase. The upper body remains erect without sideways motion, and arm swing is passive. During the swing phase, which emanates from the hip, there is flexion of the knee and ankle (plantar flexion), and when the foot lands, there is flexible heel strike followed by toe off without any slapping motion.

The following sequence is helpful in the examination: Observe the child's stance when he is completely undressed and look for symmetry of both extremities. Avoidance of heel or toe walking indicates foot problems. Check for equal levels of the iliac crests, and measure leg lengths from the anterior-superior iliac spine to the medial malleolus. It is also useful to measure thigh and calf circumferences to detect muscle wasting or hemihypertrophy. Inspect the skin for any discoloration, rash, sites of trauma or puncture, and swelling over joints. At this time, it is helpful to ask the child to point with one finger to where it hurts most. Next, observe the child in the sitting position, and again check the levels of the iliac crests from behind. Unequal leg lengths cause asymmetry of heights of the iliac crest while standing but not in the sitting position. Inspect the feet and toes for plantar lesions or lesions of the toes, such as ingrown toenails.

After evaluating joint and limb function, observe the active phase of walking, standing, and running as described above. The child is examined in the supine position, undressed except for underclothes, for passive range of motion and stability of all joints. In the knee one determines stability in the anterior-posterior and lateral-medial stressing maneuvers and examines for crepitance and pain on flexion. It is also helpful to examine the patient's shoes to determine excessive or uneven wear.

Local knee joint tenderness, joint effusion, atrophy of the quadriceps muscles, and a positive McMurray test (flexion and extension of the knee with the tibia externally rotated and internally rotated producing a palpable and painful clunking) are indications of traumatic knee injury, especially to a meniscus.

The hip joint should be passively flexed fully in the prone position. If the thigh abducts and externally rotates, it is almost pathognomonic for slipped femoral capital epiphysis. The feet should be palpated for flexibility and suppleness, and the entire region of suspected pain or dysfunction should be palpated for tenderness. Table 3 indicates the diagnoses to be considered with certain physical findings.

Hip.

Slipped Capital Femoral Epiphysis. In this condition, the laboratory findings are normal, and the diagnosis is made on clinical and radiological grounds alone. Posterior-anterior, frog leg, and lateral views must be obtained in order not to miss subtle or early findings. Initially, there is an increase in the width of the epiphysis with irregular margins. As the condition progresses, there is a

TABLE 3. CHARACTERISTICS ON PHYSICAL EXAMINATION OF VARIOUS DISORDERS OF THE LOWER EXTREMITY

Part of Body	Abnormal Physical Findings	Etiology To Be Considered
Hip joint	Abduction, external rotation on flexion	Slipped capital femoral epiphysis
	Obesity, limp, external rotation, decreased hip rotation	Slipped capital femoral epiphysis
	Trendelenburg gait/sign, decreased abduction	Congenital hip dysplasia
	Limp, limitation of internal rotation, abduction, may be thigh atrophy	Transient synovitis
	Antalgic gait, limitation of range of joint motion, decreased internal rotation and abduction, flexion contracture, atrophy and tenderness of thigh muscle	Legg-Calvé-Perthes disease
	Swelling of thigh, pain on movement of joint, systemic findings, fever, increased WBC	Septic hip
Knee	Tenderness and swelling over anterior tibial tuberosity	Osgood-Schlatter disease
	Tenderness of patella articular surface, painful crepitance	Chondromalacia patella
	Tenderness of medial condyle, limp, swelling, decreased range of motion	Osteochondritis dissecans
	Mass in popliteal fossa, painless	Baker's cyst
	Joint effusion, localized tenderness over lateral or medial joint, positive McMurray test, atrophy of quadriceps	Menisci injuries
Leg	Painless limp, compensatory scoliosis, unequal leg lengths	Congenital hip dysplasia, congenital neurofibromatosis
	Persistent pain, limp, tender or nontender mass	Tumor: osteoid osteoma, osteochondroma, osteogenic sarcoma, Ewing sarcoma
Foot	Rigidity of foot, deep arch vs absent arch	Pes cavus, pes planus

lateral movement of the femur in relation to the head, which slips medially with shearing of the epiphyseal plate. Discontinuity of the medial border of the head of the femur at the level of the epiphysis demonstrates the degree of displacement or slippage.

Transient or Toxic Tenosynovitis. Laboratory examinations are helpful only because the CBC and ESR are usually normal and, therefore, rule out other conditions. Radiographic examinations of the hip are usually completely normal but occasionally may show some widening of the joint space between the head of the femur and the acetabulum medially and, on traction views, superiorly. A bulge of the capsule is seen rarely on the lateral side, and, on occasion, alterations of soft tissue shadows are seen laterally.

Legg-Calvé-Perthes Disease. The laboratory studies reveal a normal CBC and ESR. The principal aid to diagnosis is radiography, which reveals changes that may be divided into four stages: (1) widening of the distance between the femoral head and the acetabulum, (2) collapse of the femoral head with increased density and characteristic subcapsular semilunar lucencies, (3) increase in width of the femoral neck, and (4) reossification of the femoral head and metaphysis. In early states, before radiographic changes become obvious, a technetium scan will show decreased uptake in the epiphysis, in contrast to the diffuse increase in uptake seen in transient synovitis.

Septic Arthritis. The diagnosis of septic arthritis is suspected clinically and then confirmed by appropriate laboratory tests. It is imperative to make this diagnosis as early as possible to avoid destruction of joint tissues.

Laboratory investigations demonstrate a markedly elevated WBC with a shift to the left and an elevated ESR. Although radiographs of the hip made very early in the course of the disease may be negative, they usually reveal soft tissue swelling, capsular swelling, and lateral and upward displacement of the femur. More advanced cases show subluxation and destruction of the femoral head. In neonates, whose ossification is incomplete, there may be displacement of the medial metaphysis from the acetabulum.

If the diagnosis of septic hip is suspected, needle aspiration of the joint must be performed promptly for both diagnosis and identification of the organism. Recovery of the organism from the hip joint may be unsuccessful, and a negative gram stain or culture does not exclude the diagnosis of septic arthritis. Frequently, the organism is obtained by multiple blood cultures rather than by direct aspiration of the hip.

Knee.

Osgood-Schlatter Disease. The diagnosis rests exclusively on clinical findings. Radiographic evaluation is not helpful or diagnostic and is not indicated. All tibial tubercles are irregular at this stage of development, and there are no radiographic criteria upon which to make the diagnosis. Other laboratory tests are neither necessary nor helpful.

Chondromalacia Patella. Diagnosis of this debilitating condition, which may even lead to joint effusion and weakness of the quadriceps is made primarily on clinical grounds. X-rays are usually not abnormal except in cases secondary to direct trauma. Orthopedic consultation is required for further evaluation, including arthroscopy, which may be definitive; arthrography is helpful only in very experienced hands. Treatment ranges from simple abstinence from offending activities or repositioning cleats to surgical intervention.

Trauma. The laboratory contributes little to the diagnosis of injuries to the knee, such as meniscal tears, subluxation or dislocation of the patella, and fracture of the anterior tibial spine. Arthrography and arthroscopy are usually necessary. Conventional radiographic techniques often fail to reveal the diagnosis.

Osteochondritis Dissecans. In osteochondritis dissecans, x-rays may show the subchondral bone fragment either in position or separated and lying free in the joint space.

Nontraumatic Inflammatory Conditions. The laboratory becomes particularly useful in the differential diagnosis of nontraumatic, acute inflammatory, and arthritic etiologies of limp secondary to joint involvement. We believe that the sedimentation rate is the single most useful test in determining whether or not an inflammatory condition exists and whether or not further laboratory investigation will be useful in arriving at a diagnosis.

The Laboratory Examination

Table 4 indicates laboratory tests that are useful in the differential diagnosis of limp and pain in a child. In the presence of an elevated ESR, it becomes increasingly important for the pediatrician to obtain further diagnostic laboratory determinations, including rheumatoid factor (RF), ANA, HLA-B27, serum

TABLE 4. LABORATORY TESTS IN THE DIFFERENTIAL DIAGNOSIS OF LIMP

Part of Body	Common Diagnostic Considerations	Diagnostic Tests	Results Anticipated
Hip	Slipped femoral capital epiphysis	X-ray (AP frog leg) technetium bone scan	Increased width of epiphysis, frank slip, increased uptake on the joint
	Transient synovitis	X-ray	Usually normal, occasional widening of joint space on traction
		CBC	Normal
		ESR	Usually normal or slightly increased
	Legg-Calvé-Perthes disease	X-ray	Widening of joint space
			Widening of epiphyseal line, increased density of femoral epiphysis, collapse of femoral head, increased width of neck of femur
		Bone scan technetium	Decreased uptake in FC-epiphysis initially, later increased uptake
	Septic hip	CBC	Increased WBC with shift
		ESR	Increased
		X-ray	Increased soft tissue and capsular swelling with lateral displacement of the proximal femur
Knee	Osgood-Schlatter	None	Normal
	Chondromalacia patella	X-ray arthroscopy	Usually normal, rough articular surface
	Osteochondritis dissecans	X-ray	Subchondral bone fragmentation
	Baker's cyst	Transillumination needle aspiration	Positive gelatinous fluid
	Traumatic conditions Dislocation of patella, subluxation of patella, injuries of the menisci, fracture of anterior tibial spine	Radiography Arthrography Arthroscopy	Displacement of patella, bone fragments, degeneration of patella
Leg	(Femur or tibia) osteoid osteoma	X-ray	Radiolucent nidus surrounded by sclerotic bone
	Osteochondroma	X-ray	Ossification
	Osteogenic sarcoma	X-ray	Lytic and calcified areas of bone
	Ewing sarcoma	X-ray	Lytic lesions
	Trauma	X-ray	Various fractures

complement, ASLO titer, and viral titers. As discussed above, the diagnosis of septic arthritis ultimately rests on joint aspiration with demonstration of organisms on smear or culture as well as blood cultures.

An elevated WBC and ESR associated with fever and limb pain also suggest the diagnosis of osteomyelitis. Blood cultures and radiographs should be obtained, but since x-ray findings of osteomyelitis lag 10–14 days behind symptomatology, a radionuclide bone scan is indicated to detect the condition early.

Malignancy. Leukemia also must be suspected in children with persistent lower limb pain, limp, and systemic symptoms. The laboratory diagnosis is often made by obtaining peripheral blood count and x-rays of the affected region that show osteolytic lesions, rarification of the metaphyses, and periostitis in affected joints.

Various tumors of bone, including osteoid osteoma, osteogenic sarcoma, Ewing's sarcoma, and benign exostosis of bone, are suggested by persistent pain sometimes associated with limp. In these conditions x-rays of the affected region may be diagnostic. See Table 4 for diagnostic findings.

Foot. The laboratory is not particularly helpful in conditions of the foot causing pain or limp.

MANAGEMENT

The management of many of the conditions described in this chapter involves the cooperative efforts of the pediatrician and the pediatric orthopedist. Although some of the conditions can be managed by the pediatrician with or without orthopedic consultation, and although many of the conditions require only evaluation and surveillance, the pediatrician must recognize when surgical or invasive diagnostic procedures are indicated and not hesitate to call in an orthopedist promptly. Table 5 outlines the management of various conditions considered in this chapter.

The most important role for the pediatrician is in early diagnosis, prompt and definitive shared management, and subsequent long-term follow-up and emotional support for patient and family.

Slipped Capital Femoral Epiphysis
Treatment of this condition is prompt surgical pinning of the epiphysis to prevent further slippage. Immediate hospitalization and orthopedic consultation is indicated as soon as the diagnosis is established. The pediatrician should provide long-term follow-up and

be aware of the possibility of contralateral involvement at a later date.

Legg-Calvé-Perthes Disease
The role of the pediatrician in Legg-Calvé-Perthes disease is most important in two aspects: (1) the diagnosis must be suspected and established, which requires an appropriate index of suspicion and a correct diagnostic approach, and (2) the pediatrician must participate with the orthopedist and family in carrying out a plan of treatment. Basically, the goals of treatment are to reduce weight-bearing on the affected side over a prolonged period of time, which may involve 2–4 years of continued follow-up and planning. The range of treatment may include periods of bed rest and traction, braces, crutches, or surgical intervention. Since there are many different approaches to eliminating weightbearing, which affect the child's life to varying degrees, the pediatrician must help to plan an acceptable therapeutic program.

Transient Synovitis
Treatment involves bed rest and analgesics for 3–5 days. Although traction has been used by some orthopedists to relieve discomfort, our experience is that this is rarely if ever necessary providing the diagnosis is well established.

The condition is invariably self-limited, of short duration, and usually has no sequelae, although the condition may recur. In addition, it now appears that about 5% of children with transient synovitis of the hip go on to develop Legg-Calvé-Perthes disease, and long-term follow-up studies suggest that there may also be an association with the development of osteoarthritic changes in adulthood. It is unclear at this time whether any form of treatment has a significant influence on the prevention of sequelae.

Septic Arthritis of the Hip
Treatment of a septic hip must be vigorous and combines medical and surgical approaches. Treatment must be instituted im-

TABLE 5. TREATMENT OF ORTHOPEDIC CONDITIONS

Diagnosis	Management by	Treatment
Slipped capital femoral epiphysis	Pediatrician/orthopedist	Urgent surgical pinning
Legg-Calvé-Perthes disease	Pediatrician/orthopedist	Reduce weightbearing long term
Transient synovitis	Pediatrician	Rest, analgesics
Septic arthritis	Pediatrician/orthopedist	Surgical drainage, IV antibiotics
Osgood-Schlatter disease	Pediatrician	Analgesics/decreased activity
Trauma	Pediatrician and/or orthopedist	Rest, casting, surgical reduction
Chondromalacia patella	Pediatrician/orthopedist	Decrease in activities, splinting, surgery
Osteochondritis dissecans	Orthopedist	Casting, surgical removal
Baker's cyst	Pediatrician/orthopedist	Aspiration, no treatment or surgical removal
Ligament and menisci injuries	Orthopedist	Surgical
Bone tumors		
Osteoid osteoma	Orthopedist	Surgical
Osteochondroma	Orthopedist	Surgical
Osteogenic sarcoma	Orthopedist	Surgical
Ewing sarcoma	Orthopedist	Surgical
Pes planus, hypermobile	Pediatrician	None
Pes planus, rigid	Orthopedist	Surgical/arches
Pes cavus, rigid	Orthopedist	Surgical/arches
Achilles tendonitis	Pediatrician	Rest, immobilization
Stress fractures	Pediatrician/orthopedist	Rest, immobilization

mediately following diagnosis, since articular surfaces can be severely damaged within hours. Prognosis is relatively good with proper measures, but ineffective or delayed diagnosis and treatment may result in disastrous consequences.

Osgood-Schlatter Disease

Treatment for this self-limited condition involves rest, analgesics, supportive knee bandaging, knee guards, and avoiding physical activities that may cause exacerbations. The pediatrician must counsel the adolescent and family so that they tailor the child's activities sensibly, avoiding excessive limitation of activity. In some cases a change of major sport activity may need to be advised, but usually a balance between the degree of morbidity tolerable and the amount of activity can be achieved. There are no known sequelae other than "knobby knees."

Trauma

The management of traumatic limp varies greatly depending upon the degree and location of the injury. The vast majority of lower extremity injuries can be managed by the pediatrician alone. Contusions, sprains, strain, and foreign body are far more common than severe fractures or ligamentous tears. In most instances, full function can be reestablished after an appropriate period of rest, elevation, and immobilization. Although pediatricians are becoming more knowledgeable in the management of serious trauma, these conditions should be referred to the orthopedist when there is significant bony or soft tissue destruction.

Knee

Many conditions of the knee in their early stages can be managed by rest, decreased strenuous sporting activities, and even immobilization. Chondromalacia patella and osteochondritis dissecans can be managed conservatively, as can Baker's cyst, which may resolve spontaneously. On the other hand, by the time the diagnosis is established in severe cases, surgical intervention by an orthopedist is warranted. Serious injuries to the menisci and collateral or cruciate ligaments usually require surgical intervention.

While the child with a benign bone cyst, osteochondroma, and even relatively benign osteoid osteomas may be followed by the pediatrician, most tumors or lesions of bone should be evaluated by the orthopedist and are subject to surgical excision.

Foot

Hypermobile Flatfoot and Rigid Foot Deformities.

Flatfoot is neither prevented nor improved by special shoes, arches, or other devices. The pediatrician's role is to help the parent to accept the condition as being within normal limits and to avoid useless special appliances. On the other hand, rigid foot deformities (cavus or planus) are amenable to surgical correction, and pain is often relieved by prosthetic devices.

Achilles Tendonitis. Achilles tendonitis is virtually the equivalent of Osgood-Schlatter disease in the ankle at the insertion of the Achilles tendon and should be managed identically, with rest, analgesics, warmth, and immobilization.

BIBLIOGRAPHY

Chung S: Diseases of the developing hip joint. Pediatr Clin North Am 24:857, 1977

Ferguson A Jr: Pathology and treatment of Legg-Calvé-Perthes disease. Pediatr Ann 2:272, 1978

Fields L: The limping child—a review of the literature. J Am Podiatry Assoc 71:60, 1981

Gross R: Foot pain in children. Pediatr Clin North Am 24:813, 1977

Hensinger R: Limp. Pediatr Clin North Am 24:723, 1977

Peterson H: Leg aches. Pediatr Clin North Am 24:731, 1977

Westin GW: The limping child. Pediatr Clin North Am 14:601, 1967

Cross-Reference—to *Pediatrics,* 17th ed.

SIXTEEN

Lymphadenopathy

Marc Bestak

Enlarged lymph nodes in children are a common finding. Most often, they represent a response to a transient localized infection, but sometimes such enlargement points to a variety of more serious illnesses. The purpose of this chapter is to offer an approach to accurate and efficient diagnosis and management of lymphadenopathy.

DEFINITION OF THE PROBLEM

Lymphadenopathy is the abnormal enlargement of one or more lymph nodes. When single nodes are enlarged or when several nodes are enlarged in one area, the lymphadenopathy is regional or localized. When lymph nodes are enlarged in multiple areas of the body, generalized lymphadenopathy is present. Lymph nodes may be acutely enlarged. Lymphadenopathy persisting more than a month is considered chronic.

Lymphoid tissue may enlarge at different rates in response to antigenic stimuli at different ages. Lymphoid tissue is quite significant at birth, increases in quantity steadily until the teenage years, and then decreases steadily afterward. Lymph nodes are much more commonly palpable in children than in adults. Typically, cervical, axillary, and inguinal nodes are palpable in the normal child. Occipital, postauricular, supraclavicular, popliteal, mediastinal, epitrochlear, and abdominal nodes, if palpated or visualized, signify a state worthy of evaluation.

The spleen and thymus, also lymphoid organs, may seem to be enlarged in normal children. The spleen is palpated in 1 of 7 normal newborns, and in 1 of 15 children less than 10 years of age. A chest x-ray may reveal a large thymic shadow in the first year of life, which disappears by the third year in the normal child.

Lymph nodes may be enlarged because the lymphocytes they contain have proliferated or because the histiocytes typically present in lymph nodes have increased in number. When lymphocytes increase in number, they usually do so in response to an antigen. If the antigen is catabolized to a nonantigenic substance, the lymphocyte proliferation is self-limited, and the lymph node will recede to its previous size. If the antigen persists, as occurs when it is intracellular and cannot be catabolized (as in the case of parasites), chronic enlargement may occur.

Lymph node hyperplasia, an increase in the numbers of normal elements in the lymph nodes, may occur without antigenic stimulation, as in lymphoma and hyperthyroidism. In the histiocytoses, some forms of Hodgkin's disease, and some lipid storage diseases, histiocytes may accumulate. Cells typically extrinsic to lymph nodes may infiltrate them, causing their enlargement. Infectious lymphadenitis is usually the invasion of lymph nodes by polymorphonuclear leukocytes and is a common cause of lymph node enlargement. In addition, extrinsic metastatic tumor cells or leukemia cells may invade the node, enlarging it.

ETIOLOGY

The major disease processes resulting in lymphadenopathy are listed in Table 1. A detailed discussion of each of these entities is beyond the scope of this chapter, but, a brief discussion follows of those conditions most frequently seen in children. More importantly, a reasonable approach to evaluating a child who is found to have lymphadenopathy is presented.

Bacterial Infectious Processes

Bacterial infections lead to lymphadenopathy in the region draining the infected area. *Staphylococcus aureus* is the most common cause of pyogenic infections giving rise to regional lymph node enlargement, as is seen in such conditions as cervical adenitis and skin infections. However, bacteria, such as the group A Beta hemolytic streptococcus and oral bacterial flora (both aerobic and anerobic and from humans and animals), may cause regional lymphadenitis secondary to localized infection.

Mycobacteria, both *Mycobacterium tuberculosis* and the atypical mycobacteria, may cause regional or generalized lymphadenopathy. At the present time, the atypical mycobacteria are a more common cause of cervical node enlargement than *M. tuberculosis*, which is more likely to cause pulmonary or generalized lymphadenopathy.

Viral

Both Ebstein-Barr virus and cytomegalovirus are associated with lymph node enlargement in the *infectious mononucleosis* syndrome. Cervical and axillary lymphadenopathy are common. Pharyngitis, muscle ache, headache,

anorexia, and splenomegaly and hepatomegaly are in evidence. Severe pharyngeal pain is more common in Ebstein-Barr viral infection than in cytomegaloviral infection. Hepatitis with or without jaundice is seen with both, while a vesiculopapular rash develops in patients with Ebstein-Barr virus treated with ampicillin. A number of other viruses may be associated with both regional and generalized lymphadenopathy. Some of these may be recognized by the typical syndromes that they produce, e.g., measles, German measles, varicella, roseola infection, while others have less obvious presentations, e.g., adenovirus, Coxsackie virus, echovirus.

Others

Toxoplasmosis is an infection with an intracellular protozoan that may cause either congenital infection (acquired by the fetus in vivo) or acquired infection. The classic congenital infection presents with failure to thrive, fever, hepatosplenomegaly, generalized lymphadenopathy, microcephaly or hydrocephaly, and chorioretinitis. The acquired infection may be asymptomatic, with signs limited to generalized lymphadenopathy with or without tenderness, or may closely resemble infectious mononucleosis. The diagnosis should be suspected if the patient has had a possible exposure to cat feces, since cats are known carriers of toxoplasma.

Histoplasmosis. Histoplasmosis is a fungal disease caused by *Histoplasma capsulatum*, with findings similar to those of tuberculosis. Calcified pulmonary lesions may be seen on chest x-ray and are associated with mediastinal nodes. Fever, tiredness, cough without sputum production, and failure to thrive are common. Vomiting and diarrhea are also seen. The spleen and liver are usually enlarged, and lymph nodes in regions beyond the thorax are often noted. Other possible findings include meningitis, ulcerations of the skin, mucous membranes, and eye, cardiac inflammation (endocarditis and myocarditis), and bowel disease (ulcerative colitis).

TABLE 1. ETIOLOGY: DISEASE PROCESSES

Infections
Bacterial
  Pyogenic bacterial infection (e.g., *Staphycoccus aureus,* scarlet fever, impetigo, group A β-hemolytic streptococcus, anaerobes)
  Typhoid fever
  Syphilis (See Chapter 37.)
  Tuberculosis
  Plague (bubonic)
  Brucellosis
  Chancroid (See Chapter 37.)
Viral
  Rubella
  Rubeola
  Roseola
  Cytomegalovirus infection
  Mycoplasma infection
  Adenovirus infection
  Herpes simplex infection
  Ebstein-Barr virus (infectious mononucleosis)
Others
  Toxoplasmosis
  Histoplasmosis
  Malaria
  Pediculosis
  Ringworm infection
  Chlamydial infection
  Tularemia

Malignancies
Leukemia
  Acute lymphoblastic
  Acute myeloblastic
  Others
Lymphoma
  Hodgkin's disease
  Non-Hodgkin's lymphoma
Other solid tumors
  Neuroblastoma
  Rhabdomyosarcoma

Immunologically Mediated Inflammatory Disease
Systemic lupus erythematosus (active)
Juvenile rheumatoid arthritis
Serum sickness
Autoimmune hemolytic anemia
Dilantin pseudolymphoma
Angioimmunoblastic lymphadenopathy

Immunodeficiency States with Chronic Lymphoid Stimulation
T cell deficiencies (acquired immunodeficiency syndrome, AIDS)
B cell deficiencies

Deficiencies of Neutrophil Number
Chronic benign neutropenia
Cyclic neutropenia
Drug, viral, or antibody-induced neutropenia
Others

Abnormalities of Neutrophil Function
Chronic granulomatous disease
Chédiak-Higashi syndrome
Job's syndrome
Others

Lipid Storage Disease
Gaucher's disease
Niemann-Pick disease

Diseases of Uncertain Etiology
Mucocutaneous lymph node syndrome (Kawasaki's disease)
Histiocytosis-X
Hand-Schüller-Christian disease
Letterer-Siwe disease

Immunizations
BCG vaccine
DPT and smallpox vaccines (administered to deltoid)

Pediculosis. Pediculosis is the result of infestation with pubic lice, head lice, or body lice. The body louse, in addition to causing an annoying infestation itself, is capable of carrying typhus and relapsing fever. *Pubic lice* cause itching, and the scratched skin often becomes secondarily infected (often with *S. aureus*); resultant inguinal lymph node enlargement is common. Blue spots may occur in the region or on the upper legs or lower abdomen. Nits may be seen on the hair shafts. *Body lice* live in clothing and bedding and are not often found on the skin. Poor hygiene is a necessary condition for the propagation of the nits, since laundering of clothing kills the lice. Itching is associated with wheals. Eczematization and secondary skin infection with regional adenopathy are usually seen.

Pediculosis capitis is associated with head itching. Skin infestation and occipital, postauricular, and posterior cervical adenopathy are common. Lice can most easily be found on the hairs at the back of the ears, and in the occipital region.

Malignancies

Leukemia. Leukemia in childhood occurs most frequently between the ages of 3 and 5 years and is acute lymphoblastic leukemia in 80% of cases. However, presentation may be at any age. Anemia, neutropenia, and thrombocytopenia and their consequences lead to most common presenting symptoms. Thus, lethargy, pallor, anorexia, bone or joint pain, skin or mucous membrane bleeding, and fever are often seen. Generalized lymphadenopathy, hepatosplenomegaly, and an anterior mediastinal mass upon chest x-ray tend to be seen in patients with white blood cell counts greater than 20,000 per mm^3, and teenage males are most likely to have this combination of findings. *Acute myeloblastic leukemia* may present at any age. High white blood counts (often over 50,000 per mm^3) with hepatosplenomegaly and generalized lymphadenopathy are observed even more commonly than in acute lymphoblastic leuke-

mia. In addition to the findings reviewed above common to all the acute leukemias, acute myeloblastic leukemia may also be first considered when a boy develops priapism (unremitting painful penile erection). This latter physical finding is also found in children with sickle cell anemia. The finding of gingival enlargement in a patient not using phenytoin may lead to the diagnosis of *acute monoblastic leukemia,* one of the myeloid leukemias.

There are several disease syndromes in which acute leukemia is considerably more common than in the general population. These include Down's syndrome, Von Recklinghausen's neurofibromatosis, Bloom syndrome, Wistkott-Aldrich syndrome, and ataxia-telangiectasia syndrome. Leukemia is much more likely to occur among identical twins than in the population as a whole.

Lymphoma.

Hodgkin's Disease. Hodgkin's disease is a malignant tumor of the lymphoid system primarily. In the pediatric age group it is most common in adolescents over the age of 15, but it may occur in younger children as well. Presentation is usually with an enlarged *painless* lymph node which is firm, not hard. The clavicular area is involved in 90% of patients. Other possible primary sites include the axillae, mediastinum, and inguinal regions. If lower cervical or supraclavicular nodes are involved on the right side, one quarter of these cases will also have mediastinal or hilar disease. If the left lower cervical or supraclavicular nodes are involved, the spleen and abdominal lymph nodes are more likely involved, and the mediastinum is usually spared. The nodes often change in size. Unlike other lymphomas, Hodgkin's disease rarely occurs in the tonsils or nodes of Waldeyer's ring or in Peyer's patches of the ileum or in epitrochlear nodes. Other symptoms often associated with Hodgkin's disease are tiredness, weight loss, fever, and sweating, particularly at night. Occasionally patients present with the superior vena cava syndrome (neck and face swelling, eyelid and conjunctival swelling, seizures), caused by a large mediastinal mass compressing that vessel. Only rarely do pulmonary involvement, hepatic involvement, bone, or bowel involvement cause symptoms at the time of presentation.

Non-Hodgkin's Lymphoma. This is another group of malignancies affecting the lymphoid organs, which occurs more often among teenagers than in any other group of children and in boys more than twice as frequently as girls. The non-Hodgkin's lymphomas tend to occur much more frequently in children with immune deficiency syndromes than in the general population. Thus, patients with Bruton type sex-linked agammaglobulinemia, severe combined immunodeficiency, ataxia-telangiectasia, and the Wiskott-Aldrich syndrome have a risk thousands of times as great as the general population. Patients treated with immunosuppressive agents, such as those who receive renal transplants or who are treated for systemic lupus erythematosus or for chronic renal disease, also have a higher risk of developing lymphoma. Patients taking phenytoin and mesantoin may have a reaction called "pseudolymphoma syndrome," in which lymphadenopathy, hepatosplenomegaly, fever, rash, and eosinophilia are seen. This condition usually disappears upon discontinuation of the drug, but, recently, true lymphoma has been reported following the use of phenytoin. People who receive significant radiation exposure, such as children who receive thymic irradiation, people irradiated for ankylosing spondylitis, and survivors of atomic bomb explosions all have double the risk of lymphoma.

Lymphadenopathy is the presenting finding in one quarter of patients with lymphoma. Although usually involving cervical nodes, enlargement of axillary, preauricular, epitrochlear, and inguinal nodes may be seen first. The nodes are not tender and are firm.

They are usually unilateral. Often no other symptoms are complained about. However, if the presenting tumor is in the mediastinum, symptoms may include cough, shortness of breath, and the superior vena cava syndrome. Pleural effusion is often seen with mediastinal lymphoma. Hilar node lymphoma is almost always unilateral. The gastrointestinal tract may be the primary site for presentation, with the ileum, cecum, appendix, and ascending colon being the areas involved. Pain, diarrhea, and vomiting are more common than abdominal distention or a palpable abdominal mass. Occasionally, intussusception is caused by intestinal lymphoma, and in children over 6 years old, lymphoma is the most frequent cause of intussusception.

Lymphoma in African black children is most commonly of the type called Burkitt's tumor, a malignancy causing a mass in the jaw. In Americans, Burkitt's tumor presents more often as an abdominal mass, and in one fifth of Americans with this tumor, acute paraplegia secondary to infarction of the spinal cord by pressure of retroperitoneal disease is seen.

Other sites of lymphoma involvement include the bone marrow, meninges, bones, brain, and gonads. The tonsils and Waldeyer's ring are involved in about 10% of cases.

Neuroblastoma. Neuroblastoma is a malignant tumor arising in the adrenal medulla or the sympathetic nervous system in children less than 5 years old; most occur near the age of 2. Presentation in more than 50% is in the adrenal medulla or in a retroperitoneal sympathetic ganglion. One half are calcified, and an intravenous pyelogram demonstrates an inferolateral displacement of the kidney with minimal calyceal distortion. Signs and symptoms are dependent on tumor distribution. Tumors in the sympathetic chain may compress the ureters and cause hydronephrosis. They may compress the bladder, causing frequency or inability to void. Posterior mediastinal tumors may produce dyspnea or obstruction, leading to pneumonia. Paravertebral tumors may compress the spinal cord, resulting in paraplegia. Cervical tumors may lead to eyelid droop (Horner's syndrome).

Two thirds of neuroblastoma patients present with widely metastatic disease to liver, bone marrow, bone, and skin. Generalized hard lymph node enlargement is also common. The skin may be involved with bluish nodules, which, when pressed upon, blanch for several minutes. Hepatomegaly may be massive. Skeletal involvement is most often in the skull and long bones; lytic lesions, often symmetrically placed, cause pain. Orbital soft tissue or bone involvement often produces proptosis, periorbital edema, and eyelid ecchymosis. The bone marrow has evidence of tumor in most cases of metastatic disease.

Most often the child with neuroblastoma is irritable, febrile, and has lost weight. Anemia and thrombocytopenia are also often found. Diarrhea, hypertension, opsoclonus, ataxia, and encephalopathy are other possible but less common findings.

Rhabdomyosarcoma. Rhabdomyosarcoma is a malignant tumor of striated skeletal muscle, occurring most frequently in children 1–5 years of age. It is the most common malignant tumor in children to arise in the bladder, vagina, prostate, uterus, paratesticular region, orbit, middle ear, nose, pharynx, and the soft tissues of the arms, legs, and trunk. The tumors spread locally or via the lymphatic and vascular systems. Regional nodes become enlarged with hard tumor most often if the primary tumor is pelvic or is in an extremity. Other sites of metastases are the lungs, liver, bones, brain, bone marrow, and heart. Cardiac tumor may result in congestive failure.

Immunodeficiency States

Lymphocyte disorders which result in chronic immunoglobulin deficiencies are often associated with compensatory lymph node hyperplasia, which may be massive and suppurative. Furunclosis, tonsillitis, pneumonia, otitis media, and meningitis are frequent in these syndromes. Two forms of B cell abnormalities resulting in immunoglobulin deficiency are Bruton's sex-linked agammaglobulinemia and immunodeficiency with increased IgM (and deficiency of both IgG and secretory IgA). These children with chronic infections, most often with pyogenic organisms, are usually male.

Neutrophil Abnormalities

Chronic Neutropenia. This is a group of disorders in which the number of circulating neutrophils is reduced. Infection usually does not become a major problem until the neutropenia reaches less than 500 per mm³, although children with neutrophil counts below 1,000 per mm³ may recover more slowly from their infections. Patients have varying degrees of infection with pyogenic and enteric bacteria. *S. aureus, Pseudomonas, Escherichia coli,* and other enteric species are most often found in blood, skin, and soft tissue infections. In the mouth, anaerobic organisms may constitute a serious problem for these patients. Regional inflammatory lymph node enlargement is common.

The most common forms of childhood neutropenia are *cyclic neutropenia* and *benign familial chronic neutropenia*. In cyclic neutropenia, neutrophil counts fall to neutropenic levels with a definite periodicity, ranging from 14 to 30 days. The most frequent clinical findings are fever, mouth ulceration, gingival inflammation (which usually begins when the patient's secondary teeth have evolved), skin infection, and otitis media. Regional lymphadenopathy develops frequently. During periods of normal neutrophil counts, these children are well, but the symptoms noted above become prominent during the neutropenic phase. Benign familial chronic neutropenia is a disorder resulting in mild neutrophil deficiency seldom resulting in chronic symptoms, although mild skin furuncules and mouth ulcers may develop. Again, regional inflammatory lymph node enlargement may occur.

Chronic Granulomatous Disease. This is an X-linked disorder of neutrophil bacterial killing resulting from the failure of granulocytes to produce hydrogen peroxide and other bactericidal oxidizing materials. Thus, ingested bacteria, if they do not produce hydrogen peroxide (as, for example, *S. aureus*, with no catalase system), are capable of surviving within the neutrophil. Serious persistent infection may result, most often with the following organisms: *S. aureus, Staphylococcus albus, Klebsiella, Enterobacter, E. coli, Serratia marcescens, Pseudomonas aeruginosa, Aspergillus, Candida albicans, Shigella, Salmonella,* and *Proteus.* Symptoms begin early in life, with head and neck lymph node enlargement frequently requiring repeated drainage. Pneumonia, pulmonary abscesses, skin furuncles, impetigo of the face, and stomatitis are common. Occasionally, osteomyelitis, granulomatous colitis with diarrhea, and perianal abscess may occur.

Diseases of Uncertain Etiology
Mucocutaneous Lymph Node Syndrome (Kawasaki's Disease). This newly recognized clinical syndrome was first described in 1967 by Kawasaki, a Japanese pediatrician who published a report in Japan of a number of children who appeared with a similar constellation of physical findings. Though originally noted primarily in children less than 2 years of age, there have been recent reports in the United States of apparent epidemic outbreaks that have affected older children.

The characteristic presenting findings are cervical lymphadenopathy, fever for at least 5 days and often lasting for weeks, marked bulbar conjunctival infection, a bright red erythematous rash which often begins in the more prominant skin fold areas (cervical, axillary, antecubital, and inguinal), characteristic desquamation under the fingernails and of the palms and soles after 2 weeks of the disease, marked erythema of the lips and pharyngeal area, and often in the first 5 days of the child's presentation, an indurative edema of the hands and feet.

Many etiologies for this syndrome have been hypothesized by both Japanese and American investigators, as there have now been numerous descriptions of outbreaks in the United States (Hawaii, New York, eastern Massachusetts). No singular bacterial, viral, toxic, or other underlying cause has been identified. There have been periodic reports of children with positive serology for leptospirosis, but this has not been found consistently. Pathologically, the syndrome appears to be similar to that in infantile polyarteritis nodosa.

There are no characteristic laboratory findings, except for an elevated $alpha_2$ globulin, elevated ESR, and a thrombocythemia which occurs 5–10 days into the course of this illness. The electrocardiograms are abnormal in 40% of these children during the acute course, though only a small percent have persistent cardiologic abnormalities.

The mortality appears to be 1–2%. The major cause of death being coronary arterial thrombosis and subsequent myocardial infarction and/or ruptured coronary arterial aneurysm. The coronary thromboarteritis usually appears from 10–25 days into the illness and is often manifested by the presence of coronary arterial aneurysms. These aneurysms may be detected by two-dimensional echocardiography. There should be close follow-up of those children with evidence of aneurysms, as they appear to be at risk for thrombosis or perforation and sudden death. The greatest risk of sudden death appears to be within the first 4 months after the onset of the acute phase of the illness.

Cat-Scratch Disease. Cat-scratch disease is a benign disorder that may develop after contact with, and scratch by, a cat. Initial symptoms include tiredness, fever, and muscle aches. Three to ten days later, the primary site develops a papule or pustule, and 1–7 weeks hence, this disappears. Lymph node enlargement, which may be impressive (up to 6 cm) usually begins about 2 weeks after the scratch. The regional nodes most often involved are on the head, cervical region, or axilla, and they are tender for 7–14 days. Nodal enlargement may persist for up to 2 years, and they may drain in 10% of cases. Other findings include a variety of rashes (maculopapules, petechiae, erythema nodosum), conjunctivitis and oculoglandular syndrome, encephalitis, meningitis, thrombocytopenic purpura, osteomyelitis, and atypical pneumonia. Most of these are unusual, and all patients recover without specific therapy.

Histiocytosis X. Histiocytosis X is a disorder complex which includes an acute disseminated form (Letterer-Siwe disease), a chronic disseminated form (Hand-Schüller-Christian disease), and a localized benign form (eosinophilic granuloma). Lymph node enlargement is prominent in the first two, although eosinophilic granulomata of nodes may occur rarely in the eosinophilic granuloma type.

Letterer-Siwe disease affects infants and younger children. Presentation is with massive visceral, oral, skin, and hematologic manifestations. A cutaneous eruption of scaly, crusting maculopapules begins at the hairline and spreads to involve the trunk, scalp, axillae, ears, and groin. The rash may appear hemorrhagic, and there may be petechiae. Pruritis is common. The liver and spleen are enlarged, and jaundice and hepatic dysfunction occur. Generalized lymphadenopathy is found, and there is oral gingival swelling. Very often anemia, leukopenia, and thrombocytopenia and the related symptoms of lethargy, purulent infections, and bleeding are seen. Pulmonary involvement is not unusual, and high fever is common. Bony defects of the skull and long bones may occur if

the child does not first succumb to the other manifestations of this disease.

Hand-Schüller-Christian disease is that form of histiocytosis X involving bones, organs, and soft tissues at the time of diagnosis. The classic triad of exophthalmos, bone defects, and diabetes insipidus is rarely seen, but when these problems occur, they often become chronic and debilitating. Presentation may be in childhood or adolescence but is seldom during infancy. Most frequently, a seborrheic rash, ear discharge, or signs of diabetes insipidus are the initial findings. Growth deficiency may be the result of bone disease or of pituitary compression. Younger children are more likely to have significant generalized lymphadenopathy and patchy pulmonary infiltration. The skull, flat bones, and long bones are commonly involved in this syndrome, with palpable soft tissue nodules overlying the lytic bony lesions.

Venereal Disease

Venereal diseases capable of causing lymphadenopathy include syphilis, chancroid, and lymphogranuloma venereum. They are discussed in Chapter 37.

DIFFERENTIAL DIAGNOSIS

History

The history should include careful questioning to determine the duration of nodal enlargement, whether there has been a cat scratch, a rodent bite, or a tick bite, and whether any skin lesions, abrasions, or infections have occurred in the region drained by the enlarged nodes.

The patient may easily forget trauma or infection distal to the local nodal enlargement, and information about recent systemic symptoms capable of accounting for generalized adenopathy (e.g., fever, joint pains, rashes, headache, chest pain or abdominal pain, diarrhea, pallor, jaundice, anorexia, lethargy, weight loss, and bruising) may not be volunteered.

Pelvic pain, genital discharge, or genital ulceration elicited by history may suggest venereal infection. Chronic cough and weight loss may be symptoms of tuberculosis, sarcoidosis, or histoplasmosis.

Physical Examination

The physical examination should concentrate on the location, size, and quality of the enlarged nodes. Tables 2 and 3 summarize the diagnostic categories to be considered depending on the site of lymphadenopathy.

The location of the enlarged node often helps to determine the probable etiology and may suggest the need for further evaluations. Tonsillar enlargement is most often the result of local infection (for example with β-hemolytic streptococci), and inguinal lymphadenopathy is most often the result of local infection and/or local trauma to the feet, legs, or genital region. By contrast, axillary and supraclavicular nodes, when enlarged, suggest more serious illness. The side of supraclavicular adenopathy may help determine the site of the abnormal process, particularly if a malignancy is involved. A left supraclavicular node is often enlarged when abdominal disease (e.g., Hodgkin's disease, non-Hodgkin's lymphoma, and rhabdomyosarcoma) has spread via the thoracic duct. Right-sided supraclavicular adenopathy suggests intrathoracic disease, and a search for mediastinal and pulmonary diseases must be performed. Bilateral hilar nodes without other lymphadenopathy are more likely the result of infiltration by sarcoid rather than lymphoma.

Lymph node size may be of significance, since benign hyperplastic nodes are seldom more than 2.5 cm in diameter, and nodes this size or larger should be observed and/or evaluated for an underlying disease process.

TABLE 2. ETIOLOGY: REGIONAL LYMPHADENOPATHY

Occipital region/postauricular region
  Local inflammation, e.g., impetigo of scalp
  Pediculosis capitis
  Ringworm infection of scalp
  Seborrhea
  Rubeola
  Roseola

Preauricular region
  Chlamydial infection
  Trachoma
  Lymphogranuloma venereum
  Cat-scratch disease
  Tularemia
  Adenovirus infection (type 3 or 8)
  Sarcoid

Submaxillary and submental region
  Herpes simplex gingivitis and stomatitis
  Dental caries and abscesses (with mixed oral flora)
  Infections of gums, tongue, or buccal mucosa

Cervical region
  Viral upper respiratory infections
  Bacterial infection of the upper respiratory tract
  Impetigo of the head and neck (including scarlet fever) caused by *Steptococcus pyogenes*
  Staphylococcus aureus infection
  Diphtheria
  Infectious mononucleosis
  Mycobacterium tuberculosis and atypical mycobacteria
  Sarcoidosis
  Cat-scratch disease
  Hodgkin's disease
  Cytomegalovirus infection
  Toxoplasmosis
  Mucocutaneous lymph node syndrome (Kawasaki's disease)

(continued)

TABLE 2 (*Continued*)

Cervical region (*continued*)
Histiocytosis-X (Hand-Schüller-Christian disease and Letterer-Siwe disease)
Non-Hodgkin's lymphoma
Deltoid vaccination (DPT and smallpox)
Rat-bite fever

Cervical masses of nonlymphoid origin
Cervical ribs
Thyroglossal cysts
Branchial cleft cysts
Cystic hygromas
Sternomastoid tumors
Goiters
Neurofibroma
Neuroblastoma

Supraclavicular region
Hodgkin's disease
Non-Hodgkin's lymphoma

Mediastinal region
Chronic pulmonary disease
Cystic fibrosis
Tuberculosis
Histoplasmosis
Sarcoidosis
Pneumoconiosis
Coccidioidomycosis
Lymphoma
Hodgkin's disease
Non-Hodgkin's lymphoma

Mediastinal masses of nonlymphoid origin
Ganglioneuroma
Neuroblastoma
Esophageal duplication cysts
Bronchial adenoma
Branchiogenic cyst
Teratoma
Dermoid
Substernal goiter
Pericardial cyst

Axillary region
Infection or inflammation of the arm, including impetigo
Rheumatoid arthritis
BCG vaccine
Cat-scratch disease
Rat-bite fever

Epitrochlear region
Local impetigo or skin infection of forearm and hand
Tularemia
Sporotrichosis
Secondary syphilis (part of generalized lymphadenopathy)

Inguinal region
Lymphogranuloma venereum (See Chapter 37.)
Chancroid (See Chapter 37.)
Herpes simplex
Bubonic plague
Syphilis
Rickettsial infections following insect bites of the legs

Inguinal masses of nonlymphoid origin
Hernias
Aneurysms
Lipomas
Ectopic spleen
Ectopic testicle
Inguinal edometriosis

Iliac region
Lymphoma
Iliac adenitis
S. pyogenes
S. aureus (secondary to trauma)
Appendicitis
Urinary tract infection

Popliteal nodes
Local infections of
Knee joint
Lateral lower leg
Foot skin

Abdominal and pelvic region (associated with disorders causing generalized lymphadenopathy)
Allergy
Exanthems
Typhoid fever
Infectious mononucleosis
Streptococcal pharyngitis
Yersinia infection
Acute rheumatic fever
Mesenteric adenitis

TABLE 3. ETIOLOGY: GENERALIZED LYMPHADENOPATHY

Systemic infections
  Pyogenic bacterial infection
  Syphilis
  Tuberculosis
  Toxoplasmosis
  Brucellosis
  Infectious mononucleosis
  Histoplasmosis
  Typhoid fever
  Malaria
  Scarlet Fever
  CMV
  Rubella
  Rubeola
Chronic granulomatous disease
Immunologically mediated inflammatory disease
  Active systemic lupus erythematosus
  Juvenile rheumatoid arthritis
  Serum sickness
  Autoimmune hemolytic anemia
  Acquired immunodeficiency disease (AIDS)

Lipid storage disease
  Gaucher's disease
  Niemann-Pick disease

Malignant disorders
  Leukemia
    Acute lymphoblastic
    Acute myeloblastic
  Hodgkin's disease
  Non-Hodgkin's lymphoma
  Neuroblastoma
  Rhabdomyosarcoma

Viral diseases
  Cytomegalovirus infection (CMV)
  Rubella
  Rubeola

Other
  Angioimmunoblastic lymphadenopathy
  Dilantin pseudolymphoma

The quality of enlarged lymph nodes should be carefully considered. Infected nodes may be fluctuant. They are often tender, with overlying superficial erythema. Several nodes are frequently matted together. Sinus tract formation may occur in tuberculous nodes and in those infected by aspergillosis or actinomycosis. Nodes enlarged because of an immune response to infection, but not themselves infected, are usually tender but lack other signs of inflammation. Nodes invaded by lymphoma are often firm, separate, rubbery, and movable, whereas those involved with other solid tumors are usually hard and frequently bound to each other. Nodes that are enlarged in the absence of other symptoms or signs may be infected by the toxoplasmosis parasite.

Additionally, a search should be undertaken for masses, hepatomegaly, splenomegaly, jaundice, pallor, ecchymosis, petechiae, joint inflammation, limb swelling, sites of animal bites, and wheezing or rales in the lungs.

Laboratory Investigation

Depending on the results of a complete history and physical examination, the following laboratory studies should be performed:

1. Complete blood count with differential, platelet count, and erythrocyte sedimentation rate.
2. Skin testing for tuberculosis, fungal diseases.
3. Bacterial culture of localized accessible lesions, such as the throat.
4. Chest x-ray.
5. Specific serologic tests, such as the differential heterophil for infectious mononucleosis, titers for toxoplasmosis, cytomegalovirus, and Epstein-Barr virus.
6. Lymph node puncture for culture and smear stained with gram stain and Wright's stain. This is helpful in a determination of a causative organism, and may reveal the cells causing the nodal enlargement. It is also particularly useful when malignancy is suspected. The method is

not difficult. After cleansing the skin, and without anesthesia, the physician grasps the node between thumb and index finger, and using a 20-gauge needle and a sterile syringe, pierces the node, rapidly aspirates the fluid, and removes the needle. Cultures, smears, and stains are made. It is not necessary to perform node puncture, however, if a lymph node biopsy is to be done.

7. Bone marrow aspiration and biopsy should be performed if the blood studies suggest leukemia before the node biopsy is performed.

8. Excisional lymph node biopsy is performed when the patient's symptoms and signs suggest malignancy or when the specific etiologic investigations fail to provide the diagnosis and a 2-week trial of appropriate antibiotic therapy has not resulted in regression of node size. Excisional biopsy yields tissue for histologic section, electron microscopy, and culture. In addition, imprints of the node provide exact individual cell definition. It is important that the pediatrician and surgeon agree before the biopsy is performed on the node to be biopsied based on the following:

   a. Lower cervical, supraclavicular, and axillary nodes are most likely to yield diagnostic information. Upper cervical and inguinal nodes are much less likely to be useful.

   b. The largest node is more likely to provide diagnostic material, even if it is less easily reached by the surgeon than another smaller node.

   c. The entire node should be excised in one piece.

   d. Preparation must be made for handling of the excised node. Culture materials for fungi and for aerobic and anaerobic bacteria must be available. An imprint must be made by repeated light pressure of the cut edge of the node against a glass slide. The node is then prepared for histologic section and electron microscopy.

9. If lymphoid hyperplasia or nonspecific granulomatous change is found in the biopsy material, it may be appropriate after a period of observation to perform more detailed evaluations of lymphoid and neutrophil function with the help of a hematologist or an immunologist. Further, Hodgkin's disease and non-Hodgkin's lymphoma may not be evident in the materials from a first excisional biopsy, and additional observation together with other diagnostic studies [e.g., computerized tomography, radionuclide (^{99m}Tc) scans of the liver spleen and bones and a gallium (^{67}Ga) scan] should be undertaken to provide evidence of other enlarged and perhaps involved organs and nodes.

MANAGEMENT

The initial management of lymphadenopathy is based on an evaluation of the findings of historical and physical examination.

When an infectious process is the main consideration, an assessment of whether it is bacterial or viral is made. Bacterial infections tend to be associated with regional lymphadenitis (tender, warm swelling) usually due to skin or pharyngeal involvement. Determination of the most likely bacterium associated with the infection is based on the history, with *S. aureus* and *S. pyogenes* group A being the most common organisms. Exceptions to this occur when dealing with animal bites (consider *Pasteurella multocida* with dogs) or with infections, such as sinusitis or peritonsillar abscess (consider mouth anaerobes). Treatment with β-lactamase-resistant antibiotics (oxacillin or nafcillin 100 mg/kg/day, or dicloxacillin 50–75 mg/kg/day for 10–14 days) is effective therapy for both staphylococcal and streptococcal infections. High-dose penicillin G or V (150 mg/kg/day) is effective therapy for *P. multocida* or mouth anaerobes. These medications may be given orally or intravenously depending on the patient's clinical condition. When viral infections are considered, the appropriate confirmatory tests should be done to establish a diagnosis. These include a complete blood count, serologic tests, and attempts at viral isolation.

If unusual infectious problems are suspected (e.g., patient from a different area of the world, infection not responding to usual measures, atypical *Mycobacterium*, child with a possible immunodeficiency), consultation with an infectious disease or immunology expert is appropriate.

In children with the diagnosis of Kawasaki's disease, the current management recommendation consist of the use of salicylate in a dose of 30–100 mg/kg/day for weeks to months. This regimen appears theoretically to be effective in counteracting the potentially serious sequelae which result from the coronary thromboarteritis and aneurysm formation. Salicylate should probably be used for the length of time the child appears to be at risk, i.e., while aneurysms continue to be present. As the underlying etiology of this syndrome becomes known over time, no doubt more specific therapy will evolve.

When hematologic or neoplastic problems are suspected, early consultation with a qualified subspecialist is advised. The diagnosis and treatment of these conditions often requires additional experts in the areas of radiology, nuclear and ultrasonographic imaging, and oncologic surgery.

BIBLIOGRAPHY

Knight PJ, et al.: When is lymph node biopsy indicated in children with enlarged peripheral nodes? Pediatrics 69:391, 1982

Lake AM, Oski FA: Peripheral lymphadenopathy in childhood. Am J Dis Child 132:357, 1978

Melish ME: Kawasaki syndrome (The mucocutaneous lymph node syndrome). Pediatr Ann 2:255, 1982

Melish ME, et al.: Kawasaki syndrome: An update. Hosp Prac 99, 1982

Zuelzer WW, Kaplan J: The child with lymphadenopathy. Semin Hematol 12:323, 1975

Cross-Reference to *Pediatrics,* 17th ed.

SEVENTEEN

Seizures in Infancy and Childhood

Carol Leicher

Seizures are common in the pediatric age group, their incidence in children under 5 years of age ranging from 6 to 7%. The pediatric practitioner often is the first physician consulted following the occurrence of a seizure. Therefore, he must be familiar with the differential diagnosis and initial treatment of the various types of seizures that affect children.

DEFINITIONS

Seizures are paroxysmal, uncontrolled electrical discharges, affecting the gray matter of the central nervous system, that interrupt normal function. The source of the discharge and the extent of its propagation will determine the clinical appearance of the seizure. The clinical features of seizures vary and are associated with abnormal discharges in different areas of the brain. It is important to define the general classification of types of seizures that may be encountered. The following is based on an international classification of seizure types.

Generalized seizures are bilaterally symmetrical, with no localization at onset. They include absences (alterations of consciousness with little or no motor component),

tonic-clonic seizures (loss of consciousness with bilateral motor involvement), infantile spasms (or salaam seizures), massive myoclonic jerks involving trunk and extremities, and kinetic seizures (drop attacks) with sudden momentary loss of tone, resulting in a fall.

Partial seizures are subdivided into two categories, those with elementary symptomatology and those with complex symptomatology. Partial seizures with elementary symptomatology generally have no associated impairment of consciousness. These seizures may have motor symptoms, sensory or special sensory symptoms, or autonomic symptoms. Partial seizures with complex symptomatology include the group commonly known as temporal lobe or psychomotor seizures. They are associated with impairment of consciousness and may have a host of affective, psychosensory, or automatic behavioral symptoms.

Finally, there is a group of unclassifiable seizures that represent unusual variants, which do not fall into the categories above.

The purpose of this chapter is to describe the common clinical situations in which a pediatrician encounters a seizure as a presenting symptom and to guide him toward the correct diagnosis and most appropriate

223

treatment. In addition, situations in which immediate consultation with a neurologist is necessary are defined. These include conditions in which seizures are associated with chronic or progressive neurologic disorders and intractable seizure disorders.

Neonatal seizures are not included here; for a discussion of these the reader is referred to *Pediatrics,* 17th ed.

ETIOLOGY AND CLINICAL FEATURES

A child may present to the pediatrician either at the time of a seizure or subsequently. A child in the process of having a seizure, especially one in status epilepticus, must be treated immediately to control the seizure and to maintain adequate oxygenation and circulation. Following this emergency treatment, the primary physician must obtain a history and physical examination to help separate the various diagnostic possibilities and evaluate the need for urgent consultation. In this section, the types of disorders that present with seizures as a major symptom are divided into four categories: Category 1, seizures that may be managed solely by a pediatrician; Category 2, those that may be managed acutely by a pediatrician with subsequent neurologic consultation; Category 3, those that require immediate neurologic consultation; and Category 4, those that should be managed primarily by a neurologist.

Category 1: Seizures that May Be Managed by a Pediatrician

Category 1 is comprised of conditions that the pediatrician should feel comfortable in managing without neurologic consultation. It includes:

- Meningitis
- Ingested toxin, including drugs and heavy metals (e.g., lead)
- Metabolic derangements
- Benign febrile convulsions
- Infectious causes (e.g., *Salmonella, Shigella*)

It is assumed that there is *no* focal neurologic deficit. While the seizure itself may be the cause of a transient deficit, a new neurologic deficit should lead to prompt neurologic consultation.

Meningitis. Meningitis may result in seizures that are either generalized or focal. The etiology may be multiple. The presence of inflammation in the central nervous system may produce changes in local metabolism. Alternately, there may be small infarcts due to thrombosis of small cortical veins.

Ingestion of Toxins. Ingestion of toxic substances, especially ingestion of inappropriate medication, may be a cause of seizures. It is important to ask what medications are being taken by members of the family. Asking the question in this way is more likely to be informative than asking if the child has taken any pills. On physical examination, there is usually a depressed level of consciousness. *Theophylline* ingestion may be accompanied by marked tachycardia. *Phenytoin,* although it is an anticonvulsant, can produce tonic spasms in severe overdose. Physical examination may show nystagmus and, at time, abnormalities of eye movement. If the child is awake enough to be tested, marked ataxia will be present. *Phenothiazine* ingestion may produce severe extrapyramidal effects, which may mimic toxic seizures. Table 1 lists common medications that can produce seizures in overdose. If there is a question about the contents of common household products, or their toxicity, this information can be obtained from the Poison Control Center.

Lead Ingestion. This is a special category of toxic ingestion in which the child may present with signs of increased intracranial pressure and focal or generalized convulsions. There may have been progressive lethargy, behav-

TABLE 1. COMMON MEDICATIONS AND HOUSEHOLD SUBSTANCES THAT CAN CAUSE SEIZURES WHEN INGESTED ACCIDENTALLY

Amphetamine	Boric acid
Antihistamines (diphenhydramine, chlorpheniramine, cyproheptadine, promethazine)	Caffeine
	Camphor
	Carbon monoxide
Atropine	Glutethimide
Aspirin	Phenothiazines (chlorpromazine, fluphenazine, trifluoperazine, prochlorperazine)
Ammonia	
Alkaloids (cocaine, codeine, morphine, heroin, quinine)	Theophylline
	Tricyclic antidepressants (nortriptyline, amitriptyline)
Benzene	

ioral changes, and abdominal complaints preceding the appearance of these symptoms. The acute encephalopathy of lead intoxication is more common in toddlers and occurs more often in summer months. Physical examination is remarkable for depressed consciousness. Papilledema may be present, and nuchal rigidity may also be seen.

Metabolic Derangements. Children with acute metabolic derangements may present with encephalopathy and convulsions. Seizures are particularly common with *hyponatremia, hypoglycemia,* and *hypocalcemia.* Hypernatremia can also produce seizures, usually in patients with subdural hemorrhage resulting from severe brain shrinkage. *Uremia,* when severe enough to produce an encephalopathy, may also produce seizures that may be focal or myoclonic in type. Hypoglycemia should always be suspected in a diabetic with seizures. On physical examination, there may be signs of dehydration, pallor, and sweating in a child with seizures due to hypoglycemia or uremic frost in a child with uremia.

Benign Febrile Convulsions. Benign febrile convulsions are the most frequent type of seizures seen by a pediatrician; they occur in 5–6% of all children under the age of 5.

Their significance, need for treatment, and prognosis have been the subject of much discussion through the years. Benign febrile convulsions are defined as seizures associated with fever and not associated with central nervous system infection or certain systemic infections, such as salmonellosis or shigellosis. They occur in children from 6 months to 6 years of age. They are usually brief, generalized convulsions, associated with a rapid rise of temperature.

As a result of prospective studies, certain factors have been identified that are associated with a greater risk of later development of epilepsy. These include: (1) pre-existing abnormal neurologic examination or abnormal developmental milestones, (2) prolonged convulsions (lasting 15 minutes or longer), multiple convulsions, focal convulsions, or postictal focal findings, (3) family history of epilepsy, and (4) onset at less than 1 year of age. Of these risk factors, the most significant one is a pre-existing abnormal neurologic or developmental examination. This characteristic suggests strongly that fever is a precipitating event for a seizure in a central nervous system that is already compromised and emphasizes the necessity of a good history to elicit such details at the time the child is seen.

Physical examination may be entirely normal after the seizure, although there is usually evidence of an infectious process, such as otitis media or pharyngitis. Since children with early meningitis may present with seizure before other physical findings are present, a lumbar puncture (LP) is recommended to exclude that possibility in children thought to have a febrile seizure. Similarly, routine chemical studies, such as serum glucose, calcium, and electrolytes, should be performed to rule out metabolic abnormalities. The EEG is not a helpful test initially, as there may be slowing solely on the basis of fever. An EEG may be done 1–2 weeks after the episode.

The issue of treatment is not resolved among pediatricians and pediatric neurologists. It has been established that the frequency of recurrent febrile convulsions may be reduced by maintaining therapeutic levels of phenobarbital through daily administration. Intermittent use of phenobarbital only during a febrile episode has been proven ineffective. In view of the fact that the majority of children with benign febrile convulsions have a single episode, many physicians do not treat with chronic medications. Chronic therapy is reserved for children with the risk factors listed above or for children with recurrent febrile convulsions and is generally continued throughout the age of susceptibility.

Features of Category 1 seizures are shown in Table 2.

Category 2: Seizures Managed Acutely by Pediatrician with Subsequent Neurologic Consultation

Category 2 includes isolated seizures or those unassociated with a new or progressive neurologic deficit. These patients usually will be seen first by the pediatrician, and although neurologic consultation should be obtained in most cases, the pediatrician is usually responsible also for chronic management. The pediatrician's task is to obtain a history and to recognize evidence of a neurologic deficit that would mandate immediate neurologic consultation. Many of the primary diagnostic tests can be performed by the pediatrician, and once a plan of therapy has been instituted, the pediatrician should be confident in supervising chronic therapy, using specialty consultation when necessary.

Idiopathic Epilepsy. Idiopathic epilepsy takes two forms in childhood, grand mal and petit mal. *Grand mal epilepsy* is thought to be genetically determined by dominant inheritance with incomplete penetrance. The seizures are characterized by loss of consciousness and generalized tonic-clonic motor activity. They may be accompanied by cyanosis, flushing, diaphoresis, or incontinence of bowel or bladder. The child may have postictal confusion or lethargy. There is frequently a family history of epilepsy, and the parent may have made the diagnosis from experience with other family members. There are no clear, precipitating factors, such as ingestion of a toxic substance or infection. Typically, this type of seizure begins in the second decade but may begin as early as 5 years of age. The children have no focal neurologic deficit and usually have had normal development.

Petit mal epilepsy is another form of idiopathic generalized epilepsy. It occurs typically in children from 4 to 15 years of age and is an autosomally dominant disorder. The attacks, properly known as "absences," consist of staring spells with lapse of consciousness. Typically, the child suddenly develops a blank expression and does not respond to external stimuli. These episodes last several seconds to 30 seconds. There may be minor motor manifestations, such as eye blinking or myoclonic jerks of the head or arms. There is no postictal confusion. The attacks are generally multiple. There are no associated physical abnormalities. Neurologic and intellectual development usually is normal, although mental retardation occurs in 6% of children with petit mal. The child may be brought to medical attention because his parents or teacher note that he is daydreaming or tun-

TABLE 2. CATEGORY 1: SEIZURES THAT MAY BE MANAGED PRIMARILY BY A PEDIATRICIAN

Cause	Seizure Type	Neurologic Findings	Diagnostic Tests	Radiographic Tests
Infectious	Generalized tonic-clonic	Irritability, lethargy (no focal neurologic abnormalities should be present)	LP	
Ingestions	Generalized tonic-clonic or focal motor	Lethargy to coma, no focal deficit	Toxicology screen, LP (to rule out infection)	
Electrolyte disturbances	Generalized tonic-clonic or focal motor	Change in consciousness, no focal neurologic deficit	Electrolyte and glucose determination, LP (to rule out bleeding, especially in hypernatremic states)	
Benign febrile seizures	Generalized or focal	Normal except for postictal irritability	CBC, blood culture electrolytes, Ca, glucose, LP (to rule out early CNS infection), EEG (to be performed after febrile episode resolved)	
Heavy metal intoxications	Focal	Irritability, papilledema	Lead level, do not do LP if papilledema present	Long bones (lead lines)

ing out during conversations. The family history may be helpful. The most important diagnostic test is the EEG, which shows generalized 3 Hz spike and wave complexes; these can be induced by hyperventilation. The response to hyperventilation is so marked that an attack can be observed in the office by having the child overbreathe for 3–5 minutes. If an attack occurs, the child will stop hyperventilating, stare, and will not respond to questions. Petit mal seizures generally have a good prognosis. Attacks almost always subside by the end of the second decade, although a significant proportion of these patients will develop grand mal type epilepsy.

The staring spell or absence seizure may occur in children who do not have petit mal. These children may be distinguished by a much higher frequency of mental retardation or other forms of aberrant neurologic development. They may have other types of seizures, such as drop attacks. The EEG in these children is more likely to show spike and wave at 1.5–2.5 Hz with abnormal background activity. These children should have a more intensive neurologic evaluation and may require other diagnostic procedures. In general, their seizures have a poorer prognosis and are more difficult to control.

Benign focal epilepsy of childhood is a type of seizure that occurs in the latter half of the first decade. The seizures frequently occur in sleep and consist of unilateral twitching of the face, sometimes with extension of clonic activity to the same arm and leg. They may become generalized to involve both sides of the body. There is a family history of seizures in 20% of patients. The physical and neurologic examinations are normal. These seizures must be differentiated from focal seizures discussed below under Category 3. These patients are often brought in after the parent has noted several episodes of nighttime twitching. In addition to a careful neurologic examination and history, the diagnostic work-up should include an EEG, which shows spikes originating in the centrotemporal area. These seizures are generally well controlled with carbamazepine or phenobarbital and almost always stop spontaneously by the mid to late teens. Features of Category 2 seizures are shown in Table 3.

Category 3: Seizures that Require Immediate Neurologic Consultation

Category 3 includes seizures that are associated with either an acute or a chronic neurologic deficit. In general, the investigation and treatment of these children require the active participation of a pediatric neurologist or neurosurgeon. They will be presented according to their etiology and discussed only briefly.

Infectious Causes. Several infectious processes involving the central nervous system may present with either focal or generalized seizures. Because of the high morbidity and mortality of these diseases, prompt diagnosis and treatment are of utmost importance.

TABLE 3. CATEGORY 2: SEIZURES MANAGED ACUTELY BY THE PEDIATRICIAN WITH SUBSEQUENT NEUROLOGIC CONSULTATION

Cause	Seizure Type	Neurologic Findings	Diagnostic Tests	Radiographic Tests
Idiopathic epilepsy				
Grand mal	Generalized	Normal	Electrolytes, Ca, glucose, EEG, LP (optional unless meningeal signs)	Only with a history of trauma
Petit mal	Absence	Normal	EEG	
Benign focal epilepsy of childhood	Focal	Normal	EEG	CT scan (only if persistent focal slowing on EEG)
Conditions confused with seizures				
Apnea	Loss of consciousness with or without clonic movements	Normal	EEG (normal cardiorespiratory monitoring)	
Breathholding spells	Loss of consciousness with or without cyanosis	Normal	EEG (normal)	
Syncope	Loss of consciousness	Normal	Blood sugar, EEG (normal)	

Meningoencephalitis. Bacterial or viral infection of the meninges may extend to involve the parenchyma of the brain and may present with seizures. These may be either generalized or focal, the latter reflecting a localized area of involvement (as seen, e.g., in herpes simplex encephalitis). The history is usually that of a few days of progressive confusion or obtundation, but the symptoms may be nonspecific. Physical examination may reveal signs of meningeal irritation and usually will show prominent changes in the state of consciousness and mental status. Neurologic examination may or may not reveal focal motor findings, such as hemiparesis or abnormal reflexes. If there are no focal signs and meningeal signs are prominent, a lumbar puncture should be the first diagnostic test. If there are focal signs, a mass lesion should be ruled out first with a CT scan.

Epidural Abscess. The first presenting sign of an epidural abscess may be a seizure. These abscesses result from extension of infection from a parameningeal focus, such as sinusitis, mastoiditis, or dental abscess. There is usually a history of recent infection of the sinuses or ear, which may or may not have been treated with antibiotics. Headache is a frequent accompanying complaint. The seizure may be focal or generalized. Unfortunately, the physical examination may be entirely normal at this time, and the diagnosis is often missed unless special attention is paid to possible sites of parameningeal infection, such as the sinuses, mastoids, and orbits. The neurologic examination may show evidence of papilledema or focal deficit, or lethargy or confusion may be the only manifestation. Since these children have a focal lesion which results in elevated intracranial pressure, a lumbar puncture is contraindicated. CT scan with contrast is the indicated diagnostic procedure, as well as radiograms of the mastoids and sinuses to locate the source of infection.

Subdural Empyema. Subdural empyema, or infection of the subdural space, may be associated with otorhinologic infections, underlying meningitis, or trauma, or it may occur from hematogenous spread of infection. Clinically, the patients may present with fever, seizures, and signs of increased intracranial pressure. There may or may not be a focal neurologic deficit. The most common clinical situation is recurrence of fever or seizures or both in a child under treatment for meningitis. The diagnosis may be made by CT scan or by subdural taps in a child with an open fontanel.

Intracerebral Abscess. Seizures may be due to an intracerebral abscess, formed either by hematogenous spread or by direct extension from a parameningeal focus, such as a sinus or mastoid infection. Patients with cyanotic congenital heart disease with right to left shunting are particularly susceptible to the development of a brain abscess. Clinically, they may present with seizures, which need not be focal. They also may complain of headache. Fever is not a necessary finding. On physical examination, they often have cardiac findings. The neurologic examination may reveal a focal deficit or signs of increased intracranial pressure, although early in the course the examination may be normal. The clinician must have a high index of suspicion. The diagnostic test of choice is the CT scan with contrast enhancement. Lumbar puncture is contraindicated if there are signs of increased pressure. Often it is not helpful, since the cell count, chemistries, and culture may be negative in a well-circumscribed abscess. Even after successful treatment, these patients have a significant risk of epilepsy.

Head Trauma. Trauma may be responsible for seizures in children, especially in those with open injuries or penetrating injuries to the head. In general, these seizures are divided into early posttraumatic seizures occurring within 1 week of trauma and late posttraumatic seizures occurring after 1 week or as long as 2 or 3 years later.

The prognosis in these two types of posttraumatic seizures is different. Early posttraumatic seizures are more likely to be focal motor attacks, and they have a risk of recurrence of about 20–25%. The prognosis is better in children under 16 years. Late posttraumatic seizures are more commonly generalized and associated with chronic epilepsy. Important points in the history are whether the seizure was focal or generalized and the temporal relation between the trauma and the seizure. Particular attention in the physical examination should be given to the nature of the trauma, including laceration, scalp hematoma, signs of basilar skull fracture, and the neurologic status. Any child with focal neurologic signs of depressed consciousness needs immediate evaluation by a neurosurgeon for epidural hematoma or brain contusion. Children with significant scalp laceration, swelling, and seizures need appropriate radiograms of the skull to detect depressed fractures.

Children with normal neurologic examinations and an early posttraumatic seizure may be observed without neurologic treatment. A particular group who do not require neurologic treatment are children with contact seizures, defined as generalized seizures that occur at the moment of impact and are free from neurologic deficits.

Many physicians recommend the use of prophylactic anticonvulsants in patients with penetrating wounds of the skull and in those with depressed skull fractures, even if seizures are not present. Such prophylactic therapy is thought to reduce the risk of epilepsy.

Evaluation of a patient with a late posttraumatic seizure should include an EEG. These patients should be given chronic therapy with anticonvulsants, as they are likely to have recurrent seizures.

A special category of posttraumatic seizures in young infants are those that occur in association with subdural hematomas. When there has been repeated shaking or battering of an infant's head, there can be tearing of the cortical veins with bleeding into the subdural space. The infant's head can expand to accommodate this blood for awhile. These infants are irritable, often fail to thrive, and may have focal or generalized seizures that are difficult to control. On physical examination, they may have macrocephaly, bulging fontanel, irritability, and emaciation. There may be associated focal, neurologic findings. The diagnosis may be made by CT scan or, if this is unavailable, by subdural taps, which yield proteinaceous, xanthochromic, or bloody fluid. These findings on physical examination may mimic those of meningitis in a young infant. A lumbar puncture may show xanthochromic fluid, with elevated protein. Subdural hematomas may be due to child abuse, and these children, therefore, should have radiograms of their long bones, skull, and ribs to detect other fractures.

Vascular Causes. The major vascular causes of neurologic abnormalities that produce seizures are arteriovenous malformation and cerebrovascular accidents.

Arteriovenous Malformations. These are congenital anomalies of the cerebrovasculature in which abnormal vessels form arteriovenous fistulas within the parenchyma of the brain. They can cause shunting of blood within the brain and produce localized ischemia. They may leak blood into surrounding tissue or rupture, causing a catastrophic intracerebral hemorrhage. In adults, the local damage to tissues caused by these malformations may give rise to focal seizures. This occurrence is relatively unusual in children, who generally present with hemorrhage rather than seizures. If an arteriovenous malformation is suspected, a bruit may be heard over the head or neck, indicating increased flow. Rarely is a focal neurologic deficit present in an otherwise asymptomatic patient. The diagnostic test of choice is a CT scan with contrast, followed by cerebral angiography. An EEG will show evidence of the lesion only if a seizure focus has been caused by destruction of tissue around the lesion.

Cerebrovascular Accidents. The incidence of cerebrovascular thrombosis is relatively low. Previously healthy children may have arterial occlusion that presents with hemiparesis and status epilepticus. Arterial and venous occlusion may also occur in children with sickle cell anemia or collagen-vascular disease, such as lupus erythematosus. These children may present with seizures and acute onset of a focal, persistent neurologic deficit, such as hemiparesis, field cut, or aphasia. The work-up consists of a CT scan or angiography to define the site and size of the lesion as well as the etiology. EEG may show the epileptic activity caused by the structural lesion.

TABLE 4. CATEGORY 3: SEIZURES THAT REQUIRE IMMEDIATE NEUROLOGIC CONSULTATION

Cause	Seizure Type	Neurologic Findings	Diagnostic Tests	Radiographic Tests
Acute infectious				
Meningoencephalitis	Focal or generalized	Focal deficit, lethargy	LP (after CT scan if no mass effect), viral studies, EEG	CT scan
Epidural abscess	Focal or generalized	Focal deficit, or normal	LP (contraindicated)	CT scan
Subdural empyema	Focal or generalized	May have papilledema		CT scan
Brain abscess	Focal or generalized	Focal deficit, papilledema (possibly), signs of cyanotic heart disease	EEG—slow wave focus	CT scan
Traumatic	Focal or generalized	Focal neurologic signs	EEG	CT scan, skull xray (for depressed fx)
Subdural hematoma of infancy	Multifocal	Lethargy, irritability, bulging fontanel	EEG, subdural tap, LP to rule out infectious process	CT scan, bone survey
Vascular				
AV malformation	Focal or generalized	Bruit, hemiparesis field cut		CT scan, angiography
CVA			If examination normal except for meningeal signs, LP fluid	
Neoplastic	Focal or generalized			

Neoplasm. Although neoplasm is a major cause of seizures in the midadult population, it is relatively rare as a cause of seizures in children. Therefore, unless there is persistent unexplained neurologic deficit or signs of increased intracranial pressure, extensive investigation to rule out brain tumor should not be done in a child who presents with seizures, even if they are focal. Features of Category 3 seizures are shown in Table 4.

Category 4: Seizures that Should Be Managed Primarily by a Neurologist

Category 4 includes seizure disorders with a fixed or chronic neurologic deficit and those associated with progressive neurologic deterioration. These conditions are discussed only briefly, since children with them should be handled directly by or in close consultation with a pediatric neurologist. Some of these disorders are shown in Table 5. Details of treatment are discussed in *Pediatrics,* 17th ed.

There is one broad category of seizures that present in infancy of which the pediatrician should be especially aware. From the age of 3 months to 2 years an infant may present with *infantile spasms.* These seizures consist of lightning-fast flexor spasms involving the head, trunk, and extremities. They are described as jackknife seizures because the child may fold up at the waist. Less commonly, the spasms involve extension of the legs, arms, and neck. They occur in clusters, many times a day. When questioned, the parents may relate that the child has stopped performing developmental tasks previously achieved. On physical examination, evidence of abnormal development, retinal findings such as a cherry spot in the macula, and skin lesions such as hypopigmented macules may be present. Neurologic examination frequently shows hypotonia or hypertonia. The EEG in these children shows a highly disorganized abnormal pattern known as "hypsarrhythmia." Causes of this type of seizure disorder are diverse and include inborn metabolic errors (such as aminoacidurias), neurophakoma-

TABLE 5. CATEGORY 4: STATIC OR PROGRESSIVE NEUROLOGIC DISORDERS ASSOCIATED WITH SEIZURES

Etiology

Congenital malformations
    Cerebral agenesis
    Holoprosencephaly
    Porencephaly

Degenerative diseases
    Neurophakomatoses
        Tuberous sclerosis
        Neurofibromatosis
        Sturge-Weber syndrome
        Von Hippel-Lindau syndrome
    Incontinentia pigmenti
    Alper's disease
    Leukodystrophies

Metabolic diseases
    Aminoacidurias
    Neuroaxonal dystrophies
    Ceroid lipofucinosis
    Sphingolipidosis

Perinatal trauma
    Anoxia

Postinfectious/congenital infections
    Toxoplasmosis
    Rubella
    Syphilis
    Cytomegalovirus
    Herpes simplex

toses, and severe structural abnormalities. There is also a group of children with no known etiology (so-called cryptogenic infantile spasms).

The prognosis for children with infantile spasms is generally poor. In most children the seizures are not fully controlled and lead to intractable seizures of different types. They also have a high rate of mental retardation.

DIFFERENTIAL DIAGNOSIS

The pediatrician must decide the significance of the symptoms being presented, assess the category in which they appear to be, and decide the appropriate intervention. The approach must consist of a thorough history, physical examination, and appropriate laboratory tests before accurate diagnosis is possible and proper intervention is decided upon.

There are several conditions that must be differentiated diagnostically from seizures. These includes breathholding spells, syncope, and, in the young infant, apneic episodes. Infants less than 6 months of age may present with a history of being found cyanotic and not breathing. Sometimes there may be abnormal movements associated with the cyanosis. The question that arises is whether this was a respiratory arrest of the type seen in sudden infant death syndrome (SIDS) or whether the child became apneic and cyanotic as part of a generalized seizure. Historically, it is important to get a description of the sequence of events, especially whether the cyanosis preceded the clonic movements or vice versa. In addition, a careful neurologic examination should be done as well as a developmental assessment. Consultation with a neurologist experienced in the differential diagnosis of these conditions is required. The laboratory examination should include cardiorespiratory monitoring as well as EEG. The EEG should be normal in a child with apnea as part of SIDS, and a continuous cardiorespiratory tracing should document frequent apneic periods. Any abnormalities of the neurologic or developmental examination would suggest some type of seizure disorder.

Breathholding spells of infancy and early childhood also present a diagnostic challenge. Typically, these occur in children from 6 months to 2½ years of age. There are two subcategories, sometimes called "pallid" and "cyanotic." In the cyanotic spell, the event is precipitated by obvious frustration. The child begins to wail and, after a prolonged expiration, stops breathing. He becomes progressively cyanotic and, if the spell is prolonged, may lose consciousness, sometimes having a few clonic jerks if the apnea continues for more than 30 seconds. Afterwards,

he resumes breathing and returns to normal. The pallid spell is generally provoked either by a frightening experience or a minor painful injury. The child becomes pale, stops breathing, and loses consciousness. After a brief time, breathing resumes, and the child returns to normal. By carefully questioning the parent, one may identify the precipitating episode and the typical pattern. In addition, there is often a family history of breathholding spells. Physical examination and the EEG are normal.

In the pallid type of breathholding spell, increased vagal tone has been implicated as the cause of the apnea and bradycardia. These changes can sometimes be demonstrated by light ocular compression during EKG recording. The ocular compression can cause asystole; regular rhythm returns when pressure is relieved. There is no treatment for breathholding spells, although atropine has been used in severe cases of the pallid type. Parental reassurance is especially important, since the fear and anxiety created by the episode may reinforce it.

Syncope may occur in a child of any age, but it is particularly common in adolescents. The onset of syncope is gradual, and the patient may describe dimming vision. As the patients lose consciousness, they become limp, but if the syncope is prolonged, there may be some clonic movements. Upon awakening, there should be no confusion or disorientation, but there may be diaphoresis and nausea. Urinary incontinence may occur in girls. The causes of syncope are multiple, including a vasovagal reaction to a frightening or emotional experience, cardiac arrythmias, and hypoglycemia. The pediatrician should attempt to get the best possible description of the event and any possible precipitating event, including the time of the last meal. The neurologic examination should be normal. Special attention should be paid to the cardiac examination. Laboratory work-up should include an EKG and a fasting blood glucose. EEG is normal in syncope and should be performed only if the description of the event makes seizures a more likely diagnosis.

History

A detailed history is of great importance and may provide valuable clues to the etiology. Some of the questions that need to be asked to obtain the maximum amount of information follow.

- What was the seizure like? This question must be broken down into several parts:
- Was there associated loss of consciousness? It is important to determine whether the child was completely unresponsive to the environment or seemed to be in a trancelike state. It is also important to establish if the loss of consciousness preceded or followed abnormal motor activity.
- Was there motor activity during the episode? An accurate description of movements that occurred must be sought. With generalized seizures, there may be stiffening of the entire body, including the jaw, or there may be repetitive, bilaterally simultaneous clonic movements of the extremities. Focal motor seizures may involve only one extremity or half of the body. The head or eyes may deviate tonically to one side during the seizure. During partial complex seizures, the observer may note that the patient performs automatic behaviors, such as picking at clothing, mumbling, chewing, or walking in circles.
- Was there a specific precipitating event? Seizures may be precipitated by flashing lights, loud sounds, hyperventilation, fatigue, or hunger. Breathholding spells may be precipitated by frustration or minor trauma. Syncope may be preceded by emotional upset or fear.
- How did the seizure begin? This feature frequently is not witnessed, but, if it is, it may be very helpful. An abnormal feeling may precede the seizure, and a child may describe abdominal discomfort or fright prior to onset. Similarly, the seizure may begin with focal motor activity and then progress to generalized motor activity.
- What happened after the seizure? Seizures that are generalized or involve impaired consciousness may produce amnesia for the event. More prolonged seizures will also produce a postictal state characterized by lethargy or confusion or both.
- Were there any other preceding or associated symptoms? The physician should obtain information about recent infection, fever, headache, or vomiting. It is vital to ask about exposure to toxins, such as lead, and especially about the availability of any medications in the home.
- Was there recent head trauma? Even minor head trauma may be a cause of seizures, and this information may not be offered spontaneously.
- Does the child have any other medical illnesses that might predispose him to infection or metabolic derangements? Specific inquiries should be made about past infectious illnesses, such as meningitis or viral illnesses, such as varicella or mumps, known to be associated with postinfectious encephalopathy.
- In an older child or adolescent, were there previous convulsions or febrile convulsions of infancy? Obviously, it is necessary to ask if the child has had previous seizures of any type, but it is useful to ask for a history of prolonged febrile convulsions, as these seem to have some correlation with the development of seizures later in life.
- Does the child have normal developmental milestones? A history of a developmental delay may be the only clue to a preexisting neurologic deficit. The question is particularly important in a child who presents with a seizure with fever, since the answer may influence the decision whether or not to institute treatment. Furthermore, a history of regression of developmental milestones or intellectual ability requires consideration of different categories of disease.
- Were there complications at birth or prenatally? This question also seeks evidence

of a preexisting neurologic deficit or a predisposition to certain types of seizures. Episodes of hypoxia or congenital infection are of specific interest.

- Is there a family history of epilepsy or neurologic disorders? There is frequently a family history of epilepsy in children with major motor or petit mal seizures. A history of mental retardation or epilepsy may suggest a neurologic disorder associated with seizures, such as neurofibromatosis, tuberous sclerosis, or inborn errors of metabolism. Benign febrile convulsions of infancy may also be familial.

Physical Examination

The essential points in the physical examination are presented in Table 6.

Laboratory Tests

Several laboratory tests are helpful in corroborating the correct diagnosis. The lumbar puncture, EEG, and CT scan represent the three most imporatnt resources when used appropriately. Tables 2, 3, and 4 summarize their appropriate use and the results anticipated in specific conditions.

MANAGEMENT

The pediatrician must play a role in deciding the appropriate therapy for those conditions that should be managed without consultation. In addition, however, the practitioner must be aware of appropriate therapy for those more complex situations where a consultant is required. Tables 7, 8, and 9 summarize the recommended therapy for the conditions already described under the three categories. Dosage schedules for the commonly used anticonvulsants are shown in Table 10.

It is appropriate here to discuss the problem, not uncommon, of a child with a single generalized seizure. Historically, there may

TABLE 6. PHYSICAL EXAMINATION IN A CHILD WITH SEIZURES

Physical Examination	Diagnostic Considerations
Vital signs	
Fever	Infections such as meningitis or meningoencephalitis, benign febrile convulsions of infancy
Increased blood pressure	Increased intracranial pressure or hypertensive encephalopathy
Skin	
Petechiae/purpura	Meningitis (meningococcal), collagen-vascular disease
Hypopigmented/hyperpigmented lesions	Neurocutaneous disorders, such as tuberous sclerosis, neurofibromatosis, incontinentia pigmenti
Capillary hemangioma	Sturge-Weber (encephalofacial angiomatosis)
Head	
Microcephaly	Congenital malformations, intrauterine infections
Macrocephaly	Degenerative disease, hydrocephalus
Bruit	Arteriovenous malformation
Battle sign (bruise over mastoid) or external abrasions	Head trauma

(continued)

TABLE 6 (*Continued*)

Physical Examination	Diagnostic Considerations
Eyes	
Abnormal funduscopic examination	
Papilledema (swelling of optic disc, hemorrhages around disc, venous engorgement with lack of venous pulsations)	Increased intracranial pressure from mass lesion, e.g., tumor, abscess, trauma, hypertensive encephalopathy
Macular changes (cherry red spot)	Tay-Sachs disease
Chorioretinitis	Congenital infections
Visual abnormality	
Decreased acuity	Optic atrophy
Hemianopsia	Structural lesion
Strabsimus (acute onset)	Ocular muscle paresis secondary to increased pressure
Raccoon sign	Discoloration around lids may indicate basilar skull fracture
Ears	
Battle sign	Discoloration over mastoid may indicate basilar skull fracture
Neck	
Stiff neck, positive Kernig or Brudzinski sign	Meningeal irritation secondary to acute infection or hemorrhage
Heart	
Murmur, cyanosis	Brain abscess in child with cyanotic heart disease, cerebral embolism from acute bacterial endocarditis
Abdomen	
Organomegaly	Degenerative diseases of childhood, such as Gaucher's, Niemann-Pick, or Krabbe's disease
Abdominal tenderness	Acute intermittent porphyria
Extremities	
Asymmetry (disparity in size of thumbnails, size or length of extremities)	Indicative of chronic lesion affecting opposite cerebral hemisphere
Neurologic examination	
Acute change in personality or affect or change in level of alertness	Diffuse encephalopathic process in intoxications, infection, or electrolyte disturbances
Fixed focal neurologic deficit (hemiparesis, hemisensory loss, reflex asymmetry)	Underlying structural abnormality, such as static encephalopathy, porencephaly, infarction, or trauma
Transient neurologic deficit	Secondary to seizure itself (Todd's paresis)
Multifocal abnormalities	Toxic metabolic encephalopathy

be nothing to suggest an infectious process, recent head trauma, or ingestion of a toxic substance, and the family history is negative. Physical examination is normal. The routine diagnostic blood tests and EEG show no abnormalities. The need for treatment in such a child with a single episode, a negative history, normal physical examination, and normal laboratory findings is controversial. Pediatric neurologists who argue against treating such a child with anticonvulsants believe that it may be more deleterious to label the child as

TABLE 7. TREATMENT OF CATEGORY 1 SEIZURES

Cause	Therapy
Infectious	Antibiotics Fluid restriction Phenobarbital 10–15 mg/kg loading dose IM *or* diphenylhydantoin 10–15 mg/kg loading dose IV or po
Ingestions	Specific antidotes if possible Anticonvulsants (as above)
Electrolyte disturbances	Correct electrolyte disturbance Administer glucose Anticonvulsants (usually these will be ineffective if electrolyte disturbances are not corrected)
Benign febrile seizures	Antipyretics Phenobarbital (optional; see text)
Heavy metal intoxications (lead)	Chelating agents

TABLE 9. TREATMENT OF CATEGORY 3 SEIZURES

Cause	Therapy
Acute infectious	
Meningoencephalitis	Appropriate antibiotics if bacterial Diphenylhydantoin, phenobarbital ara-A (for herpes)
Epidural abscess	Neurosurgical consultation Drainage of abscess
Subdural empyema	Neurosurgical consultation Anticonvulsants
Brain abscess	Neurosurgical consultation
Traumatic	
Subdural hematoma of infancy	Neurosurgical consultation
Vascular	
AV malformation	Neurosurgical consultation, diphenylhydantoin
CVA, neoplastic	Neurosurgical consultation

epileptic than to risk a second episode. Advocates of treatment suggest that the convulsion is frightening for the child and parent and that the risk of a second episode warrants preventive therapy. There is no firm evidence to provide a general answer to this problem. The role of the pediatrician in this instance is to help the pediatric neurologist evaluate the feelings of the patient and the family and to determine the best treatment for that specific child.

Status Epilepticus

Although in most cases, the pediatrician will not be the sole doctor responsible for a child who presents with major motor status epilepticus, he often is the first doctor on the scene and should be prepared to provide initial therapy.

Status epilepticus is defined as either recurrent seizures in a patient who does not regain consciousness between seizures, or a single seizure lasting 20–30 minutes. During status epilepticus, the brain and body are in a hypermetabolic state, requiring increases in glucose and oxygen. In addition, the clonic-tonic activity may interfere with efficient res-

TABLE 8. TREATMENT OF CATEGORY 2 SEIZURES

Cause	Therapy
Idiopathic epilepsy	
Grand mal	Phenobarbital Diphenylhydantoin
Petit mal	Ethosuximide Valproate
Benign focal epilepsy of childhood	Phenobarbital Carbamazepine

TABLE 10. COMMONLY USED ANTICONVULSANTS

Seizure Type	Drugs	Usual Daily Dosage mg/kg	Therapeutic Serum Concentration μg/ml	Plasma Half-Life
Tonic-clonic (generalized or focal)	Phenytoin	4–7	10–20	7–42 hr
	Carbamazepine	20–30	6–12	Acute: 12–30 hr Chronic: 7–12 hr
	Phenobarbital	3–5 8 in infants	15–30	2–6 days
	Primidone	10–25	6–12	3–12 hr
Absences (petit mal)	Ethosuximide	20–30	40–100	36–72 hr
	Valproic acid	30–60	50–100	8–15 hr
	Clonazepam	0.0–0.02	0.013–0.072	18–15 hr
	Trimethadione	10–25	—	12–24 hr
Partial complex (psychomotor or temporal lobe seizure)	Same as tonic-clonic but often must use combinations; valproic acid may be used			

(*From: Adapted from the Medical Letter on Drugs and Therapeutics.*)

piration, producing hypoxia. The end result is that major motor status epilepticus creates a neurologic emergency that may result in brain damage or death. Rapid and effective treatment is required.

When presented with such an emergency the physician should proceed as follows:

I. Maintain respiration and circulation
   A. Establish an adequate airway, suction and intubation if necessary, administer oxygen
   B. Place an intravenous line
   C. Determine blood levels of glucose, calcium, electrolytes, urea, and anticonvulsants
   D. Reduce fever if present
II. Administer 25% dextrose IV (1 g/kg)
III. Give anticonvulsants.

The drugs administered are listed below. The choice of drug is based on personal preference and experience.

Valium. Valium is given intravenously in a dose of 0.3–0.5 mg/kg over several minutes; this may be repeated every 15 minutes if necessary. The maximum single dose is 2.5 mg in infants, 10 mg in older children.

The major drawbacks of Valium are the depressive effect on respiration and the short action of the medication. One can control respiration artifically if necessary, so the respiratory depression or arrest is a manageable problem. The duration of action of Valium is about 15–20 minutes. Unless the child is treated with a long-acting anticonvulsant, the seizures may recur at the end of this time.

Phenobarbital. Phenobarbital is given intravenously in a dose of 10 mg/kg over several minutes. An additional dose of 5 mg/kg may be given in 20 minutes if seizures persist (total 15 mg/kg). In a child less than 10 years old, 5 mg/kg may be given after another 20 minutes for persistent seizures (total dose 20 mg/kg). Status epilepticus should not be treated with phenobarbital intramuscularly.

The major side effects of phenobarbital are respiratory depression, hypotension, and sedation. The respiratory depression may be particularly severe if Valium has been used also. As with Valium, the physician should be prepared to intubate and ventilate artifically if necessary.

Phenytoin. Phenytoin is given intravenously in a dose of 15 mg/kg in normal saline over 20 minutes. The rate should not exceed 25–50 mg/minute. This drug may cause cardiac arrythmias, so cardiac monitoring is necessary when it is being infused. There is no respiratory depression. Phenytoin should not be used intramuscularly, as it is poorly absorbed and causes sterile abscesses.

Paraldehyde. Paraldehyde in a 4% solution diluted 10 ml in 90 ml isotonic saline can be given intravenously, titrated to the patient's needs. Alternatively, 0.15 ml 4% solution/kg mixed with an equal volume of vegetable oil can be given per rectum (maximum dose 5 ml).

The drawbacks of paraldehyde are the effects on acid-base balance and the irritation to the respiratory system. It will interact with plastic IV bags and tubing and deteriorates on exposure to light, making it a difficult substance to handle. The major side effect of rectal administration is proctitis.

BIBLIOGRAPHY

Dodson WE, Prensky AL, DeVivo DC, Goldring S, Dodge PR: Management of seizure disorders, Part I and II. J Pediatr 89:527, 695, 1976

Epilepsy Foundation of America: Basic Statistics on the Epilepsies. Philadelphia, Davis, 1975.

Livington S: Comprehensive Management of Epilepsy in Infancy, Childhood and Adolescence. Springfield, Ill, Thomas, 1972

O'Donohue NV: Epilepsies of Childhood. Boston, Butterworths, 1979

Penry K, Newmark: Antiepileptic drugs. Ann Intern Med 90:207, 1979

Solomon GE, Plum WB: Clinical Management of Seizures. Philadelphia, Saunders, 1976

Swaiman KF, Wright FS: The Practice of Pediatric Neurology. St. Louis, Mosby, 1975

Cross-Reference to *Pediatrics,* 17th ed.

EIGHTEEN

Sore Throat

Andrew P. Mezey

Sore throat is one of the most common complaints brought to the attention of the pediatric practitioner. Usually the complaint is secondary to a self-limited illness and of little consequence. There are, however, a number of conditions that, although uncommon, are potentially life threatening. These conditions must be recognized and dealt with promptly. The less serious, but much more common, causes of sore throat, must also be identified and treated appropriately.

INCIDENCE

It has been estimated that in the first 6 years of life children have 6–8 illnesses per year, at least half being associated with evidence of an upper respiratory infection with an inflamed pharynx. Although the annual incidence of episodes of disease drops to 3–4 after 6 years of age, the incidence of sore throat remains about the same. It is, therefore, the most common acute illness among children of school age.

DEFINITION

It is difficult to define the entire clinical spectrum of sore throat. A verbal child usually complains of pain on swallowing; on examination a red pharynx is seen. In a nonverbal child, the suspicion that a sore throat may be present is usually based on changes in behavior. Often, however, the symptoms of illness do not match the physical signs. Some individuals complain bitterly of a painful throat but have little in the way of physical findings. At other times, the practitioner sees a beefy red, obviously inflamed pharynx, but the child states there is little or no pain in the throat.

ETIOLOGY

An etiologic diagnosis can be made on the basis of the history and physical examination in only a few specific instances, where the lesion is pathognomonic of the illness (Table 1). However, these conditions make up a small minority of patients who complain of sore throat. In the great majority, the infection is of unknown origin. A specific organism can sometimes be implicated by knowing which disease is most common at the time, especially at times of the year when influenza A and B, parainfluenza, respiratory syncytial virus, and adenovirus are being identified in epidemologic surveys. However, the most important cause of sore throat in children is that due to the group A beta-hemolytic streptococcus. A diagnosis is easily made by means of a throat culture, a procedure that most clinics and private offices are prepared to do

TABLE 1. ETIOLOGY OF SORE THROAT

Etiologies Recognizable on Physical Examination	Etiologies Not Recognizable on Physical Examination

Bacterial
  Scarlet fever (group A beta-hemolytic strepto-coccus)
  Acute epiglottitis (*Haemophilus influenza* type b)
  Peritonsillar abscess (mouth anaerobes)
  Retropharyngeal abscess (*Staphylococcus, Streptococcus,* anaerobes)
  Diphtheria (*Corynebacterium diphtheriae*)
Viral
  Herpetic gingivostomatitis (herpes simplex type I)
  Herpangina (Coxsackie virus A)
  Hand, foot, and mouth disease (Coxsackie virus A)
  Pharyngoconjunctival fever (adenovirus)
  Measles
  Varicella
Other
  Kawasaki syndrome (mucocutaneous lymph node syndrome)
  Mycoplasma pneumoniae
	Bacterial
	  Strep throat (group A beta-hemolytic strepto-coccus)
	Viral
	  Infectious mononucleosis (Ebstein-Barr virus)
	  Flu syndrome (influenza A and B)
	  Laryngotracheitis (parainfluenza virus, respiratory syncytial virus)
	  Adenovirus
	Allergy

and interpret on the premises. What follows are descriptions of the more important and frequent infectious causes of sore throat in children. Table 2 provides guidelines that the pediatric practitioner can follow in assessment.

Group A Beta-hemolytic Streptococcal Pharyngotonsillitis (Strep Throat)

Strep throat is the diagnosis that pediatric practitioners must rule out. Its *common* suppurative sequelae are not life threatening (cervical adenitis, otitis media), and its very *serious* suppurative sequelae (pneumonia, septicemia, osteomyelitis) fortunately are very uncommon in developed countries. Prevention of the nonsuppurative sequelae, acute rheumatic fever (ARF) and acute glomerulonephritis (AGN), is the major rea-

son for the serious efforts that are made to establish the diagnosis and to treat the primary disease appropriately. Early treatment will prevent the appearance of ARF, whereas this probably does not apply to AGN. However, early treatment does prevent spread of a nephritogenic strain to others in whom AGN otherwise might develop.

There are situations that make it more likely that the child has a streptococcal pharyngitis.

1. Children under 1 year of age rarely have strep throat. When present, the infection is usually associated with symptoms of a URI, with or without otitis media. Sometimes impetiginized skin lesions are seen spreading out from around the nares.
2. Children under 3 years of age are less likely to have strep throat, though between 2

TABLE 2. COMMON SIGNS AND SYMPTOMS IN PATIENTS WITH SORE THROAT

Cause	Severity of Sore Throat	Fever	Severe Systemic Signs	Drooling
Viral	Mild to moderate	37–40+	Rare	Rare
Streptococcal pharyngitis	Mild to severe	38–40	Common	Unusual
Infectious mononucleosis	Mild to severe	37–40+	Variable	Infrequent
Peritonsillar abscess	Severe	38.5–40+	Common	Frequent
Epiglottitis	Severe	38.5–40+	Invariable	Frequent

and 3 years of age the incidence starts to increase, and symptoms and signs begin to resemble those of the older child.

3. Most children with strep throat have a temperature over 38.5C, with or without sore throat as an initial symptom. However, in most instances, a throat culture *will be required to rule out group A beta-hemolytic streptococcal infection.* It has been shown that dependence on history and physical examination alone is unreliable in differentiating bacterial from nonbacterial sore throat. We recommend that a throat culture be taken, therefore, on every child over the age of 2 years who presents with sore throat, fever, vomiting and abdominal pain not associated with diarrhea, or any combination of these symptoms.

4. The classic symptoms and signs of severe strep throat are the abrupt onset of fever from 39.5–40.5C associated with a severe sore throat, abdominal pain (with or without vomiting), and a beefy red pharynx and tonsils with enlarged, somewhat tender, anterior cervical nodes. Less well known, but a frequently present physical sign, is a palatal enanthem and a bright red uvula. If the child is seen within the first few hours of the onset of the fever, the pharynx may not be very red at all. If the child is examined after the first 24 hours, exudate on the tonsils usually will be seen. The abdominal pain can be so severe that acute appendicitis is a considera-

tion. With this presentation, the child is very uncomfortable. If the illness is untreated, the symptoms will subside over a period of 3–5 days, usually without complications.

5. Scarlet fever should be discussed, since it is nothing more than a strep throat with a rash. Historically, scarlet fever was a severe illness, occurring in epidemics and associated with major systemic manifestations and an appreciable rate of mortality. Though the illness became milder in character prior to the introduction of penicillin, the use of the term "scarlet fever" still has an ominous ring to many people. It is important for the pediatric practitioner to realize that the presence of the rash no longer bears any relationship to the severity of the illness. The rash is recognized by its characteristic appearance: an erythematous, sunburnlike background, often associated with a rough sandpapery feel, circumoral pallor (area about the lips is spared of rash), with a progression of the rash from the groin and axilla to the rest of the body. An increased pigmentation in the antecubital fossae (Pastia's lines) is sometimes seen, as are petechiae, especially if a tourniquet is used to draw blood. Peeling of the skin occurs 1–2 weeks after the rash and is most prominent on the hands and feet. This condition can be confused with Kawasaki's disease (see below).

Acute Epiglottitis

At present, acute epiglottitis is the most ominous cause of sore throat in the young child (diphtheria having been all but eradicated). The average age of onset is 3–4 years, though a child of any age may be affected. Initially the child complains of a sore throat, is febrile, and seems sicker than patients with the usual sore throat. Drooling is a very important early sign and should be looked for and asked about in every child presenting with sore throat and fever. The child usually leans forward, sitting up, trying unconsciously to maximize an airway compromised by an inflamed supraglottic area. Tachycardia, out of proportion to the elevation in temperature, is present. Occasionally, the heart rate is so rapid that it may suggest a supraventricular tachycardia.

Acute epiglottitis is almost always caused by infection with *Haemophilus influenzae* type b. If the diagnosis is suspected, and the child is willing to open his mouth, one can look for the enlarged, brightly inflamed, so-called cherry red epiglottis. A tongue blade should not be used to help view the pharynx. The rapidity of progression of symptoms may be a clue to the diagnosis, for the average time from the onset of the illness to hospitalization is 8 hours. Acute epiglottitis should be suspected in any toxic-appearing child presenting with a sore throat. This toxicity is due to the fact that in almost all cases a positive blood culture for *H. influenzae* type b is present.

Peritonsillar Abscess

This is another cause of serious sore throat; it presents with fever, sore throat, trismus, and drooling. Trismus, defined as difficulty in opening the mouth, is secondary to inflammation of the internal pterygoid muscle. The soft palate on the side of the peritonsillar abscess bulges forward, and the uvula is deviated to the opposite side. The usual causative organisms are mouth anaerobes. Children over 10 years of age are most commonly affected. Complications include airway obstruction, spread to the parapharyngeal space, mediastinum, or pericardium. Many people believe that the disease tends to recur and that tonsillectomy, therefore, is indicated following therapy for the acute episode.

Infectious Mononucleosis

This disease is due to infection with the Ebstein-Barr virus. It is associated with pharyngeal inflammation, often with an exudate and palatal petechiae. In its most spectacular form, the tonsils are markedly enlarged, the patient complains of severe sore throat, drools because swallowing is very painful, and has markedly enlarged anterior and posterior cervical nodes, an enlarged spleen, and generalized lymphadenopathy. The enlargement of the posterior cervical nodes in infectious mononucleosis helps differentiate it from a streptococcal infection. Definitive diagnosis is made by finding a positive heterophil test or rising Ebstein-Barr virus blood titers. Since streptococcal pharyngitis and infectious mononucleosis often occur together, a throat culture should be obtained.

Liver function tests in a child with infectious mononucleosis usually show evidence of parenchymal involvement, with elevation of aminotransferases and, less frequently, the total bilirubin. These tests always return to normal with time. A number of complications have been seen in infectious mononucleosis, including thrombocytopenia, meningoencephalitis, Bell's palsy, Guillain-Barré syndrome, and ruptured spleen. The last complication is limited to young adults, since the capsule of the child's spleen is more resistant to rupture.

Herpetic Gingivostomatitis

This illness deserves special consideration, since it can be very severe, especially for the younger child. It is due to a primary infection with herpes simplex virus type 1 and is easily recognized by the presence of shallow, round ulcers (aphthous ulcers) of both the anterior and posterior oral cavity, including the tongue. Symptoms begin with fever, proceed to an inflammation of the gums, and then progress to the classic ulcers. In the most severe form of illness, the fever can persist for 7–10 days, the pain is so severe that liquids are refused (especially by the younger child), and hospitalization for intravenous fluids may be necessary to avoid dehydration. Fortunately, the usual case is much milder and easily managed.

Kawasaki Disease (Mucocutaneous Lymph Node Syndrome, MLNS)

Although rare, this disease deserves consideration, for it is usually quite spectacular in its presentation. First described by Kawasaki in 1967 in Japan, since 1974 it has been diagnosed and reported in increasing numbers in the United States. Though the etiology is still unknown, a recent report from Japan suggests the possibility of a rickettsia-like organism borne by a mite.

It begins initially with fever, and progresses to include a bright red pharynx, red, cracked lips, swollen cervical nodes, conjunctivitis, and a generalized erythematous rash, associated with swelling and redness of the hands and feet. The fever lasts for over a week, and the rash resolves with desquamation, especially prominent around the fingertips. In its most flagrant form, the rash resembles scarlet fever, being bright red and confluent, though not with the same sandpaper feel nor the perioral pallor of scarlet fever.

Antibiotics are not helpful in controlling the symptoms and signs, and the disease relents after 10–14 days. The major complication is sudden death secondary to myocardial infarction due to coronary arterial aneurysm rupture or thrombosis. This event occurs in about 2% of patients, usually within the first 2 months after the illness. Hydrops of the gallbladder, causing bilious vomiting, also occurs and may suggest an acute abdomen.

Sore Throat Secondary to Allergy

This type of sore throat is most often associated with mouth breathing. The lack of humidification of inspired air when nasal breathing is obstructed causes drying of the posterior oropharynx with resultant morning sore throat. It is not associated with fever or other systemic signs. Within an hour or so after arising, the sore throat usually disappears, due to rehydration of the pharynx with ingested fluids and normal secretions. There may be a marked seasonal variation, associated with exacerbations of allergic symptoms. Management is initially directed toward humidification of the air in the bedroom. Attempts should be made to decrease exposure of the child to antigens in the home. Antihistamines may also be helpful.

DIFFERENTIAL DIAGNOSIS

History

The first contact with the patient with sore throat is often over the telephone or by triage personnel in a clinic or emergency room. It is important, therefore, that the initial questioning be directed to ascertain the seriousness of the problem.

- Is the child drooling? Drooling is due to pain so severe that the child cannot swallow his saliva. It should make one think of epiglottitis, peritonsillar abscess, severe infectious mononucleosis, retropharyngeal abscess, herpetic gingivostomatitis, or foreign body.
- Does the child have difficulty in opening and closing his mouth? Trismus is due to inflammation of the internal pterygoid muscle and is associated with inflammation in the peritonsillar or parapharyngeal space.
- Is the child having any difficulty in breathing? Enlargement or inflammation

of any of several structures in the mouth or pharynx can cause difficulty in breathing. Epiglottitis, peritonsillar abscess, retropharyngeal abscess, diphtheria, and severe infectious mononucleosis can all cause acute airway obstruction.

- Has there been any change in the child's voice? Hoarseness is often associated with laryngitis or laryngotracheobronchitis (croup).
- How long has the child had a sore throat? The longer the duration of symptoms, the less likely it is that the sore throat is associated with one of the critical conditions requiring immediate care.
- Is the child febrile and, if so, does he appear sick? Sore throats most often are due to viral infections, especially in the younger child, presenting with high fever but with minimal toxicity (e.g., herpangina, hand-foot-and-mouth disease).
- Is the sore throat present mainly in the morning, improving as the day proceeds? In this case, it is most likely caused by sleeping with the mouth open due to a cold or to allergy.
- Are the glands in the neck swollen, and are they tender? The presence of enlarged tender, anterior cervical nodes, associated with fever, in the appropriate age group (over 3 years) increases the likelihood or group A beta-hemolytic streptococcal infection.
- Are there any other symptoms or signs? The presence of cough, runny nose, inspiratory stridor, or hoarseness make the diagnosis of viral infection more likely. Abdominal pain, vomiting, elevated temperature, or rash associated with sore throat are often symptoms of a streptococcal infection. Sore throat followed by lower respiratory disease, especially wheezing, is often seen with *Mycoplasma pneumoniae* infections.
- Has any one else in the family, or close to the family, been sick recently, or is anyone sick now? This question is obviously helpful in establishing a diagnosis.

Physical Examination

Usually the only finding on physical examination of a child complaining of sore throat is a reddened posterior pharynx. Sometimes no evidence of inflammation is seen. Physical examination, therefore, is usually not helpful in making the diagnosis, although there are a number of diseases in which it does suggest a specific diagnosis.

1. Elevated temperature with aphthous ulcers on the posterior soft palate, just lateral to the uvula, is diagnostic of herpangina, a condition due to infection with Coxsackie virus group A.
2. Palatal ulcers, associated with a vesicular rash on the palms and soles, is diagnostic of hand-foot-and-mouth disease, associated also with Coxsackie virus group A.
3. The acute onset of aphthous ulcerations on the buccal mucosa, gingiva, and posterior palate, associated with fever, is diagnostic of herpes simplex gingivostomatitis.
4. The constellation of beefy red tonsils, a bright red, often petechial, palatal exanthem, an elevated temperature, and enlarged anterior cervical nodes is characteristic of infections caused by group A beta-hemolytic streptococcus. Tonsillar exudate develops only after symptoms have been present for 2–3 days and, therefore, is usually not seen if the patient is examined soon after the onset. However, the symptoms and signs of disease in most cases are much less prominent than those described here.
5. A diffuse maculopapular rash associated with sore throat suggesting streptococcal infection is diagnostic of scarlet fever. The rash begins in the groin and axilla, looks like sunburn, and often feels rough, like sandpaper. A similar rash is seen with mucocutaneous lymph node syndrome. However, the rash in the latter condition is somewhat different in that it is associated with redness and

swelling of the palms and soles and does not spare the circumoral area, a characteristic of the rash of scarlet fever. In addition, it usually does not have the rough, sandpapery feel of the scarlet fever rash.

6. Enlarged tonsils with or without exudate, palatal petechiae, enlarged anterior but especially posterior cervical nodes, with or without generalized lymphadenopathy, splenomegaly, or hepatomegaly, should suggest a diagnosis of infectious mononucleosis.

7. Bulging of the posterior soft palate, with deviation of the uvula to the opposite side, is diagnostic of peritonsillitis or peritonsillar abscess.

8. A white coating on the tongue associated with similar plaques on the buccal mucosa and posterior soft palate is diagnostic of oral thrush secondary to a monilial infection.

9. Bulging of the posterior oropharynx is seen in patients with retropharyngeal abscess (now a rare diagnosis).

10. A swollen, cherry red epiglottis is diagnostic of epiglottitis.

Laboratory Diagnosis

Laboratory examinations by the pediatric practitioner are limited to the identification of streptococcal infections of the pharynx and the presence of heterophil antibodies for infectious mononucleosis in the blood.

Inexpensive, commercially available 5% sheep's blood agar plates are used for throat cultures. The technique for obtaining material for culture is relatively simple to describe but not always simple to perform in an uncooperative child. When possible, swabs are taken of both tonsils, the posterior edge of the soft palate, and the uvula, using a sterile cotton-tipped applicator. The specimen is plated, using another sterile cotton applicator to streak out the plate and incubated at 37C for approximately 24 hours and at room temperature for another 24 hours if it is negative initially. It is not difficult to recognize beta hemolysis and the typical morphology of colonies of streptococci. Sometimes a bacitracin disc is used to help differentiate group A from other beta-hemolytic streptococci, since it selectively inhibits the growth of group A beta-hemolytic streptococci. Therefore, there will be no evidence of beta hemolysis in the area surrounding the bacitracin disc on culture plates positive for streptococcal growth. Although the fluorescent antibody technique is more accurate, it requires sending the culture to an outside laboratory. Most pediatric practitioners prefer, therefore, to use the culture method, since it combines convenience and low cost with reasonable realiability.

Commercial kits are available for the identification of heterophile antibodies to aid in establishing the diagnosis of infectious mononucleosis. These are slide or spot tests, readily adaptable to both office and hospital use and characterized by their reliability, easy performance, and rapid results. People tend to overinterpret the tests, calling them positive when they are not, but this tendency can be reduced by including a control when in doubt. The slide or spot tests use horse or sheep red blood cells, with or without guinea pig kidney absorption. In an office or small laboratory, we recommend a test kit that uses horse red blood cells with guinea pig kidney absorption because of its reliability and simplicity. The time of doing the test is important; it is negative very early in the disease, generally becoming positive by the end of the first week. If it is negative the first time, it can be repeated after 7–10 days. Children with atypical or minimal disease are less likely to have positive heterophil antibody tests than are those with more typical symptoms and signs of infectious mononucleosis. If more specific tests are required, the child's blood can be analyzed by a hospital laboratory. These tests include, in addition to the standard white blood count and blood smear for atypical lymphocytes, serologic tests for the Ebstein-Barr virus.

Other laboratory tests, such as blood counts, cold agglutinins, blood culture, culture of the epiglottis, and viral cultures, are rarely indicated. Measurements of cold agglutinins (for *Mycoplasma*) are usually reserved for patients with lower respiratory disease, often associated with wheezing. Blood cultures and culture of the epiglottis are done on the patient with epiglottitis who is being managed in the hospital. Viral cultures are usually done only for epidemiologic purposes.

X-ray examinations should be limited to a lateral neck view in cases where the diagnosis of epiglottitis cannot be made on the basis of history and physical examination alone. With a little experience, it becomes easy to recognize the signs of supraglottic swelling on x-ray. We keep a demonstration x-ray in our pediatric emergency room to aid the house staff.

MANAGEMENT

The management of the child with sore throat proceeds logically after the appropriate history, physical examination, and laboratory examinations have been done. In most instances, the pediatric practitioner will be able to carry out the plan of treatment without help from a consultant.

General Principles

At this point in evaluation of the patient, some basic decisions are required.

- Is the child seriously ill?
- What should be done, and is consultation needed?
- Have the patient and family been made aware of the concern?
- If the child is not seriously ill, is there sufficient information to proceed with treatment?
- If not, what further examination or diagnostic tests must be done?

- Have the patient and family been advised sufficiently, and do they understand the instructions?

We recommend beginning therapy with penicillin (erythromycin in the child allergic to penicillin) in any child suspected of having a sore throat that may be due to streptococci while waiting for the results of the culture. An exception would be if a sibling had a recent illness and had a negative throat culture. Recommending treatment prior to positive culture is controversial. It is based, however, on our firm clinical impression that symptoms and signs of strep throat respond within hours of starting penicillin and that prompt treatment of children with streptococcal infection is important, whereas a short period of treatment of patients with other infections not affected by penicillin is not harmful. By the time a positive culture is reported, the child with a strep throat is no longer contagious. Early treatment reduces absenteeism for both the child and the parents, both of whom may work outside the home and rely on day care, nursery school, or public school attendance for their children. Even if one parent does not work, decreasing the duration of illness and reducing the period of contagion are worthwhile goals. Early treatment may not prevent poststreptococcal acute glomerulonephritis, and the incidence of acute rheumatic fever, though reduced by early treatment, is probably not altered significantly by a delay of 24 hours in instituting therapy. Prevention of these two diseases, therefore, cannot be used as an argument in favor of early treatment.

The diagnosis of viral pharyngitis is made after streptoccal infection has been ruled out by a negative throat culture or when a specific diagnosis is made on the basis of the history and physical examinations described above. Viral pharyngitis accounts for the great majority of children and adults with sore throat. Treatment is aimed at alleviating the symptoms. Lozenges, hard candy, fluids, gargles, aspirin, and acetaminophen are all acceptable and effective. Analgesics stronger than aspirin or acetaminophen are almost never indicated. Antipyretic usage for fever is discussed in Chapter 9. Oral decongestants or antihistamine-decongestant mixtures are sometimes recommended, but our experience is that they are overprescribed and probably ineffective. In addition, these medications are often associated with irritability or sleepiness in children, and, therefore, they should not be given. Since viral pharyngitis is a self-limited illness, with an average duration of 3–4 days, a little patience on the part of the physician, the patient, and the parent is the best medication.

Streptococcal Pharyngotonsillitis

The treatment and management of this illness has been standard for many years. Basic therapy is with penicillin. Erythromycin is reserved for individuals allergic to penicillin. The oral cephalosporins and clindamycin are also effective drugs but are reserved for the rare individual who is unable to tolerate either penicillin or erythromycin. The sulfonamides and the tetracyclines are not acceptable as alternative forms of treatment.

Recommended treatment regimens are as follows:

- Oral: Phenoxymethyl penicillin potassium (penicillin V) 250 mg tid × 10 days. Erythromycin 20–40 mg/kg up to 1 g divided qid × 10 days. Both these regimens effect a cure rate of 85–90%.
- Intramuscular: Benzathine penicillin G (Bicillin) 600,000 U IM in children under 6 years or under 60 pounds; 1.2 million U IM in children over 6 years or over 60 pounds. Benzathine penicillin G (600,000 U) is usually combined with 600,000 U of procaine penicillin. This combination decreases pain at the injection site. Recently a preparation composed of 900,000 U benzathine penicillin and 300,000 U procaine penicillin was introduced. It is effective therapy for

children up to adolescence and has markedly reduced the need for the 1.2 million U benzathine penicillin G dosage form.

We believe the choice between oral and parenteral forms of penicillin rests mainly on the assessment of compliance. Which form one uses requires an individual judgment; the regimens are equally effective. It is difficult to remember to take an oral medication 3 times a day for 10 days, especially when the patient feels well within 24–48 hours. However, most pediatric practitioners in private practice use the oral form of treatment, resorting to intramuscular penicillin when there is a relapse or recurrence. Physicians in hospital clinics and emergency rooms generally use intramuscular therapy because it is believed that many of the patients will not comply with oral treatment.

Symptomatic recurrences after adequate therapy (assuming compliance) are thought to be due to one of two possibilities: (1) organisms are not completely eradicated during the 10 days of therapy, possibly because of a small focus of infection within the tonsils, or (2) reinfection occurs from another member of the family, a friend, or a pet. Our experience is that the most common cause for relapse is failure to eradicate the organism from the throat of the index case.

In summary, a reasonable approach to management is the following:

1. For a first infection (following throat culture) give oral penicillin for 10 days.
2. If there is a symptomatic recurrence (usually within the first month after discontinuing treatment), repeat the oral course or give intramuscular penicillin.
3. If there is a second symptomatic recurrence, repeat the intramuscular treatment, and culture all members of the family and the family dog. (Fighting with cats to obtain a culture is not worth the risk of losing a finger.) If any of the family has a positive throat culture, he should be treat-

ed orally for 10 days. If there is another symptomatic recurrence in the index case, it is not worthwhile bothering the asymptomatic family members again. If the child continues to have recurrences of symptomatic disease, we prefer to treat them as they occur rather than to consider tonsillectomy. (See end of chapter for a discussion of the indications for tonsillectomy.) The asymptomatic carrier state, on the other hand, is not necessary to treat.

There have been a number of studies advocating changing medications to erythromycin, cephalosporins, or clindamycin in patients with persistent or recurrent infections. Our experience is that the use of these agents is no more effective than persisting with penicillin. Use of a β-lactamase-resistant penicillin has also been advocated, on the possibility of β-lactamase-producing staphylococci residing in the nasopharynx and interfering with the efficacy of penicillin. We do not believe that this regimen offers any benefits over penicillin. Despite this extensive but necessary discussion of the treatment of persistent or recurrent infections, it should be clear that the great majority of children with streptococcal sore throat respond quickly and completely to treatment with penicillin.

Infectious Mononucleosis

Despite its great notoriety, infectious mononucleosis is usually a mild, self-limited illness, and management consists primarily of rest. In the younger child, the period of restricted activity is usually limited to the duration of the fever. The older child may have malaise and lethargy for 1–2 months, though usually symptoms subside earlier. Children should be encouraged to return to school early but to refrain from contact sports until the spleen and liver are of normal size. It is not necessary to rely on the presence or absence of heterophil antibodies in determining the resumption of activities. In the child with infectious

mononucleosis whose airway is compromised or in one with severe toxicity, adrenocorticosteroids are beneficial in rapidly reducing the symptoms. Since streptococcal pharyngitis and infectious mononucleosis often occur together, a throat culture should be obtained. In the seriously ill child, penicillin should be started before the results are available.

Kawasaki's Disease (Mucocutaneous Lymph Node Syndrome, MLNS)

The major concern in the management of the child with MLNS is the possibility of sudden death because of myocardial infarction. All children with this disease should be evaluated for the presence of coronary arterial aneurysms, using two-dimensional echocardiography. If present, it is recommended that a course of low-dose aspirin (30 mg/kg/day) should be initiated in order to decrease platelet aggregation and be continued until the aneurysms resolve. The state of our knowledge at the present time is not complete enough to know whether this therapy changes the natural history of cardiac disease in patients with MLNS. Some individuals recommend starting high-dose aspirin initially (serum level of 20–25 mg%) in order to decrease the severity of symptoms, such as fever and malaise. Our own thoughts on this issue are ambivalent. While high-dose aspirin therapy will shorten the duration of fever by 1–2 days, recent concerns about the use of aspirin at this dosage possibly contributing to the onset of Reye's syndrome have made us more cautious.

Hydrops of the gallbladder, when it occurs in MLNS, should be managed conservatively. The diagnosis can be made when severe abdominal pain develops, which is usually but not always worse in the right upper quadrant. The signs may resemble an acute abdomen, but sonography demonstrates a markedly enlarged gallbladder. Physical examination of young children with severe abdominal pain is often difficult, so that it may not be possible to appreciate the distended gallbladder by palpation. With conservative management (intravenous fluids and nasograstic drainage if indicated), the symptoms and signs subside after 3–5 days.

Acute Epiglottitis

All pediatric practitioners should be familiar with the protocol for the management of acute epiglottitis. They should also make sure that their otolaryngology and anesthesia consultants and the emergency room personnel at their hospital are also familiar with this protocol. An understanding of the proper way to manage this disease may make the difference between life and death. Table 3 provides a step-by-step outline of management when the diagnosis is suspected. Under no circumstances should the child be forced to open its mouth. A tongue blade must never be used. There are numerous instances of sudden cardiorespiratory arrest after attempts at forceful visualization of the posterior pharynx in children with acute epiglottitis.

If the child is willing to open its mouth, the swollen, cherry red epiglottis may be visualized. If there is doubt about the diagnosis and the child's condition allows it, a lateral x-ray of the neck can be taken. This will demonstrate swelling in the supraglottic area, even in early cases of acute epiglottitis, when the epiglottis may not yet be markedly inflamed. It should be understood that the child must be accompanied to the x-ray suite by someone prepared to establish an airway quickly should the need arise. A sudden disturbance, precipitating gagging or vomiting, can cause an acute arrest. Since most of these children hypoventilate because of the severe pain, they may have been hypoxemic and acidemic for some undetermined time. If a cardiorespiratory arrest does occur, it is unlikely that resuscitation can be accomplished without neurologic damage. It is imperative that everyone concerned understand this, so that the importance of being calm and proceeding systematically is recognized. With the diagnosis of acute epiglottitis, two consultants are called immediately and simultaneously: an anesthesiologist adept at endotracheal intu-

TABLE 3. PROTOCOL FOR THE MANAGEMENT OF ACUTE EPIGLOTTITIS

Steps in Management

Presumptive diagnosis made on clinical grounds by initial observer

Minimal disturbance of child (nothing by mouth, no blood drawing)

Anesthesiologist and otolaryngologist emergently summoned to emergency room

Child moved to operating room when everyone arrives, consider lateral neck x-ray

Slow face mask general anesthesia given with child sitting upright

Preliminary oral translaryngeal intubation accomplished

Diagnosis confirmed by inspection of epiglottis

CBC, blood culture, surface cultures, arterial blood gas obtained

Intravenous cannula placed

Ampicillin 100 mg/kg/24 hr and chloramphenicol 100 mg/kg/24 hr begun intravenously

Nasotracheal intubation accomplished if possible

Consider tracheostomy if concern about translaryngeal intubation

Transfer to intensive care area

Extubation accomplished at 48–72 hours, consider operating room site

Continue ampicillin or chloramphenicol for 10 days as indicated by antibiotic sensitivities

bation of children and an otolaryngologist or pediatric surgeon capable of performing a tracheostomy if necessary. These consultants should be called prior to obtaining an x-ray of the neck. The operating room should be notified and made ready. No unnecessary manipulations are done, such as starting intravenous fluids or instituting some form of inhalation therapy. The child is made comfortable, seated leaning forward, and brought to the operating room suite with everyone in attendance: pediatric practitioner, anesthesiologist, and otolaryngologist. Anesthesia is induced, an intravenous line is inserted, and cultures of the surface of the epiglottis and of the blood are taken. Ampicillin 100 mg/kg and chloramphenicol 50 mg/kg are given intravenously as an immediate intravenous bolus, followed by intravenous ampicillin 200 mg/kg/24 hours, given in divided doses every 4 hours, and chloramphenicol 100 mg/kg/24 hours, given every 6 hours. Adrenocorticosteroids are not of benefit. While these procedures are being done, nasotracheal intubation is attempted by the anesthesiologist. Most of the time this procedure will be successful. If it is not, an oral endotracheal tube is placed. Since oral endotracheal tubes are more easily displaced than are nasotracheal tubes, a decision must then be made whether to leave it in place or perform a tracheostomy. This decision is based on an assessment of whether nursing care is expert enough to prevent self-extubation for at least 48 hours. After the procedure is completed, the child is brought to an intensive care area. Extubation may be attempted after 48–72 hours, usually in an operating room, with the surgeon and the anesthesiologist present. If the epiglottis looks normal, the child is extubated and observed for another 24–48 hours. Results of culture and antibiotic sensitivities should be available, allowing one of the antibiotics to be discontinued. Intravenous antibiotics are given for 24 hours after extubation, followed by oral therapy for a combined total of 10 days. One week after discharge, the child should be seen for

follow-up. In addition to discussing the medical and surgical aspects of the hospitalization, it is important at that time to explore the feelings of both parent and child about this frightening episode. It should be clearly stated that this was a one time occurrence and will not recur, since acute epiglottitis is caused by a single organism, with sustained immunity resulting after only one exposure.

Peritonsillar Abscess

In the management of peritonsillar abscess, it is necessary to obtain consultation with an otolaryngologist to determine the need for surgical drainage. Early in the course of the illness, there may only be cellulitis (peritonsillitis), and in this case antibiotic therapy without drainage is adequate. If indicated, drainage is important to provide more rapid resolution of a potentially serious infection.

As soon as the diagnosis of peritonsillitis or peritonsillar abscess is made, the child should be hospitalized, drainage performed if fluctuance is noted on palpation of the tonsil, and intravenous antibiotics begun. Since the usual causative organisms are mouth anaerobes, penicillin G 200,000–300,000 U/kg/24 hours divided q4h is the antibiotic of choice. Less commonly, Group A streptococcus, staphylococci or *H. influenzae* type b is the causative organism. Therefore, if the child appears very toxic or if there has been compromise of the airway or if the infection has spread to the parapharyngeal tissue, as evidenced by swelling of the neck or submandibular areas, treatment with ampicillin, chloramphenicol, and a beta-lactamase-resistant penicillin is indicated after local and blood cultures have been obtained.

Tonsillectomy

It is appropriate in this chapter to mention the indications for tonsillectomy. Our opinion at this time is that tonsils need to be removed very rarely and that beliefs about enlarged or kissing tonsils causing everything from bad breath to juvenile delinquency are in the main unfounded. Indications for adenoidectomy with or without tonsillectomy will not be discussed, since that subject is covered in Chapter 8.

Reasons given for not parting with one's tonsils include the probability that they serve some useful purpose and that an increase in allergic symptoms or other undefined deleterious effects may occur after their removal. In the past, an increase in the incidence of bulbar poliomyelitis was associated with tonsillectomy. Though controversial, Hodgkin's disease has also been linked with tonsil removal.

Our recommendations for performing a tonsillectomy are limited to a few uncommon situations. Extremely rarely, the tonsils hypertrophy to such a great extent that they interfere with swallowing or breathing. Cor pulmonale as a consequence of hypoventilation with resultant hypoxemia secondary to obstructive tonsillar hypertrophy does occur but is very rare. If either of the above are demonstrated unequivocally to exist, tonsillectomy is indicated. In our experience, peritonsillar abscess tends to recur. Although not everyone agrees on this point, we advise tonsillectomy following the first episode of peritonsillar abscess based on our concern about the potential seriousness of this disease.

Though some physicians consider recurrent or chronic tonsillitis of any etiology an indication for tonsillectomy, we strongly disagree with this point of view. Some physicians will recommend tonsillectomy when recurrent tonsillitis occurs secondary to the group A streptococcus. We do not agree with this point of view either. An extensive experience in the private practice of pediatrics has convinced us that recurrent tonsillitis of any etiology usually disappears with time without recourse to tonsillectomy. The morbidity and mortality from the surgery, though small, is real, and we believe that even this risk is not warranted.

BIBLIOGRAPHY

Battaglia JD, Lockhart CH: Management of acute epiglottitis by nasotracheal intubation. Am J Dis Child 129:334, 1975

Faden HS: Treatment of haemophilus influenzae type B epiglottitis. Pediatrics 63:402, 1979

Kaplan EL: The group A streptococcal upper respiratory tract carrier state: An enigma. J Pediatr 97:337, 1980

Katz HP, Clancy RR: Accuracy of a home throat culture program: A study of parent participation in health care. Pediatrics 53:687, 1974

Melish ME: Kawasaki syndrome (The mucocutaneous lymph node syndrome). Pediatr Ann 2:255, 1982

Peter G, Smith AL: Group A streptococcal infections of the skin and pharynx. (First of two parts) N Engl J Med 297:311, 1977

Peter G, Smith AL: Group A streptococcal infections of the skin and pharynx. (Second of two parts) N Engl J Med 297:365, 1977

Cross-References to *Pediatrics,* 17th ed.

PART III

Behavioral and Developmental Problems

NINETEEN

Depression and Suicide during Adolescence

S. Kenneth Schonberg

Death from suicide is now the third most common cause of mortality among older adolescents and young adults. Only accident and homicide lead to greater loss of life in this age group, and even within these categories of traumatic death, self-destructive intent may play a role. Each year some 5,000 young people between the ages of 14 and 24 die from suicide. A much larger number seriously attempt to end their lives but are not successful. Detecting the depressed teenager at risk of suicide and addressing the needs of the adolescent who has already made such an attempt has become an unavoidable concern for those health professionals who care for youth.

DEFINITION

The annual death rate from adolescent suicide is now over 12 per 100,000, and, although not as high as in older age groupings, it recently has been escalating. The reason for the increase in the number of both deaths from suicide and unsuccessful attempts remains unclear. A variety of explanations have

been proffered, including the nuclear age, the increased stress of current day life, and the dissolution of traditional family structure with divorce and separation. None of these theories adequately explains the acceleration of the rate of suicide among young people.

Among those youth who die from suicide, males outnumber females in a ratio of 4:1. However, among those who attempt suicide, females account for the large majority. This disparity is explained in part by differences in the methods used to attempt suicide. The vast majority of young women attempt suicide by self-poisoning and present for medical attention with remediable dysfunction or minimal physiologic compromise. Although most young men similarly attempt self-poisoning, a significant number utilize hanging, firearms, and jumping from buildings and bridges. These latter methods often result in death prior to any possible medical intervention.

The *actual number* of deaths per year from suicide among young people almost certainly *exceeds 5,000*. As noted previously, other traumatic deaths, particularly those involving automobile accidents, are secondary to willful self-destruction. In addition, fatal drug overdoses among experienced drug users are frequently marked by a lack of prior

[1]Supported in part by Grant 7254 from the Robert Wood Johnson Foundation.

concern by the deceased regarding self-preservation. Despite these provisos, the published number of adolescent deaths from suicide remains fairly accurate. No such statement can be made regarding the number of suicidal attempts. Various authors have suggested that there are between 50 and 200 attempts for every fatality. There are currently some 40 million individuals in the United States between the ages of 14 and 24. Hence, the 5,000 deaths per year translates to 1 fatality for every 8,000 individuals. Using a modest estimate of 100 attempts for each fatality results in a calculation of 1 attempt for every 80 adolescents each year. The application of these calculations to the number of teenagers within a given community or a specific school yields a more poignant understanding regarding the current level of concern about adolescent depression and suicide.

ETIOLOGY

A wide range of mental disorders and untoward circumstances are etiologic of suicidal attempts. Although it is often difficult or impossible to ascertain the cause of a self-destructive act at the moment of presentation, the determination of the operative etiology in a particular teenager during the ensuing days is crucial in mangement and disposition. At one extreme are young people with organic psychosis, and at the other are adolescents with no prior history of mental dysfunction who have suffered an overwhelming psychic insult. The large majority of teenagers who attempt suicide lie between these two extremes and may be roughly categorized as suffering from borderline personality disorders or chronic situational depressions.

Psychosis

There is a small minority of teenagers, in our experience some 5% of those who make an attempt, whose suicidal behavior is secondary to a psychotic disorder. The biologically based depressions, including both unipolar (depressive episodes only) and bipolar depressions (depressive and manic episodes), may first manifest themselves during adolescence and come to medical attention after a suicide attempt. Although these disorders are increasingly thought to be genetically determined neurochemical dysfunctions which may be manifest even in preteens, they are most often noted only in retrospect in adults with repeated episodes of depression. In adolescents, such episodes are more frequently attributed to a reaction to untoward circumstances, and the existence of an underlying biologic depression is not appreciated.

Schizophrenia also frequently begins during the teen years, and episodes of psychotic behavior may include self-destructive acts. *Command hallucinations* may occur, in which God, a relative, or other voices instruct the individual to attempt suicide or to perform a death-defying act. The hallucinating individual is usually identified easily and represents a serious and acute risk of continuing suicidal behavior.

Borderline Personality

Far more common than psychotics among suicide attempters are teenagers with borderline personalities. This nebulously defined category of mental illness in fact represents a variety of disorders that share in common an inability to cope adequately with the demands of life. Some of the circumstances that result in borderline personality disorders are now achieving definition, while others remain poorly understood. Some of these teenagers, although not psychotic, have defects in the machinery of thought or, in other words, an organic, physiologic, or structural etiology to their personality deficit. Minimal brain dysfunction, impaired intellect, hyperactivity syndromes, and specific learning disorders are all examples of persistent abnormalities that may result in deficiencies in the ability to deal with the stresses of life. Other adolescents, although not inherently damaged, have experienced a childhood characterized by great deprivation or repetitive mental trauma and enter adolescence with emotional disorganization, which places them at risk for a variety of negative behaviors including suicide. Regardless of the etiology of the borderline personality, be it inherent to the individual or an outgrowth of his or her childhood surroundings, these teenagers will have great difficulty accomplishing the developmental tasks of adolescence and emerging as functional adults.

Chronic Situational Depression

In contrast to the young person with a borderline personality who enters adolescence with an inherent vulnerability, there are individuals with no underlying disorder who are impacted upon by repetitive, adverse circumstances in their environment. Although borderline personality and chronic situational depression are presented here as two distinct entities, the reader must appreciate that it is often difficult to determine if an adolescent who has attempted suicide has an inherent emotional disorganization or, alternatively, has intact mental machinery but has been subjected to extremes of stress. However, despite the difficulty, attempting to differentiate between these two etiologies is important in dispositional planning.

Some understanding of the tasks that must be accomplished during adolescence, and hence the opportunities to experience failure, are prerequisite to a full understanding of the causes of chronic depression during the teenage years. During a period of less than a decade, the child must become an adult. Physical, psychosexual, social, and intellectual goals must be attained. The young person must undergo a period of rapid physical maturation, with marked increases in height and weight and the development of secondary sexual characteristics. The child must mature to an adult not only in appearance but also in function. Young people must emerge from isosexual groups and progressively move through those learning experiences that result in adult sexual attitudes and practices. The adolescent must advance from a position of dependence upon family to a status of emancipation and independence. Educational and vocational goals must be established and accomplished. The adolescent must develop his or her own self-image with the confidence and ability to be emotionally and financially independent of parents. Adult cognitive abilities must be developed, with the capability for abstraction replacing the concrete thinking of childhood.

There is great variation in the age of onset and rapidity of accomplishment of these developmental tasks. The adolescent may progress rapidly in one developmental sphere while lagging behind in another without this dyssynchrony being evidence of pathology. The teenager may achieve physical maturity quite early and adult sexuality quite late, without any indication of dysfunction. However, there is much opportunity for failure and, of greater importance, the *perception* of failure, in the quest to accomplish these developmental tasks. It is when the adolescent perceives failure that stress and depression may ensue. The magnitude of such failure, particularly as measured by adult standards, is of little importance. It is the adolescent's perception of lack of accomplishment, inability to effect a positive change in life circumstances, and feelings of decreased self-worth that may be precipitants of depression and self-destructive behavior.

At times factors intrinsic to the teenager, such as chronic illness, may lead to failure to complete the tasks of adolescence. More often it is factors within the adolescent's environment that either prevent success or, alternatively, fail to support him or her adequately as the unavoidable difficulties of the teenage years are encountered. As such, these intrinsic and extrinsic circumstances may be viewed as risk factors for the development of chronic depression, antisocial and self-destructive behavior, and suicidal ideation and action.

The single factor most frequently associated with suicidal behavior in adolescents is severe family disruption. Approximately 75% of teenagers who attempt suicide come from families where either one or both natural parents are absent from the home because of divorce, separation, or death. More often than not, the teenager has lived outside of the home for extended periods of time in either foster placement or with relatives. A large majority of such teenagers view their family conflicts as extreme. Areas of conflict most often include school performance, choice of friends, sexual behavior, drug use, unwillingness to perform chores, and inability to please their parents in general. These teenagers find themselves in an environment that is not only nonsupportive in their need for guidance but also additive to their difficulties by producing feelings of guilt, isolation, rejection, and decreased self-worth. It is not at all surprising that family disruption emerges as the single, most common theme among teenagers who attempt suicide.

As is commonly known, a family history of suicide makes it more likely that a teenager will exhibit self-destructive behavior. Approximately 20% of teenagers who attempt suicide have a parent who has attempted suicide, and this percentage doubles if close relatives are included. Parental histories of alcoholism or mental illness are also common. These associations may in part be due to the familial nature of biologic depressions and other mental illness or the disruption of family that is inherent to the situation where a parent or close relative has committed suicide, is suicidal, or is mentally ill.

Academic stress has been mentioned frequently as a precipitant of suicidal behavior in adolescents. Suicide rates are higher among students at selective and highly competitive colleges. However, some surveys have indicated that suicide rates are greater among nonstudents than they are among students, and few differences can be detected between communities with highly competitive high schools versus those with less demanding environments. The relationship between academic stress, depression, and suicide remains unclear. It would appear that the highly competitive academic situations offer one type of opportunity for perceived failure, while noncompetitive, nonsuccess-oriented situations offer other opportunities for feelings of defeat.

In contrast to circumstances in which depression arises out of a failure of the environment to support the teenager, there are instances in which the adolescent is suffering from conditions that place additional demands upon both the teenager and significant others within his or her environment. Chronic physical illness is such a circumstance. It may interfere with the normal progression through adolescence in numerous ways. Physical growth and development may be delayed. Independence may be stymied, and the development of social and psychosexual skills may be made more difficult by the incapacities, therapeutic restrictions, and cosmetic deformities of the illness. Educational and vocational goals may be curtailed. The abnormality of illness, at a time when it is so important to be normal, may impact severely on the development of a healthy self-image. It would appear that chronic illness during adolescence is a greater risk factor for depression and suicide among males than among females. This finding has been attributed to the interference produced in reaching vocational and academic goals and achieving the competence necessary for masculine identity. The teenage girl is more likely to tolerate chronic illness in that such disability frequently induces care and support from important persons in her life. When the illness becomes a cause of rejection and loss of family support, the female is placed at higher risk.

It should be noted that acute, mild, and transient depression is quite common among teenagers and is most often a healthy mechanism of coping in response to adverse circumstances. One would not be surprised or alarmed to encounter aspects of depression in an adolescent who had suffered a romantic defeat, lost a job, failed an examination, been rejected by a college, been cut from a team, or been subjected to the myriad other traumas that are part of becoming an adult or being an adult. It is only when the depression is unremitting and does not respond to either the tincture of time or the adolescent's efforts to alleviate the adverse situation that suicidal thoughts and actions become a concern. It is in those instances where factors intrinsic to the adolescent or within his or her extrinsic environment prevent remediation of adverse circumstances that chronic depression and its consequences may eventuate.

Acute Reactive Depressions

Acute reactive depressions rarely result in suicidal attempts, except in those instances when there is a major insult to a fragile adolescent with limited healthy mechanisms of coping. Most adolescents are able to tolerate major psychic insult without becoming suicidal. Hence, the death of a parent or some other loved one would be likely to result in depression but not suicide. Exceptions to this rule may occur in instances of rape or incarceration. The perceived magnitude of these insults is such as to precipitate suicidal attempts in previously stable adolescents. Hence, the degree of psychic trauma experienced by the teenager who has been a victim of sexual assault is at least as important as the physiologic consequences of the attack. Similarly, those responsible for the care of adolescents who have been incarcerated must be sensitive to the frequency with which self-destructive acts occur within a prison setting.

EVALUATION

When an adolescent comes to medical attention because of a suicidal attempt, the need to conduct a psychosocial and developmental history is explicitly clear. It should be equally clear that the detection of young people in difficulty, some of whom will be depressed and at risk of suicide, is accomplished through the routine inclusion of similar historical information in the evaluation of all teenagers who present for care. This is particularly true not only for those adolescents complaining of the more traditional depressive symptoms of decreased appetite, weight loss, constipation, and insomnia but also for young people with a variety of functional complaints, including abdominal pain, headaches, chest pain, dizziness, and insomnia. It is noteworthy that over half of the adolescents who attempt suicide have made contact with a physician in the month preceding their attempt.

Although recognition of the depressed teenager may be difficult, the routine assessment of mood, academic achievement, vocational goals, family relationships, social progress, sexual practices, and drug use habits will detect most youths who are exhibiting deviant and disturbing behavior. At times, adult symptoms of depression will be elicited, including apathy, sleep disturbances, and decreased appetite. More frequently depression during adolescence is manifested by nonadult symptomatology. The young person exhibits a variety of troubling behaviors, termed "depressive equivalents," that are indicative of underlying dysfunction. These depressive equivalents include not only the previously noted functional somatic complaints but also acting-out behavior, running away, boredom, and difficulty concentrating.

Acting-out behavior, including delinquency, truancy, running away from home, temper tantrums, and sexual promiscuity, is always a sign of a young person in difficulty and frequently is indicative of underlying depression. This behavior often defends the adolescent against coming to grips with feelings of inadequacy and emptiness. Such action is substituted for thinking, and for as long as the action continues, the teenager avoids the pain of depression. A poor self-image may be temporarily improved by the sense of bravery, cleverness, and independence necessary to accomplish antisocial and defiant acts. Unfortunately, such acts serve to alienate the young person further from available systems of support and ultimately to increase rather than to alleviate the underlying depression.

Running away from home, one form of acting-out behavior, requires special emphasis. Approximately half of the teenagers who attempt suicide have a history of having run away. Such a history indicates not only that the teenager is in difficulty but also that the home situation is perceived as hostile and nonsupportive. Unfortunately, there are few safe places where a teenager may seek refuge. These young people most often find themselves in environments that are more hostile and threatening and less supportive than the home from which they fled, and they may become victims of exploitation and abuse. Therefore, the adolescent who is running away from home represents a behavioral emergency.

The depressed teenager is often bored and restless and may exhibit short-lived intense interest in a particular project, with quick abandonment of that activity and a return to boredom. The great enthusiasm for a hobby, a sport, or another diversion serves as an escape from the intolerable boredom that accompanies depression. However, such relief is temporary, and depression returns as interest wanes. In addition to boredom, teenagers complain of difficulty concentrating, and a deterioration of performance at school or work may be the first sign of depression. These adolescents note that as hard as they may try to apply themselves to their studies, they are unable to absorb information or complete tasks. More than 70% of depressed teenagers report difficulty concentrating and diminished academic performance.

The teenager suspected of being depressed must be questioned for any evidence of the classic adult signs of depression as well as the depressive equivalents more common to the adolescent population. Such questioning should include not only a search for the

vegetative signs of depression (such as insomnia, decreased appetite, weight loss, and constipation) but also an appraisal of the broad spheres of academic, vocational, social, recreational, and sexual activities.

- Recent school performance should be assessed in search of evidence of failed courses, declining grades, and truancy.
- For the adolescent who is no longer in school, information should be sought regarding meaningful employment, attendance and tardiness at work, and frequency with which jobs have been changed.
- Within the social sphere, does the teenager enjoy interactions with peers, or, alternatively, is he or she a loner who no longer participates in group activities?
- What does the adolescent do for fun?
- Are there activities that have sustained interest over long periods of time, or, in contrast, is the teenager's life devoid of recreation or marked by brief spurts of interest in projects that are then quickly abandoned?
- Does the teenager date?
- Is he or she sexually active?
- Is promiscuity with transient, superficial relationships an issue?
- How are things at home?
- Is the family intact?
- Does the teenager get along well with parents and siblings, or is life in the household a constant adversarial relationship?
- Has the teenager ever run away from home?
- Has the adolescent engaged in delinquent behavior or been arrested?
- Is the adolescent using or abusing drugs?
- To what extent is intoxication or the lifestyle of the drug abuser interfering with the accomplishment of adolescent tasks?
- Has the teenager ever experienced an "accidental" drug overdose?

All of the above explorations will serve not only to detect the teenager who is in difficulty and at risk but also to provide an understanding of the etiologic factors that are causing disruption. The understanding of both the nature and etiologies of disruption is crucial to management. In addition, having detected an adolescent in difficulty, an assessment of urgency must be made. As noted previously, the teenager who is running away from home is at great risk. Similarly the adolescent who is being abused must be protected quickly.

- Is a suicide attempt imminent, likely, or a distinct possibility? Direct questions regarding suicidal ideation are indicated at any time depression is suspected.
- Has the adolescent ever contemplated hurting himself?
- How would he hurt himself?
- How often and in how much detail has suicidal planning taken place?
- Has he ever acted on these plans in any way?
- Has he actually made a prior suicidal attempt?
- Is there evidence of hallucinations or other manifestations of psychosis?
- Does the teenager ever hear voices?
- Have the voices ever advised self-destructive behavior?

Such questioning will serve either to allay or to increase the clinician's fear of an impending suicidal attempt. Often teenagers report that they never have thought and never will think of harming themselves. At other times psychotic behavior or suicidal planning is active and acute and mandates an urgent response.

The evaluation of the adolescent who comes to medical attention after a suicidal attempt includes an exploration of all the aforementioned areas of behavioral function. Clearly, this evaluation is urgent and is motivated by the need for dispositional planning rather than the detection of a young person at risk. Assessment of continued suicidal ideation is critical and impacts upon the immediate management. The presence of hallucinations or other evidence of psychosis

is of similar import. An additional area of exploration is a search for the immediate cause of the suicidal attempt. The most frequent precipitating events noted by adolescents include a family fight, a romantic conflict, the loss of a loved one through death or departure, a dispute with peers, and a pregnancy.

Eliciting the precipitating event is more helpful in quantifying the adolescent's threshhold for suicidal behavior than it is in clarifying the underlying circumstances that led to the self-destructive behavior. As noted previously, it is rare that a single event causes a suicidal attempt. Most frequently, the precipitant is the final straw superimposed upon the burden of chronic depression or prolonged behavioral disruption. Hence, the clarification of the acute cause of the suicidal behavior is useful in determining the level of psychic insult that was required to initiate the attempt. At greatest risk are those adolescents who cannot identify any immediate cause for their behavior or who attempted suicide after what would be regarded by others as minimal trauma. In general, teenagers who became suicidal only after a major loss, a rape, or a monumental psychic insult have a more favorable prognosis.

Other circumstances surrounding the suicide attempt also need to be explored.

- Was the method chosen for self-destruction likely to result in death, or, conversely, was it certain to cause little or no risk to the individual? It should be noted that few teenagers have sufficient knowledge of toxicology to predict the outcome of a specific drug overdose. At times that which is perceived by the clinician as a gesture, where true physiologic compromise would be impossible, was intended by the adolescent to be fatal.
- Did the teenager tell anyone about the suicidal act or was he or she found, and saved, only by chance?

Such questioning is not intended to separate those adolescents who are at risk from those whose behavior can be safely ignored. All teenagers who attempt suicide are at risk of repeating the behavior with a subsequent fatal outcome. An understanding of the circumstances that were immediate to the attempt is additional information needed for short- and long-term therapeutic decisions.

The importance of gaining a full understanding of the behavior of the adolescent who attempted suicide and the family and social environment that gave rise to such behavior most often requires the involvement of other health professionals. Psychiatric consultation is mandated whenever there is a question of psychosis and in almost all other instances where suicide has been attempted. Similarly, the appraisal of family circumstances and interactions is facilitated by social workers, psychologists, and other behavioralists with an understanding of family dynamics. The teenager thought to be depressed, at risk of suicide, or, for that matter, evidencing any significant disruption will also profit from such consultation.

MANAGEMENT

As the search for the depressed and potentially suicidal adolescent is, in fact, a search for the young person who is evidencing behavioral disruption, management is directed toward correction of that disruption. The urgency of intervention is determined by the clinician's sense of the immediacy of the crisis, with little regard to the nature of the perceived crisis. Certainly, an impending suicidal attempt demands an immediate response, but so too would running away from home, out-of-control substance abuse, serious acts of delinquency, and a variety of other behaviors characterizing an adolescent at risk. Management is directed toward the further delineation of the etiologies of depression and the remediation of these root causes. As noted previously, consultation with a psychiatrist, a psychologist, or a social worker is most often necessary for both evaluation and therapy. The nature of the specific disruptive factors in the life of the teenager will determine the direction of therapeutic intervention. For the minority of adolescents who are found to be psychotic, psychiatric care and possible hospitalization must be considered. For the majority of suicidal teenagers who evidence family disruption, family therapy should be attempted. Addressing issues of substance abuse, sexual promiscuity, school failure, vocational ineptitude, social retardation, and delinquency is integral to the management of the depression. Therapy must be attempted within the constraints of the possible. Borderline adolescents will exhibit inherent limitations in their ability to achieve up to the standards of society. Setting goals too high may increase rather than alleviate feelings of poor self-worth. Similarly, families suffering from significant disruption cannot readily be turned into well-functioning units. Chronic depression is not alleviated in a few days or by simple, short-term counseling. The objectives of therapy are twofold: (1) the adolescent must be provided with mechanisms for dealing with stress and depression that are less destructive than a suicidal attempt, and (2) the stresses and failures in the life of the teenager should be remediated to the extent possible. Behavioralists, family workers, teachers, relatives, and friends may all play a role in the therapy of these adolescents.

The management needs of the teenager who comes to medical attention after a suicidal attempt are much the same. However, the possibility that the adolescent soon will make another attempt to die imparts an urgency to evaluation and management. As most teenagers who attempt suicide arrive in the physician's office or the emergency room with little or no physiologic compromise, hospitalization for evaluation and management is not mandatory. However, the complexity of the required evaluation, the frequency with which such teenagers are suffering from environmental disruption, and the possibility that another attempt will be made dictate inpatient care in almost all instances. It should be regarded as dangerous to discharge immediately a young person back to the same circumstances that led to a suicide attempt. A brief hospitalization on either a general medical or a psychiatric unit, where behavioral consultation can be obtained, is almost always the best course of action. An immediate concern is the detection of continued suicidal ideation or hallucinations. The patient who is hallucinating, is acting bizarrely, or continues to express a wish to die must be provided with the external controls to prevent further injury. Physical or pharmacologic restraint may be necessary, as well as constant observation. Patients who continue to act in a self-destructive manner may require transfer to a secure and protected setting.

Most adolescents who attempt suicide are not psychotic, are not hallucinating, and do not continue to express a wish to die. In fact, quite often the suicide attempt relieves the immediate crisis, and the teenager expresses regrets for the action and promises it will never occur again. Unfortunately, despite the expressed regrets, these adolescents remain at risk of a subsequent suicide attempt weeks or months later, when unavoidable stresses again give rise to depression. Careful evaluation and dispositional planning must precede the release of these teenagers from care.

There are many dispositional alternatives for the adolescent who has attempted suicide. For some, psychiatric hospitalization will be required. At the other extreme are young people who can be discharged home with periodic behavioral support. As with the teenager who is found to be depressed but has not yet attempted suicide, an effort will need to be made to address the stresses and failures of the particular adolescent. Most frequently, teenagers who have attempted suicide can be discharged to home with arrangements for ambulatory psychiatric care. Often such care requires the participation of the family as well as the adolescent. At other times, the extent of familial disruption precludes discharge to home, and the teenager needs to receive behavioral support while residing with relatives, foster parents, or in a group home. Often, finding an appropriate setting for the teenager unable to return home is difficult because of a paucity of suitable alternative living arrangements for this age population. Frequently, finding such an appropriate setting requires both patience and cooperation between health care providers and child protective agencies.

There is little information available regarding the long-term prognosis for teenagers who attempt suicide. Information that is available indicates that 5% of adolescents who attempt suicide subsequently die from suicide within 5 years. Although survival bears some relationship to the seriousness of the initial attempt, even those teenagers who were judged to have made less intense gestures made a significant contribution to the subsequent death rate. Clearly, all adolescents who have made a suicide attempt or who are found to be depressed and at risk of suicide deserve efforts at evaluation and management that might impact upon this behavior, which now ranks among the leading causes of death in young people.

BIBLIOGRAPHY

Inamdar, SC et al.: Phenomenology associated with depressed moods in adolescents. Am J Psychiatry 136:156, 1979

Marks A: Management of the suicidal adolescent on a nonpsychiatric unit. J Pediatr 95:305, 1979

McIntire MS et al.: Recurrent adolescent suicidal behavior. Pediatrics 60:605, 1977

Petzel SV, Cline DW: Adolescent suicide: Epidemiological and biological aspects. Adolescent Psychiatry Developmental and Clinical Studies, Vol VI, Chicago, University of Chicago Press, 1978, pp. 239–266

Rosen DM: The serious suicide attempt: Five

year follow-up study of 886 patients. JAMA 235:2105, 1976

Schrut A: Some typical patterns of behavior and backgrounds of adolescent girls who attempt suicide. Am J Psychiatry 125:107, 1968

Teicher JO: Children and adolescents who attempt suicide. Pediatr Clin North Am 17:687, 1970

Weinberg S: Suicidal intent in adolescence: A hypothesis about the role of physical illness. J Pediatr 77:579, 1970

Cross-Reference to *Pediatrics,* 17th ed.

TWENTY

Common Behavioral Problems in Preschool Children

Esther Wender

The topic of this chapter is the assessment and management of the behavioral problems most commonly encountered in the preschool child. Some physicians question the need to take responsibility for these problems, and a few words about this issue seem appropriate. The parent does seek advice from the primary care physician on these matters. Many studies indicate not only that parents wish to discuss such issues with the physician but also that satisfaction with health management is influenced by the quality of this aspect of care.

Physicians often argue that problems with behavior should be referred to mental health professionals who receive more training than the physician in normal development and behavioral management. However, during the preschool period the physician is often the only professional who has established a relationship with the family. Therefore, the parent more comfortably turns to the physician for initial advice. In addition, biologic factors may contribute significantly to behavioral symptomatology and may be overlooked by specialists not trained in medicine. Parents are frequently concerned about the possible biologic contribution to their child's behavior and seek medical advice because of these concerns.

Though these arguments may be convincing, it is unfortunate if the primary care practitioner accepts the role of behavioral problem counselor as a necessary, but not very desirable, obligation. This attitude often stems from a simplistic notion that behavior becomes a problem only when the parents are either naive or malevolent. Instead, problem behavior often occurs as the result of either normal or pathologic development or is one of the consequences of disease. Even when parent-child interaction is at fault, the parent's behavior is understandable, and the interaction is treatable in ways that are very rewarding to the practitioner.

This chapter will cover only the most common behavioral problems encountered in the first 6 years of life. The focus is on prevention and the early stages of management. Appropriate referral is encouraged, and general guidelines for this are discussed. Each specific problem is reviewed in a similar manner. First, an outline of the important developmental considerations gives the clinician a perspective on the problem and highlights the important preventive approaches to counseling. Second, a discussion of the psychodynamic issues—usually those affecting the parents—provides the clinician with reasons why normal, as well as pathologic, development poses problems for some parents. The third section reviews relevant medical considerations. Finally, these three approaches are synthesized to yield recommendations for management.

Two aspects of management, talking to young children and modification of behavior, are common to all of the problems discussed in this chapter and are, therefore, reviewed below.

TECHNIQUES OF MANAGEMENT

Behavioral Modification

This management technique has been developed by psychologists, based on the science of behavioral conditioning. Through careful study of the antecedents and consequences of specific behaviors, behavioral scientists have built a body of knowledge describing how the probability of a designated behavior occurring can be increased or decreased. These principles, initially discovered with animals, also apply to human behavior and constitute the guidelines for behavioral management. Conditioning theory is covered in many other books, and the reader is referred to these for additional information. In this section, some of the basic guidelines will be reviewed briefly, since they are referred to repeatedly in the management sections of this chapter.

First, most parents view reward and punishment in moralistic terms. In conditioning theory, a reward is anything that results in an increase in, and punishment is any response that decreases, the occurrence of a behavior. The additional notion that the child should be made to feel good by a reward and feel bad as the result of punishment is not relevant to a behavioral management approach. It has been shown, for example, that just paying attention to a behavior increases its occurrence, and, conversely, ignoring a behavior can quite effectively make it disappear. Therefore, the parent who tries to punish by yelling at the child may be rewarding the behavior with attention, and the seemingly benign approach of walking away from the child who is misbehaving may very effectively punish, if by punishment is meant that the behavior decreases in frequency. Many parents' notions of appropriate reward and punishment do not accurately consider the child's developmental level. For example, the parent who rewards the 5 year old by saying that tomorrow he will be able to go to the park fails to appreciate the limited time frame of the average child of this age. An important step in behavioral management is to analyze the specific ways parents are now responding to a behavior and then helping them devise more appropriate deterrents to unwanted behaviors and more effective ways of encouraging desirable performance.

A second principle relates to immediate response and follow-through. Parents and teachers often delay their reaction to a behavior or fail to carry out their threatened response. The reaction to a child's behavior that is immediate prevents the child from delaying his own response. Verbal threats to respond can be ignored, while a behavioral reaction cannot. Immediate response and follow-through are difficult, since the adult *must* interrupt his own activity or train of thought in order to respond to the child. The experimental psychologist who is attempting to shape the behavior of the laboratory animal is aware of these principles and stays poised and alert to respond. The adults who live with children, by contrast, pursue their own activities and must shift their focus of attention when they wish to affect the child's behavior. Therefore, when trying to help the parent develop new management techniques, the usual response to behavior must be analyzed in detail to see if the parent is reacting immediately and following through. If, for example, the parent is concerned that the child does not get dressed in the morning, and her usual approach is to demand that the child dress himself and then to leave the child alone while preparing breakfast, the recommendation would be for the parent either to remain with the child until dressing is complete or to have dressing take place in the kitchen where the parent can be present.

A third important principle is that rewarding desirable behaviors can be a very effective method of reducing misbehavior. However, this approach requires the parent to observe even the smallest signs of desired behavior. If, for example, the issue is fighting with other children, the parent must learn to watch the child's play and notice whenever the child shares a toy or plays appropriately even for a few minutes. It is much more natural for the parent to ignore quiet play and pay attention only to conflict. The parent's ability to observe appropriate behavior often can be determined in an interview by asking the parent to describe the child's desirable behaviors. The parent who can only remember the misbehavior has probably lost, for now, the ability to observe appropriate performance.

In summary, much can be accomplished in behavioral management if the parent can adopt three basic techniques that affect conditioning of behavior. First, rewards and punishment should be broadly defined as responses that either encourage or discourage behavior, and disciplinary measures should be carefully analyzed to insure that they are doing just that. Second, immediacy of reaction and follow-through to completion should be a goal of each parental response. Third, parents should learn to notice and then respond to desirable behaviors rather than attending only to misbehavior.

Talking to Young Children

The skilled and persistent employment of conditioning techniques can powerfully affect performance. Animals can be taught remarkable feats of behavior, e.g., the rat who learns to press a bar a thousand times for each pellet of food, or the chicken who learns to turn around and around in a whirling dervish dance when the experimenter institutes a gradual behavioral shaping program. Children, however, are not experimental animals, a truth that can easily be forgotten in the first blush of enthusiasm for behavioral modification techniques. Behavioral modification is a technique for shaping behavior, not a method for understanding it. Understanding behavior is accomplished by understanding normal development, being aware of common psychodynamic issues, and being able to talk to children.

Talking to the young, preschool child is difficult for many adults. Children at this age say things that make little sense from the adult point of view. A preschool child's perspective is limited, and he will frequently relate an experience as if the listener knows all the background information that he fails to give. Children at this age have little sense of cause and effect, and they fail to distinguish between real and make-believe. It is common, for example, for young children to believe that television cartoons are real.

The adult skilled at talking to preschool children makes guesses as to what the child is thinking. This skill is put to use in the art of active listening. Active listening means not only hearing the child's words but acknowledging the feelings underlying those words. For example, if the 4-year-old child has been told he must accompany his mother on an errand, and he responds by crying and refusing, the adult who is skilled in active listening will consider possible reasons for that refusal from the child's perspective. Is he afraid of something in the car or at the site of the errand? Did something happen the last time he went to this place? An active listening response will acknowledge the child's refusal along with a guess as to the underlying feeling. The following hypothetical exchange will illustrate this technique:

Susan is a 4 year old whose mother has just said that she is going to the department store and Susan will come with her.

Susan: "I don't like that store."
Mother: "There's nothing wrong with that store."
Susan: "I don't want to go."
Mother: "You must. I don't have anyone to leave you with."
Susan: (crying) "No."

At this point the mother recalls that the last time they went to this store, there was entertainment in the form of life-sized Sesame Street characters, and Susan was frightened by them.

Mother: "Big Bird and Oscar are gone. They went to another store."
Susan: "They're gone?"
Mother: "Yes. They were scary, weren't they?"
Susan: "Yes."

This brief vignette illustrates the thought processes involved in active listening responses. It is tempting for the adult to respond only to the child's refusal, as the mother begins to do in this example. Using behavioral modification techniques to force compliance in this type of situation could be emotionally harmful.

Children at this age frequently ask repeated questions when they are really trying to make a statement. This following interchange between a 4 year old and his doctor will illustrate this point.

Doctor: "I'm going to put this around your arm to check your blood pressure."
Jimmy: "Why?"
Doctor: "So I can tell if everything is all right."
Jimmy: (looking apprehensive) "Why?"
Doctor: "It's just one of the things doctors do. It won't hurt. It just squeezes a little."

Jimmy: "Why?"
Doctor: "Because that's the way you check blood pressure."
Jimmy: (pulling back) "I don't want to."
Doctor: "Sometimes kids think this lets all the blood out. It doesn't. It just pushes on the skin. I bet you thought it would do something else."
Jimmy: (looking relieved) "It just pushes on the skin?"
Doctor: "Yes."

Being able to guess the child's thoughts requires an understanding of how children this age think. Selma Fraiberg's classic book, *The Magic Years*,[7] has done much to help adults understand the thinking of preschool children, and is recommended for further reading.

SLEEP PROBLEMS

Developmental Issues

Sleeping behavior normally shows great fluctuation during the first 4 months of life, and there are wide variations in the establishment of sleeping patterns. In the average infant, there is a considerable change in sleep patterns between birth and 3 or 4 months of age. Parmelee et al.[8,9] have shown that at 1 and 2 months of age, the average infant sleeps 15.4 hours in each 24 hours. By 4 months, the total sleep in 24 hours decreases a small amount to 14.8 hours. A big change occurs, however, in the distribution of that sleep. At 1 month, the longest sleeping period in an average day is 4.6 hours, while at 4 months, the longest sleeping period is 8.4 hours. During the first 2 weeks of life, infants sleep the same number of hours during the day and night. By 5 weeks of age, 66% of normal infants show a diurnal cycle, and by 3 months, 98% sleep much longer at night than during the day. These changes are accompanied by EEG changes in the proportion of active and quiet sleep within sleep cycles. In the first 2 weeks, quiet and active sleep are equal, but by 8 months, quiet sleep is twice as long as active sleep.

The young infant who does not sleep is usually crying. Even when there is no illness and hunger has been satisfied, young infants cry. This phenomenon is often explained as due to neurologic immaturity. Prematures show more nonspecific crying than do full-term infants, an observation that supports the neurologic immaturity explanation.

By 4–5 months of age, the average child establishes a fairly regular pattern of sleeping 2–4 hours after each feeding and 6–7 hours at night. Periods of quiet and attentive wakefulness gradually increase after feedings during the day and before the next sleeping period. By 6 months of age, the pattern emerges of two naps during the day after meals and awake times in between. At around the age of 1 year–15 months, the morning wakeful period lengthens, and the morning nap is dropped. Then the pattern of one long afternoon nap emerges and continues for the next 2 or 3 years. These general patterns are widely variable, of course.

At the age when stranger and separation anxiety first appear, a different type of sleeping variation emerges. The infant is either reluctant to go to sleep and cries at being put to bed, or else he goes to sleep but awakens and cries at night after being asleep 2 hours or so. This problem is thought to be due to separation anxiety, since it stops readily when the child is put to bed with the parent or older sibling, and, as the child becomes verbal, he will call out for the parents or siblings. This behavior usually fades, if it has been a problem, as verbal ability becomes firmly established between ages 3 and 4.

Finally, children between ages 3 and 5 seem initially prone to night terrors, which are seen in about 2% of children of this age.[10] A night terror, unlike the nightmare which is seen more frequently in older children, is a phenomenon that apparently occurs during the transition from stage 4 to lighter stages of sleep (stages 1 and 2). The child usually sits up or gets up and either talks or, more likely, cries or screams. Often there are physiologic signs of terror, i.e., widely dilated eyes and rapid pulse. The child is not responsive at the time and has no memory for the event when later awakened. The child's apparent terror and anxiety are upsetting to the caretaker, especially since the child is unresponsive and, therefore, cannot be comforted. Typically, such episodes occur infrequently (once every few weeks or months) and decrease as the child gets older.

Psychodynamic Considerations

Parents normally experience a strong need to comfort the crying infant, a behavior obviously well adapted to effective infant care and survival of the species. Success in their efforts to quiet the crying infant is accompanied by satisfaction and a sense of competence. Conversely, inability to comfort is for many parents a source of intense frustration. Yet, the nonsleeping crying of the first 4 months is often difficult to stop by the usual comforting techniques. Many factors accentuate this inherently frustrating situation, the most common one being ignorance of the normal amount of crying and nonsleeping of this period. Therefore, the problem is worse in the new parent and the parent with little support from experienced, knowledgeable friends or relatives. As Frodi and Lamb have shown,[11] parents vary a great deal in their emotional and even physiologic response to the infant cry. Less tolerance would be expected in the tense, high-strung individual and in the parent who experiences strong ambivalence toward or even dislike of the infant.

The wakeful, crying infant puts considerable stress on the parents' own need for sleep. Even the most enthusiastic and prepared mother and father are often surprised by the irritability and anger that arises in them as sleepless nights and demanding days combine to stress their adaptability. This is felt most strongly by very young parents who also experience conflict between the demands of the infant and their own need for personal gratification.

A more pathologic reaction is for the parent to view the infant's inconsolable crying as personally aimed at making him or her look bad as a parent or as an attempt by the infant to manipulate the parent's behavior. This kind of thinking often underlies acts of child abuse.

The wakeful crying that appears during the period of normal separation anxiety evokes a different kind of parental response. Often the separation anxiety of the infant stimulates a similar reciprocal emotion in the parent which, if exaggerated, leads to overprotection. At this stage of development, the infant's cry is directed personally toward the parents, who may be inclined to give up their own needs (for example, for privacy) for those of their child. This interaction is accentuated by any factors that make the parent's feel less secure about the infant's attachment, e.g., adoption or prolonged illness in the newborn period. The problem for the parents at this stage is to acquire an appropriate amount of emotional distance that allows them to tolerate frustrating and disappointing their child.

Medical Considerations

Any medical condition that affects the central nervous system either prenatally or at the time of birth is likely to prolong and accentuate the irregularity of sleep–wake cycles during the first few months. Table 1 is a partial list of such conditions. It is less widely recognized that decreased sleep time and increased crying in early infancy are often seen in children with attention deficit disorder (hyperactivity, minimal brain dysfunction). The cluster of temperamental traits designated as "the difficult child" by Thomas, Chess, and Birch[15] consists, in part, of poor adaptability, irregularity of biologic rhythms, and

TABLE 1. CONDITIONS THAT MAY RESULT IN EXCESS CRYING DURING INFANCY

Prematurity
Hypoxia during delivery
Toxemia
Fetal alcohol syndrome
Neonatal seizures
Drug addiction in the mother
Small-for-date infant

intensity, a combination that is often manifested by excessive crying in infancy. The child with colic also cries frequently and may sleep less than the average infant.

Excessive crying and poor sleep may be a general manifestation of many acute illnesses in infancy. Therefore, the physician must always remain alert to other signs of illness whenever sleep problems are reported. Of particular concern is that irritable crying may be the first manifestation of increased intracranial pressure. The measurement of head circumference, the examination of fontanels, and the use of transillumination will help detect this problem.

Management

As the previous remarks indicate, management depends upon the age at which sleeping problems are reported. In infancy, it is important at first to document the sleeping pattern, since parents may lack knowledge of what is normal and often exaggerate the amount of crying time. The parents should be instructed to keep track of the actual time the infant cries during one or two 24-hour periods. Brazelton[12] has shown that during the first 2 months of life, normal infants cry between 2 and 3 hours a day. By 3 months, this drops to an average of 1 hour a day, and the variation among infants is less. Between 2 and 6 weeks, there is great variation among infants, with some crying as much as 3½ hours a day and others as little as 1½ hours. If the pattern is normal, explaining this to parents may be all that is needed. However, sleeping problems are often reported by parents who are having difficulty tolerating their infant's crying, and this issue needs to be explored, sympathetically reviewing the issues described in the section on Psychodynamics. Often, just uncovering these mechanisms in a sympathetic, nonjudgmental way is sufficient to help the parent control them. If the physician senses, however, that the empathtic listening has not affected the process, referral should be considered. If only one parent is experiencing the problem, it is helpful to suggest ways that the other parent can help with critical aspects of the infant's care.

If the amount of nonsleeping crying appears excessive, the infant's developmental pattern needs to be evaluated, including a careful neurologic assessment. The family history, focusing on developmental disorders, such as those listed in Table 2, needs to be reviewed. If there is a prominent family history of one or more of these disorders, it is likely that the child may be displaying early signs of a similar developmental disorder. However, it is important to keep in mind the danger of overprognosticating during infancy. Many infants look suspect at this age but turn out to have no problems later on. The art of counseling during this period is to give possible explanations of the infant's behavior while discouraging the parent from overinterpreting these explanations as predictors of later problems. The overly concerned parent may behave in a way that shapes the infant's future into a self-fulfilling prophecy.

If the infant appears to be developmen-

TABLE 2. COMMON DEVELOPMENTAL DISORDERS

Mild or borderline mental retardation
Attention deficit disorder (hyperactivity)
Learning disability
Developmental delay of speech

tally immature, management consists primarily of emotional support of the parents and providing suggestions that help them adapt to the behavior. Such measures include alternating the caretaker roles of the parents and obtaining mature, reliable babysitters who can give the parents relief. The crying of these infants is often temporarily controlled by motion. Therefore, when the infant is old enough, the automatic swing may be very helpful. During particularly difficult times of the day, the infant may be quiet when carried about the house, pushed in the carriage, or driven in the car.

If the crying and difficulty with sleep appear during the last part of the first year, the management issues are quite different. Once the characteristic pattern has been identified, the parent needs to try letting the child cry for specified times to see if the child will return to sleep on his own. Specific guidelines for this procedure are outlined in Spock's *Baby and Child Care*.[13] For the parent who finds it psychologically difficult to refrain from comforting the infant, an important instruction is to time the length of crying by the clock. To this parent, 5 minutes may seem like 2 hours. Usually, if left to cry for 2 or 3 nights in a row, the infant with this problem will quickly resume sleeping through the night. Some infants, however, are particularly resistant to this kind of conditioning procedure. In these cases, it is helpful to assess the infant's temperamental style and the parent's general approach to the demands of the infant's crying. Interactions uncovered by such inquiry may explain persistent problems and suggest alternative approaches. The infant who tends to cling may be particularly prone to this type of night crying. Such children often resist other caretakers during the day, quickly ask to be picked up or comforted if something startles them, and are easily frightened. Such children may be helped by keeping a light on in the bedroom or sleeping in the same room with siblings. These children are often brought to the parent's bed because this effectively controls the crying. Unfortunately, sleeping with the parent is a habit that is then extraordinarily difficult to break and often becomes a source of contention as the parents face the conflicting needs for privacy and for a quiet child.

The parents who find it very difficult to disappoint their infant are also at high risk for this type of sleeping problem. This discomfort can be detected by sensitive interviewing centering around daytime issues that require saying "no" to the infant. The most common issue at this age is teaching the child to stay away from breakable or potentially dangerous things. The typical pattern is for the parent to say "no" and then give in as the infant starts to cry. These parents may respond too quickly to the fussy, irritable crying of the tired infant. If the parent demonstrates these patterns, the problems may be helped by the brief counseling involved in simply identifying the issue in a supportive interview. If this is insufficient, a referral for more prolonged counseling may be necessary. Often, such parents are affected by issues, such as their lack of confidence as parents, or more serious problems, such as ambivalent feelings about being a parent toward this particular infant.

The third type of sleep problem, the night terror, responds very well to explanation. Parents find it especially difficult to tolerate the fear that is often obvious in the child's facial expression. Once they understand that the child is only semiconscious, they can usually learn appropriate management, which is to keep trying to waken the child by talking to him and attempting physical comfort, such as hugging or stroking. Once the child is awake, he will quickly become quiet and usually fall right back to sleep. Night terrors very seldom need any other management. Occasionally, however, the older child (5 years and over) may become fearful of going to sleep if night terrors are frequent, e.g., two or three episodes a week. It may be appropriate to treat such children

with a dose of diazepam (0.15 mg/kg) just before bed, which is usually quite effective in preventing the terrors. If medication is used, it should be gradually withdrawn after 1 month.

FEEDING PROBLEMS

Developmental Issues

Three developmental issues significantly affect the emergence of feeding problems: (1) the development of self-feeding motor skills, (2) the reduction in appetite that accompanies slower growth rates at the end of the first year, and (3) increasingly finicky food preferences that develop during the preschool years.

Self-feeding skills gradually emerge out of normal motor development during the first year of life. At about 6 months of age in the normal infant, there is a convergence of (1) the ability to sit, which changes the child's visual perspective to what is in front of him (rather than above him), (2) the ability to visually guide hand movements, and (3) the skill of purposefully grasping and holding. The child at this age accordingly begins to put things in his mouth, including food. Anything that affects normal motor development may produce feeding problems. In the retarded infant, for example, this developmental sequence will be slowed. As the child reaches 9 months, he develops the ability to voluntarily release a handheld object, a new skill that is practiced often, like all new motor skills. Therefore, the child at this age enjoys dropping and throwing things, including food. Though the self-feeding of solid foods, such as crackers, begins at 6–7 months, it is not until 12–15 months that most children can manage a spoon sufficiently to even begin the more civilized consumption of soft foods. By the age of 1 year, however, most children are very interested in self-feeding of even the soft foods that they cannot yet manage without considerable mess. The process of self-feeding may be significantly affected if this messy stage is constrained by psychologic or biologic factors.

The second developmental issue stems from the relatively dramatic reduction in growth rate that occurs towards the end of the first year. The average infant, for example, gains 3 pounds 10 ounces between the ages of 3 and 6 months but only 2 pounds between the ages of 9 and 12 months and 1 pound 6 ounces between 15 and 18 months. This change is usually accompanied by a significantly reduced appetite.

The third developmental issue has not been well studied. During the preschool period many children become increasingly finicky and rigid in their food preferences. The degree to which this is learned vs a biologic phenomenon is not known. It seems reasonable to speculate that this change is greater in our Western culture due to the wide variety of foods available in combination with the lack of rigid social control over what foods are served. Children, therefore, have considerable opportunity to choose what they eat.

Psychodynamic Considerations

Enthusiastic eating is a commonly accepted indication of good health. Most parents take pride in their child's appetite and are genuinely concerned when he shows little interest in food. Therefore, the normal reduction in appetite during the latter part of the first year may set the scene for feeding problems as the parent pushes food on the reluctant child. The problem is often exacerbated by relatives and friends who share the belief that a robust appetite is a sign of health. Enthusiastic eating is also viewed as a sign of good parenting. An indication of this attitude can be seen on pediatric wards, where nursing personnel often view the child who is reported to eat poorly as a challenge to their nursing skill. Some cultures emphasize these issues more than others. For example, enthusiastic eating and weight gain are particularly important in the Jewish culture, and Mexican parents consider themselves failures if their child has a significant feeding problem. During the developmental phase of autonomy (2–3 years old), children may refuse food. Parents who can accept rebellion on other issues may overreact to the refusal to eat, since food is seen as such a basic need.

The fastidious parent is particularly troubled by the messy transition toward self-feeding. All parents must be able to tolerate the stage when food is on the face and spread over the highchair and the floor before tidy eating gradually becomes possible. The parent who has particular difficulty with this stage may report feeding problems, though the child is developmentally normal.

Finicky tastes present great problems for some parents and none for others. The important variable is the parent's attitude toward this issue. Some parents feel that the child who refuses specific foods is spoiled and see rigid tastes as a problem requiring discipline. If both parent and child are unyielding, this issue can become a serious, chronic battleground that may affect other areas of parent-child interaction.

Medical Considerations

In the attempt to sort out medical and psychosocial issues, the physician must first determine whether the child is thriving. The best judge of whether the child is thriving is the measure of growth rate over time. If growth rate is consistent for the child's stature, appetite can be considered appropriate for that child's growth whether judged to be small or great by the parent. If, however, the child is growing at a rate slower than predicted for his age and stature, the differential diagnosis of failure to thrive must be considered. (See Chapter 24.) Of particular importance in the assessment and management of feeding problems are those disorders that result in a slowed growth rate because there is an intrinsic lack of response to growth factors at the cellular level or because of a developmental delay in growth. An example of the former is constitutional short stature, which is seen in many congenital syndromes associated with mental retardation. Developmental delay in growth is an inherited pattern consisting of slower growth rates during the first 3 or 4 years of life, resulting in stature that is below norms of the child's age. Through the rest of childhood, yearly growth increments are usually normal but stature remains small until a longer than average growing period during adolescence and even early adulthood results in normal adult stature. Both patterns require no medical treatment. Gastrointestinal function is normal in these children. However, appetite is poor, since caloric requirements are low. If these patterns are not recognized, feeding problems frequently ensue because parents pressure reluctant children to eat. If the child is failing to thrive, and developmental delay or congenital syndromes are not suspected, failure to thrive may be due to psychologic factors.

Most recent surveys of children hospitalized with failure to thrive estimate that 50% of cases are produced entirely or in part by psychosocial factors. The most commonly encountered problem is psychologic neglect stemming from ambivalent feelings toward the child. This factor may be difficult to assess, since parents may not be consciously aware of such feelings. These issues are reviewed in Chapter 24.

Obviously, feeding problems can develop as the result of gastrointestinal disorders. Particularly, the physician may overlook two conditions that can affect feeding in subtle ways. If the child cannot eat normally during critical periods of development, feeding behavior may be profoundly affected once normal feeding is possible. This critical period is not clearly defined but generally covers the first year of life. Thus, for example infants who cannot suck because of a large cleft palate and lip or Pierre Robin syndrome may suck poorly when normal function is restored by surgery. Children who have been fed par-

enterally for long periods because of intractable diarrhea may refuse to self-feed when the problem is resolved. Whenever gastrointestinal problems of this type occur during the first year, every attempt should be made to preserve at least some part of the normal feeding process.

Any disorder that involves the neuromuscular control of the chewing and swallowing process may result in the child refusing to self-feed. Such problems are more likely to appear in retarded children but may occur in normal children with movement disorders, such as cerebral palsy or dystonias. At times, this problem may be suspected but very difficult to detect. Often, such neuromuscular difficulties are accompanied by drooling, dysarthria, or both. Referral for a specialized evaluation is usually required.

Management

If the physician has judged that the child is thriving, the feeding problem, by definition, is due to a problem in parent-child interaction. Of course, the physician should explain normal growth and the developmental reasons for reduced appetite despite normal weight gain. He should look for indications that the child is refusing food as one method of establishing his own autonomy and counsel the parents to ignore this behavior. However, if a significant feeding problem has developed, it is usually despite these explanations. The next step is to consider and to uncover by skillful interview the dynamic factors mentioned above. If the parents can acknowledge the feelings that result when the child eats very little or their emotional response to the messy eating of the young child, the problem may improve. If the parent cannot perceive these reactions or if no improvement is seen following exploration of these feelings, referral should be considered. If the parent can accept a need to explore these dynamic issues, referral for psychotherapy is indicated. If, however, as is more likely, the parent is reluctant to accept his own contribution to the problem, success is more likely if the referral is to a professional experienced in developing a behavioral modification program, and the referral is explained in terms of the need for the parent to learn new, specialized feeding techniques.

If there are medical reasons for a significantly reduced appetite, i.e., constitutional short stature or developmental delay in growth, these conditions need to be explained, and tolerance of poor appetite needs to be empathically supported.

If there is a problem with neuromuscular coordination, referral to an occupational therapist can be helpful. These professionals employ techniques that help the patient become more aware of and then obtain control of muscles they seldom use.

If the child has missed normal feeding experiences because of gastrointestinal disease, both the rehabilitation training provided by the occupational therapist and a behavioral modification program may be helpful. The behavioral modification program needs to be specifically tailored to provide incentives for the child to self-feed.

Finally, if the feeding problem is due to battles over the child's rigid and finicky tastes, the parent needs to confront his need to control this issue. It has been my experience that the problem seldom develops in homes where eating is carefully controlled by the parents, i.e., the only food available is that prepared by the parent. Instead, the problem occurs when children have access to the kitchen and the freedom to choose their food. Parents who present this issue as a problem have conflicting attitudes. They like to allow their children free access to food but are also angered by the child's finicky tastes. Sometimes, the problem can be solved by confronting the parent with the kind of behavioral modification program that would be required to alter the child's behavior. This confrontation would require the parent to restrict children to the foods prepared only for meals. Most parents would object to these restrictions.

The parent might then choose to live with the finicky tastes. Parents should be assured that the range of food preferences will enlarge as the child gets older.

DISCIPLINE

The term "discipline" is very broad and refers to the whole range of children's behavior and parents' attempt to control and socialize the child. In this section, the focus will be on the common types of misbehavior expected at different stages of the preschool period and the typical parental reactions to those behaviors. This approach will uncover issues that are common to all discipline problems.

Developmental Issues

Often, the first disciplinary actions are aimed at the child's crying. Young children cry easily and frequently. An important component of normal development is the gradual increase in tolerance to frustration and pain, and thus a decrease in crying that comes with age, and the ability to verbalize. Both experience and biology affect this process, but most adults (including physicians) are more impressed by the environmental than the biologic contributions. When a child is crying, for example, people usually ask, "What does he want?" or "Is he upset?" or "What did I do wrong?" rather than explain the crying by the fact that he is 2 years old and 2 year olds cry easily. Two common biologic contributors to excess crying are variations in temperament and developmental disorders. The temperamental pattern of the "difficult child" includes the tendency to withdraw from rather than approach new situations and a style of intense emotional reactions. These two traits lead to excessive crying. Children with developmental delays often manifest their developmental deviation by an increase of crying in response to frustration. It is this characteristic that leads adults to describe these children as emotionally immature.

As the child develops, the next disciplinary actions are usually in response to the child's increasing motor skills, which normally lead to exploration and, therefore, potential for destructiveness and danger. There is considerable variability among children in their activity level and their response to fear—either fear of the unknown as they explore, or fear of the disapproval of adults. Children who are hyperactive usually begin to manifest that problem at this age, both in their excess activity level and in their fearlessness and resistance to disciplinary techniques.

As children enter into the well-known "terrible 2s," the disciplinary issue becomes the parent's response to the child's assertion of independence. This behavior is manifest most typically in the child saying "no" to the requests or demands of his parents and the temper tantrum, which is a more diffuse, nonverbal "no." This assertiveness is normal and is thought to be an important developmental phase because it helps the child separate from overdependence on the caretaker. If this phase is too firmly controlled, the child may have difficulty acquiring independence, including the ability and interest in developing relationships with other children and adults.

Three year olds, like 2 year olds, provoke disciplinary responses because of crying and assertiveness, though both behaviors are usually diminishing by this age. In addition, caretakers begin to respond to the selfishness that is normal at this age. The play of 3 year olds, like the rest of their cognitive development, is very egocentric, and these children are characteristically reluctant to share toys or play cooperatively.

During the 3–5 year period, three types of normal behavior often provoke disciplinary action. First, children at this age frequently go through a stage when they try out the use of bad language and seem to enjoy the reaction that this provokes. For similar reasons, i.e., experimentation without an understanding or acceptance of social prohibition, they often engage in sexual play consisting of exploring each other's genital organs. Second, children at this age often have quite unrealistic fears that relate directly to their level of cognitive development. They do not yet think in cause and effect terms and, therefore, attribute magical properties to many phenomena. For example, children this age see the make-believe characters on television as real. They may be genuinely frightened by people in costumes. They are often afraid of dolls that are broken or balloons that pop. The adult who does not understand normal development may interpret this as unreasonable or "sissy" behavior and feel it should be disciplined. Finally, 3–5 year olds may be shy, and the adult caretaker may feel that shy behavior should be disciplined. Though the origins of shyness are still somewhat controversial, most experts believe shyness is a temperamental trait that begins to clearly manifest itself at this age.

Psychodynamic Considerations

Crying in the newborn period is seen by most parents as the infant's way of indicating hunger or other discomfort. A change in the parent's perception occurs sometime during the first year, when crying, at times, is seen as manipulative and the parent begins to be concerned about spoiling the child. Once this change in attitude occurs, crying becomes, for that parent, a disciplinary issue. Parents vary enormously in their reaction to this issue, and there are socioeconomic and cultural differences that contribute to this variation. Probably the greatest amount of the variance is due to the parent's own rearing experiences as a child. Studies have repeatedly shown that the more punitive adult received more punishment during his own childhood. Parents who respond early and strongly by punishing crying so that the child will not be spoiled usually feel a strong need to control. If inner thoughts are revealed, such parents often think that they will lose the upper hand and fantasize no longer being able to control their child. If this pattern characterizes the parent, excessive discipline may first show up in response to crying but will probably continue in response to all of the behaviors described under Developmental Issues.

Another issue that may underlie excessively punitive behavior is the fantasy that the child will turn out badly. This fantasy may stem from the child's resemblance to a relative that the parent characterizes as "bad." Because of physical resemblances or personality similarities, the parent may attribute to their child traits that they dislike in a relative. The child may also be seen as "bad" if he manifests behavior that represents an unresolved issue for the parents. For example, the normal sexual exploration of the 3–5 year old may provoke anxiety in the parent who sees any overt sexual play as "wicked" because of his own childhood experiences.

An issue that may lead to inappropriately lax discipline is the parent's fear that the child will dislike him. This parent has felt the rejection of discipline in the past and projects this feeling onto his own child. The parent's fantasy, which may be subconscious, is that, "If I punish you, it means I don't love you." The parent who, because of his own history, feels this message strongly has difficulty disciplining the child. The parent with low self-esteem is particularly prone to these feelings.

At particularly high risk for all of these problems is the young parent with few supports who is unsure of himself and knows little about normal child development. If this parent also experienced a harsh or negligent upbringing, the risk for parenting problems is very high.

Medical Considerations

Developmental disorders result in focal areas of immaturity. Discrepancies in maturation, e.g., normal intellect but immature social behavior, are very difficult for parents to accept. The most common developmental disorders are listed in Table 2. Any of them may result in some behaviors that are characteristic of the younger child.

Children who are sick frequently will regress emotionally, usually for limited periods of time. However, the parent who does not understand this phenomenon may contact the physician regarding behavior that is upsetting. Chronic disease often produces a more prolonged regression in development, and one of the challenges of management of chronic disease is to minimize or prevent this phenomenon.

Management

Parents usually seek the advice of a physician because they feel their child is behaving inappropriately, or else they complain that the child is resistant to a disciplinary technique that they feel should have been effective. They do not usually seek help because they believe their discipline technique is faulty. Therefore, the physician should listen to their concerns about the child and begin to judge whether the behavior is stage related and if the parent's expectations are unrealistic or whether the child may, because of a developmental disorder, be showing an excessive amount of certain behaviors.

At the same time, the physician should be assessing the disciplinary technique employed by the parent. This latter task requires skill in interviewing and in analyzing human interaction. Discipline technique is usually described by the parent in general terms. The adult typically summarizes the disciplinary interaction, distorting the report in subtle ways that emphasize his point of view. For example, the parent may portray himself as very stern, while an outside observer would say that he did not seem stern. The best way to evaluate discipline is to observe it directly. However, this is not usually possible. A much more accurate account of the disciplinary encounter can be obtained if the event is analyzed step by step. The parent may relate, for example, that as the episode began the child was playing. The interviewer should ask for specifics: "What was he doing? Whom was he with?" The parent may then say he heard the child arguing with his playmate, and he told them to stop. At this point, the interviewer might query: "Where were you at the time? What were the words that you used? Were you angry at this point?" This detail yields important information of the type that was discussed in the Techniques of Management section. It provides information, for example, about how immediately the parent responded, whether follow-through was possible, whether incentives were used, and whether the punishment or incentives were appropriate for the child's age. Following this type of interview, specific suggestions can be made.

The clinician needs to remember, however, that the parent is much more likely to accept a suggestion if it is one the parent thought of, so that giving advice should be preceded by asking the parents what ideas they have already considered. They may have tried what you are about to advise. Giving advice should be done without implying that the parent was inept. This is easier if the clinician has genuine empathy with the parent's role as disciplinarian and can acknowledge that the techniques the parent has tried are those that are in common use by many parents.

If the behavior is age appropriate and the parent's expectations are unrealistic, this information should be given, also in a manner that does not make the parent feel ignorant. It helps to precede the information by a statement, such as, "Many parents don't realize that children of this age don't yet have an understanding of cause and effect, so children believe things that seem ridiculous to adults."

The most difficult task for the physician is to assess whether the behavior is appropriate for that age. The behavior seen in the most common developmental disorder is not abnormal in quality but is, instead, an exces-

sive quantity of that behavior for that age. The best way to judge the appropriateness of behavior is to compare it to the behavior of other children known to be normal. If the parent's concerns are corroborated by babysitters or relatives who have experiences with other children that age, one can be more certain that the behavior is inappropriate. The most helpful corroboration comes from experienced nursery school teachers. If the behavior is only mildly excessive or if the child's behavior is excessive in some settings and not others, it is best to follow the child with later appointments but deemphasize the potential diagnoses that behavior suggests. If, however, the behavior seems definitely deviant, the best approach at this stage is good behavioral management. The parents may need more help than the primary care physician can realistically give, in which case referral to specialists who handle behavioral management is advisable. At the same time, children with definite problems, as well as normal children, should experience the positive feelings of adults who try to understand how they feel, an approach emphasized in the section on Talking to Young Children.

If the child has been recently ill or if he has a chronic disease, these factors must be considered. In the case of regression following a recent acute illness, patience must be urged. The immature behavior should be tolerated and only mildly disciplined, since most children will improve with time. In the case of chronic illness, the physician must explore the family's attitude toward the illness. The developmental regression seen in chronic illness often stems from parental response, usually due to feelings of guilt, which results in attempts to protect the child from the discomfort and pain of needed medical procedures, e.g., injections, physical therapy, and exercises. Another common response that provokes developmental regression is the fear that the appropriate disciplinary action will make the child worse or even result in death. This reaction is particularly likely if the illness is cardiac or respiratory in nature. Another issue that affects this process is the child's temperament. Children who are by nature cautious and fearful and children who feel less in control of what happens to them are particularly prone to the developmental regression produced by chronic illness. The physician needs to evaluate these features by skillful interview. Sometimes, improvement is seen when these feelings are revealed and the parent experiences the physician's empathy. However, if the pattern of parental overreaction continues, referral to a mental health resource early in the course of the chronic illness is advisable. Many parents resist such referral and may be helped by groups composed of parents of children with the same or similar disorders.

SIBLING RIVALRY

Developmental Issues

It is normal for children to be affected by new, competing involvement of the parent's time and attention. The extent to which the child will be affected depends, in part, on the developmental stage he is at when parental attention is distracted elsewhere. The usual source of distraction is the birth of a sibling, but other possible sources include a serious illness in another family member that is emotionally involving for the parent or a new job that takes the parent's time and attention. The arrival of a new sibling is, however, an ongoing source of emotional competition, and one can observe not only the initial impact but the changing effects as the child develops. Sibling rivalry also gradually evolves in the younger child toward his older siblings as he becomes developmentally ready for this type of emotional reaction.

Before 1 year of age, little rivalry occurs, and the infant responds primarily to whether his basic needs are being met. Once the infant begins to distinguish between caregivers (i.e., begins to develop stranger anxiety between 7

months and 1 year), he becomes theoretically capable of noticing and reacting to the attention that the adult gives to others. Children vary a great deal in when and how intensely they respond to competing attention. By age 2, however, most children react when the parent's attention is diverted elsewhere. At this age, frustration tolerance is also very low, and the attention given to siblings often results in frustrating their own needs for immediate gratification. Reaction to competing parental attention continues and may even worsen at age 3, when children are particularly egocentric. By the age of 4, the rivalry is often less obvious. Most children this age have entered a stage in which they are more verbal and like to imitate the behavior of their parents, including child care. Therefore, they begin to control their jealousy through helpful behaviors, such as bringing the clean diapers. They also work out their rivalrous feelings in play, and 4 and 5 year olds are often seen parenting their dolls or pets. As children reach school age, they more easily disregard the presence of a new sibling as they become involved in their own peer relationships and their own play. However, at this age competition becomes a real factor as the child strives to learn new skills and is quite conscious of his own performance compared to others. Sibling rivalry can become quite intensified at this age, particularly in the child who feels he is not competing well.

Psychodynamic Considerations

Parents frequently feel that sibling loyalty is an important value. These feelings lead them to punish sibling rivalry, which they see as a threat to family solidarity. Such feelings are most likely in the parent with low self-confidence or the one who did not experience much support in his own nuclear family.

Parents may also prefer one child to another, and this show of preference will affect the development of rivalrous feelings. It may be difficult for the physician, who has only a superficial knowledge of the family, to accurately detect this problem. Parents usually hide their preference for one child because society admonishes them not to play favorites. Children often accuse their parents of favoring another child when such accusations are really their way of justifying their own feelings of inadequacy. A skillfully conducted family interview may reveal the true nature of these feelings and relationships.

Though some sibling jealousy is probably felt by all children, the extent of these feelings is strongly affected by the child's temperament and his own self-esteem. As a toddler, the child who is emotionally labile and easily frustrated will show the most sibling rivalry. Therefore, children with attention deficit disorder are particularly susceptible to rivalrous feelings and aggressive behavior toward siblings. Any child whose self-esteem is low will experience strong feelings of sibling jealousy. The common developmental disorders, such as learning disability and attention deficit disorder, often result in low self-esteem, and sibling rivalry is likely to be more pronounced in these children. If the parent prefers one child, the emotionally neglected sibling will gradually develop low self-esteem and accentuated jealousy toward the preferred child.

Medical Issues

A serious illness or the conception and birth of an unwanted child can markedly affect the development of sibling rivalry. The physician shows recognition of these issues when he urges the parent of a sick child to also attend to the emotional needs of the well children at home or when he advises contraception to avoid unwanted pregnancies. When managing illness, it is important for the physician to remain aware of the total family in order to advise appropriate preventive measures to minimize the development of sibling rivalry.

As mentioned previously, the common developmental disorders affect the severity of sibling rivalry. Such disorders should be detected early, and appropriate preventive measures should be instituted.

Management

It is important for parents to understand the distinction between the child's feelings of jealousy and his expression of those feelings in actions. Ginott's book, *Between Parent and Child,*[5] is very helpful in making this point. Though it is normal for the child to feel jealous, aggressive expression of those feelings should not be allowed. The skill of active listening can be used effectively to acknowledge the child's feelings, which may also help him to control their expression. If, for example, the 3 year old is reaching over to pinch his 1-year-old sibling who has just been bathed and readied for bed, the parent might say, "I know sometimes you wish your baby sister would go away, but I won't let you hurt her. Go get a story book, and I'll read it to you before bed time." The response acknowledges the child's feelings, clearly limits his behavior, and promises fulfillment of some of his own needs.

The naive parent may underestimate the harm that an older sibling, especially between ages 2 and 4, may inflict on an infant. As a regular part of anticipatory guidance, the physician should explore the parent's attitude toward and management of toddler-aged siblings at the time of an infant's well child visits. The infant needs to be protected from the impulsive acts of the older sibling, who may hit or otherwise harm the infant when jealous feelings are aroused.

If sibling rivalry appears to be excessive, the factors described under Psychodynamic Considerations should be explored. If one finds a parent who punishes jealousy, these feelings should be explored through an empathetic, nonjudgmental interview. If the attitude remains unaffected, referral to a mental health resource should be explored. If one suspects that the parent prefers or has negative feelings toward a particular child, those attitudes may be altered if they are identified and acknowledged during a supportive interview. If the physician senses, however, that such feelings are firmly entrenched, the parent may need more intensive psychotherapy, which the primary care physician can encourage through his own identification of the issues. The parent is not likely to acknowledge a need for such help, but he may gradually do so if the physician identifies his perception of the problem in a frank and neutral manner. He might say, for example, "I notice things that make me think that deep down inside you feel much more warmly toward Susan than toward Jim. It's easy to understand how these feelings might have developed, but I fear they will be harmful to both children's development. I would recommend that you take some time to explore your feelings with someone who may help you understand them, which may also help you change them." Such frank confrontation can be helpful if the parent knows that the physician feels warmly toward her and will remain involved in the child's health care.

If the physician suspects a developmental problem in the child, more severe rivalry behaviors can be anticipated. Much can be accomplished if the parent understands this and takes extra care to bolster the self-esteem of such a child and protect him from comparisons with more successful siblings. Such children need to have their own special talents acknowledged and encouraged. They need to be protected from unfavorable comparisons to their siblings, such as the teacher who says, "I don't know what's the matter with you. Your sister did very well in this class." Often, such children are helped by encouraging individual sports and activities rather than group efforts that invite unfavorable comparisons. Children with developmental disorders often control their emotions poorly, and parents should avoid either putting them under the supervision of older siblings or having them supervise younger siblings. Both situations are often handled poorly by such children. Finally, any situation that can be anticipated to produce rivalrous feelings will probably do so more strongly, and the parents must be prepared to respond with greater skill and effort.

Parents often ask about the appropriate method of settling fights between siblings. A basic beginning principle is that children must not be allowed to hurt each other and that it is usually difficult to determine the cause of the conflict. Often, for example, the child who strikes out is the one who has difficulty controlling his emotions, but the conflict may be instigated by the sibling who provokes the emotional response. If the parent recognizes this pattern early in the conflict before a fight begins, he may successfully prevent the battle by identifying and punishing this early stage of interaction. For example, he may identify that one sibling is provoking and then isolate that child unless he stops. Usually, however, the parent hears the battle and not the preliminaries. In this case, it is best to isolate the children from each other if they are physically fighting or else remain neutral if they are trying to work out the conflict but also attempting to solicit the parent's support. Isolation should be accomplished by sending both children to a time-out location, their own bedrooms, for example. If they share bedrooms, other time-out locations need to be identified just for such occasions.

REFERENCES

1. Chamberlin RW: Management of preschool behavior problems. Pediatr Clin North Am 21:33, 1974

2. Smith EE, VanTassel E: Problems of discipline in early childhood. Pediatr Clin North Am 29:167, 1982

3. Drabman RS, Jarvie G: Counseling parents of children with behavior problems: The use of extinction and time-out techniques. Pediatrics 59:78, 1977

4. Patterson GR, Gullion ME: Living with Children! New Methods for Parents and Teachers. Champaign, Il, Research Press, 1968

5. Ginott HG: Between Parent and Child. New York, MacMillan, 1965

6. Gordon T: P.E.T.—Parent Effectiveness Training. New York, New American Library, 1975

7. Fraiberg S: The Magic Years. New York, Scribner's, 1959

8. Stern E, Parmelee AH, Ariyama Y, et al.: Sleep cycle characteristics in infants. Pediatrics 43:65, 1969

9. Parmelee AH, Wenner WH, Shulz HR: Infant sleep patterns: From birth to 16 weeks of age. J Pediatr 65:576, 1964

10. Keith PR: Night terrors. J Am Acad Child Psychiatry 14:477, 1975

11. Frodi AM, Lamb ME: Fathers' and mothers' responses to the faces and cries of normal and premature infants. Dev Psychol 14:490, 1978

12. Brazelton TB: Doctor and Child. New York, Dell Publishing Co., Inc., 1978

13. Spock G: Baby and Child Care, (Rev). New York, Wallaby Pocket Books, Simon & Schuster, 1972

14. Palmer S, Thompson RJ, Linscheid TR: Applied behavior analysis in the treatment of childhood feeding problems. Dev Med Child Neurol 17:333, 1975

15. Thomas A, Chess S, Birch HB: Temperament and Behavior Disorders in Children. New York, New York Univ Press, 1968

Cross-Reference to *Pediatrics,* 17th ed.

TWENTY-ONE

Constipation

Steven P. Shelov

DEFINITION

Constipation is defined as a condition in which the stools are hard, infrequent, and difficult to pass. These complaints are heard frequently by pediatric practitioners, and it is important to respond with full knowledge of the range of possible underlying causes, from the most common to the esoteric.

A logical, systematic approach should be used in evaluating and treating children with constipation. Only rarely is referral to a consultant required. It is tempting to prescribe a cathartic medication without a complete evaluation, but this is poor practice and may increase rather than decrease the time required for proper care.

CAUSES OF CONSTIPATION

Constipation in Infancy

Underfeeding. This is the most common problem leading to the complaint of constipation in infants. Usually, however, the infant is not truly constipated. When the stools are soft and the only complaint is of decreased frequency, the history will reveal that intake is less than desirable. Counseling to increase the volume of feeding will usually result in increased frequency of stool.

Formula Feeding. Infants fed proprietary formulas, especially those with iron, often have hard stools and may even appear to strain with bowel movements. The hard stools may be accompanied by decreased frequency. The cause of this form of constipation is probably multifactorial. It is termed "functional constipation" and probably is the result of increased water absorption in the rectum, resulting in the formation of a harder and smaller fecal mass. The problem appears to be familial and is aggravated by the increased content of calcium salts and casein in milk formulas and in whole milk. It has been shown that these children have increased colonic pressure wave patterns associated with the increased water absorption. In addition, they do not respond with propulsion activity when challenged with a parasympathomimetic. This form of functional or constitutional constipation is not serious, but it may cause much anxiety.

Breastfeeding. Breastfed infants have a variable stooling pattern. Parents often consider that their infant is constipated when the intervals between each small, soft stool are 1 or 2 days. This stool pattern is normal for a breastfed infant, even if the interval occasionally is as long as 5 days. The long intervals are due to the fact that breast milk is nutritionally excellent, and it is digested completely, with a resultant lack of residue and bulk.

Hirschsprung's Disease. This condition is secondary to an aganglionic segment of the colon, due to malformation of the parasympathetic system of ganglion cells of the submucosal (Meissner's) plexus and myenteric (Auerbach's) plexus. This abnormality results in a failure of proper propulsion of stool, with functional obstruction of the distal colon. The entire rectum is usually involved. The degree of involvement at the proximal colon is variable, but at least one half of the patients have aganglionosis up to the midsigmoid colon. The usual time of presentation is in the newborn. This is an extremely rare condition, but it must be considered, especially in male children who present with severe constipation (i.e., intervals of 5–7 days or more between bowel movements). Additional characteristics found in children with Hirschsprung's disease are shown in Table 1. For a further description of Hirschsprung's disease, see *Pediatrics*, 17th ed.

Meconium Ileus, Cystic Fibrosis. The majority of infants with cystic fibrosis of the pancreas (CFP) will present in early infancy with poor weight gain, steatorrhea, increased stool volume and bulk, and recurrent pulmonary symptoms. Only 15% of children with CFP manifest symptoms in the newborn period of meconium ileus. However, should a newborn present with no stool formation within 24 hours, the diagnosis of meconium ileus must be considered, and an evaluation for cystic fibrosis should ensue.

Hypothyroidism, Diabetes Mellitus. Only rarely will constipation be the only presentation for children with hypothyroidism and diabetes mellitus and other neuromuscular disorders. Each of these conditions results in an ileus and failure to have normal propulsion of stool to the distal intestine. In most cases,

other signs and symptoms would be suggestive of the underlying problem.

Anal Fissure. Frequently, young infants with functional constipation develop a small tear in the anal mucosa. This may cause pain on defecation, which often makes the infant withhold stool and further aggravates the preexisting constipation. Application of petroleum jelly over the fissure and softening of the stool, as described later, are usually curative of this cause of constipation.

Constipation after Infancy

There are four major categories of constipation in the older child.

Uncomplicated Minor Constipation. This is most common in active, vigorous, preschool or school-aged children who are often too busy to go to the bathroom and go 1–2 days between bowel movements. This is not true constipation. Before the pediatric practitioner advises any intervention, an accurate assessment of the severity must be made. If it appears to be a mild form with hard stools but only 1–2 days between each stool, attention should be directed to the composition of diet. This condition will often be corrected with the addition to the diet of bulk laxatives that are hydrophilic or the addition of stewed fruit, such as prunes. Occasionally, there is the additional problem of a hypotonic colon that will require some form of treatment with a peristaltic stimulant. This hypotonicity, resulting in increased transit time, will probably persist through the individual's life and always require some form of occasional assistance.

Functional Stool Retention. Beginning around the time of toilet training, some children develop a pattern of stooling that can lead to a chronic form of constipation. The circumstances surrounding the child's ease at toilet training should be discussed.

TABLE 1. CHARACTERISTICS OF AGANGLIONIC MEGACOLON

Prevalence	1:25,000 births
M:F	9:1
Constipation in newborn period	Almost always*
Onset of symptoms	Newborn or before 2 years
Stool size	Often thin ribbons
Stool frequency	Markedly reduced
Abdominal pain	Rare, except when obstructed
General appearance	Often chronically ill
Failure to thrive	Common
Obstruction	Common
Abdominal distention	Common
Stool in ampulla	Diminished to absent
Plain x-ray	Narrow rectum
Corroborative history	No urge to defecate found in older children

*Occasionally the diagnosis is made in a preschool child who gives a clear history of not having an urge to defecate. In this instance, the aganglionic segment usually is short. *(From Hoeckelman R, et al.: Principles of Pediatrics, 1978, p. 717. Courtesy of McGraw-Hill, Inc.)*

- Was bowel control easy to accomplish, or was it a major source of conflict between child and parent?
- Was there a great amount of fear generated in the child about the process of toilet training?
- Was bowel control ultimately attained, or was it intermittent with periods of incontinence or soiling?
- Was there any evidence of early stool withholding that has persisted?

Positive answers to these questions are often obtained in toddlers or preschool children who have shown significant constipation characterized by stool withholding. This pattern is illustrated by the following vicious cycle:

1. The child has the urge to defecate.
2. Upon sensing the urge, for a variety of different reasons, the child voluntarily withholds the stool. This action may be the result of some previous fears about stool expulsion, previous painful stool expulsion due to an anal fissure, or some minor associated event, the significance of which is not recognized. The voluntary nature of this withholding of stool is often observed by the parent, who sees the child become stiff, tighten his or her leg muscles, perhaps grimace, and then relax once the urge to defecate has passed.
3. As result of this withholding, the stool mass becomes larger and harder as water is absorbed.
4. With the next urge, the voluntary withholding persists and now is aggravated by the larger mass of rectal stool, the passage of which would be very painful.
5. The result of this cycle is a child with significant constipation, abdominal pain, and occasional abdominal distention. Further characteristics of these children are listed in Table 2.

These children often present with soiling, due apparently to overflow incontinence. The soiling is actually from soft, loose, distal colonic material passing around a large, hard mass of stool that has caused the rectum to become dilated and to function poorly.

TABLE 2. CHARACTERISTICS OF CHILDREN WITH FUNCTIONAL STOOL RETENTION

Prevalence	1.5% of 7-year-old females
Sex prevalence	86% female
Retention as newborn	Rare
Problems with bowel training	Common
Toilet avoidance	Common
Stool size	Large, may clog toilet
Frequency of defecation	Variable
Obstruction	Rare
Stool in ampulla	Increased in volume, rock hard
Abdominal pain	Common
General appearance	Healthy

(From Hoeckelman R, et al.: Principles of Pediatrics, 1978, p. 719. Courtesy of McGraw-Hill, Inc.)

Therapeutic intervention is directed toward interrupting this vicious cycle.

Constipation Due to Emotional Disturbances. These children appear to be alternately constipated and encopretic. Rectal examination reveals the presence of soft stool with a nondilated rectum rather than a rock hard stool. There is usually a clear history of encopresis (defined as the passage of normal stools at inappropriate times, such as into pants or pajamas). Clear differentiation from functional constipation, however, is often not possible at first. Some observers feel that a significant proportion of these children have some degree of stool withholding, and thus the initial approach to these children should be the same as to those with documented hard rectal masses due to functional stool retention. In cases in which this approach is not productive, more significant psychopathology will often have become more apparent to the pediatric practitioner. If so, and if bowel retraining exercises are not effective, referral to a proper consultant is indicated.

Hirschsprung's Disease. Hirschsprung's disease is described under Constipation in Infancy.

DIFFERENTIAL DIAGNOSIS

History

The differential diagnosis in an infant or a child with a chief complaint of constipation depends on how constipation is defined by the parents and on the age of the patient. The following complaints are common at different age periods.

Newborn and Young Infant.

I. The baby has not passed any meconium. Failure to pass meconium within 24 hours suggests the possibility of meconium plug syndrome, which has a high correlation with cystic fibrosis. These infants should have sweat chloride measurements.

II. The newborn infant had normal, dark, thick stools for several days; they then became seedy and yellow, and now, at 5 weeks of age, the stools are much less frequent. The handling of the complaint depends upon the answers to the following questions.

A. Is the baby being breastfed? Breastfed infants often have 1–2 or more days between each stool and the stool is usually soft or semisolid. This stool pattern is normal for a breastfed infant and is not constipation.

B. Is the baby fed a formula, but only 3–4 times per day? If formula is fed too infrequently, the stools are often infrequent and hard. Pointing this out and counseling to increase intake to approximately 5 ounces/kg/day can relieve the baby's constipation. While checking the frequency of the feedings, careful questioning as to the method of milk preparation is important.

C. Does the baby being fed formula appear to strain during bowel movements although the stool is *not* hard? This is normal behavior in young infants and should not be construed as constipation.

D. Is the baby taking an iron-containing formula? These babies may have infrequent, hard stools, accompanied by straining. Although this association is commonly noted, it cannot be attributed to a definable cause.

E. Is the baby growing well and seeming to be well nourished but having infrequent, hard stools passed with difficulty? This complaint is seen most frequently in babies less than 6 months of age. It indicates a functional condition and should not be viewed with great concern. This type of constipation most often resolves in the early toddler period but occasionally may herald a similar functional condition in childhood and adulthood. The major complication is the production of a fissure in ano.

F. Has this 2-month-old infant been placed on cow's milk? The temptation to the parent to place infants on whole milk as early as possible is common. The tendency is often difficult to counteract, but, as one deterrant, the pediatric practitioner may use the fact that cow's milk with its increased concentration of casein and calcium salts may contribute to constipation.

III. Rarely, the frequency of stool may be such that periods of days to a week occur between stools. Children with this history often are not thriving and may appear to have a slightly distended abdomen. Vomiting is a common additional finding. This history would point to one of the rarer causes of severe constipation in infancy, which include aganglionic megacolon (Hirschsprung's disease), hypothyroidism, and severe cerebral palsy or other neuromuscular disorder.

Toddlers and Children. Evaluation of constipation in this age group should begin with questions concerning the frequency and consistency of the stools and whether or not there is associated pain. In addition, an understanding of the dietary pattern is essential. From this initial evaluation, the practitioner should have a clear idea concerning the severity of the problem, the need for laboratory investigation, and the degree of intervention required. It is important to remember that in toddlers and school-aged children, stool patterns can be quite variable and yet be within normal limits. Adults often consider daily bowel movements to be a highly desirable state. However, they must accept the fact that, in children, intervals of 1 or 2 days are common and should be considered normal. Occasional hard stools in a child whose stools are usually soft should also be considered as normal. Periods of illness accompanied by decreased intake and changes in diet are often accompanied by a variable stool pattern, which should not be interpreted as constipation. Fiber and bulk are not prominent food items of the diet in children, and their deficiency may contribute to the stools being hard and infrequent. If, after considering all of these variants in stool patterns, it is believed that actual constipation is present, some form of intervention may be needed, depending on the degree of severity and chronicity.

Physical Examination

Complete examination, including a neurologic evaluation, is an important part of the initial assessment. Positive findings and corresponding diagnostic considerations are shown in Table 3.

Laboratory Evaluation

Constipation in Infants. Rarely is any specific laboratory or radiographic evaluation helpful. In those newborns with meconium ileus, work-up for cystic fibrosis should be done. In the rare infant in whom Hirschsprung's disease is being considered, two types of radiographs should be performed: (1) a plain film to show a dilated colon and a narrow visualized rectum and (2) a barium enema, which should be performed without bowel preparation and reveals a ribbon-narrow rectum due to the collapsed aganglionic segment, with a large dilated colon proximal to the aganglionic segment. In newborns, a helpful radiographic sign is retention of barium for more than 24 hours. Further corroboration of this diagnosis can be obtained by suction biopsy of the rectum. Absence of the parasympathetic plexuses would confirm the diagnosis of Hirschsprung's disease.

Constipation in Toddlers and Children. The history and physical examination should enable the pediatric practitioner to categorize the type of constipation. In children who are stool withholders, a plain film will demonstrate the large amount of stool in a large dilated rectum. This plain abdominal radiograph serves the dual purpose of comparison with a postevacuation film to confirm that all stool has been removed following a course of

TABLE 3. PHYSICAL FINDINGS IN CONSTIPATION

Abnormal Findings	Diagnostic Considerations
Face	
Coarse features	Hypothyroidism
Abdomen	
Distended, wrinkled due to decreased musculature	Prune-belly syndrome (Eagle-Barret)
Distended with much stool palpated	Functional constipation Hirschsprung's disease Constipation due to stool withholding
Rectum and anus	
Fissure in ano	Withholding of stool due to pain
Abnormal anal wink reflex	Decreased innervation of rectum, possible neurologic dysfunction
No stool palpated, upper rectum fits like sleeve over finger	Hirschsprung's disease
Hard stool palpated in ampulla	Retained rectal mass due to stool withholding
Nervous system	
Hypotonia and sensory abnormalities in T12-S3 distribution	Deficit in innervation

laxatives. Further laboratory work-up is not helpful, beyond routine hemogram and urinalysis.

THERAPEUTIC INTERVENTION

Constipation of Infancy

Given the usual causes of this problem, remediation should be low-keyed. The frequency of the problem in the population should be emphasized, and parents should be reassured that in most cases, with increasing age and the addition of more bulk and variety to the diet, the constipation will be alleviated.

The following therapeutic intervention should be employed in the order given for children with functional constipation.

1. In infants less than 4 months old, ½ to 1 teaspoon of dark Karo syrup added to each of four bottles of formula per day should result in a softer stool in 2–4 days. If not, soup of malt extract (Malt Supex) may be tried. It comes as a molasses preparation or as a powder, which is easier to get into solution. Addition of 1 teaspoon to each of four bottles for 3–4 days should result in a softer stool. At that time, the frequency of addition of this sugar can be reduced to 1–2 times per day.
2. In infants 4 months or older, a stool softener, such as Colace, which acts to retain water in the rectum and soften stool, may be tried. A solution of Colace containing 10 mg/ml should be given in a dosage of 2 mg/kg/day.
3. In infants 6 months or older, a small amount of a laxative may be beneficial. Senokot syrup in a dosage of ¼ teaspoon/day may yield good results. More intensive treatment for this problem is probably not warranted and probably would be overtreatment of a condition that is usually transient.
4. Finally, in infants older than 1 year of age,

discontinuing constipating foods, such as bananas and rice cereal, may be helpful. In addition, 15–30 ml of prune juice given each day may act as a mild laxative by stimulating colonic contraction.

Constipation in Toddlers and Older Children

In this age child, constipation that requires intervention is usually accompanied by stool withholding and often is accompanied by encopresis as well. The approach to these children should be a combination of three efforts.

1. An initial evaluation performed in a supportive and understanding fashion. If the child is verbal, a clear attempt must be made to have the child understand the problem and to educate the child about the response to the urge to defecate. Understanding and support are crucial.
2. An attempt to remove the large stool volume by catharsis and/or enemas.
3. A long process of reeducation and retraining to help introduce normal training and stooling patterns. This reeducation process is accompanied by the liberal use of mineral oil administered in the fashion popularized by Davidson et al., as shown in Table 4.

Only occasionally will there be clear evidence of a severe emotional disturbance or of family disruption. In such cases, referral to a proper consultant is in order.

USE OF CONSULTANT

All infants with constipation should be managed initially by the pediatric practitioner. In those rare cases where the diagnosis of Hirschsprung's disease, hypothyroidism, cystic fibrosis, or neuromuscular disorder is sus-

TABLE 4. MEDICAL MANAGEMENT OF SIGNIFICANT CONSTIPATION WITH OR WITHOUT ENCOPRESIS

Treatment Phase	Treatment Program	Comments
Initial counseling	1. Education and demystification of problem 2. Removal of blame 3. Establishment and explanation of treatment plan	Include drawings, review of colonic function, joint observation of x-rays
Outpatient	1. High normal saline enemas (750 ml bid) 3–7 days 2. Bisacodyl (Dulcolax) suppositories bid 3–7 days 3. Use of bathroom for 15 min after each meal	Patient admitted when 1. Retention very severe 2. Home compliance likely to be poor 3. Parents prefer admission 4. Parental administration of enemas inadvisable psychologically
Home	1. In moderate to severe retention, 2–4* cycles as follows: Day 1: hypophosphate enemas (Fleet adult) twice Day 2: Bisacodyl (Dulcolax) suppositories twice Day 3: Bisacodyl (Dulcolax) tablet once 2. In mild retention, senna or danthron, 1 tablet for 1–2 weeks	1. Dosages or frequency may need alteration if child experiences excessive discomfort 2. Admission should be considered if there is inadequate yield
	Follow-up abdominal x-ray to confirm adequate catharsis	
Maintenance	1. Child sits on toilet twice a day at same times each day for 10 min each time 2. Light mineral oil (at least 2 tablespoons) twice a day for at least 6 months 3. Multiple vitamins, 2 a day, between mineral oil doses 4. High roughage diet	1. Kitchen timer may be helpful 2. Chart with stars for sitting may be good for children under 7 3. Bathroom reading encouraged 4. Mineral oil may be put in juice or cola or any other medium 5. Vitamins to compensate for alleged problems with absorption secondary to mineral oil 6. Diet should be applied but not to the point of coercion
Follow-up	1. Visits every 4–10 weeks, depending on severity, need for support, compliance, and associated symptoms 2. Telephone availability to adjust doses when needed 3. In case of relapse: Check compliance Trial of oral laxative (e.g., Senokot) for 1–2 weeks Adjust dosage of mineral oil 4. Counseling and/or referral for associated psychosocial and developmental issues	1. Duration of treatment program may be as long as 2–8 yr or as short as 6 months 2. Signs of relapse: Excessive oil leakage Large-caliber stools Abdominal pain Decreased frequency of defecation Soiling 3. Physician should spend time alone with child 4. In case slow to respond, physician should sustain optimism, persistence cures almost all cases eventually

*All dosages and frequencies are calculated for an average sized 7-yr-old child. Appropriate adjustments should be made for smaller and larger patients. *(From Levine MD: In Hoeckelman R, et al.: Principles of Pediatrics, 1978. Courtesy of McGraw-Hill, Inc.)*

pected, referral to the appropriate pediatric subspecialist is required.

The vast majority of older children with constipation should be managed by the pediatric practitioner. Only in the case of an accompanying severe emotional disorder should referral be made to a mental health professional. It is our opinion that such referral should be for the whole family. The pediatric practitioner should work together with the mental health professional to optimize the intervention and help improve both the symptomatology and the function of the child in the family.

REFERENCES

Apley J: The Child with Abdominal Pains. Oxford, Blackwell, 1974

Brazelton TB: A child-oriented approach to toilet training. Pediatrics 29:121, 1962

Davidson M, Kugler MM, Bauer CH: Diagnosis and management in children with severe and protracted constipation and obstipation. J Pediatr 62:261, 1967

Hoekelman R, Blatman S, Brunell P, Friedman S, Seidel H: Principles of Pediatrics. New York, McGraw-Hill, 1978

Cross-Reference to *Pediatrics,* 17th ed.

TWENTY-TWO

Delayed Gross and Fine Motor Development

David L. Diamond

The basis of any discussion of developmental delay in pediatric practice is the understanding of normal child development and its underlying mechanisms. A thorough knowledge of normal development makes the clinician sensitive to the presence and significance of deviation.

Development refers here to changes in the function of the organism from conception to maturity. Although no two children follow exactly the same pattern of development, a certain sequence emerges in the pattern of healthy, normal children, which is intimately related to the maturation of the nervous system. Thus, no amount of practice can cause a child to walk before his nervous system is ready. It is important also to note that the *sequence* of development is the same in all children; it is the *rate* of development that varies from child to child.

Arnold Gessel first systematically studied the sequence of development in large numbers of children. In order to facilitate discussion and understanding of the developing child, he divided the developmental sequence into five fields.

1. Gross motor—includes control of head, trunk, and extremities, sitting, standing, creeping, and walking.

2. Fine motor—pertains to achievement of the control of fine and purposeful movements of the fingers.
3. Language—includes the production of sounds, single words, combinations of words, and facial expressions used as a vehicle for communication with an understanding of others.
4. Adaptive—refers to manipulation and exploitation of objects, the use of motor capacities in such practical situations as pencil grasping, block building, and so on. (Gessel states that intelligence is based largely on adaptive behavior.)
5. Personal-social—has the widest variations of all the fields and depends to a large extent on culture and environment.

In this chapter, the focus of discussion is in the areas of gross and fine motor development. Table 1 lists the developmental norms within each field of development at crucial ages. The sequence within each developmental area is fixed, although the development of one field may not run parallel with the others. For example, a child with cerebral palsy involving only the lower extremities may be delayed in walking, but if his intelligence is normal, his fine motor development, adaptive skills, and language may be normal or even

TABLE 1. DEVELOPMENTAL NORMS

Age	Motor Behavior	Adaptive Behavior	Language	Personal and Social Behavior
Under 4 weeks	1. Makes alternating crawling movements 2. Moves head laterally when placed in a prone position	1. Responds to sound of rattle and bell 2. Regards moving objects momentarily	1. Small, throaty, undifferentiated noises	1. Quiets when picked up 2. Impassive face
4 weeks	1. Tonic neck reflex positions predominate 2. Hands fisted 3. Head sags but can hold head erect for a few seconds	1. Follows moving objects to the midline 2. Shows no interest and drops objects immediately	1. Beginning vocalization such as cooing, gurgling, or grunting	1. Regards face and diminishes activity 2. Responds to speech
16 weeks	1. Symmetrical postures predominate 2. Holds head balanced 3. Head lifted 90° when prone on forearms	1. Follows a slowly moving object well 2. Arms activate on sight of dangling object	1. Laughs aloud 2. Sustained cooing and gurgling	1. Spontaneous social smile 2. Aware of strange situations
28 weeks	1. Sits steadily, leaning forward on hands 2. Bounces actively when placed in a standing position	1. One-hand approach and grasp of toy 2. Bangs and shakes rattle 3. Transfers toys	1. Vocalizes "m-m-m" when crying 2. Makes different vowel sounds (e.g., "ah," "eh")	1. Takes feet to mouth 2. Pats mirror image
40 weeks	1. Sits alone with good coordination 2. Creeps 3. Pulls self to standing position	1. Matches two objects at midline 2. Spontaneously rings bell 3. Uses thumb and index finger for prehension	1. Says "da-da" or equivalent 2. Responds to name or nickname	1. Responds to social play such as "pat-a-cake" or "peekaboo" 2. Feeds self cracker and holds own bottle

(*continued*)

TABLE 1 (*Continued*)

Age	Motor Behavior	Adaptive Behavior	Language	Personal and Social Behavior
52 weeks	1. Walks with one hand held 2. Stands alone, briefly	1. Tries to build tower of two cubes 2. Attempts to imitate scribble	1. Beginning expressive jargon 2. Gives a toy on request	1. Cooperates in dressing
15 months	1. Toddles 2. Creeps upstairs	1. Builds tower of two cubes 2. Imitates a scribble	1. Says three to five words meaningfully 2. Pats pictures in book 3. Shows shoes on request	1. Points or vocalizes wants 2. Casts objects in play
18 months	1. Walks, seldom falls 2. Hurls ball 3. Walks upstairs with one hand held	1. Builds a tower of three to four cubes 2. Scribbles spontaneously and imitates a stroke	1. Says 10 words, including name 2. Identifies one common object on picture card 3. Names ball and carries out two directions ("put on table" and "give to mother")	1. Feeds self in part, spills 2. Pulls toy on string 3. Carries or hugs a toy (e.g., a doll)
2 yr	1. Runs well, no falling 2. Kicks large ball 3. Goes upstairs and downstairs alone	1. Builds tower of six to seven cubes 2. Aligns cubes, imitating train 3. Imitates vertical and circular strokes	1. Uses three-word sentences 2. Carries out four directions	1. Pulls on simple garment 2. Domestic mimicker 3. Refers to self by name
3 yr	1. Rides tricycle 2. Jumps from bottom step 3. Alternates feet going upstairs	1. Builds tower of 9 to 10 cubes 2. Imitates a three-cube bridge 3. Copies a circle and imitates a cross	1. Gives sex and full name 2. Uses plurals 3. Describes what is happening in a picture book	1. Puts on shoes 2. Unbuttons buttons 3. Feeds self well 4. Understands taking turns

(*continued*)

TABLE 1 (*Continued*)

Age	Motor Behavior	Adaptive Behavior	Language	Personal and Social Behavior
4 yr	1. Walks down-stairs one step per tread 2. Stands on one foot for 4–8 sec	1. Copies a cross 2. Repeats four digits 3. Counts three objects with correct pointing	1. Begins to name colors, at least one correctly 2. Understands five preposi-tional direc-tives ("on," "under," "in back," "in front," "be-side")	1. Washes and dries own face 2. Brushes teeth 3. Plays cooper-atively with children
5 yr	1. Skips, using feet alterna-tely 2. Stands on one foot for more than 8 sec	1. Copies a square 2. Draws a recog-nizable man with a head, body, and so on 3. Counts 10 ob-jects accurately	1. Names the primary col-ors 2. Names coins: pennies, nick-els, dimes 3. Asks meaning of words	1. Dresses and undresses self 2. Prints a few letters 3. Plays compet-itive games

(*From Wasserman E, Slobody L: Survey of Clinical Pediatrics, 6th ed., McGraw Hill, 1974, p 15*)

advanced for his age (Table 2). Illingworth has used the term *dissociation* for this lack of parallelism between different fields of development.

DEFINITION

In the early stages of development, motor function is the main behavior available for judging neurologic integrity. There is pro-gression in a cephalocaudal direction from generalized reflex muscular activity in infan-cy (Fig. 1) to specific, individual, well-orga-nized functional responses in the child.

In the development of locomotion, each child goes through an orderly sequence from the development of head control to mature

TABLE 2. DISSOCIATION PHENOMENA IN DEVELOPMENTAL DISABILITIES

Developmental Area	Mental Retardation	Cerebral Palsy	Deaf ness
Motor			
Gross	V	D	N
Fine	V	D	N
Problem solving	D	V	N
Language			
Receptive	D	N	D
Expressive	D	V	D
Personal-social	D	V	V

D, delayed; N, normal; V, variable. (*From: Accardo PJ, Capute AJ: The Pediatrician and the Developmentally Delayed Child: A Clinical Textbook on Mental Retarda-tion. University Park Press, 1979, p 124*)

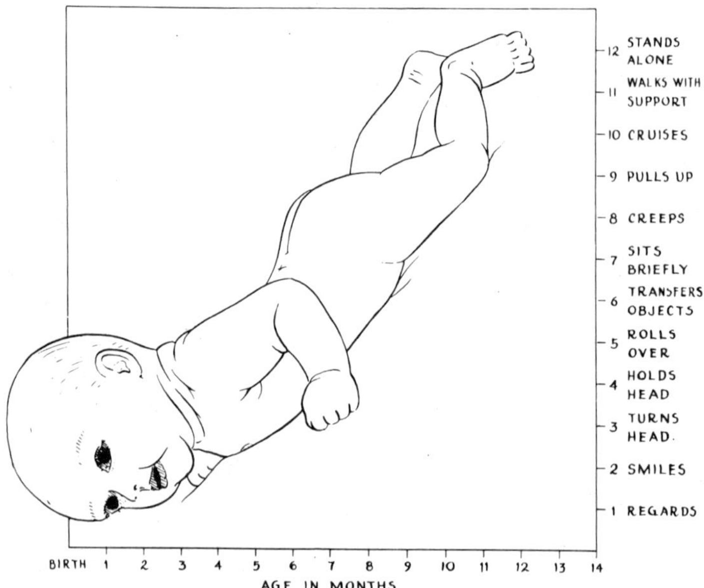

Figure 1. Developmental diagram for the first year of life. The infant's figure represents a diagonal line on which is plotted the progress of behavior (right of the diagram) against chronologic age. The cephalocaudal pattern of behavior is diagrammatically illustrated by position of the figure. (*Reproduced with permission from Lowry GH: Growth & Development of Children, 7th ed. Copyright © 1978 by Year Book Medical Publishers, Inc., Chicago. (After Aldrich CA, Hewitt ES: Outlines for well baby clinics: Development for the first twelve months, Am J Dis Child 71:131, 1946.)*

walking to running and skipping (Table 1). This development can be observed when the infant is held in ventral suspension, when he is placed in the prone position, and when he is pulled to sitting. Subsequently, gross motor development is observed in the sitting and upright position.

Fine motor function or manipulation skills proceed from primitive to voluntary grasp responses, thereafter moving through several states from the ulnar grasp to radial grasp and, ultimately, the finger-thumb or pincer grasp. Increasing development of fine motor skills, visual motor coordination, and perception can be tested in the preschool child by cube play (tower, bridge building), manipulation of pellet and bottle, and the use of a crayon.

ETIOLOGY OF DELAYED MOTOR DEVELOPMENT

Delayed motor development can be due to a multiplicity of entities, ranging from environmental and sociologic factors to a wide array of organic etiologies. The entity can be classified as either static or progressive, dependent on etiology and clinical course.

A full review of each clinical entity is beyond the scope of this chapter, and we provide a brief review of the common clinical conditions and relevant discussion concerning clinical diagnosis.

Familial Factors

The age at which children begin to walk may be genetically determined. Questions asked of parents as to when they walked or the age of walking of the patient's siblings may modify concerns of motor delay. In order to make this diagnosis, evaluation must reveal a positive family history, normal neurologic examination, and normal development in language and adaptive areas.

Environmental Factors

Most of the literature devoted to environmental deprivation has studied its affect on intelligence or language. Children who have been brought up in an institutional setting and those who have suffered environmental or social deprivation from early infancy have been found to be delayed in motor development. These children have a positive history of severe deprivation, with associated delays in other areas of development. They have no specific neurologic abnormality. They benefit greatly from intensive intervention and therapy, if it is initiated early.

Blindness

Blind children have to be taught to walk. A blind child's motor development may be retarded because, out of fear of bodily harm, he is not given the same chance to learn to walk as a normal child.

Mental Retardation

Mental retardation is defined as significantly subaverage general intellectual functioning, originating during the developmental period and associated with impairment of adaptive behavior, learning, and social adjustment. Table 3 lists the characteristics of varying degrees of mental retardation.

The majority of retarded individuals fall into the mild or borderline range, presenting with essentially normal physical and neurologic examinations. This group is being recognized with increasing frequency at younger ages due to early developmental assessment and screening.

The child presenting at a very young age with significant delay in motor development due to mental retardation will usually be functioning in the moderate to severe range. Delays in all areas of development should be observed. A positive history or direct observation of developmental delay with associated risk factors (Table 4), as well as observance of physical stigmata (Table 5) or disturbances of the growth pattern, may be noted.

Since this delay is global in nature, the actual sequence of motor development is dependent on the level of intellectual functioning. The severely retarded youngster may present with early motor delay, and, in contrast, the child diagnosed as mildly retarded may never demonstrate evidence of motor delay. It is important to note that motor delay presents as only part of the clinical picture in a child with mental retardation.

Cerebral Palsy

Cerebral palsy is a disorder of posture and movement due to a static lesion of the brain, with the insult occurring prenatally, perinatally, or in early childhood. It is a motor disorder with associated cognitive, sensory, visual, and auditory impairment. There are numerous clinical classifications (Table 6), each with different diagnostic criteria and prognoses.

Spastic Cerebral Palsy. Spastic cerebral palsy is due to involvement of the upper motor neurons and is characterized by increased tone of the involved musculature, exaggeration of the deep tendon reflexes, clonus, and abnormal postural reflexes.

Dyskinetic Cerebral Palsy. Dyskinetic cerebral palsy implies an impairment of volitional activity by uncontrolled and purposeless movements. These movement disorders are usually related to lesions of the basal ganglia, the most common type being athetoid cerebral palsy.

TABLE 3. CHARACTERISTICS OF VARYING DEGREES OF MENTAL RETARDATION

I.Q.=M.A./C.A.		SD	Function	Physical Findings
Borderline	70–84	−1.01 to −2.00	Basic academic skills, "slow learner"	Essentially normal
Mild	55–89	−2.01 to −3.00	Educable (vocational training)	
Moderate	40–54	−3.01 to −4.00	Trainable	Increasing frequency of neurologic deficits, stigmata of dysmorphism
Severe	25–39	−4.01 to −5.00	Dependent	
Profound	<25	−5.00	Totally dependent	

MA/CA, mental age/chronological age; MR, mental retardation; SD, standard deviation.

TABLE 4. HIGH-RISK FACTORS PREDISPOSING TO MENTAL RETARDATION

Family history
1. Deafness, blindness, neurologic diseases, cerebral palsy, epilepsy
2. Congenital malformations (including congenital dislocation of the hip)
3. Mental disorder
4. Elderly or very young mother

Prenatal
1. Rubella and other viral infections contracted in early pregnancy
2. Toxoplasmosis
3. Hyperemesis
4. Threatened abortion
5. Severe illnesses in the early months necessitating chemotherapy or major surgery
6. Exposure to radioactive substances during pregnancy
7. Blood group incompatibilities
8. Maternal diabetes mellitus
9. Maternal thyrotoxicosis and toxemia
10. Uterine hemorrhage
11. Hydramnios
12. Multiple pregnancy

Perinatal
1. Premature birth (39 weeks and earlier)
2. Low weight at birth in relation to gestational age
3. Postmature birth (42 weeks and later)
4. Abnormal presentation
5. Prolonged, precipitate, or instrumental labor
6. Birth asphyxia
7. Neonatal jaundice
8. Presence of any congenital abnormality
9. Induction of labor

Postnatal
1. Difficulties in sucking and swallowing
2. Convulsions
3. Cerebral palsy
4. Meningitis or encephalitis
5. Any serious illness or infection in first few months of life

Symptomatic group
1. Mother's suspicion that the child is blind, deaf, retarded, or otherwise abnormal
2. Inattention to sound or to visual stimuli
3. Delayed motor development
4. Delayed development of vocalization and speech

(*From: Sheridan:* Monthly Bull Minist Health (London) *21:238, 1962.*)

Family History of Mental Retardation	Socio-cultural Factors	Prevalence (%)		Therapeutic Goals
		MR	Total Population	
+	4+	67	13	Basic academic and social skills to be capable of selfsupport and independent living in community
+	3+	22	2.7	
Only in cases due to genetic disorders	0	6	0.2	Self-care skills involving activities of daily living and sheltered workshop
	0	3	0.1	Protective care at home or group home
	0	2	0.05	Custodial care

Ataxic Cerebral Palsy. Ataxic cerebral palsy, the least common type, is characterized by ataxic phenomena related to a static lesion of the cerebellum and its pathways.

The clinical presentation and prognosis are variable, depending on type, extent of involvement, existence of associated cognitive deficit, and therapeutic intervention.

Degenerative and Demyelinating Diseases

The progressive diseases of the nervous system present clinically with a wide diversity of symptoms, depending on anatomic site and type of disease (Table 7).

Loss of motor accomplishments is suggestive of degenerative or demyelinating disease but is not specific. Associated positive family and parental consanguinity may be present. Physical and neurologic examination may reveal funduscopic findings, macrocephaly, hepatosplenomegaly, neurocutaneous lesions, muscle weakness, or hypoflexia (Table 7).

In undertaking any evaluation of a child with delayed motor development, these diseases must be considered when indicated, and necessary consultation must be obtained.

Diseases of the Motor Units. Any abnormality of the motor unit, comprised of the motor neuron, neuromuscular junction, and muscle, will affect motor development. Neurologic examination and proper application of laboratory techniques are needed to make a proper diagnosis.

An example of an entity affecting the motor neuron is infantile spinal muscular atrophy. The clinical picture is that of reduced muscle power, decreased spontaneous movement, and symmetrical muscle weakness. Muscle atrophy and markedly reduced or absent deep tendon reflexes are present. The patient has no sensory loss and has normal intelligence on psychologic testing. Diagnosis is made by abnormal findings on electromyelogram and nerve conduction studies.

Myasthenia gravis is the principal disorder of the neuromuscular junction. Though this entity is rare in children, the transient neonatal and persistent neonatal forms can present with delayed motor development.

TABLE 5. PHYSICAL STIGMATA OFTEN ASSOCIATED WITH MENTAL RETARDATION

Head
  Asymmetry
  Microcephaly
  Macrocephaly
  Frontal bossing
  Flat or prominent
    occiput
Facial appearance
  Odd
  Coarse features
  Expressionless
Hair
  Alopecia
  Hirsutism
  Synophrys
  Kinkiness
Mouth
  Micrognathia
  Cleft lip and palate
  Prognathia
  Macroglossia
Chest
  Shieldlike
  Pectus excavatum
  Deformed
  Short or webbed
    neck

Skin
  Abnormal dermato-
    glyphics
  Hemangiomata
  Cafe au lait spots
  Increased elasticity
Eyes
  Abnormal slant
  Blue sclera
  Epicanthal folds
  Brushfield spots
  Cataracts
  Ptosis
Teeth
  Absent or supernu-
    merary
  Enamel hypoplasia
  Staining
  Malposition
  Delayed eruption
Abdomen and
  genitourinary
  Umbilical hernia
  Ambiguous genitalia
  Hypospadias
  Cryptorchidism
Extremities
  Short metacarpals
  Polydactyly, clino-
    dactyly
  Short metatarsals
  Rocker bottom
  Toenail dysplasia
  Syndactyly, equi-
    novarus or equino-
    valgus

TABLE 6. CLINICAL CLASSIFICATION OF CEREBRAL PALSY

Spastic cerebral palsy
  Spastic hemiplegia
  Spastic quadriplegia
  Diplegia
    Spastic
    Atonic
  Spastic paraplegia
  Monoplegias and triplegias
Dyskinetic cerebral palsy
  Athetosis
  Other forms
Ataxic cerebral palsy
Mixed syndromes

servation of a positive response to cholinesterase-inhibitor drugs and abnormal findings on EMG.

Normal muscle function can be affected by a large number of degenerative, metabolic, and inflammatory disorders. Any entity interfering with muscle function has the potential to interfere with normal motor development.

Clinical and laboratory findings helpful in the consideration of muscle disease are a positive family history, abnormalities of muscle tone and strength, and muscle atrophy or hypertrophy. Abnormal posturing and toe walking may be seen, as well as a variability of deep tendon reflexes. Elevation of serum enzymes (CPK, SGOT) and abnormal findings on EMG will help make the diagnosis.

DIAGNOSIS

A useful assessment tool in the initial stage of an evaluation is the Denver Developmental Screening Test. This tool provides a well-organized, reliable listing of developmental norms for history taking and assessment. It is not an intelligence test and does not establish a diagnosis. It serves as a screening device for the detection of deviation from normal devel-

These children may present with weak cry, difficulty in swallowing and sucking, and generalized hypotonia. Progressive weakness on repetitive or sustained muscle contraction is noted. Deep tendon reflexes are usually normal but may disappear after repeated elicitation. Diagnosis can be made by the ob-

TABLE 7. DEGENERATIVE AND DEMYELINATING DISEASES

Disease Site	Skin and/or Systemic Findings	Ocular Findings	Neurologic Findings
Gray Matter			
Tay-Sachs	Normal	Cherry red macula	Early paresis Hyperacusis Late spasticity
Neimann-Pick	Hepatosplenomegaly, xanthema of skin	Cherry red macula	Spastic paresis
Gaucher's	Hepatosplenomegaly	Normal	Strabismus Spastic paralysis
White Matter			
Krabbe's	Normal head size	Optic atrophy	Spastic paresis Head retraction
Metachromatic leukodystrophy	Head enlarges late	Late optic atrophy	Combined upper and lower motor signs, blindness, deafness
Canavan's	Head enlarges early	Optic atrophy	Hypotonia, spastic diplegia

opment by history and direct observation of the child.

History

In taking the developmental history, open-ended, specific questions generate the most useful information. The history is of particular importance in those children who present with variation in their development, thus providing clues to the clinician as to any temporal pattern of delay.

Preceding the specific questions con-cerning developmental milestones, a thorough birth, medical, and family history is indicated. Table 4 is one of the many possible illustrations of risk factors that may lead to a high index of suspicion for developmental delay. A family history of any sibling or parent with delay in acquisition of motor milestones is of significance. Important information regarding the familial rate of motor development may be obtained from a parent's casual comments, such as, "My older child didn't walk, till almost 2 years either."

Relevant developmental questions in the newborn period are those regarding head and body movement and feeding behavior.

- "Does he lift his head?"
- "Are there feeding difficulties?"
- "Does he suck strongly?"

Table 8 lists specific developmental questions at crucial ages from infancy to preschool in the areas of locomotion (gross motor) and manipulation (fine motor). These questions are designed to alert the physician to specific quantitative and qualitative delays in development.

- "Does he roll from front to back?"
- "Does he pivot when sitting?"
- "Does he run well without falling?"

Questions relating to quality of motor function include:

- "When he crawls, does he use both legs and hands equally well?"
- "Does he walk on his toes?"
- "If he falls, does he get up easily?"
- "Does he still drool a lot?"

It is important to point out that motor abilities have the weakest correlation to general function. In fact, early acquisition of certain skills should lead to suspicion of possible pathology. For example, a mother boasts that her 2-month-old baby "can turn over." She

TABLE 8. DEVELOPMENTAL QUESTIONNAIRE

Age	Posture and Locomotion	Manipulation	Age	Posture and Locomotion	Manipulation
3 months	A. Does he support himself on forearms when lying? B. Does he hold his head up steadily while on his stomach?	A. Are his hands usually open at rest? B. Does he pull at his clothing?	2 years	A. Does he run well without falling? B. Does he walk up and down stairs alone?	A. Does he turn book pages one at a time?
6 months	A. Does he lift his head when lying on his back? B. Does he roll from back to front?	A. Does he transfer a toy from one hand to the other? B. Does he pick up small objects?	2½ years	A. Does he jump, getting both feet off the floor? B. Does he throw a ball overhand?	A. Does he unbutton any buttons? B. Does he hold a pencil or crayon adult fashion?
9 months	A. Does he sit for long periods without support? B. Does he pull up on furniture?	A. Does he pick up objects with his thumb and one finger? B. Does he finger-feed any foods?	3 years	A. Does he pedal a tricycle? B. Does he alternate feet (one stair per step) going upstairs?	A. Does he dry his hands (if reminded)? B. Does he dress and undress fully including front buttons?
12 months	A. Is he walking (alone or with hand held)? B. Does he pivot when sitting?	A. Does he throw toys (objects)? B. Does he give you toys (let go) easily?	4 years	A. Does he attempt to hop or skip? B. Does he alternate feet going downstairs?	A. Does he button clothes fully? B. Does he catch a ball?

(continued)

TABLE 8 (*Continued*)

Age	Posture and Locomotion	Manipulation	Age	Posture and Locomotion	Manipulation
18 months	A. Does he walk up-stairs with help? B. Can he throw a toy while standing without falling?	A. Does he turn book pages (two or three at a time)? B. Does he spoon and feed self?	5 years	A. Does he skip, alter-nating feet? B. Does he jump rope or jump over low obstacles?	A. Does he tie his own shoes? B. Does he spread with a knife?

(From Accardo PJ, Capute AJ: The Pediatrician and the Developmentally Delayed Child: A Clinical Textbook on Mental Retardation. University Park Press, 1979, p 110)

may be telling the clinician that the infant has severe tension of the spinal musculature secondary to cerebral palsy. Another example is of the child who "is definitely right-handed" at 6 months of age. Normal infants do not establish dominance until 18 months or later. An infant who seems to prefer one hand over the other should be suspected of having weakness of the opposite extremity.

Physical and Neurologic Examination

Subsequent to developmental history and assessment, physical and neurologic examinations are performed. Areas of particular concern on physical examination are evidence of deviation of normal growth patterns, physical stigmata (Table 5), or congenital defects.

All aspects of the neurologic examination are of value in the identification of a motor abnormality. In infants under 6 months of age, the following areas of importance.

- Observation of asymmetric movements. Asymmetry of movements in neonates and babies of 1–2 months of age may be indicative of a lower motor neuron problem, such as peripheral nerve palsy, rather than an upper motor problem as suggested in children over 3 months of age.
- Observation of the expected disappearance of primitive reflexes at about 3–4 months, with the eventual emergence of secondary or postural responses related to the achievement of motor milestones. Table 9 lists the most frequently observed primitive and acquired reflexes and the approximate age when they can be observed. Persistence of the tonic neck or Moro reflex past 3–4 months of age or the observation of an obligatory tonic neck reflex at any time is indicative of motor pathology.

Achievement of secondary or postural responses, listed in Table 9, can be used as predictors of eventual motor function.

Molnar et al. have shown that sitting posture can be predictive of walking skills in children with delayed development. A child who sits by 2 years of age will eventually ambulate.

The completion of the neurologic examination to determine abnormalities of gait, symmetry of muscle tone, and deep tendon reflexes, as well as the presence of intact cerebellar and sensory function, is vital in determining the etiology of delayed motor development at any age. (A full discussion of this is presented in Chapter 13.)

TABLE 9. INFANTILE REFLEXES AND AUTOMATISMS

Response	New-born	1	2	3	4	5	6	9	12
Primitive responses									
Moro	+	+	+	70%	+	±	0	0	0
Rooting and sucking	+	+	+	+	+	+	+	0	0
Palmar grasp	+	+	+	+	+	0	0	0	0
Asymmetric tonic neck	+	+	+	50%	±	±	±	0	0
Plantar grasp	+	+	+	+	+	+	+	0	0
Placing	+	+	+	+	+	+	+	Decreased but persists to 24 months	
Stepping	+	+	+	+	+	0	0	0	0
Supporting reaction	±	50%	+	+	+	+	66%	100% True supporting	
Secondary responses									
Neck righting reactions									
Head	0	0	+	+	+	+	+	+	+
Body	0	0	0	+	+	+	+	+	+
Body derotative	0	0	0	0	+	+	+	+	+
Body rotative	0	0	0	0	0	0	0	+	+
Parachute reaction									
Downward	0	0	0	0	+	+	+	+	+
Sideways (propping)	0	0	0	0	0	0	+	+	+
Forward	0	0	0	0	0	0	0	+ (At 7 months)	−
Backward	0	0	0	0	0	0	0	+	−
Landau	0	0	0	0	0	0	42%	+ To 24 months	−

(From Baker D, Vanace P: Motor and Intellectual Development In Kaye R, Oski FA, et al. (eds.) Core Textbook of Pediatrics JP Lippincott Co., 1978, p 38)

The greatest number of children presenting with delay in motor development have no discernible neurologic abnormalities. These delays are due to the variation in the individual patterns of normal development. However, before any decision can be made by a clinician that the child is normal in his development, i.e., "He'll grow out of it," all etiologies of delay in motor development must be considered and ruled out.

DIFFERENTIAL DIAGNOSIS OF DELAYED MOTOR DEVELOPMENT

This differential diagnosis is based on an integration of history, physical examination, and laboratory findings. However, it is important to note that not all criteria listed are needed to make specific diagnoses. It is for this reason that a check list is provided to act as a guide in the differential diagnosis.

Mental Retardation

- Positive history of developmental delay
- Presence of risk factors
- Presence of morphologic stigmata
- Possible disturbances of growth patterns
- Qualitative differences in each area of development
- Delays in all areas of development
- No specific evidence of asymmetry of tone or reflexes on neurologic examination (difficulty will arise in the presence of combined deficits, which is often the case)
- Primitive reflexes will usually not be observed
- Delay in the acquisition of postural responses is noticed
- Motor development will be dependent on level of intellectual functioning
- Presence of associated sensory deficits

Cerebral Palsy

- Positive history of delay
- Presence of risk factors
- Delay in motor development and function
- Asymmetry of muscle tone, presence of hypertonia or hypotonia
- Hyperreflexia associated with spasticity
- Presence of pathologic reflex, i.e., clonus, persistence of Babinski reflexes
- Persistence of primitive reflexes
- Delay in acquisition of normal postural responses
- Presence of associated handicaps

Diseases of the Motor Neuron

- Reduced muscle power
- Decreased spontaneous movement
- Symmetric muscle weakness
- Muscle atrophy
- Reduced or absent deep tendon reflexes
- No sensory loss
- Normal intelligence
- Positive findings on EMG and nerve conduction series

Myasthenia Gravis

- Weak cry
- Difficulty in swallowing and sucking
- Generalized hypotonia
- Progressive weakness on repetitive or sustained muscle contraction
- Response to anticholinesterase drugs
- Positive findings on EMG
- Tendon reflexes are usually normal but may disappear after repeated elicitation

Muscle Disease

- Positive family history
- Delay in motor development
- Abnormalities of muscle tone and strength
- Muscle atrophy
- Muscle hypertrophy
- Abnormal posturing
- Toe walking
- Defective intellectual development
- Variability of deep tendon reflexes
- Elevation of serum enzyme
- Positive findings on EMG
- Positive finding on muscle biopsy

Familial Factors

- Positive family history
- Normal neurologic examination
- Normal development in language and adaptive areas

Environmental Factors

- No specific neurologic abnormality
- Positive history of severe deprivation
- Associated delays in other areas of development

MANAGEMENT

Once a diagnosis is made, the specific modes of management are as variable as the clinical entities presented. A common element in all management is the need for a multidisciplinary approach to provide all aspects of the diverse treatment required and ongoing re-evaluation. For example, children who have been diagnosed as having cerebral palsy may require active physical and occupational therapy, close follow-up by a number of physicians (pediatrician, neurologist, psychiatrist), as well as school placement by trained psychologists and educational specialists.

Early detection of mental retardation may uncover a preventable etiology, as congenital hypothyroidism or PKU, requiring active metabolic management. Other aspects of mental retardation management may require infant stimulation programs, special education, parent groups, and genetic counseling.

Myopathies and neurologic entities require close medical management, including seizure control, prevention of associated disabilities when possible, and counseling of parents regarding prognosis.

A single professional may be able to identify the existence of a problem and guide the family to the appropriate referral center for diagnosis and management. Specific management requires a multidisciplinary approach, with all professionals interacting on behalf of the patient. The pediatrician can and must maintain a focal point in decision making and parent counseling in order for this process to work and for management to be most effective.

SUMMARY

Normal gross and fine motor development are important elements of pediatric practice in the young child. Early detection of delay is crucial in order to achieve maximum results of treatment, intervention, and parent counseling. Thorough understanding of normal development, accurate history taking, and careful neurologic examination will provide the necessary data for diagnosis.

Relevant clinical entities were reviewed to provide a frame of reference for further diagnostic evaluation and referral when indicated.

BIBLIOGRAPHY

Accardo PJ, Caperte AJ: The Pediatrician and the Developmentally Delayed Child: A Clinical Textbook on Mental Retardation. Baltimore, University Park Press, 1979

Baker D, Vanace P: Motor and Intellectual Development. *In* A Core Textbook of Pediatrics. Kaye, Oski, Barnes (eds). New York, Lippincott, 1978 p 31

Holt KS: Developmental Pediatrics, Post Graduate Pediatric Series, Apley J (ed). Butterworth Pub, 1977

Illingworth RS: The Development of the Infant and Young Child, 7th ed., New York, Churchill Livingstone, 1980

Lowrey GH: Growth and Development of Children, 7th ed. Chicago, Yearbook Medical Pub, 1978

Menkes JH: Textbook of Child Neurology, Lea & Febiger, 1974 p 463

Molnar GE: Analysis of motor disorder in retarded infants and young children. Am J Ment Defic 83 (3): 213, 1978

Molnar GE, Gordon SV: Cerebral Palsy: Pedictive value of selected clinical signs for early prognostication of motor function. Arch Phys Md Rehabil 57:153, 1976

Nelson KB, Ellenberg JH: Neonatal signs as predictors of cerebral palsy. Pediatr 64(2):225, 1979

Taft LT, Barabas G: Infants with delayed motor performance. Pediatr Clin North Am 29:1, 1982

Cross-Reference to Pediatrics, 17th ed.

TWENTY-THREE

Nocturnal Enuresis

Steven P. Shelov

Wetting the bed at night has been a common problem in children over the centuries. Reports as early as the sixteenth century indicate that parents and physicians have struggled for years, with little success, to understand the causes and treatment of nocturnal enuresis in children. In his treatise on this subject in 1900, Bierhoff concludes, "In view of its widespread prevalence and distressing character, this condition, trivial though it may seem, deserves greater study than it has received in the past." Over the years, multiple attempts to answer the questions of why children are enuretic and what is the best way to manage them has led to some increased knowledge. However, the condition remains a common one of extreme annoyance, although, for the most part, of little physical consequence. A sensible approach to the problem of enuresis is a prerequisite for optimal care of children with this disorder.

DEFINITION

Enuresis is defined as involuntary passage of urine, which may be nocturnal or diurnal. An important distinction is made between primary and secondary enuresis, each of which may be due to either functional or organic causes. Primary enuresis connotes that the child has never had a prolonged period (greater than 4 weeks) when he or she has been dry. Secondary enuresis refers to a child who has been dry for a period of at least 3–6 months. Primary nocturnal enuresis, which is usually functional, is the most common form of nocturnal enuresis. It is defined here as a condition in which a child 4 years of age or older urinates in bed at night at least once per week. In this discussion, the term enuresis, unless otherwise specified, refers to primary, functional, nocturnal enuresis.

The reported prevalence has varied. In a large household survey of a metropolitan area, 13% of 6 and 7 year olds and 3% of 13 and 14 year olds were still wetting their beds more than once per month. Of 1,275 6–13 year olds brought in for routine medical examinations, 20% wet the bed at least once a week. In an additional collaborative study done through a questionnaire, 346 of 1,435 children 4 years or older were continuing to wet the bed at night at least once per week.

DIFFERENTIAL DIAGNOSIS

History

A number of important questions must be asked in assessing a child with enuresis.

- Has the child ever been dry? The detailed answer to this key question distinguishes the condition as either primary or secondary.

- Is there a history of bedwetting in the family? Enuresis is often familial.
- What is the urinary pattern during the day? Is there daytime incontinence or constant dribbling throughout the day? These symptoms suggest an organic abnormality of the bladder or an ectopic ureter.
- Is the daytime pattern one of a frequent need to void but not one of excessive volume? Several studies have suggested that many enuretic children have this type of urinary pattern because of a small functional bladder capacity.
- Is the child dry when he sleeps at another house? Children with primary enuresis often are dry when sleeping away from home.
- Is there any burning, pain, or discomfort when urine is passed? Secondary enuresis may be due to urinary tract infection.
- Is there a history of diabetes mellitus in the family? The polyuria of diabetes mellitus can present as secondary enuresis.
- Is there a history of sickle cell disease in the child or in the family? Children with sickle cell anemia have a concentrating defect with a high rate of urinary flow that may cause secondary enuresis.
- How is the family responding to this problem? In some families with enuresis, the child is viewed in an extremely negative role and blamed for disrupting the family equanimity. Other families deal with the problem in a much calmer, less punitive fashion. As a result, the child is not identified as a bad person and probably experiences less damage to his self-image.
- How is the child reacting or responding to his situation? Is he secretive and embarrassed and frightened to talk about it? Enuretic children often think they are particularly strange or unique.

Physical Examination

The focus of the physical examination is determined by an evaluation of the history. Nevertheless, even when functional enuresis is suggested by the history, and positive findings on physical examination are not expected, special attention should be paid to certain specific aspects. Rarely is anything significant found on physical examination. In a large study of enuretic children, the paucity of physical findings was apparent, even in the careful examination of the genitourinary and perineal area. Spina biffida occulta, vulvitis in girls, and circumcision in boys have been shown to have no causal association with enuresis. A thorough neurologic examination must be performed, including pinprick sensation around the perineal area. Any abnormal neurologic finding might suggest further evaluation and is discussed subsequently.

EVALUATION OF THE CHILD ON THE BASIS OF HISTORY AND PHYSICAL EXAMINATION

Primary Nocturnal Enuresis

Investigation of the child with primary nocturnal enuresis should include a urinalysis and urine culture. If negative, further laboratory work-up at this initial stage is not necessary, and the condition should be presumed to be functional. This approach has been confirmed by the most recent report of the Committee on Radiology of the American Academy of Pediatrics. It was the Committee's opinion "that a critical review of the available data supports the position that routine radiologic studies are not indicated for enuretic children with normal examinations and cultures."

The pathogenesis of primary nocturnal enuresis has been debated, but it appears that it is a functional condition that may be related to a combination of an immature arousal mechanism from stage 3–4 (non-REM) sleep and a small bladder capacity. Attempts to relate the condition to abnormal EEG patterns, excessively deep sleep, severe psychiatric disturbances, or other causes have not yielded convincing evidence. Psychologic disturbances in the child and difficulties experienced by the family appear to be more a result of the condition than a cause, and they often require as much attention as the symptom itself.

An extensive family and psychosocial history should be elicited and a determination made of the impact the symptom of enuresis is having upon the family. Is the child identified as a bad child? Does the enuresis appear to be an additional manifestation of a generalized acting-out, disruptive type of behavior? If the answer to those questions are "yes," probably a more intensive psychosocial investigation and perhaps some form of therapeutic intervention are indicated. If the situation is being handled well by the child and the family and they are aware of the functional, self-limited nature of the problem, a more nonintervening, supportive role on the part of the physician is wiser.

Primary nocturnal enuresis associated with daytime dribbling and incontinence suggests an organic etiology. In addition to a urinalysis and urine culture, the investigation should include a radiographic evaluation, including an IVP and VCU done in consultation with a urologist, as discussed below.

Secondary Enuresis

The child over the age of 4 years who has been dry for at least 6 months and then begins wetting the bed again should have a urinalysis, with particular attention to glycosuria and specific gravity, a urine culture, and a sickle cell preparation.

An extensive evaluation of the psychosocial environment is as important as the laboratory investigation in a child with secondary enuresis. The family structure, the role of the child in the family vis-à-vis parents, siblings, and friends, sleeping arrangements, and any recent trauma should all be explored. Has the child been hospitalized, or has some significant family member been sick, hospitalized, or left the home? Secondary enuresis is more often due to a psychosocial disturbance than to an organic condition. Often, uncovering of the situation or termination of a psychologically traumatizing event (such as hospitalization) is accompanied by disappearance of the symptom.

Less frequently, secondary enuresis is the presenting symptom in certain organic conditions. Urologic or radiologic investigation is indicated in patients with abnormal voiding patterns, dribbling, daytime incontinence, or symptoms suggestive of infection. Evaluation of concentrating capacity is indicated in children with polyuria. In these instances, the polyuria of nephronophthisis, diabetes insipidus, diabetes mellitus, and sickle cell disease must be considered.

Table 1 summarizes the approach to differentiating between primary and secondary enuresis.

MANAGEMENT BY PRIMARY CARE PEDIATRICIAN

Primary Functional Enuresis

The approach to therapeutic intervention should follow a specific sequence. If the child is between 3 and 4 years of age, the pediatrician should try to reduce the anxiety of the patient and the family about the symptom. The source of the pressure by the family should be identified and attempts made to reassure everyone that enuresis is most often a self-limited problem. It should be pointed out that fluid restriction, punishment, shame, or other vigorous measures might have appeared to the parents to be appropriate and necessary but that they have been quite uniformly unsuccessful and must be strongly discouraged.

Reassurance. If the family and child do not seem inordinately bothered by the bedwetting, further support and reassurance are appropriate. Knowledge that there is a 14% annual spontaneous cure rate can be reassuring.

TABLE 1. DIFFERENTIATION BETWEEN PRIMARY AND SECONDARY ENURESIS

Findings in History or Physical Examination	Primary Enuresis	Secondary Enuresis	Other Diagnostic Considerations
Child never dry since birth, no daytime wetting	+		Usually functional, psychosocial disturbances usually secondary, small bladder capacity
Voiding frequently but in small volumes	+		
Child is dry when sleeping away from home	+		
Child dry for 6 months, then began wetting		+	Severe primary psychosocial difficulties, urinary tract infection, diabetes mellitus, sickle cell anemia
Daytime incontinence with stress		+	GU anomaly—ectopic ureter
Child is a boy	+		
History of sickle cell disease		+	Sickle cell disease
Burning on urination, previously dry		+	Urinary tract infection
Abnormal neurologic examination		+	Possible intraspinal tumor, early neurogenic bladder

Bladder Stretching Exercises. If the patient and the family are eager to do something active and the child is 6–8 years old and still wetting the bed, bladder stretching exercises might be useful. Even though the value of this approach has not been uniformly established, it appears to be harmless. The mother is asked to measure the urine output of several voidings. A volume greater than 4 ounces indicates that the child does not have a small functional bladder capacity. If the amount voided is less than 4 ounces, it can be suggested that a small functional bladder capacity might be playing a role in causing enuresis and that bladder stretching exercises

might be useful. The procedure, as described by Starfield, for parents, is as follows:

1. Once every day have your child hold his urine as long as he can before going to the bathroom. This way he will learn to hold more and more water in his bladder. On school days, the best time for him to hold his urine is when he comes home after school.
2. Have the child drink a lot of water, milk or juice while he is holding his urine in his bladder. This will help stretch the bladder faster.
3. Use a cup or jar that has ounces marked on

it and ask the child to urinate into the cup so it can be measured. Remember, he should do this AFTER he has held his urine as long as he can.

4. Use a calendar to write down the number of ounces of urine the child voids after he held it as long as he could. Do this each day right after the urine is measured. Also, on the calendar you should put a check in the space for wet or dry, or give a gold star for being dry.
5. Sometimes it will be hard for your child to hold the urine in his bladder for a long time. Sometimes it will hurt. The hurting will be less and the time will go faster if you help the child to keep busy while he is holding his urine. To help him, try television or play games like Bingo, or draw or read to him.

Conditioning. If the bladder stretching exercises are not successful, a second intervention is to establish a conditioning response using the enuresis alarm (formerly called a bell and pad device). There has been extensive experience in England with this approach, and Turner has written a detailed review. He showed that in the experience of many clinicians using the apparatus, enuresis ceased in 65–100% of patients. A certain number relapse, but the overall cure rate for selected, cooperative populations is about 75%.

The rationale for the use of such conditioning devices is for the child to transfer the bladder-contracting reflex induced by his being awakened by the alarm to a similar arousal and bladder-contracting reflex when there is subliminal sensation of bladder fullness or contraction while asleep. Cures are attained slowly with the use of these alarms.

The course of treatment progress is a fairly predictable one. Initially, the child awakens after a complete void has occurred. Gradually, over the ensuing several weeks, the child awakens more quickly as less and less urine is passed. Eventually (and this may take 1–2 months), the child awakens in response to the sensation of the filled bladder rather than the alarm. It is usually necessary to wear the alarm for about 1 month after wetting has stopped.

In contrast to the older, more cumbersome bell and pad devices, there are currently two new enuresis alarms available. These new products provide certain advantages over the older devices.

1. They are lightweight and portable and depend only on a hearing aid battery for proper functioning.
2. They are relatively inexpensive. Each costs approximately $30.
3. They do not require massive bed and sheet preparation. No special conducting pad is required.
4. The electrode or sensors are attached to the child's underwear and the circuit is transistorized.
5. The buzzer wakes only the child. One new device, Wet-Stop* has a buzzer attached to the pajama collar, while the second new device, Nytone,† has a buzzer attached to the wrist.

Even though these newer conditioning devices have made this method of therapy relatively more convenient, success requires a somewhat older child (8 years at a minimum), significant motivation, and good cooperation between parents and child. In addition, as relapses do occur with this as well as other modes of therapy, encouragement to persist for an additional period of time is often necessary.

How are these alarms best used? Table 2 indicates a simple set of guidelines for proper use of these alarms. Close communication between physician and parent is important, es-

---

*Palco Laboratories, 5026 Scotts Valley Drive, Scotts Valley, CA 95068.

†Nytone Medical Products Inc., Salt Lake City, UT 94119.

**TABLE 2. DIRECTIONS FOR USE OF
ENURESIS ALARMS**

Be sure the child sets the alarm

The child should void completely before going
to sleep

Trigger the buzzer several times to make sure
the battery is working

Put a flashlight near the bed or leave a light
on

Before going to sleep, the child simply says to
himself that he will stop urinating when the
alarm goes off

Once awakened in the night, the child should
get up and go to the bathroom and finish
voiding

The child goes back to bed, having dried off
the electrodes and reset the alarm

pecially in the beginning when the child and family can easily become discouraged.

Medication. If the patient continues to be enuretic after trials of bladder stretching exercises and attempts to condition dryness have failed, a trial of medication may be tried. Imipramine (Tofranil) is the only drug used for enuresis that has been studied extensively. The mechanism of action appears to be a combination of local constriction at the bladder neck and a central effect to decrease deep sleep and improve arousal. Continence appears to be achieved in 75–80% of children. However, there are several disadvantages in the use of this approach.

1. There is an extremely high relapse rate (50% of those initially cured).
2. Once there is a relapse there is much discouragement on the part of the child and family. Compliance then becomes more difficult.
3. The medication has potent complications when taken in excessive dosages. Each year, several children die as a result of imipramine overdose. One troublesome case report described two children with noc-

turnal enuresis for whom imipramine had been prescribed. Both boys took an overdose of the medication, believing that more of the drug would cure their bedwetting. The patient and the family must understand thoroughly these very serious potential complications.

Treatment with imipramine is initiated with a dose of 25 mg hs. This is increased stepwise to the maximum dose as indicated in Table 3. Therapy should be maintained for 2 months after success has been achieved. If dryness continues, the dosage should be tapered over a 1-month period.

Other agents have been used. Pseudoephedrine (Sudafed) has been tried with only equivocal results. Oxybutynin (Ditrupan), a new antispasmodic agent, which reduces detrusor muscle contractions, has been used in several studies. Though it appears to have some initial benefit, further studies are indicated. Desmopressin (DDAVP), an analog of vasopressin has also been used. Once again, however, extensive results with large numbers of patients have not been published.

In using and evaluating any of these interventions, it is important to remember that each year 14% of enuretic children will spontaneously become dry. Thus, by age 12, only 3% of children who had been enuretic at 4 years are continuing to wet the bed. This fact must be considered carefully before subjecting patients to the inconvenience of active intervention. However, in many instances, the attitude of the patient and the family requires some form of intervention, and in these in-

**TABLE 3. MAXIMUM IMIPRAMINE DOSAGE
FOR BEDWETTING**

Age	Dose
4–6 years	25 mg hs
6–8 years	50 mg hs
> 8 years	75 mg hs

stances, it should be provided with the safeguards described.

Secondary Enuresis

Secondary enuresis is often associated either with severe psychosocial disturbances or with organic pathology. Therapy is based on the specific etiology (Table 4).

Active children between the ages of 4 and 8, particularly boys, occasionally wet their pants during the day, often during times of prolonged play when interruptions for urinating are delayed due to excitement, leading to a miscalculation and an occasional accident. This is common and need only be minimized. This form of daytime enuresis usually stops when increased social pressure makes these accidents unacceptable.

Some children will void with great frequency during the day but have neither diurnal nor nocturnal enuresis. This condition, pollakiuria, is probably a result of increased tension and nervousness but is thought to be of no consequence.

Some children, especially girls, have slight urinary incontinence when laughing or giggling, so-called giggle incontinence. No true weakness in the bladder outlet has been demonstrated in these children, and this condition should not be of concern. It seems to stop as the child enters early adolescence.

ROLE OF PRIMARY CARE PEDIATRICIAN IN DIFFERENTIAL DIAGNOSIS AND TREATMENT OF CONDITIONS REQUIRING CONSULTATION

When should a specialist be consulted? The majority of children with the diagnosis of primary, functional, nocturnal enuresis, with a normal physical examination and laboratory evaluation, can be managed by the primary pediatrician without consultation. Most children with secondary enuresis due to urinary tract infection can also be managed by the pediatric practitioner.

Daytime and Nighttime Enuresis with Dribbling

Constant dribbling suggests the possibility of an ectopic ureter or other anatomic abnormality. Referral should be made to the urologist.

Enuresis and Encopresis

Encopresis may indicate significant psychopathology in a child who has a completely normal neurologic examination. Referral in this case is both for diagnostic evaluation and probable therapeutic intervention.

TABLE 4. THERAPY OF SECONDARY ENURESIS

Etiology	Therapy
Severe psychosocial disturbance	Appropriate form of psychotherapy
Family disruption	Thorough uncovering of family or individual problem, short-term counseling
Urinary tract infection	Antibiotic therapy and urologic evaluation (*Pediatrics,* 17th ed.)
Glycosuria	Evaluation for diabetes mellitus (*Pediatrics,* 17th ed.)
Isosthenuria due to sickle cell disease	Reassurance, management of sickle cell disease

Enuresis as Consequence of Repeated Urinary Tract Infections

Children with recurrent infections may have ureteral reflux or other urologic abnormalities. Referral to a urologist should be made.

Secondary Enuresis due to Significant Family Disruption or Severe Behavioral Problems

A psychiatrist or psychotherapist with skills in family intervention should be consulted for diagnostic evaluation and possible therapeutic intervention. Some typical situations that provoke the development of enuresis include:

1. Divorce in the family, with strong attachment of the child to the departing parent.
2. Inability of the child to participate in normal peer-related activities (school, play, or sibling).
3. Behavior of the child that becomes the focus of the anger and hostility of one or both parents. Family relationship in turmoil.

Persistent Functional Enuresis in Child Older than 12 Years Old

The child who is 12 years old or older and who has had some or all the medical treatment described under primary functional, nocturnal enuresis, with little permanent success, should be referred to a consultant. In most cases, a referral to a psychiatrist or psychotherapist is the appropriate course. It is usually most effective to urge the family that they be seen as a unit, since there are often problems, secondary to the persistent enuresis, that need discussing, and the dynamics of the family interaction may be playing a large role in the persistence of the problem.

It should be stressed, however, that even at this point the primary care physician should be optimistic about the problem, which usually resolves spontaneously even when it persists into adolescence.

BIBLIOGRAPHY

Bakwin M: Enuresis in children. J Pediatr 58:806, 1961

Bierhoff F: On enuresis and the irritable bladder in children. Pediatrics 10:161, 1900

Cohen MW: Enuresis. Pediatr Clin North Am 22:545, 1975

Esperanca M, Gerrard JW: Nocturnal enuresis: studies in bladder function in normal children and enuretics. Can Med Assoc 101:324, 1969

Forsythe WI, Redmond A: Enuresis and spontaneous cure rate. Arch Dis Child 49:259, 1974

Hallgreen B: Enuresis II. A study with reference to physical, mental and social factors possibly associated with enuresis. Acta Psychiatr Neurolog. Scand 31:405, 1956

Hallman N: On the ability of enuretic children to hold urine. Acta Paediatr Scand 39:87, 1950

Hicks WR, Barnes EH: A double blind study of the effect of imipramine on enuresis in 100 normal recruits. Am J Psychiatry 120:812, 1969

Kolvin I, MacKeith RC, Meadow SR: Bladder control and enuresis. Clin Develop Med 48:195, 1973

Maxwell C, et al.: Imipramine in the treatment of childhood enuresis. Practitioner 207:809, 1971

McKendry JB, et al.: Enuresis: a study of untreated patients. Appl Therapy 10:815, 1968

Olness K: The use of self-hypnosis in the treatment of childhood nocturnal enuresis. Clin Pediatr 14:273, 1975

Poussaint AF, Ditman KS: A controlled study of imipramine (Tofranil) in the treatment of childhood enuresis. J Pediatr 67:283, 1965

Schmitt BD: Nocturnal enuresis: an update on treatment. Pediatr Clin North Am 29:21, 1982

Shelov SP, Edelmann CM: Nocturnal enuresis. Pediatric Basics 25:4–7, 1980

Shelov SP, et al.: Attitudes of Patients toward Enuresis, presented at the 18th Annual Scientific Meeting, April 1978, Ambulatory Pediatric Association. Abstract published.

————.:Enuresis: a contrast of attitudes of parents and physicians. Pediatrics 67:707, 1981

Starfield B: Enuresis: its pathogenesis and management. Clin Pediatr 11:343, 1972

Starfield B: Functional bladder capacity in enuretic and non-enuretic children. J Pediatr 70:777, 1967

Stemmerman E, et al.: Frequently seen symptomatic problems in a private pediatric practice. Personal communication.

Turner RK: Conditioning treatment of nocturnal enuresis: Present status. *In* Kolvin I, MacKeith RC, et al. (eds), Bladder control and enuresis. Clin Prov Med

Wagner W, et al.: A controlled comparison of two treatments for nocturnal enuresis. J Pediatr 10:302, 1982

Cross-Reference to *Pediatrics,* 17th ed.

TWENTY-FOUR

Failure to Thrive

Janna Collins and Andrew P. Mezey

Failure to thrive (FTT) is a problem that has been recognized since the beginning of recorded civilization. Its causes often are obscure, and unraveling the genetic and environmental factors involved may be difficult.

Complex issues may be associated with FTT. For example, an infant with intra-uterine nutritional deprivation who is small for gestational age often grows at a rate more than 2SD below the mean for age, while his head circumference may increase along the 25th percentile. His family treats him differently from his siblings. His appetite is modest, he has his share of acute upper respiratory and gastrointestinal illnesses, and he enters puberty later than his peers. Inevitably, the conscientious pediatrician will question how deeply to delve into this child's FTT at each developmental state.

This chapter concentrates mainly on the determination of whether or not FTT exists and deals less extensively with the factors that may be involved in its pathogenesis.

DEFINITION

The diagnosis of failure to thrive implies that an infant or child has suboptimal growth in weight or height or both. In order to establish the diagnosis of FTT, all available data concerning the child's height, weight, and head circumference must be plotted on an appropriate growth chart (Figs. 1, 2, 3, and 4), permitting an accurate determination of whether or not a deviation from normal exists. Growth velocity is also plotted, if sufficient information is available. The diagnosis of FTT is made when (1) a child is growing along a curve that is more than 2 SD below the mean for age and sex (i.e., below the 3rd percentile), (2) a child has had actual weight loss or is falling to lower percentiles for weight, (3) growth velocity is less than 5 cm per year for children 3 years of age to puberty, or (4) a child's height crosses down percentile curves.

Several cautionary statements must be made about these definitions. Growth charts are derived from samples of certain populations, such as middle class, white children from a particular geographic area. A growth chart for white or black American children does not accurately predict growth for other populations, such as minority ethnic groups (e.g., Oriental and Hispanic children). Of the normal children in a particular population, 2.5% percent by definition will be more than 2 SD above the mean for height or weight, and 2.5% will be more than 2 SD below the mean, without implying FTT.

Recognizing the limitations of these graphic standards for height and weight, and calculation of growth velocity, especially for children growing at or below the 3rd percentile or for children from population groups

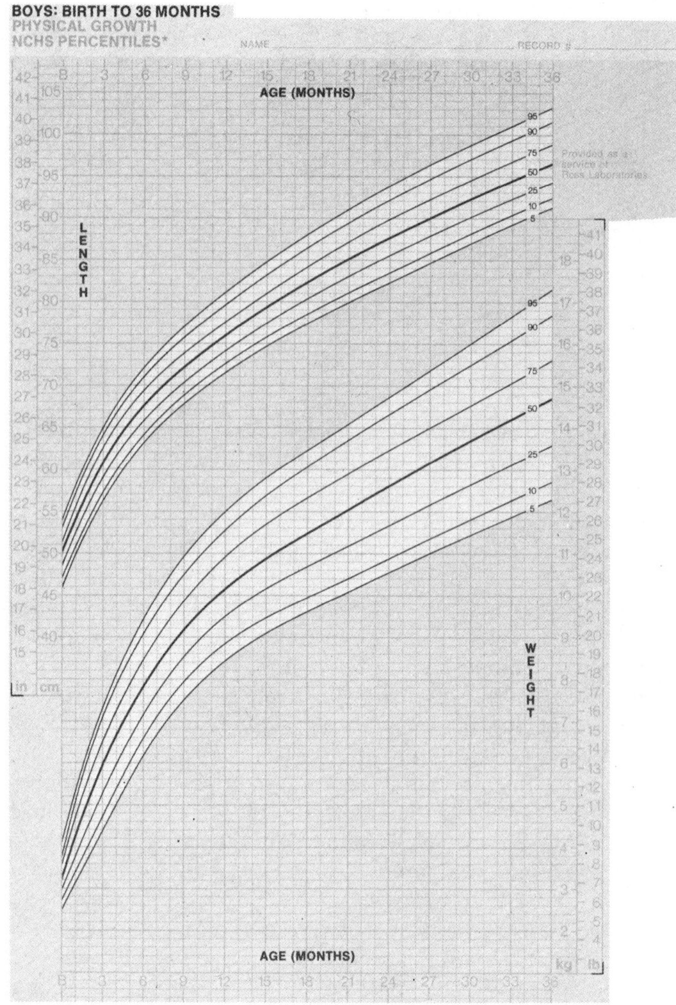

Figure 1. Physical growth in boys from birth to 36 months. (*Adapted from: National Center for Health Statistics: NCHS Growth Charts, 1976. Monthly Vital Statistics Report, Vol. 25. No. 3, Supp. (HRA) 76. Health Resources Administration, Rockville, Maryland, June, 1976. Data from The Fels Research Institute, Yellow Springs, Ohio.)*

for whom we lack normative growth data, provides a sensitive indicator of FTT. Linear growth velocity should be calculated over 3–12 month intervals and expressed as centimeters per year. Weight velocity curves can be computed in the same fashion.

Other data helpful in evaluating growth include parental stature and head circumference, and patterns of growth of siblings. Since growth of the brain is most resistant to both organic and nonorganic causes of FTT,

the head circumference often can be used as a predictor of optimal weight gain and linear growth.

ETIOLOGY

Chronic illness involving any organ or body system may be associated with FTT. In most instances, the underlying cause—such as congenital heart disease, renal insufficiency, or a

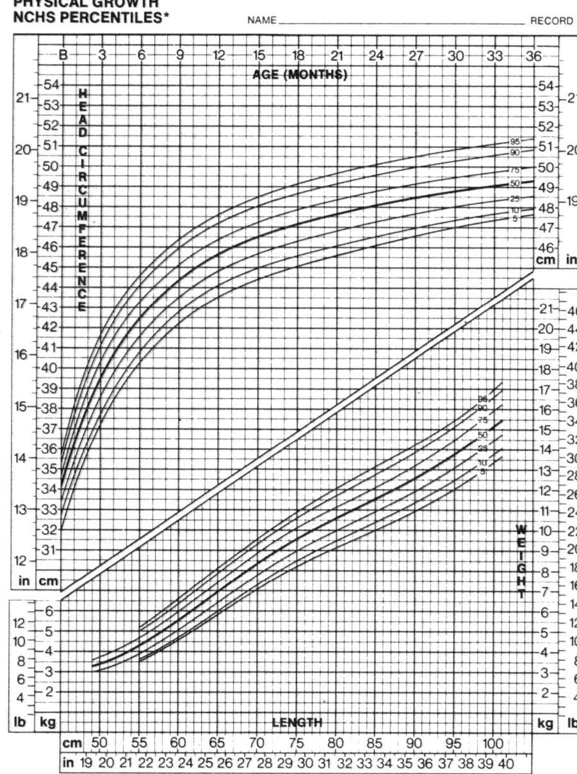

Figure 2. Physical growth in girls from birth to 36 months. *(Adapted from: National Center for Health Statistics. NCHS Growth Charts. 1976. Monthly Vital Statistics Report. Vol. 25, No. 3, Supp. (HRA) 76. Data from the National Center for Health Statistics.)*

metabolic disorder—is easily recognized. In such instances, the primary condition becomes of paramount concern, there is no problem of differential diagnosis, and the FTT is only of secondary importance. These disorders will not be considered further in this chapter.

FTT is found in many children with mental retardation. It may be impossible to determine whether the cause is related to the central nervous system abnormality per se or is due to nonspecific feeding difficulties.

There are other organic disorders that may present as FTT in an otherwise seemingly healthy child. These conditions must be considered carefully so as not to miss the correct diagnosis.

Finally, nonorganic causes of FTT, in-cluding parental neglect, parental ignorance, and other psychosocial disorders, must be considered as possible etiologies (Table 1).

Disorders of Growth
Nonorganic Failure to Thrive. The dynamics of the mother-infant relationship play a major role in the ability of the infant to thrive emotionally and nutritionally. The ability of the infant to ingest sufficient calories to grow normally can easily be disturbed by a variety of problems, including (1) poor interaction in and around the feeding time, which allows the parent to withdraw from the child or vice versa, (2) the inability of the parent to develop an attachment to the infant, resulting in infant withdrawal, (3) actual abuse or neglect of the infant, and (4) ignorance on the part of

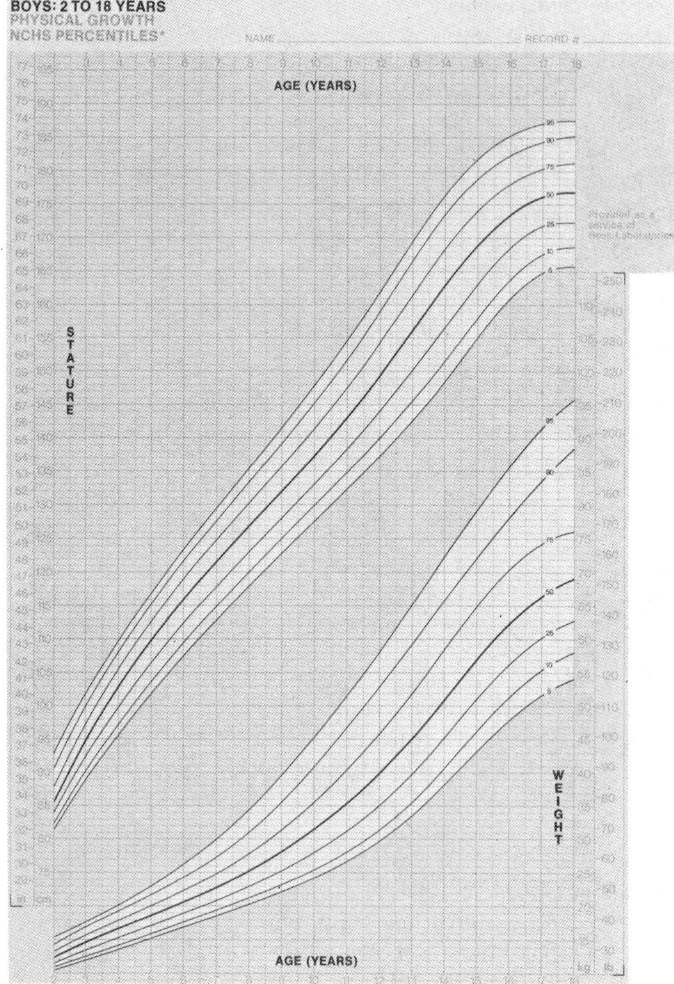

Figure 3. Physical growth in boys from 2 to 18 years. (*Adapted from: Hamill PVV, Drizd TA, et al.: Physical growth: National Center for Health Statistics percentiles. AM J CLIN NUTR 32:607, 1979. Data from the Fels Research Institute, Wright State University School of Medicine, Yellow Springs, Ohio.*)

the parents as to the correct manner in which to feed the infant and the appropriate types and quantities of food to be given.

Sills reviewed a series of 185 children admitted to Buffalo Children's Hospital with FTT. In 85%, nonorganic factors were thought to be causative. Moreover, in the small minority found to have an organic etiology, all were previously suspected on the basis of the history and physical examination to have an organic cause for FTT. Only 1.4%

of the laboratory examinations performed were positive. Similar findings have been reported by others.

Infants with nonorganic FTT appear to have characteristic interactive behavioral patterns. Rosenn et al. examined three small groups of children 6–16 months of age. One group had the diagnosis of nonorganic FTT, one group consisted of children with organic FTT, and the third group was comprised of hospitalized controls. Using a behavioral

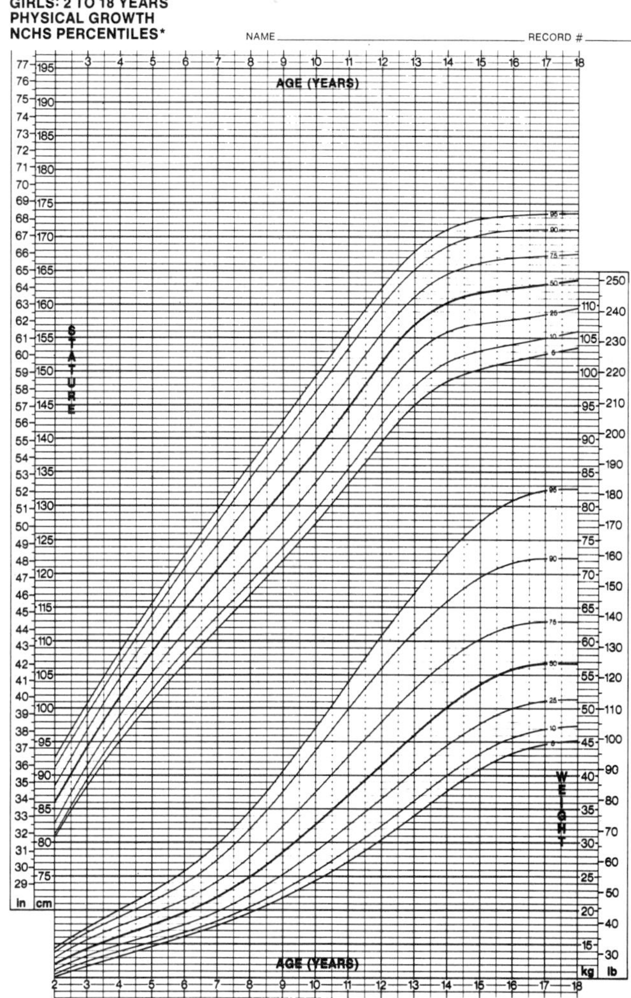

Figure 4. Physical growth in girls from 2 to 18 years. *(Adapted from: National Center for Health Statistics: NCHS Growth Charts, 1976. Monthly Vital Statistics Report. Vol. 25, No. 3. Supp. (HRA) 76. Health Resources Administration, Rockville, Maryland, June, 1976. Data from the National Center for Health Statistics.)*

scale that assessed the infants' response to close and distant objects, they found that children with nonorganic FTT favored distant objects. The closer such objects got, the more uncomfortable the children became. Infants with organic FTT and the hospitalized controls, on the other hand, were more comfortable with closer objects. When the infants with nonorganic FTT were stimulated and given close attention, some demonstrated a shift in response, with a preference for close objects. Within 48–72 hours of this change in behavior, weight gain was noted.

Organic Failure to Thrive.

Genetic Short Stature and Constitutional Delayed Growth. So-called genetic short stature and constitutional delayed growth (Chapter 27) are difficult diagnoses conceptually, because they imply that there is no true FTT but simply a pattern of growth that is different from what is defined as normal. For

TABLE 1. COMMON CAUSES OF FAILURE TO THRIVE IN INFANTS, CHILDREN, AND ADOLESCENTS

Cause	Infant	Child	Adolescent
Nonorganic	Feeding problem, neglect, abuse	Psychosocial dwarfism, neglect, abuse	Depression, bulimia, anorexia nervosa
Organic			
Gastrointestinal*	Disorders of suck, swallow, and esophagogastric motility Chronic diarrhea and malabsorption syndromes, Hirschsprung's disease	Malabsorption syndromes, parasitism	Peptic ulcer disease, inflammatory bowel disease
Metabolic/genetic	Cystic fibrosis, juvenile diabetes mellitus, storage disorders (carbohydrate, fat, lipid, and mucopolysaccharide)	Diabetes mellitus	
Endocrine	Hypothyroidism, adrenal insufficiency	Hypo- and hyperthyroidism Growth hormone deficiency, panhypopituitarism, diabetes insipidus	
Allergic/immunologic	Chronic and recurrent infection		
Genitourinary	Chronic and recurrent infection, chronic renal failure, renal tubular acidosis, rickets—vitamin D dependent or resistant		
Miscellaneous	Malignancy Congenital heart disease	Malignancy	Malignancy
		Disorders of bone growth, gonadal dysgenesis, genetic short stature, constitutional delayed growth	

*Primary neurologic and cardiac disorders with FTT usually fit into this category and are associated with inadequate intake of nutrients.

these children, caloric intake, although tending to be low (even relative to the size of the child), is adequate for their metabolic needs. They have no abnormal losses by emesis or in the stool or urine. Their growth curves parallel those of normal children.

Genetically short children have a bone age that corresponds to their chronologic age, and they can be expected to be short adults. Constitutional growth delay is accompanied by a correspondingly delayed bone age, the pubertal growth spurt occurs at a later chronologic age than in other adolescents, and adult height is normal. There is a need to make these two diagnoses and to exclude *disorders of bone growth* and *gonadal dysgenesis,* so that the child and family can receive accurate information about expectations for future growth and can be supported in dealing with secondary psychologic problems related to short stature.

Disorders of Suck, Swallow, and Esophagogastric Motility

These disorders usually are apparent in early infancy and include such conditions as cleft palate, disorders of muscle tone (either primary neurologic or muscular), and gastroesophageal reflux. Infants with disordered suck or swallow are more likely to have an underlying neurologic disorder than are those with gastroesophageal reflux. However, both groups are at risk for additional nonorganic components to their FTT if the feeding problem disrupts the mother-infant relationship.

Malabsorption Syndromes

These disorders may be either acute or chronic and may be genetic or acquired. The onset and severity of symptoms dictate the way the FTT is analyzed. However, regardless of etiology, adequate growth requires that nutrient intake compensate for abnormal stool losses. These patients present when nutrient intake is insufficient, whether on the basis of decreased intake because of de-

creased appetite, self-restriction (discomfort), or when the caregiver can no longer provide adequate calories to keep up with excessive loss.

Inflammatory Bowel Disease

At the time of diagnosis, inflammatory bowel disease is associated with short stature, varying degrees of protein-calorie malnutrition, or failure of sexual maturation in 15–30% of cases. Growth failure is the chief complaint in many of these patients, with minimal evidence or no history of gastrointestinal symptoms. A history of frequent abdominal pain, abnormal bowel pattern (either constipation or diarrhea), and occult or visible rectal bleeding suggests inflammatory bowel disease as the etiology of FTT. In some cases, the differential diagnosis between Crohn's granulomatous enterocolitis and anorexia nervosa cannot be made with certainty.

Miscellaneous Disorders

Cystic fibrosis of the pancreas, a genetic disorder, and *peptic ulcer disease,* an acquired disorder, are usually associated with normal linear growth. However, a mild degree of protein-calorie malnutrition can be detected by the subnormal weight-to-height ratio in some patients with peptic ulcer, who have anorexia secondary to pain, and in many patients with cystic fibrosis, who have pancreatic insufficiency causing malabsorption. Ordinarily the complaint of FTT is accompanied by other significant complaints of abdominal pain, abnormal stool production, or, in the patient with cystic fibrosis, pulmonary disease.

Acquired *hypothyroidism, juvenile diabetes mellitus,* and *storage disorders* may present as subnormal linear growth with relative preservation of weight gain. More recently *immunodeficiency syndromes* have been recognized as occasionally presenting as FTT, especially with chronic diarrhea as a major symptom. Both weight and height can be affected, with subnormal weight being the most obvious.

DIFFERENTIAL DIAGNOSIS

History

In addition to obtaining information that might support certain diagnoses, the pediatric practitioner has three specific goals in taking a careful history:

1. Establishing whether or not significant FTT exists
2. Evaluating intake and output and, by inference, utilization of nutrients
3. Gaining insight into the psychodynamic and socioeconomic influences on the child

Answers to the following questions are the most informative:

- How long has poor growth been a problem? FTT results from prolonged (chronic) pathology. The growth chart should be filled out at this time and examined in detail to relate weight loss or failure to gain weight or height to specific events in the history.
- When did the child last outgrow his shoes or change to the next size in clothes? These questions, in addition to growth data, can help establish the presence of FTT.
- What are growth patterns in the family? What are the heights and body types of parents and siblings? By age 2–3, children's genetic growth pattern (in the absence of pathology) can be discerned. The short child who, in addition to a family history of short stature, has another complaint, such as asthma or recurrent abdominal pain, presents a difficult problem of dissociating genetic factors from organic disorders that might be associated with inadequate nutritional intake or abnormal losses through vomiting or malabsorption. The family is often more able than the doctor to separate the short stature per se from an extraneous complaint. If other diagnoses are made, the pediatrician should critically assess the child's pattern of growth to determine if it is altered by treatment. This is best done by comparing growth velocity just prior to and in the several months following introduction of the specific treatment.
- What is the usual intake; what did the child eat in the last 24 hours? Adequate caloric intake ranges from 70–120 kcal/kg/d in infants. Protein intake is approximately 2 g/kg/d. Intake derived primarily from formula is simple to calculate:

$$\frac{(\text{ounces/feed}) \times (\text{number of feeds per day})}{\text{kg body weight}}$$

$$\frac{\times (20\ \text{kcal/ounces})}{} = \text{kcal/kg/day}$$

The dietary history for older patients can be scanned for adequacy and compared to other children of similar size and age. Are there one or two sources of protein each day in addition to milk? Are there yellow and green vegetables, some fruit, and some fat? If children are allowed to choose their own diet, the remainder of their diet consists largely of a mixture of simple and complex carbohydrates to meet energy requirements. Calculations using diet manuals are not usually necessary and are often inaccurate, but one can get some idea of adequacy by having patients keep a dietary record with approximations of portion sizes and frequency of feeding.
- Does the child have difficulty with drinking or eating? Disorders of suck or swallow, choking, regurgitation, or prolonged feeding time can be clues to central nervous system disorders and congenital anomalies of the head, neck, and thorax.
- Does the patient vomit? If so, when and how often? Primary gastroesophageal reflux may cause an overflow type of regurgitation beginning during a feed, whereas pyloric stenosis is associated with later projectile emesis of curdled milk. Increased intracranial pressure is associated typically with early morning, even preprandial, emesis. An estimate of caloric loss with vomiting, whether large or small, should be made in relation to caloric intake.

- Does the child sweat excessively, have a pounding heartbeat, rapid breathing, or frequent fever? What is his activity level? These questions may provide evidence for hypermetabolic states that require higher than usual caloric intake (e.g., hyperthyroidism, congenital heart disease, chronic infection, pheochromocytoma). Other disorders may reduce the efficiency of utilization of nutrients (e.g., glycogen storage disease, diabetes mellitus) and thus increase caloric requirements until treatment is instituted. Very active children and children medicated for hyperkinesis may have excessive muscular activity, tachycardia, and diminished sleep requirement, all of which increase energy expenditure. They may be too busy to eat food carefully and tend to miss meals entirely or in part. A secondary parental response to avoid the conflict and give food only upon request adds inadequate intake to the problem of excessive utilization.
- Does the child have dysuria, polyuria, cloudy urine, wetting, or a bad perineal odor? Congenital and acquired disorders of the urinary tract resulting in eventual loss of renal parenchyma and uremia are associated with inadequate nutrient intake (anorexia) and hypermetabolic states (e.g., fever and stress with chronic and recurrent infections). Diabetes insipidus or diabetes mellitus are important considerations with the constellation of polyuria, polydipsia, and FTT.
- What are the frequency, consistency, and odor of the stools? Has rectal bleeding been noted? Malabsorption syndromes often are not associated with loose stools but rather with more than the usual number of stools, which are foul smelling, tenacious, and sticky. Infrequent stools supervene when intake secondarily becomes inadequate. For example, a patient with undiagnosed celiac disease becomes anorectic to avoid painful cramping related to gluten ingestion. Hirschsprung's disease in children

may be detected by a history of FTT with infrequent and unpredictably irregular stools, usually without painful defecation. (See Chapter 21: Constipation.)
- How does the parent respond to the patient's symptoms? Does the mother avoid holding her vomiting baby? Is the vomiting child given oversolicitous attention? Does the infant's diarrhea or constipation disrupt the entire family? Is the older child required to have a parent inspect his emesis, urine, or stool? Is the child or adolescent participating normally in school, athletic, and social activities?
- The psychodynamic factors need to be separated out. An assessment should be made as to the strength of parent-child bonds and the adequacy and appropriateness of family support systems. It is also important to distinguish the disruption in a family that results from a chronic medical problem from a primary disturbance in the family that has taken the form of excessive preoccupation with a symptom (e.g., vomiting), which was not terribly important in the first place.
- Who is the child's caretaker? Is there adequate food in the home, and is it prepared on a regular schedule? The issues of maternal-infant bonding and parental-child relationships must be explored in depth and on more than one occasion. Nonorganic causes of FTT range from overt child abuse to inadvertent neglect due to lack of knowledge. For example, a mother who nurses her infant exclusively for 10–12 months may fail to provide solid foods or supplemental vitamins and iron. Since successful bonding is believed to require that the infant respond appropriately to the parent, secondary disturbances leading to nonorganic FTT often supervene in children who have a primary disorder (e.g., congenital anomalies, mental retardation, recurrent vomiting) and are unable to provide a reciprocal response. An iatrogenic contribution to FTT is exemplified by the child

with chronic diarrhea who is routinely placed on glucose-electrolyte solution, then half-strength formula, then rice, chicken, and banana. Since his diarrhea has frequent exacerbations, his caloric intake may be excessively and inappropriately restricted by the physician or parents or both. The FTT becomes a result of inadequate intake, only distantly related to the original problem.

Finally, as families eat more of their meals in restaurants and from take-out establishments, it is increasingly common to encounter homes in which there are insufficient supplies of nutritious food—only snack-type foods that are more expensive than nourishing. At all socioeconomic levels, the potential exists for food deprivation in the home because an adult is not present most of the time or because neither parent is committed to providing three good meals a day in addition to snacks.

Additional questions should be directed to adolescents and their families:

- At what age did pubertal development begin; how advanced is sexual development? Is or was the patient sexually active? For girls, the menstrual history of other family members may be relevant to her own pattern. Delayed puberty is associated with many chronic diseases, particularly inflammatory bowel disease (most commonly Crohn's granulomatous enterocolitis). It is also a sign of gonadal dysgenesis (Turner's and Noonan's syndromes) and other endocrine disorders. Secondary amenorrhea can be the result of rapid and severe weight loss, such as occurs with inflammatory bowel disease, bulimia, anorexia nervosa, or even extreme physical training.
- What are the parent's academic and social aspirations and achievements? Is there disparity between goals and reality? Do the parents and patient have common goals, or are there significant areas of conflict? The adolescent should be permitted to give his

history in the absence of family and be encouraged to take an active part in analyzing his problem.

Physical Examination

The physical examination provides an opportunity to assess nutritional status, to detect signs consistent with growth failure, and often to determine what systems bear the responsibility for FTT. Although the physical examination may permit the diagnosis of a specific organic disorder, such as congenital heart disease, most children appear entirely normal or exhibit only nonspecific and questionably significant abnormalities.

The physical examination also allows the pediatrician to observe the parents' and patient's behavior toward one another, the amount of reassurance given the child, and its effect. Much has been written about the behavioral characteristics of children with FTT due to emotional deprivation: they lie with elbows flexed and hands close to the head, legs flexed and abducted, with whimpering, watchful, frightened appearance, making no attempt to resist the examination. This apathetic, protective posture is seen commonly in patients who have been chronically ill from infancy, whether at home or in an institution, and is not specific for nonorganic FTT. Ordinarily, when it is present, the FTT is obvious, and the objective of the physical examination is to include or exclude specific systems and organic disorders (Table 2).

Laboratory Examination

Laboratory tests may be indicated to determine the etiologic basis of FTT. However, the majority of patients who present with FTT have a history suspicious for nonorganic causes and no specific abnormalities will be noted on physical examination. For these patients, environmental intervention should begin immediately, and laboratory tests should be deferred. If an underlying systemic illness is suspected, laboratory investigation is indicated immediately, as shown in Figure 5.

TABLE 2. PHYSICAL EXAMINATION OF CHILD WITH FTT

	Possibly Significant	Significant	Considerations
Vital signs			
Blood pressure	Decreased		Life-threatening hypothyroidism, adrenal insufficiency, or malnutrition in crisis
Blood pressure	Increased		Essential hypertension, renal disease
Heart rate, respiratory rate, temperature	All low		Increased metabolic requirements
Height/length	Note abnormal body proportions		Endocrine disorders and genetic diseases
Weight	Less than 3rd percentile	Significantly less than 3rd percentile	20–30% loss may be fatal
Head circumference	Less than 3rd percentile		Microcephaly and congenital disorders *or* normal
Skin	Pallor		Anemia, allergy
		Edema	Hypoalbuminemia, renal and cardiac disease
	Chronic mucocutaneous infection		Immunodeficiency
	Eczema, seborrhea		Allergy, histiocytosis
	Erythema nodosum		Vasculitis, ulcerative colitis
		Jaundice, angiomas, xanthomas	Liver disease
Head		Hair loss or abnormal texture	Protein-calorie malnutrition, stress, hypothyroidism
Fontanelle		Craniotabes	Osteomalacia, rickets
ENT	Otitis media, serous or purulent nasal congestion, tonsillar/lymphoid inflammation		If chronic or recurring, may be allergic/immunologic problems often with inadequate nutrient intake
Eyes		Cataracts	Galactosemia and other genetic diseases, intrauterine acquired viral disease
		Papilledema	Increased intracranial pressure
	Redness (uveitis, conjunctivitis)		Hypoparathyroidism, systemic inflammatory diseases

(*continued*)

TABLE 2 (*Continued*)

	Possibly Significant	Significant	Considerations
Head			
Mouth	Cheilitis, stomatitis, aphthous ulcers, thrush		Acutely cause anorexia; when recurrent associated with systemic disorders
Teeth		Delayed eruption	Corresponds to bone age delay
		Multiple caries	Abnormal structure (protein matrix or calcification), neglect by caretaker
	Mottled discoloration		Systemic stress in pre-eruptive period (usually early infancy)
Neck		Thyroid enlargement or nodule	Thyroid disease
Chest		Wheezing, rales, kyphosis	Obstructive lung disease, e.g., bronchial asthma, cystic fibrosis
Cardiovascular	Flow murmur	Stenotic murmur, acrocyanosis, clubbing, delayed femoral pulses	Anemia, A-V shunts, congenital heart disease
Abdomen	Bowel sounds, rushes	Distended visible peristalsis	Malabsorption syndromes, Hirschsprung's disease
	Tenderness	Rebound, direct or referred	Pyelophlebitis, abscess
		Organomegaly	Infection, tumor, storage disorders
		Other masses, including fecaloma	Benign and malignant tumors, inflammatory bowel disease, Hirschsprung's disease
Genitourinary tract		Visible anomalies	Associated endocrine or urologic disorders
		Poor hygiene	Neglect
	Rashes		Immune and diarrheal disorders
Rectum		Fistula, tenderness, bleeding	Infection, inflammatory disorders
		Empty ampulla	Hirschsprung's disease

(*continued*)

TABLE 2 (*Continued*)

	Possibly Significant	Significant	Considerations
Back	Scoliosis	Wasting of buttocks	FTT of many etiologies
Extremities	Diminished muscle mass, tone, or strength		Malnutrition, various CNS and neuromuscular disorders
		Clubbing, pruritic changes	Chronic pulmonary or liver disease
		Wrist swelling and tenderness	Rickets
Neurologic reactions	Abnormal DTRs		Primary CNS disorders
	Delayed motor milstones		May be primary or secondary to nutritional inadequacy
		Cranial nerve palsy, poor suck, swallow	These abnormalities restrict intake
General behavior	Inappropriately submissive or uncooperative		Emotional factors as primary in FTT; management as a first priority

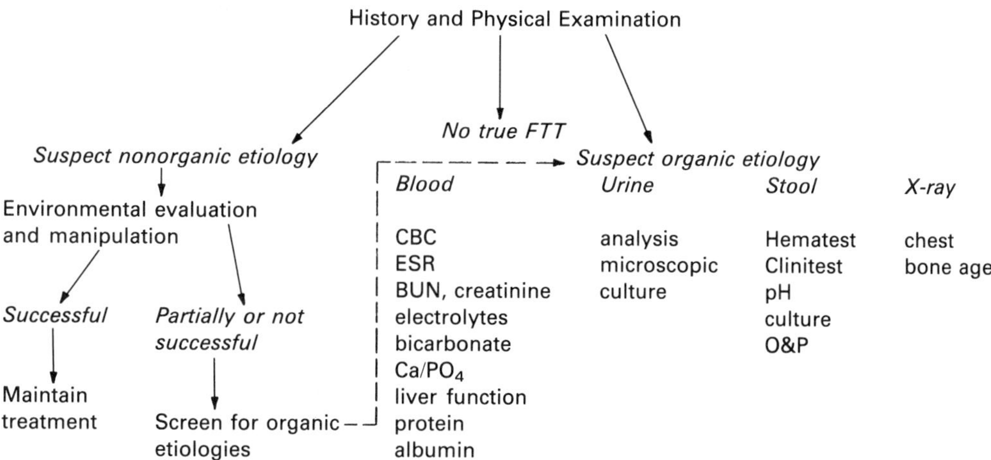

Figure 5. Laboratory tests to determine the etiologic basis of FTT. Abnormal results from these tests will direct the pediatrician to more specific studies, such as a sweat test and immunoglobulin determination if the chest x-ray shows bronchiectasis, barium enema and proctosigmoidoscopy for rectal bleeding, and so on.

MANAGEMENT

General Approach

The apparently healthy child, on the basis of information learned from the history, plotting of the growth chart, and the physical examination, can be tracked in two directions: (1) toward a diagnosis of nonorganic failure to thrive, or (2) toward laboratory evaluation of specific etiologic diagnoses. The first group includes the majority of patients, and the pediatrician or general practitioner, often in conjunction with a mental health professional, may have the responsibility of caring for an entire disrupted family. These children often are referred to a variety of specialists: the endocrinologist, gastroenterologist, allergest, nephrologist. Referrals can be selective if the practitioner performs his own screening tests for FTT. The specialist will be most valuable in confirming or revising the pediatrician's provisional diagnosis and in developing an individualized treatment plan based on his greater experience with the disorder.

In the second group, the pediatrician's challenge is to decide whether the primary diagnosis itself provides an adequate explanation for growth retardation or if there are aspects of intake, utilization, and abnormal losses than can be treated. For example, a child with chronic lung pathology (cystic fibrosis, right middle lobe syndrome, or bronchopulmonary dysplasia) need not have growth failure if the malabsorption syndrome is appropriately managed, pulmonary toilet is vigorous, and intake of nutrients is adequate for utilization. Acute exacerbations will usually be accompanied by anorexia, which leads to failure to meet increased nutritional requirements during stress. Failure to thrive follows only if exacerbations are more common than periods of good symptomatic control and alternative nutritional regimens or methods of delivery of nutrients are not found.

Nonorganic Causes of FTT

Infants and Children. Immediate management is directed to the patient with kwashiorkor, marasmus, or cachexia in malnutrition crisis. The cachectic infant, with subnormal body temperature, bradycardia, hypotension, lethargy, and little subcutaneous tissue, requires immediate hospitalization for resuscitation, management of possible infection in the face of inadequate host defenses, and nutritional repletion. The marasmic infant may appear hyperactive and excessively alert; the infant with kwashiorkor who has edema, scaly skin rash, and hepatomegaly, may be alternately irritable and lethargic. These children also require hospitalization for evaluation for infection and treatment. Unlike the cachectic patient, those with marasmus and kwashiorkor may receive nutritional therapies by the enteral route, using special formulas and often special techniques of delivery to counteract poor suck or delayed gastric emptying.

For the neglected infant, hospitalization is usually advisable on an elective rather than an emergent basis, bringing the parents into the medical setting where they can participate in the care of their child to the extent that they are able. During hospitalization, a developmental assessment should be made, and an interdisciplinary team should participate in evaluation and management, planning the supportive services that will continue following discharge. Usually these services include provision of a psychiatric social worker or psychiatrist for the parent who is not functioning normally, obtaining social service benefits (such as Medicaid, WIC program for infant formula), and referral to pediatric subspecialists in neurology and child development to evaluate the intellectual and behavioral deficits that are common concomitants of FTT.

The abused infant or child should be hospitalized immediately for his protection. In addition to signs of neglect, such as poor hygiene and dirty clothing in poor repair, he may have bruises and burns in suspicious locations, swelling and bone pain, and aberrant behavior. The Bureau of Child Welfare should be notified.

During hospitalization it is advisable to compare the patient's behavior in the absence and presence of his family, his eating habits, and his ability to gain weight in the new environment. Psychosocial assessment of the family is designed to identify primary psychopathology (schizophrenia, manic-depressive personality) and neuroses, to evaluate sources of conflict (e.g., marital instability, alcohol and drug abuse), and to ascertain economic and educational needs (e.g., to plan and to prepare meals). The child and family need access to ongoing therapy, as well as counseling and support from the pediatrician, mental health, and social service personnel and parent support groups, which furnish a hotline for acute crisis intervention.

Adolescents. Both bulimia and anorexia nervosa should be distinguished from other causes of anorexia, vomiting, and weight loss (such as peptic ulcer disease and Crohn's disease) by screening tests and barium swallow with small bowel x-rays. Bulimia is ordinarily treated on an outpatient basis by a psychiatrist or psychologist who deals with the underlying personality traits that led to the symptom. Behavioral modification to reduce frequency of vomiting requires close supervision. Medical complications requiring hospitalization are rare but include Mallory-Weiss tears of the distal esophagus or actual perforation of esophagus or stomach during forced emesis. Hypokalemia may be a metabolic complication of prolonged emesis.

Anorexia nervosa is also an emotional disorder but of life-threatening severity, and hospitalization is indicated when chronic starvation leads to the equivalent of marasmus and cachexia in the infant. Both parenteral nutrition and special techniques of enteral feeding with elemental diets may be necessary for survival. Long-term psychiatric care by someone with special expertise in anorexia nervosa should be sought as soon as the diagnosis is made.

These entities are described more extensively in Chapter 25.

Organic Causes of FTT
Gastrointestinal etiology. Disorders of deglutition and esophagogastric motility often are not evaluated extensively as long as strategies for feeding can be devised that improve caloric intake, minimize vomiting, and avoid complications of obstructive apnea and aspiration pneumonia. Since these disorders are symptomatic from the neonatal period, obstructing lesions, such as pyloric stenosis and intestinal malrotation and the H-type tracheoesophageal fistula, are considerations. The most valuable studies include cranial nerve evaluations, examination of the palate and larynx (indirect laryngoscopy), and a barium swallow with fluoroscopic control to evaluate pharyngeal, esophageal, and then lower esophageal sphincter function. Additional studies, such as direct laryngoscopy, esophagoscopy, esophageal pH and motility studies, and ^{99m}technetium scintiscan to study gastric emptying, may be recommended by otolaryngology or gastroenterology consultants. Treatment of disordered reglutition requires special feeding techniques, best discussed with the physical therapist. Poor esophageal motility and reduced lower esophageal sphincter tone may respond to Urecholine, while gastric motility can be improved with metaclopramide. These disorders also respond to special feeding techniques and positioning of the patient.

Chronic diarrhea, if caloric intake is normal, should not cause failure to thrive because there is usually no malabsorption of nutrients, simply a failure of colonic reabsorption of water and sodium, with perhaps some excessive loss of mucus from goblet

TABLE 3. MANAGEMENT PLAN FOR DISORDERS ASSOCIATED WITH FTT

Diagnostic Category	Acute Concerns	Medication	Additional Procedures	Consultant
Nonorganic FTT				
Infant and child	Observation	—	Denver Developmental Examination	
Feeding problem	Isolate maternal from patient etiology		Estimate daily intake, weigh frequently, consider special feeding techniques	
Neglect	Elective hospital admission	—	Family interview and observation	Multidisciplinary support team, including nurse, social worker, child development, and neurology services
Abuse	Emergency hospital admission, prevent further physical injury, evaluate for sexual abuse, assess neurodevelopmental status	—	Skull, long bone, rib x-rays, throat, genital cultures for gonorrhea	As above, plus Bureau of Child Welfare
Adolescent				
Depression	Distinguish endogenous from exogenous depression			
Bulimia	Assess nutritional status, exclude peptic ulcer and medication abuse		Barium swallow, monitor weight and frequency of emesis, behavioral modification therapy OR	Psychologist, psychiatrist
Anorexia nervosa	Hospitalize to treat cachexia (below), marasmus		Consider possibility of Crohn's or other organic etiology	Psychiatrist
Malnutrition of any etiology	Emergency hospital admission			
Kwashiorkor	Infection, provide protein and calories (enteral route), repair specific vitamin, mineral, and fatty acid deficiencies	Appropriate antibiotics	Urine, blood, and stool cultures, tuberculin test	Nutritional support team

(*continued*)

TABLE 3 (*Continued*)

Diagnostic Category	Acute Concerns	Medication	Additional Procedures	Consultant
Marasmus	Same	Same	Often requires supplemental parenteral nutrition, elemental formula, and nasogastric tube feedings	Same
Cachexia	Protective isolation, monitor vital signs, consider possibly adrenal insufficiency	Same	Total parenteral nutrition	Same
Organic FTT Gastrointestinal Sucking and swallowing disorders	Obstructive apnea, aspiration pneumonia		Cranial nerve testing, x-rays of airway and barium swallow, laryngoscopy, skull x-rays, brain CT scan	Neurologist, otorhinolaryngologist, gastroenterologist, child development team
Esophagogastric motility disorder	Same, exclude inflammatory obstructing lesions	Sedation, antispasmodic, Urecholine, metaclopramide	Barium swallow endoscopy, esophageal pH monitor and manometry	Gastroenterologist
Malabsorption syndromes	Distinguish from chronic diarrhea without malabsorption		Sweat test, sugar tolerance tests or breath hydrogen analysis, vitamins A, D, E, carotene, serum concentration of prothrombin time, duodenal aspiration jejunal biopsy, Schilling test	Gastroenterologist
Inflammatory bowel disease (ulcerative and granulomatous)	Cachexia, abscess, toxic megacolon, exclude infectious etiologies	Sulfasalazine, prednisone	Proctosigmoidoscopy, biopsies, barium enema, small bowel x-rays, exclude amebiasis, *Clostridium difficile, Yersinia, Campylobacter* infections	Gastroenterologist

(*continued*)

TABLE 3 (Continued)

Diagnostic Category	Acute Concerns	Medication	Additional Procedures	Consultant
Metabolic/genetic Cystic fibrosis	Cachexia, pulmonary failure	Pancreatic enzymes, broad-spectrum antibiotics (esp. vs *Staphylococcus* and *Pseudomonas*)	Sweat test (duodenal aspirate for trypsin activity)	Diagnosis should be confirmed and patient followed at a regional CF center
Juvenile diabetes mellitus	Hyperglycemia, ketoacidosis (highly variable), hypoglycemia	Insulin	24-hour urine testing for ketones and glucose	Endocrinology or metabolism
Storage disorders	Cachexia, seizures, aspiration	Individualized	May require soft tissue biopsies, confirmed by specific enzyme assays	Genetics/metabolism, neurology
Endocrine Hypothyroidism	—	Thyroxine	T3, T4, TSH, TBG	Endocrinology
Adrenal insufficiency	Adrenal crisis, maintain VS			
Growth hormone deficiency or panhypopituitarism	—	Specific hormone replacement	GH stimulation tests, skull x-rays, thyroid, cortisol, FSH/LH	
Diabetes insipidus	Hypernatremia, hypovolemia	Water	Skull x-rays, pituitary hormones, water deprivation, vasopressin, serum osmolality	Endocrinology, nephrologist
Allergic/immunologic	Infection usually pulmonary but also chronic	Specific antibiotics	Immunoglobulin, absolute eosinophil count, tuberculin test, consider specific viral and bacterial and fungal infections, allergen testing, TB cell typing	Allergy/immunology
	Suppurative, otitis, sinusitis, intestinal and skin infections, occasionally chronic visceral (e.g., abscess)			
Genitourinary	Treatment of renal failure, urinary tract infection, or hypertension		See Chapter 31	

cells. If the diarrhea is on the basis of malabsorption of a specific nutrient (lactose intolerance being the most common example) or infection (e.g., giardiasis), the diagnosis usually can be made on the basis of the screening tests indicated in Figure 5 (stool O and P, pH, Clinitest) and treatment instituted. If the etiology of malabsorption is not obvious, a gastroenterologist can recommend further studies (e.g., breath hydrogen analysis, biopsy of small intestine, or Enterotest capsule).

Other Etiologies

The management of children with other organic etiologies of FTT is usually done in conjunction with an appropriate consultant. The immediate concerns, steps in management, and diagnostic procedures indicated in many of these conditions are outlined in Table 3.

BIBLIOGRAPHY

Backwin H: Emotional deprivation in infants. J Pediatr 35:512, 1949

Goldbloom RB: Failure to Thrive. Pediatr Clin North Am 29:151, 1982

Hutton IW, Oates K: Nonorganic failure to thrive: A long-term follow-up. Pediatrics 59:73, 1977

Kohler EE, Good TA: The infant who fails to thrive. Hosp Pract 4:54, 1969

Krieger I, Mellinger RC: Pituitary function in the deprivation syndrome. J Pediatr 79:216, 1971

Mitchell WG, Gorrell RW, Greenberg RA: Failure-to-thrive: A study in a primary care setting. Epidemiology and follow-up. Pediatrics 65:971, 1980

Rosenn DW, Loeb LS, Jura MB: Differentiation of organic from nonorganic failure to thrive syndrome in infancy. Pediatrics 66:698, 1980

Sills RM: Failure to thrive. The role of clinical and laboratory evaluation. Am J Dis Child 32:967, 1978

Whitten AF, et al.: Evidence that growth failure from maternal deprivation is secondary to undereating. JAMA 209:1675, 1969

Cross-Reference to *Pediatrics,* 17th ed.

TWENTY-FIVE

The Underweight and Overweight Adolescent

S. M. Coupey and M. A. Boeck

EXCESSIVE THINNESS IN THE APPARENTLY HEALTHY ADOLESCENT

Significant loss of weight or excessive thinness, particularly in an adolescent female, is a common symptom encountered in clinical practice. It may or may not be the presenting complaint. Usually, however, the weight loss is acknowledged by the patient when pointed out by the physician, and it may be a complaint of the parent. Often, a sign or symptom secondary to the extreme thinness is the focus of the patient's and the family's attention. For example, the cessation of menstrual periods, delayed pubertal development, syncope, and cold bluish hands (sometimes misinterpreted as Raynaud's phenomenon) are common reasons for seeking medical help.

Definition

For the purpose of this chapter, excessive thinnesss is defined as a weight that is 20% less than the ideal weight for height. The patient's height is plotted on an appropriate growth curve; the weight for age that falls on the same percentile as the height is taken as the ideal weight.

Etiology and Differential Diagnosis

There are relatively few clinical conditions that produce excessive weight loss in an apparently healthy teenager. Cachexia due to an indolent infectious process, such as tuberculosis, or an acute metabolic derangement, such as juvenile diabetes mellitus, is usually accompanied by other signs and symptoms, for example, fever, pain, cough, or polyuria. There are, however, a few conditions that can produce dramatic weight loss with no other signs or symptoms or only minimal findings. If the patient is an adolescent girl, the most common of these conditions is anorexia nervosa. This syndrome primarily affects girls in the 13–20 year age group. It has been described as a biopsychosocial illness, implying multifactorial etiologies. With the prevailing standard of feminine beauty emphasizing thinness, we are experiencing a period of high social vulnerability for the development of anorexia nervosa. The prevalence of the syndrome in Britain in middle and upper-middle class girls aged 16–18 was found to be 1 case per 100. There are no reliable figures for North American adolescents, but indications are that the incidence of anorexia nervosa is increasing, especially in the higher socioeconomic strata.

Other disorders that occasionally produce extreme weight loss without other phys-

[1]Supported in part by grant no. 5438 from the Robert Wood Johnson Foundation.

ical signs include severe endogenous depressive illness (rare in adolescents) and impending psychosis. Malabsorption syndromes, in particular chronic inflammatory bowel disease, can lead to impressive weight loss with few associated signs or symptoms. Very rarely, hyperthyroidism or a malignancy, such as lymphoma, has unexplained weight loss as a primary symptom.

The diagnosis of anorexia nervosa, endogenous depression, or psychosis usually can be made by history and physical examination alone. The diagnosis of a malabsorption syndrome, malignancy, or hyperthyroidism is suggested by the history and physical examination and confirmed by specific laboratory tests.

History

At the beginning of the interview, questions designed to determine the amount of weight loss, the time course over which the weight loss has occurred, and the patient's estimate of previous high and low weights are most helpful. Even if the teenager's chief complaint is that of a symptom secondary to weight loss, such as primary or secondary amenorrhea, the experienced clinician initially will direct the questioning to the weight problem. This can be done easily by saying to the teenager: "I notice that you are very thin. Sometimes the problem you are complaining of can be caused by extreme thinness. How long have you been this way?" In the next set of questions, the clinician should attempt to determine the mechanism of weight loss. Has the adolescent been dieting? Does she vomit? Does she have disturbed bowel function, such as diarrhea or constipation? At this point, it is also very helpful to inquire about the teenager's own concept of her appearance. Does she agree that she is too thin? Would she like to gain weight, or does she feel that she would look better if she lost a few more pounds?

Patients with inflammatory bowel disease, malignancy, and even those with endogenous depression usually cannot offer an adequate explanation for their weight loss and will admit that it is puzzling to them. They wish to put on weight and often state that they are just not as hungry as they used to be, but they do not know why. Patients with hyperthyroidism report eating considerable quantities and yet they still lose weight. Patients with anorexia nervosa, on the other hand, always feel as if they are still fat, even though they are thin, and usually will report this to the clinician. Occasionally, they will nod and agree with the questioner that, yes, they think they are thin, although this statement is not usually made in a very convincing manner. One of the ways to explore the issue further is to ask: "Yes, you agree you are thin, but what do you think about your thighs?" Virtually every patient with anorexia nervosa will state that she thinks her thighs are fat. Girls with other diagnoses think this is a strange question.

Following questioning about body image, it is useful to take a detailed dietary history. The clinician instructs the patient to recall every item of food and drink that she had on the previous day for breakfast, lunch, dinner, and snacks. When the diagnosis of anorexia nervosa is being considered, it is important to question the patient in minute detail in order to avoid overestimating the daily caloric intake. For instance, if she says she had a tunafish sandwich for lunch, ask specifically: "Was that with one or two slices of bread? Was it thin sliced bread or ordinary bread? Did you put butter on the bread? Was there mayonnaise in the tunafish?" If the adolescent reports drinking soda, ask: "Was that a diet soda?" If the patient had popcorn for a snack (a favorite of patients with anorexia nervosa) inquire whether it was air-popped or popped in oil? Using this very careful line of questioning, a reliable estimate of the amount of calories consumed by the patient on the previous day can be made.

A daily consumption of less than 1,500 calories will lead to weight loss in the normally active teenager. Patients with any of these diagnoses, except those who are hypermetabolic, tend to have a low caloric intake.

However, the patient with Crohn's disease usually eats regular foods but is not very hungry. She may report having a cheeseburger for lunch but state that she could eat only half of it. In marked contrast, the patient with anorexia nervosa actively attempts to reduce her caloric intake and often goes to extreme lengths to do so. For example, one patient reported eating sardines for lunch. On closer questioning, it emerged that they were sardines packed in oil. On even closer questioning, she admitted to washing them under the kitchen tap and patting them dry with paper towels to remove all traces of oil before eating them.

Patients should be asked if they ever lose control and eat large quantities of food in a short period of time. This symptom is known as bulimia. They should also be asked how often they vomit. If they report vomiting frequently, they should be asked whether they induce this themselves and how.

The thin adolescent should be questioned carefully regarding bowel symptoms and habits. Patients with occult inflammatory bowel disease often have loose bowel movements and some crampy abdominal pains, whereas those with endogenous depression and those with anorexia nervosa are constipated. Patients who are constipated should be asked how often they use laxatives, since girls with anorexia nervosa frequently abuse laxatives as an additional method of losing weight.

Careful questioning regarding the timing of the growth spurt and pubertal development, including a detailed menstrual history, is important, since these developmental features are often delayed. Questioning about the amount of exercise the patient does is important. Girls with anorexia nervosa tend to exercise excessively as another method of losing weight. It is helpful to ask if they regularly exercise at home in their room, if they take dancing lessons (how often and for how long), if they run track or jog (how much and how often). Patients who are depressed or who have a malabsorption syndrome or malignancy are often fatigued and are unlikely to do much exercise. Patients with hyperthyroidism, on the other hand, are often hyperactive.

For all teenage patients, a careful social history needs to be taken; this is particularly useful in this group of patients. Adolescents who are depressed withdraw from social contacts, spend a lot of time alone, do poorly in school, and in general present themselves as isolated individuals. Those with hyperthyroidism often have behavioral disturbances, are irritable, and get into altercations with friends, family, and teachers. Those with malabsorption syndrome or malignancy often are socially normal, although they may be fatigued, and this may interfere with their socialization. Teenagers with anorexia nervosa tend to be loners. They usually have little interest in dating or sexuality but do interact socially with their family. Often, they cook and prepare meals for the family, although they will not eat themselves. They are generally excellent students and are very meticulous and obsessive in completing assigned tasks.

Physical Examination

Patients who are very thin because of anorexia nervosa, depression, malignancy, or malabsorption syndrome are usually hypometabolic and hypothermic. Because of this, those with anorexia nervosa in particular often wear several layers of clothing, which serves to camouflage the degree of their emaciation. The less astute clinician can be fooled into thinking that the patient is heavier than she really is, especially if she is not required to undress completely for the physical examination. Patients who are hypothermic have peripheral vasoconstriction, with icy cold hands that are mottled and reddish blue in color.

As aids in assessing the severity of the emaciation, the patient should be examined for the amount of muscle mass, the presence or absence of an adequate amount of subcutaneous fat, redundant skin folds on the thighs, buttocks, and arms, and bruising over the bony prominences of the shoulders and hips (due to lack of subcutaneous padding).

Tanner staging of secondary sexual characteristics is mandatory, as there is often pubertal delay or arrest in malnourished adolescents.

Patients with anorexia nervosa characteristically have a bradycardia with a heart rate of 60 beats per minute or less, whereas patients with malabsorption syndrome have a normal to mildly elevated heart rate, and those with hyperthyroidism often have a sinus tachycardia. Blood pressure is usually in the lower ranges of normal in all of these conditions except hyperthyroidism, where it may be in the high range of normal or elevated. Extremely cachectic patients with anorexia nervosa may have lanugo on the back and chest and also may have edema of the lower extremities. These signs indicate severe malnourishment, and patients who exhibit them should be admitted to the hospital for immediate nutritional support.

Laboratory Data

In the patients with anorexia nervosa, laboratory data are most often surprisingly normal given the degree of cachexia. In spite of their poor nutritional intake, they are not anemic. The white blood cell count, erythrocyte sedimentation rate, and concentrations in blood of total protein, albumin, and minerals are usually within normal limits. Although serum concentrations of sodium, potassium, and bicarbonate are usually normal, they may be low in patients with significant vomiting, severe laxative abuse, or water intoxication. Patients with malignancy or malabsorption syndrome, in contrast, frequently have mild anemia, and those with chronic inflammatory bowel disease have an elevated erythrocyte sedimentation rate and often a thrombocytosis.

Patients with anorexia nervosa frequently have an elevated serum carotene concentration, whereas those with cachexia of other etiologies always have a low serum carotene concentration. The cause of the hypercarotenemia in anorexia nervosa is unclear, but it is probably secondary to an acquired enzymatic defect.

Tests of endocrine function are usually abnormal in severely starved patients, including those with malabsorption syndromes and anorexia nervosa. However, these tests need not be performed routinely, since they add little to the differential diagnosis or management of these conditions. In particular, however, thyroid hormone levels are low in starved patients and elevated, of course, in those with hyperthyroidism.

Patients with malabsorption syndromes are often mildly dehydrated due to excessive fluid loss and thus have high urine specific gravities and may have an elevated concentration of urea in blood. However, patients with anorexia nervosa, although they are often dehydrated and may have elevated blood urea concentrations, usually do not have high urine specific gravities, since they may have an acquired renal concentrating defect.

Anorexia nervosa is known to occur with increased frequency in girls with gonadal dysgenesis and the mosaic variants of this syndrome. Therefore, a buccal smear and karyotype should be considered, especially in those girls with short stature.

When malabsorption syndromes are being considered, a stool sample should be tested for ova and parasites, and, if none are found, barium studies of the large and small bowel should be done to find the typical malabsorption pattern or features suggestive of Crohn's disease, ulcerative colitis, or lymphoma. Patients with long-standing anorexia nervosa occasionally show evidence of gastric atony in barium studies of the upper gastrointestinal tract.

Management

If, after a detailed history and physical examination, the clinician considers that either endogenous depression or impending psychosis is the most likely reason for the teenager's weight loss, a psychiatric consultation should be sought immediately. Patients with hyperthyroidism should be referred to an endocrinologist for management. Adolescents with marked weight loss who are suspected of having a malabsorption syndrome or a malignancy are best admitted to the hospital for diagnostic work-up and institution of therapy. Appropriate consultation with a gastroenterologist or oncologist should be sought.

Patients with anorexia nervosa require a team of professionals for optimal management. This team should consist of a physician, who may be the primary care pediatrician, and a psychotherapist, preferably one with special training in the therapy of adolescents and the management of eating disorders.

In general, all patients with anorexia nervosa who have lost 30% or more of their ideal weight or who experience syncope or have peripheral edema should be admitted to the hospital immediately. Adequate nutrition must be established in these severely starved patients before psychotherapy or behavioral modification techniques have any chance of success. Adolescents with anorexia nervosa who are less emaciated can be treated as outpatients.

The teenager and her family should be referred to an appropriate therapist for diagnostic consultation and therapeutic planning. The physician should continue to see the patient on a weekly basis for weighing and nutritional monitoring. The physician and psychotherapist should communicate frequently and should agree on the behavioral management of the patient and her family.

Anorexia nervosa is a serious, chronic illness with a small but significant death rate. However, with appropriate therapy, the outcome is good to excellent in about one half of the patients and adequate in an additional one third.

Summary

Excessive thinness is a relatively common symptom encountered in clinical settings that care for adolescents from the middle and upper-middle classes. A comprehensive and detailed history and meticulous physical examination will suggest the correct diagnosis in the large majority of cases. The symptom occurs most often in girls, and the most frequent diagnosis is anorexia nervosa. Other clinical conditions can present with the primary symptom of marked weight loss and are more equally distributed in the adolescent population between boys and girls and lower and upper socioeconomic classes. Pediatricians have a major role to play in the diagnosis and nutritional support of adolescents with anorexia nervosa. These teenagers with failure to thrive can develop significant physiologic complications of malnutrition, including death, if not properly identified and appropriately treated.

THE OVERWEIGHT ADOLESCENT

Obesity is a condition of multifactorial origin involving genetic, environmental, biochemical, and psychologic components. Approximately 25% of children in the United States are overweight. Most obese children become obese adolescents, and most obese adolescents become obese adults. It is estimated that if an obese eighth grader has not reduced his or her weight by the end of adolescence, the odds against this occurring during adulthood are 28:1. Obesity in the childhood and adolescent age group is associated with hypertension, abnormalities of glucose tolerance, and hyperlipidemia. It is also associated with orthopedic disorders, such as slipped capital femoral epiphysis and Blount's disease (tibia vara).

In a society that idolizes slimness, the psychologic and social consequences of obesity are often of great magnitude. Studies have shown that even small children, when shown pictures of children with various deformities, are likely to state that they would prefer a physically handicapped child to an obese child for a friend. Discrimination also exists against the obese teenager in educational settings. It is not surprising that obese teenagers have a poor self-image and difficulties with peer interaction.

Definition

Obesity is usually defined as a weight that is 20% greater than ideal for height, and morbid obesity as a weight 50% greater than ideal weight. A variety of methods that vary in sophistication and complexity are used to determine obesity. The method most commonly used in an office setting is the nomogram that relates normal weight to age, sex, and height. The shortcomings of this method include failure to take into account ethnic differences and variations in body frame and inability to distinguish weight due to muscle from that due to fat. The most reliable office measure of body fat is the triceps skinfold thickness. Measurements obtained with standardized calipers are compared with norms for age and sex.

Etiology

Endogenous Obesity. Only a small fraction of obese adolescents have endogenous obesity due to genetic or endocrine abnormalities. These few patients can usually be readily identified by history and physical examination, since nearly all of the causes of endogenous obesity are characterized by growth failure. They are usually less than the 5th percentile in height, and their bone age is delayed. The exogenously obese child, in contrast, is almost always at the 50th percentile or greater in height and has a bone age that is normal or advanced.

Hypothyroidism. The hypothyroid teenager can be plump with myxedema and usually has a dull facial expression, dry skin, constipation, short stature, and retarded bone age. Hypothyroidism by itself, however, seldom causes massive weight gain.

Hypercortisolism (Cushing's Syndrome). Adolescents with Cushing's syndrome are short, with truncal obesity and moon facies. They may have characteristic purplish striae of the skin resulting from thinning of dermal connective tissue, and they may be hypertensive. The excessive cortisol is due to malignant or benign adrenal tumors, primary overproduction of adrenocorticotropic hormone (Cushing's disease), or prescription of exogenous hormone.

Froelich's Syndrome. A teenager with this rarely encountered condition has a hypothalamic tumor with resulting polyphagia, obesity, and hypogonadism.

Laurence-Moon-Biedl Syndrome. This is a genetic syndrome that includes obesity, mental deficiency, polydactyly or syndactyly, retinitis pigmentosa, and hypogonadism. The patient is usually shorter than average but may not be markedly so.

Prader-Willi Syndrome. This genetic syndrome is marked by obesity, small hands and feet, mental deficiency, hypogonadism, and cryptorchidism. Patients have a neonatal history of hypotonia, feeding problems, and delayed milestones. They may have a characteristic facial appearance, with almond-shaped eyes, strabismus, and a narrow bifrontal diameter. These patients are usually quite short.

Exogenous Obesity

Exogenous obesity is a poorly understood syndrome with multiple etiologies. Although it is the result of long-term caloric intake greater than metabolic demand, it is overly simplistic to blame the patient for eating too much.

Genetic and Environmental Influences. When both parents are obese, approximately 75% of their children will be obese. This incidence drops to 40–50% when one parent is obese and falls to less than 10% when neither parent is obese. Studies of twins and adoptees have had equivocal results. Genetics probably plays an important role in the development of the adipose organ.

Metabolism. Hyperinsulinemia in obesity is well documented. Insulin both increases subjective feelings of hunger and is lipogenic. It also increases hepatic synthesis of triglycerides and cholesterol and inhibits lipolysis. While true primary hyperinsulinemia leading to obesity is rare in teenagers, secondary hyperinsulinemia is common and undoubtedly contributes to maintenance of the obese state.

The role of physical activity in the development of obesity is unclear. A study of children and teenagers using movies to document the extent of physical activity indicated that obese youngsters were less active than their peers. Another study, which converted measures of activity into caloric expenditure by measuring oxygen consumption, found that obese boys actually expended more calories through activity than nonobese boys. It is thus unclear whether inactivity is a cause or a consequence of obesity. Within 24–48 hours after caloric restriction, both obese and lean individuals experience a 15–30% decrease in basal metabolic rate. Thus, caloric restriction without an increase in physical activity may not result in continued weight loss.

Differential Diagnosis

History. The history should include birth weight, early feeding history, growth pattern during the first year (with records of heights and weights if available), and developmental history. One should inquire about the age of onset of excessive weight gain or obesity and any identifiable precipitating events or circumstances. Note should be made of the presence of chronic health problems, previous starvation, abdominal surgery, or prolonged bed rest, all of which have been associated with onset of excessive weight gain. The family pattern of weight gain and history of obesity-related conditions, such as diabetes, high blood pressure, and heart disease, should be elicited.

Further questioning about the family's attitude toward obesity, eating patterns, and the relationship between eating and various moods and life stresses is important in gaining a perspective on which therapeutic strategies have the best probabilities of success. It is important to assess the adolescent's motivation to lose weight. Is he or she self-motivated or, alternatively, coerced by parents or school authorities into seeking treatment? Why is the teenager choosing to address the problem at this particular time?

Patterns of eating should be investigated, including the number of meals and snacks per day, the rate of eating, food preferences, degree of hunger and satiety, and the occurrence of binges and nocturnal eating. The adolescent should be questioned regarding previous efforts at weight loss, including the type of weight reduction program employed, the duration of the effort, amount of weight lost, and the reason for terminating the attempt.

The impact of obesity upon social function, including peer relationships, leisure time activities, school performance, and employment, should be assessed. An estimate of the teenager's energy expenditure can be made by reconstructing the pattern of a typical weekday and weekend day, including amount of sleep, time spent in school, the number of stairs climbed, and other indices of physical activity.

Physical Examination

The physical examination should include careful measurement of height and weight, with plotting of these values on a growth chart. Patients with exogenous obesity have increased height for age, or, in the case of short patients, the individual is taller than expected for the family. Triceps skinfold measurements should be made with standardized calipers. To determine triceps skinfold thickness, the distance between the olecranon and acromial process is measured in the nondominant arm of the standing patient, and the midpoint is determined. At the midpoint, a full fatfold is grasped, away from the underlying muscle, and the calipers are applied below the fingers to the fatfold for 2–3 seconds. The triceps skinfold measurement is read from the meter on the calipers. Two or three independent measurements should be made and the mean figure used for the final skinfold value. The value is then compared with standardized norms for age and sex (Table 1).

Vital signs, including blood pressure (with a thigh cuff if necessary), should be obtained. One should take note of the distribu-

TABLE 1. OBESITY STANDARDS FOR CAUCASIAN AMERICANS

Age (Years)	Skinfold Measurements*	
	Males	Females
5	12	14
6	12	15
7	13	16
8	14	17
9	15	18
10	16	20
11	17	21
12	18	22
13	18	23
14	17	23
15	16	24
16	15	25
17	14	26
18	15	27
19	15	27
20	16	28
21	17	28
22	18	28
23	18	28
24	19	28
25	20	29
26	20	29
27	21	29
28	22	29
29	23	29
30–50	23	30

*Minimum triceps skinfold thickness in mm indicating obesity. (*From Seltzer CC, Mayer J: Postgrad Med 38:A101, 1965.*)

tion of body fat, hirsutism, acne, and color of striae. Pink or red striae are common in obesity, while brown-purple striae are present in Cushing's syndrome.

Special attention should be paid to examination of the thyroid gland, breasts, abdomen, back, and weightbearing joints. There is an increased incidence of certain orthopedic disorders, including slipped capital femoral epiphysis and tibia vara, in the obese. An assessment of pubertal development should be made. Patients with exogenous obesity have normal or slightly advanced sexual development. Male patients with exogenous obesity should have a normal-sized phallus. Although the buried phallus in obese patients often gives the misleading impression of being small, size can be obtained by measuring from the phallic base. Patients with genetic syndromes in which obesity is a component have hypogonadism.

Laboratory Tests

Because obesity in the adolescent may be associated with abnormal glucose tolerance, hyperinsulinemia, hypercholesterolemia, and hypertriglyceridemia, fasting levels of glucose, cholesterol, and triglycerides should be obtained. Other laboratory tests are not indicated unless the patient is hypertensive, is of short stature, or has other clinical evidence of an endocrinologic disorder. Because decreased thyroid function can have a subtle presentation, the short obese teenager should be screened with serum thyroxine and thyroid-stimulating hormone levels. Because patients with Cushing's disease may have growth failure and obesity without other signs of excessive cortisol secretion, this diagnosis should be considered in teenagers who are short and obese.

Management

A variety of approaches to the treatment of obesity exists, including dietary counseling, behavioral modification, exercise, pharmacotherapy, and surgery. None of these approaches has proved to be particularly successful for either weight loss or for maintenance of weight. Thus, the pediatric practitioner should make every effort in his practice to prevent the problem of obesity before it occurs. While they may not eliminate the problem of overweight, medically sound practices include promotion of breastfeeding and delayed introduction of solid foods, encouragement of physical activity, and discouragement of the inappropriate use of food as punishment, reward, bribe, or substitute for meaningful interpersonal relationships.

Once it has been determined that the obesity is exogenous, the general pediatrician, with few exceptions, is in an excellent position to design and monitor a weight reduction program. As with other illnesses with a poor prognosis for complete cure, the probability of poor outcome in obesity should not be used as a rationale to avoid treating the patient.

Dietary Counseling

The treatment for obesity most frequently employed by adolescents, with or without the advice of a physician, is dieting. Very low caloric diets should not be used by teenagers until they reach Tanner Stage 4. A frequently employed approach is to tell the adolescent simply to "eat less of everything." The assumption is made that this diet will have fewer calories, will remain nutritionally balanced, and will encourage compliance through allowing the teenager to continue to eat his or her customary variety of conventional foods. While intuitively an attractive approach, it rarely has been successful. Many teenagers do not exhibit an orderly regimen of eating. A frequent pattern is to skip both breakfast and lunch and then to eat almost continuously from after school until bedtime. Their diet is frequently high in fat and concentrated sweets and low in fruits and vegetables. Retaining palatable, high caloric foods in the diet serves as a constant source of temptation to the teenager.

In many of the popular dietary regimens, dieters do not count calories but are told to drastically restrict certain categories of food, usually carbohydrate or fat. This, over the short run, usually results in an automatic decrease in calories because the individual does not totally compensate by increasing the amounts eaten in the other two food groups. While a decrease in palatability of foods makes adherence to a diet easier for some individuals, for others this makes long-term compliance impossible. Restrictive diets low in carbohydrate may result in ketosis. Although extra energy is required to excrete ketone bodies in the urine, this rarely exceeds 2–3% of the total daily energy requirement. Ketosis, however, at times is accompanied by nausea and malaise and, hence, may impair appetite.

The use of very low calorie liquid diets high in protein content ("supplemented fasting") has been associated with sudden death in physically healthy individuals. In one analysis of such fatalities in obese individuals who died of ventricular arrhythmias, the deaths were not related to lack of medical supervision, lack of potassium supplementation, or the nature of the biologic quality of the protein used. On autopsy, all victims had evidence of myocardial atrophy, a condition fairly specific for protein calorie malnutrition. For this reason, we recommend that diets providing fewer than 700 calories per day be restricted to research centers.

A rational, nutritionally sound, dietary approach is to utilize food exchanges, such as those devised by the American Diabetic Association. Foods are divided into six categories: milk, vegetable, fruit, fat, meat, and bread. Each food within a given category has an equal amount of carbohydrates, protein, fat, and calories and thus may be substituted for any other food in the same category. This allows the teenager flexibility in the choice of foods eaten without counting calories. The distribution of protein, fat, and carbohydrate is important in order to lose the maximum amount of adipose tissue with a minimum loss of nitrogen. The number of food exchanges is determined such that 15–20% of the calories are from protein, 30–35% from fat, and the remaining 45–50% from carbohydrates, preferably ones that supply vitamins and minerals and are high in fiber. Adolescents who are consuming a diet providing fewer than 1,200 calories per day should take a daily multivitamin pill.

Before the dietary program begins, it is important that the teenager have a realistic expectation about the rate of weight loss. Initial rapid weight loss in the first 1–2 weeks of dieting results from a large loss of water. After this period, it takes an energy deficit of 3,500–3,600 kcal to lose 1 pound of body weight. In other words, the teenager needs to take in 500 calories per day less than he or she utilizes in order to lose 1 pound per week.

Compliance with these new dietary habits for a prolonged period in order to attain and maintain weight losses is a major difficulty. Teenagers should be encouraged to use the concept of calorie banking, i.e., planning ahead and saving some calories in advance to be used at a later date for special parties or holidays. Weigh-in and counseling sessions on a weekly basis are essential initially, with subsequent weekly or biweekly reassessment required for many during both weight loss and maintenance.

Behavioral Treatment. Behavioral programs focus on how to eat on the assumption that eating habits must change in order to maintain weight loss. Teenagers are asked to keep a diary of all food eaten and the circumstances surrounding its consumption: time, place, activity, and mood. This identifies specific behaviors to be targeted for change by the program. Programs may focus on slowing down the rate at which food is eaten, using smaller plates, eating mainly in certain areas, and avoiding other activities while eating (e.g., watching TV, reading a book). Several studies on the effectiveness of behavioral treatment indicate that its advantage is not in the amount of weight loss but rather in the

maintenance of weight once loss has occurred.

Exercise. An exercise program should be a part of every weight reduction plan. In fact, weight loss following exercise is generally greater than would be expected through the direct expenditure of energy alone. There is some evidence that increased activity in the obese individual may decrease appetite while it increases the metabolic rate. Compliance with exercise programs in teenagers is poor, however, with various studies reporting a 25–75% dropout rate. Reasons for this poor compliance include embarrassment, lack of transportation or money, and pressures of time. Buddy systems and rewards for attendance at exercise sessons may be of help. It is important to recommend kinds of exercise, such as walking and climbing stairs, that do not require elaborate, expensive facilities. Obese individuals might benefit from special physical education classes within the school curriculum in which they could participate, with less embarrassment, with others having similar skills and stamina.

Pharmacotherapy. Several drugs that were used in the past for weight control have no role in weight reduction today. These include thyroid preparations, digitalis, diuretics, methycellulose, and human chorionicgonadotropin. Anorectic drugs are not often prescribed for adolescents because of their side effects and potential for abuse. When they have been used, the fact that they have been less successful than in adults has been attributed to noncompliance. Until safer and more effective pharmacologic agents are found, we do not recommend drug therapy for weight reduction in teenagers.

Surgery. Surgical methods for weight reduction include jaw wiring, intestinal bypass, gastric bypass, and gastric plication. Gastric bypass has been used in carefully selected adolescents with exogenous obesity and with Prader-Willi syndrome. Weight loss occurred without interruption of growth in height or significant morbidity in these carefully selected patients. The other surgical methods are not recommended.

Summary

Exogenous obesity is a common problem in adolescents. The greatest likelihood of success in treating mild to moderate obesity is a program including diet, behavioral modification strategies, and exercise individually tailored to each patient. Long-term monitoring of progress in a group or individual setting is of great importance. The physician should pay special attention to dieting teenage girls who are only mildly overweight; this may signal the onset of anorexia nervosa. Surgery is an option for carefully selected, morbidly obese, late adolescents who have failed to lose weight using other treatment modalities. While current therapeutic modalities fall far short of success, it is hoped that results of basic and clinical research will lead to more promising strategies for the future. The pediatrician should play a major role in addressing the psychologic and sociocultural issues which impact upon the obese teenager.

BIBLIOGRAPHY

Abraham S, Nordsieck M: Relationship of excess weight in children and adults. Public Health Rep 75:263, 1960

Burbige EJ, Huang SS, Bayless TM: Clinical manifestations of Crohn's disease in children and adolescents. Pediatrics 55:866, 1975

Golden MP: An approach to the management of obesity in childhood. Pediatr Clin. North Am 26:187, 1979

Hsu LKG, Crisp AH, Harding B: Outcome of anorexia nervosa. Lancet 1:61, 1979

Lucas AR: Toward the understanding of anorexia nervosa as a disease entity. Mayo Clin Proc 56:254, 1981

Maddox GL, Bach KW, Liederman VR: Overweight as social deviance and disability. J Health Soc Behav 9:287, 1968

Maloney MJ, Farrell MK: Treatment of severe weight loss in anorexia nervosa with hyperalimentation and psychotherapy. Am J Psychiatry 137:310, 1980

Soper RT, Mason EE, Printen KJ, Zellweger H: Gastric bypass for morbid obesity in children and adolescents. J Pediatr Surg 10:51, 1975

Stunkard AJ (ed): Obesity. Philadelphia, Saunders, 1980

TWENTY-SIX

School Failure

Frances Cerullo, David Diamond, and Ruth Gottesman

Approximately 10–30% of school-aged children are unable to meet the expected standards of school achievement. A majority of these children show a specific learning disability, the effects of which plague them not only during their school years but throughout their entire lives. Most children with learning disabilities manifest problems in language, motor skills, and behavior well before they encounter difficulties in school, and yet the problems remain undetected, or else they are misdiagnosed even during their school years. It is of utmost importance that these children be recognized as early as possible and provided with appropriate educational intervention and counseling for them and their parents. With proper help and support, learning disabled children will be better able to deal with the academic and other demands of life that face them.

DEFINITION OF PROBLEM

The concept of learning disabilities as a specific and identifiable entity apart from mental retardation, neurologic impairment, or emotional disturbance has come about only in the past 10–15 years as a result of the increasing interest and concern about children who, despite apparently adequate intellectual ability, were failing in school. In 1975, Congress passed Public Law 94-142, the Education for the Handicapped Act, which recognized and defined learning disabilities as a handicapping condition. This law mandated that learning disabled children receive special educational help in all public schools throughout the country. The law's definition of learning disabilities, widely accepted among specialists in education, psychology, and medicine, is as follows:

Those children who have a disorder in one or more of the basic psychological processes involved in understanding or in using language, spoken or written, which disorder may manifest itself in imperfect ability to listen, think, speak, read, write, spell, or do mathematical calculations. Such disorders include such conditions as perceptual handicaps, brain injury, minimal brain dysfunction, dyslexia, and developmental aphasia. Such terms do not include children who have learning problems which are primarily the result of visual, hearing, or motor handicaps, or mental retardation, or emotional disturbance, or environmental, cultural, or economic disadvantage.

In recent years, pediatricians have shown an increasing concern about learning disabled children in their practice. This may be due, in part, to the recognition that learning disabilities in children are manifestations of dysfunction of the central nervous system, adversely affecting their psychosocial development and general well-being. Also because of Public Law 94-142, more parents are bringing their children to their pediatric practitioners with complaints of school problems. Pediatric practitioners may be uniquely qualified to play an important role in the management of learning disabled children. As ongoing providers of care, pediatric practitioners may have more continuity with a child and the family than has any other professional. More than any other specialist, pediatric practitioners have a working knowledge of family values and styles of coping and also have substantial input into medical decisions made by the family.

ROLE OF THE PEDIATRIC PRACTITIONER

While pediatric practitioners are seldom the only specialists involved in the management of learning disabled children, their role may include the following responsibilities.

Identification

Through ongoing care to patients, often beginning in infancy, pediatric practitioners may uncover developmental delays or identify behavioral characteristics that place children at risk for learning disabilities.

Differential Diagnosis

Pediatricians can rule out sensory impairment, neurologic disorders, or other medical problems that may account for school failure. They can also determine if the school failure is due primarily to a specific learning disability or if it may be more closely related to mental retardation, an attentional deficit disorder, emotional problems, adverse environmental factors, or a combination of some of these factors.

Child Advocate

Pediatricians often can intercede as objective persons to help bring the school and the parents together on behalf of the child.

Management

Pediatricians can counsel parents on issues of child management and can investigate and treat psychosomatic problems accompanying learning disabilities, such as enuresis and encopresis, abdominal pain, and headache. Pediatricians can prescribe medication for children with problems of attention and hyperactivity.

Referral

When children need to undergo further diagnosis to clarify learning difficulties, pediatricians are able to guide the parents to an appropriate specialist, based on their own assessment.

Information Source

Pediatricians can offer a perspective to parents, teachers, and other members of the community on such issues as allergies, optometric training, diet, sensory integration therapy, and other controversial strategies of intervention offered to children with learning disabilities.

ETIOLOGY AND DESCRIPTION OF CHARACTERISTIC BEHAVIOR

Learning disabilities seldom result from a single etiology. Instead, they are thought to stem from a combination of genetic, constitutional, neurodevelopmental, environmental, and emotional factors. Adverse events of pregnancy, birth, and prenatal and postnatal development, for example, or other circumstances leading to dysfunction of the central nervous system may result in a learning disability.

Characteristics of learning disabilities

are easier to identify than are causes and can be helpful in pointing up areas of strengths and weaknesses within a learning disabled child. They are grouped below in five general areas: (1) deficits in abilities underlying academic learning, (2) behavioral disorders, (3) motor incoordination, (4) poor social adaptive behavior, and (5) problems of orientation. (Table 1). Through observation of the child, interview with the parent, and information gained from school personnel, a pediatrician can determine whether the child in question has some of these characteristics. It must be noted that not all of these characteristics are found in all learning disabled children, although very often they are found in clusters.

PEDIATRIC ASSESSMENT OF THE LEARNING DISABLED CHILD

The pediatric assessment described here focuses on guidelines for an interview of the parent, school report, and examination of the child to help in the identification, evaluation,

TABLE 1. CHARACTERISTICS OF LEARNING DISABILITIES

Characteristic	Description of Behavior
Deficit in abilities underlying academic learning	
Receptive language	Misunderstands multiple meanings of words.
Word knowledge	Shows poor grasp of instructions or directions.
Auditory comprehension	Comprehends little when reading. Retains little information.
Expressive language	Mispronounces, substitutes, or omits sounds.
Articulation	Cannot come up with exactly the right word.
Word finding	Describes the function of an object rather than
Syntax	the object's exact name. Has an immature vo-
Sequencing	cabulary. Uses incomplete sentences. Is unable
Vocabulary	to correct sequence facts. Cannot express an idea clearly. Has difficulty with written expression.
Perception	Cannot distinguish between sounds (big and pig
Auditory	sound alike). Has poor sound/symbol associa-
Visual	tion. Is unable to blend isolated sounds into words. Has trouble analyzing visual information. Is unable to discriminate between visual forms. Views visual information as parts rather than wholes. Confuses letter forms and letter order (e.g., b = d, was = saw).
Memory	Has difficulty remembering personal and general
Auditory	information (e.g., address, phone number,
Visual	days of the week). Is unable to remember classroom instructions, directions. Has difficulty recalling details of a story. Has trouble recalling number facts, time tables, spelling words. Has problem retaining visual details. Cannot remember letter names and numbers. Is unable to recall whole words.

(*continued*)

TABLE 1 (*Continued*)

Characteristic	Description of Behavior

Behavioral disorders
  Attentional deficits
    Distractibility
    Lability
    Poor concentration
    Impulsivity
    Hyperactivit
	Is unable to concentrate even for a short period of time. Cannot tune out extraneous stimuli (restless, fidgety). Has disorganized approach to work, careless. Has problems completing a task. Is unable to delay gratification, impatient. Has difficulty moderating emotions (poor self-control). Has problems sitting still—always on the move.

Motor incoordination	Shows poor coordination, is clumsy and awkward. Has poor sense of balance. Has problems learning how to tie, button, zipper. Has problems using a scissors, pencil. Is unable to copy forms accurately. Has difficulty coloring, writing within the lines. Forms letters poorly without regard for consistency in their size or for spacing between them.
Problems of orientation	Shows confusion about temporal relationships, e.g., soon, tomorrow, next week. Has poor spatial relationships, e.g., next to, in front of, in the middle. Cannot easily get around neighborhood, school. Is confused as to directions, left/right.

Poor social adaptive behavior
  Peer relationships
  Inappropriate behaviors
	Avoids or is disinterested in peers. Is disliked or isolated by peer group. Often plays with younger children. Shows poor judgment. Overreacts in social situations. Cries easily. Disregards feelings of others.

and management of a learning disability. This type of assessment enables the pediatrician to be a more effective liaison between parent and school. The assessment, however, cannot be completed in a conventional office visit. It may be necessary to allow additional time for both interviewing the parent and evaluation of the child. More specifically, the goals of this office visit are:

1. Identification if child is at risk for or has a learning disability.
2. Ruling out other causes for the child's school difficulties, such as sensory impairment, mental retardation, environmental or emotional factors.
3. Observation and description of the characteristics of learning disabilities in the child.
4. Determination if and what kind of referrals are needed for further clarification or treatment of the child.
5. Development of a management plan for the child and the family, which may include counseling for the parents or medication for the child.

Interview of Parent

The interview of the parent should include taking a history, obtaining information about the child's present functioning in school and at home, and determining how the family and the child are reacting to and coping with the problem. Many children with learning disabilities have problems not only in school subjects but in behavioral and social adjustment as well. Therefore, pediatricians have to explore all of these areas with the parents in order to appreciate the nature and extent of the disability.

While the discovery of a specific etiology of the learning problem may not be possible, the history can provide helpful information toward that goal.

Birth history should be taken to obtain specific information regarding possible pathologic entities that may occur during pregnancy, labor, or delivery. These entities may include bleeding, toxemia of pregnancy, late deceleration, fetal distress, prematurity, small for gestational age, hypoxic episodes, and so on.

Detailed questions regarding the patient's developmental milestones and early school experience may reveal variations of normal development which may be precursory of school failure. An example of this is the child with delayed language development and subsequent language-based learning disability. Patients with early delay in motor development who appear normal on neurologic examination may reveal subtle deficits in motor coordination. Questions regarding social development may be the first clues to understanding a child with hyperactive or withdrawn behavior.

A detailed family history of school failure is important in determining a genetic etiology. Each parent should be questioned as to his level of academic achievement and those of the patient's siblings. Family history of associated disabilities, such as mental retardation, emotional disturbance, and deafness, is also of importance. Pediatricians will most likely be aware of this history if they are providing primary medical care to the family.

In assessing the current status of the child's problem, parents should be asked to describe the difficulties the child is having in school. Questions that might help elicit this kind of information include:

- Were there any problems noted before the child started school?
- What kind of problems is he having in school?
- How long has he had them?
- How long has the parent been aware of them?
- Has the school spoken to the parents about the problems?
- Has your child attended more than one school?
- What kinds of teachers did he have?
- Has the school offered any help or given any suggestions?
- Have the parents taken any steps to help the child?
- Is the child a behavioral problem at school?
- Does he like to go to school?
- Does he get along with his teachers and the other children?

Often parents report that the child does not present any problems at home or that he is a different child during vacations and holidays. The following questions are helpful in obtaining more information about behavior at home.

- How does the child behave at home?
- Is behavior immature for his age?
- How do his parents manage his behavior?
- Does he understand what is expected of him?
- Does he follow through on directions he is given?
- Does he seem to understand and/or remember what is said to him?
- Does he respond to questions appropriately?
- How does he get along with other members of the family?
- How does he get along with peers in neighborhood?

Pediatricians should also focus upon the child's ability to attend to and complete tasks and might want to ask questions, such as:

- Can the child sit and watch a TV program without playing with something?
- Can he sit and complete homework?
- Can he sit through a meal?
- Can he sit through reading a story or being read to?
- Can he play board games and take turns?

Parents should be encouraged to describe the child's strengths, weaknesses, and areas of interest.

Information from School

Pediatricians will find that information from the child's teacher is an indispensable part of the assessment. Sometimes, a teacher's report differs greatly from that of the parents, who may exaggerate a problem or have unrealistic expectations or may not be paying enough attention to their child's difficulties or deny them altogether. Similar input from both parents and teacher serves to corroborate a learning disability. School contact may be done on an informal basis, such as a phone call, or through a written report from the teacher (Fig. 1.) Information about a child's functioning at school should include his level of achievement in reading, writing, arithmetic, and other subject areas in comparison with the teacher's expectations for him. Of interest is the teacher's appraisal of the child's language comprehension and usage and fine and gross motor coordination compared to those of his peers. Teachers should be asked if the child is aggressive, hyperactive, disobedient, nervous, shy, impulsive, or distractible in the classroom. Behavior in recess and social behavior are also significant areas to investigate. Other questions that a pediatrician could ask a teacher are:

SCHOOL REPORT

Date: _____________

Child's Name: _____________________________________ DOB: _____________________

School: _________________________________ Present Class Placement: _______________

Regular (Grade) ___________________ Slow _______________ Special (Name) _______________

  I. Attendance: Full-Day ______ Half-Day ______

                  Good ______ Fair ______ Poor ______

 II. Academic Achievement:

    A. Please indicate competency in each of these areas

	GRADE EQUIV.	RATING					COMMENTS
		EXCELLENT	GOOD	FAIR	POOR	UNSATISFACTORY	
Word Recognition Skills							
Reading Comprehension							
Numerical Skills							
Spelling							
Writing							
Others							

Figure 1. School Report.

B. Overall Academic Achievement: Better than expected _____
About what was expected _____ Less than expected _____

C. Suggestion of perceptual problems? Yes _____ No _____
If yes, what? ____

III. Speech and Language:

a. Is child bilingual? _____ Is second language better than English? _____

b. Speech: Unintelligible _____ Difficult to understand _____
Some articulation errors _____ Normal _____
Comments: ____

c. Comprehension: Does child appear to understand what is said to him? _____
Comments: ____

d. Language: Does child use complete sentences? _____ Age appropriate vocabulary? _____

e. Hearing: Suspicion of hearing loss? _____
What makes you suspicious? _____________________________________

f. Coordination: Rate Fine Motor: Excellent _____ Good _____ Fair _____
Poor _____ Very Poor _____
Rate Gross Motor: Excellent _____ Good _____ Fair _____
Poor _____ Very Poor _____

IV. Behavior: (Check all appropriate descriptions)

a. Aggressive _____ Hyperactive _____ Nervous _____ Shy _____ Uncontrollable _____
Quiet _____ Disobedient _____ "In a world of his own" _____ Sad _____ Impulsive _____
Fearful _____ Talkative _____ Angry _____ Slow _____ Happy _____ Persevering _____
Hypoactive _____ Other (specify) ___________________________________

b. Please describe any instances of deviant behavior: ____

V. Peer Relationships: check appropriate descriptions
Initiates contact _____ Disinterested in other children _____ Provokes other children _____
Disliked by other children _____ Mixes in the group _____ Has friends _____
Plays with younger/smaller children _____ Comments: _______________________________

VI. Has child been referred for special services? If yes, specify _____
Special Educational Services Received:

Current	In the past	Speech therapy
Remedial reading		Perceptual training
Other		

VII. Proposed school placement (for next semester) (Indicate grade and type of class): _____________

VIII. Comments:

a. What makes this child "different" from others in the classroom?

b. Do you feel this child needs special educational facilities?

c. Other comments: (Please feel free to elaborate on any of the above points or to make any other comments.)

Signature ____________________________________ Title ___________________________________
Thank you for your cooperation.

- How well does the child relate to others in the class?
- How well does he relate to peers outside of the class group?
- Does he have friends, or is he disliked by children his own age?
- Does he play with younger children, as a rule?
- Does the teacher feel that the child is different from other children in the classroom; if so, in what ways?
- Are there special services in the school that may be available for the child?

With this information, along with that obtained from the parent, the pediatrician is in a better position to appraise if the child has a serious learning problem and can also judge if the parent's and the school's expectations for the child are realistic.

EXAMINATION OF THE CHILD

The pediatrician's examination of a child with school failure includes not only an evaluation of the child's physical health but also an assessment of his emotional status, academic achievement, and underlying skills and abilities. This comprehensive evaluation, the components of which are the interview, the physical and neurologic evaluation, and the developmental assessment, enable the pediatrician to integrate and reconcile information received from the parent and teacher with his own impressions of the child. It also helps to clarify any diagnostic issues that are outstanding.

Interview

An interview can reveal much about the actual experiences a child is undergoing in school, such as how he perceives his teacher, peers, or work. Often a child reports traumatic or embarrassing experiences or insults from peers that color his attitude about school and his capabilities and achievement. Sometimes the interview reveals a child's unrealistic expectations or fears, immature or inappropriate behavior, or faulty judgment. Finally, the pediatrician can assess how school failure has affected the child's sense of himself and his ability to relate to others.

Questions one can ask the child include:

- Are you having any trouble at school? at home?
- What kind?
- When did it start?
- Do you know why you are having this problem?
- How do you feel about it?
- How do you feel about school? about your teacher?
- How do you feel about family? school friends? neighborhood friends?
- What do you like about school? What is the best thing about it?
- What is the worst thing about it?
- What are your special interests? hobbies?

Observation of the child's behavior during interview and testing is an essential part of the examination. Behaviors to be observed include:

- Concentration, attention
- Distractability, fidgetiness
- Cooperation
- Mannerisms
- Perseverance
- Impulsivity
- Orientation in space

Physical and Neurologic Evaluation

A complete physical examination is part of the evaluation of a child with learning problems. Though the actual yield of positive finding is low, a search for sensory impairment, underlying medical problems, or physical factors must be performed.

Extensive description of the physical or neurologic examination is beyond the scope of this chapter. Application of principles of physical examination, with emphasis on physical measurement and major or minor stigmata, is of importance. Appropriate laboratory testing when indicated is part of the medical screening.

The neurologic examination in most children with school failure is expected to be normal. However, on rare occasions, it will uncover localized central nervous system deficits. Subtle neurologic findings may be the first indication of progressive neurologic disease.

The neurologic examination has two parts: the standard neurologic examination and the examination for soft signs. The standard examination includes the usual techniques for the evaluation of gait, cranial nerves, cerebellar functions, muscle tone, symmetry of movement, deep tendon reflexes, and sensory function.

A more controversial aspect of the neurologic assessment is the examination for soft signs. The value of this examination is often overemphasized as the main aspect of the pediatrician's contribution to the assessment of school failure. Positive soft signs were at one time considered the diagnostic hallmark of the learning disabled child. School systems unfortunately still look for positive neurologic signs to label children as having an organic disorder as a criterion for the provision of service.

Since many of the items tested on the examination of soft signs are age related, information regarding neurologic maturity as well as development of motor skills can be obtained during this examination. Aspects of this assessment include testing in the areas of gross and fine motor performance as well as corticosensory function. Specific tests used may include the following.

Gross Motor Coordination.

- Ball playing
- Standing on one foot: left foot, right foot
- Broad jump

- Hopping: left foot, right foot
- Tandem gait: forward, backward
- Heel walking
- Toe walking

Fine Motor Skills and Observations of Motor Impersistence.

- Opposition of thumb to forefinger: right hand, left hand
- Serial opposition of thumb to alternate fingers: right hand, left hand
- Diadochokinesis: right hand, left hand
- Squeezing: right hand, left hand
- Prechtl (standing with feet together and hands stretched out)
- Oromotor coordination (stability of tongue movements)

Corticosensory Function.

- Double simultaneous stimulation: ipsilateral; right, left; contralateral
- Position sense: right side, left side
- Graphesthesia: right side, left side
- Stereognosis: right side, left side
- Finger agnosia: right side, left side (used to test child's ability to perceive and be aware of finger position without visual cues)

Right/Left Awareness.

- On self
- On examiner

It is important to understand that an isolated poor performance on any of the above tests has little meaning. Many students with normal academic achievement show positive findings, and students with significant learning difficulty may be normal. The presence of multiple signs in a particular patient may be helpful in the diagnosis.

Developmental Assessment of School-related Skills. In the developmental assessment of school-related skills, the pediatrician

observes and appraises some of the abilities and skills related to and reflective of school achievement, such as a child's competency in language, visual perceptual and visual motor development, memory, reading, mathematics, and social adaptive behavior. If a child shows deficiencies in more than one of these areas, there is a strong probability that he has a learning disability. Conversely, if his performance is uniformly at or above age level, failure in school more likely is related to motivational or attitudinal factors or unrealistic expectations on the part of the family or school staff.

Language. Through informal observation of a child's responses to questions and his spontaneous speech, the pediatrician gains insight into a child's comprehension and use of language. He is able to judge how well a child understands verbal information and whether his responses are appropriate. Answering "What?" to every question posed, irrelevant answers, and extreme confusion between similar words, such as "who," "what," "where," "when," and "why," may indicate that the child has a problem in comprehension. Expressive language difficulties include faulty pronunciation of sounds and words, dysfluent speech, and overuse of gestures. The content, quality, and organization of verbal output can be assessed by analyzing a child's language, as follows:

- Are responses concrete, functional, or abstract? Is an orange described by a child over 8 years of age as "something round" rather than "something to eat" or "a fruit?"
- Are responses tangential or to the point?
- Are there word-finding or word-naming difficulties? (Instead of saying the word "cup," a child can only say, "you know the thing we drink with.")
- Are there excessive grammatical or sequencing errors ("I wants to come," or "pasgetti" for "spaghetti").

- Is the organization of a sentence or of a more extended speech sample disorganized or difficult to follow?

Table 2 provides a brief sample of language milestones selected from published sources of normative data for ages 4 through 10 years. These milestones reflect concept formation and general information as well.

Visual-Perceptual and Visual-Motor Development. Visual perception refers to the organization and interpretation of visual information, and visual motor functioning refers to the integration of visual perception and motor movements. Both play an important role in the acquisition of reading, writing, and mathematical skills, especially in the early grades. Difficulty with using scissors or coloring within the lines or recognizing the alphabet letters may be early signs of problems in this area of development. Confusion of similar looking letters or words or problems with handwriting may be noted in the early grades.

Table 2 provides a sample of a developmental sequence of visual-perceptual and visual-motor performance. The tasks are primarily visual-motor in nature, with the assumption that poor performance suggests problems in both areas. Two widely used measures of these abilities are the copying of geometric figures and the drawing of a human figure. The latter task is also a global measure of mental maturity through a child's perception of body concepts.

Memory. Short-term memory deficits frequently are found in children with school learning problems. They forget instructions, seem bewildered or overwhelmed by a series of statements or directions given by their teacher, have difficulty remembering the order of words and letters within a word in both reading and spelling, and have problems remembering numerical facts.

TABLE 2. DEVELOPMENTAL ASSESSMENT OF SCHOOL-RELATED SKILLS

Age and Grade	Language	Visual Perceptual/ Visual Motor Development	Memory	Reading	Mathematics	Social Adaptive Behavior
4 years	Answers: "What do we do with our eyes?" Answers: "What do we do with our ears?" Tells what to do if sleepy, hungry, cold Names 4 colors Defines (by use): fork, horse, table, pencil, chair	Draws a person with 4–6 items including head, arms, legs, eyes Copies a cross	Repeats: 3 digits (said at 1-second intervals) Repeats: "We are going to buy some candy." Carries out 3 commission commands			Buttons coat or dress Washes hands unaided Plays cooperatively
5 years Kindergarten	Defines (by use): ball, hat, stove Understands most of these concepts by pointing to pictures or objects showing them: forward, first, center, widest, whole, nearest, beginning	Copies a square Draws a person with 6–8 items including the above, plus some of the following: nose, mouth, body, legs, hair, hands, and feet	Repeats: 4 digits Repeats: "Jane wants to build a big castle in her playhouse."	Prints first name Recites alphabet in order Recognizes and prints letters Reads few simple words: *stop, see, dog*	Concept of ½ Counts 1–10 Identifies and names: penny, nickel, dime	Dresses self except tying Uses pencil or crayon for drawing Plays games like jump rope, marbles, or tag
6 years First grade	Pronunciation and grammar almost without error Defines: orange, envelope, straw, puddle Answers: "How are a bird and a dog different?" Answers: "How are a slipper and a boot different?" Completes sentence: "A bird flies, a fish ______."	Copies a triangle Draws a person with 8–10 items including the above plus fingers and two dimensional arms and legs	Repeats: "Tom has lots of fun playing with his sister."	Reads these monosyllable words: *cat, was, him, work* Compound words: *basketball, household* Gives initial consonant sounds Short vowels (end 1st grade) Can read and talk about the following story: A little boy had a dog. It was brown. The dog ran down the street.	Simple addition and subtraction Counts 1–20 Tells time by hours Gives value of penny, nickel, dime	Plays simple table games like checkers Uses skates, sled, or wagon Is trusted with money

(continued)

TABLE 2 (*Continued*)

Age and Grade	Language	Visual Perceptual/ Visual Motor Development	Memory	Reading	Mathematics	Social Adaptive Behavior
7 years Second grade	Defines: balloon, tiger, football Answers: "How are an apple and peach alike?" Answers: "How are a ship and automobile alike?"	Prints letters legibly Copies a diamond Ties shoelaces Draws a person with 10–14 items including the above plus some of the following: arms down, neck, eyebrows, clothing (1–2 items)	Repeats: 5 digits Repeats: "Mama asked Nancy to bring the brown dog in the house."	Reads: *deep, even, spell, awake* Short vowels, silent e Vowel combinations Can read and talk about the following story: My Daddy took me out in the country to see a large farm. I saw some sheep, a donkey, a horse, and a mother pig with four babies.	Counts by 2s Counts to 100 Tells time by ½ hour Adds and subtracts 2-digit numbers without regrouping	Goes to bed unassisted Uses table knife for spreading Uses pencil for writing
8 years Third grade	Answers: "How are a baseball and orange similar and different?" Answers: "How are an airplane and kite similar and different?" Names: days of week in order Defines: 4 of the following words: tap, gown, roar, eyelash, Mars, juggler	Writes letters and words in script Draws a person with 14–16 items including the above plus some of the following: ears and clothing (2–3 items) Copies:	Repeats: 3 digits in reversed order Repeats: "Fred asked his father to take him to see the clowns in the circus."	Reads: *felt, stalk, cliff, lame, struck* Reads orally 2-syllable words: *finger, weather* Can read and talk about the following story: Once there was a cat named "Tiger." His fur was yellow with black stripes. He liked to chase mice. His favorite food was milk. If he saw a dog, he would climb a tree and jump on top of the house.	Counts by 5s and 10s Complex addition, subtraction, simple multiplication Tells time to quarter hour	Tells time to quarter hour Combs or brushes hair Participates in pre-adolescent play

9 years Fourth grade	Describes absurdity in these sentences: Bill Jones' feet are so big that he has to pull his trousers over his head. The fireman hurried to the burning house, got his fire hose ready, and after smoking a cigar put out the fire.	Draws a person with 14–20 items, including some of the following: 5 fingers and shoulders Copies:	Repeats: 6 digits forward Repeats: 4 digits in reverse order Repeats: "Bill has made a beautiful boat out of wood with his sharp knife."	Reads: *imply, humidity, urge, approve* Recognizes: 3–4 syllable words, *quality* Alphabetizes Can read and talk about the following story: On June 15, 1836, Arkansas became the 25th state to join the United States of America. Arkansas took its name from a tribe of Indians. The name means "people who live downstream." The rich soil of Arkansas produces rice, cotton, soybeans, peaches, strawberries, and lots of trees.	Simple division Two-digit multiplication Adds and subtracts fractions with common denominator	Uses tools or utensils Does routine household tasks Bathes self unaided
10 years Fifth grade	Answers two of the following questions: What is pity? curiosity? grief? surprise?	Draws a person with 20+ items, including ears, nostrils, two dimensional lips, elbows, knees	Repeats: "Mama brought Susie a chocolate ice cream cone after the movie yesterday."	Reads: *abuse, collapse, exhaust, bulk* Can read and talk about the following story: The helicopter is a most unusual aircraft. It can rise straight up, descend straight down, fly forward, or fly backward. It can also fly very slowly and even remain in one place while still in midair. These special flying features of the helicopter make it valuable in search and rescue missions, as it has the ability to take off and land in a small amount of space. Helicopters are also used for fire and police patrols, crop dusting, and for passenger transportation. They range in size from one person models to those which can carry more than fifty people.	Division with remainders Adds, subtracts, and multiplies with decimals	Makes minor purchases Writes occasional short letters Makes telephone calls

A widely used method of appraising memory is the presentation of an increasingly longer series of numbers and/or a series of sentences increasing in length and complexity. While factors, such as anxiety, inattentiveness, and lack of motivation, may affect a child's performance, the results give an estimate of a child's ability to retain auditory information or instructions. See Table 2 for memory milestones.

Reading. Through the screening of a child's reading skills, the pediatrician can obtain information about a child's ability to recognize and pronounce individual words and to comprehend what he has read. A child must be competent in both these areas in order to be considered an efficient and thoughtful reader. Identification of words requires the adequate perception of word configurations and the understanding of letter/sound relationships. Some words must be within the child's vocabulary in order to be pronounced correctly. Reading comprehension, a more complex task than word recognition, requires, at the minimum, underlying abilities in language, memory, vocabulary concepts, and sequential thinking, in addition to sustained attention and motivation. Table 2 provides sample words and short paragraphs appropriate for children at different grade levels.

Mathematics. Not all learning disabled children have difficulties with mathematics. Indeed, some children with reading disabilities have an excellent concept of numbers. However, other children who are experiencing school failure are deficient in a variety of mathematical skills, including number order, computation, and the understanding of concepts related to time, space, size, and money. See Table 2 for a sample of graded mathematical problems.

Social Adaptive Behavior. Under the umbrella of learning is included the learning of social competence. Children show a progressive capacity in social development, which results in independence in adulthood. Often, children with school learning difficulties have difficulties in various aspects of social adaptive behavior, leading to alienation from their peers and resulting in isolation and loneliness. See Table 2 for guidelines in obtaining a rough estimate of a child's social adaptive development.

DIFFERENTIAL DIAGNOSIS

Although this chapter has focused upon learning disabilities, there are other conditions and situations causing school failure that the pediatrician must explore. The pediatrician's referral to other specialists, recommendations regarding educational programs and classroom management, and the kind of suggestions for counseling given to parents all depend upon his ability to make a correct diagnosis. The most frequent causes for school failure, described below, are not mutually exclusive and can occur in any combination. In most cases, a pediatrician can make a diagnosis with the information obtained through the interview of the parent, examination of the child, and the school report.

Specific Learning Disabilities

Specific learning disabilities are characterized by deficits in the acquisition of reading, spelling, writing, or arithmetic skills in children of near average, average, or above average intelligence. Deficits in memory, language comprehension, and perceptual motor abilities may also be present. The learning disability may be accompanied by disorders of attention, perseverance, impulsivity, or equivocal neurologic soft signs.

Parents usually report that their child has a history of school failure. Upon questioning, they may remember delayed language milestones or excessive clumsiness and poor fine motor coordination. They may describe reversals in letter writing and confusion with similar looking or similar sounding words.

The school may note areas of specific academic weaknesses in contrast, for example, to strengths in abstract reasoning, good listening skills, or expressive language. Behavior may be variable, but often a child is described as immature, unable to do independent work, and poorly organized.

The examination reveals substantial deficits in reading, writing, or spelling in a child who may seem otherwise unimpaired. The child may show gaps in general information, i.e., he may not be able to tell time, make change, recall the months of the year, or name the state in which he lives. Low self-esteem and a negative self-image may be evident.

Attentional Deficit Disorder

Attentional deficit disorder is characterized by (1) signs of inattention that are developmentally inappropriate for age and (2) impulsivity with or without hyperactivity appearing in a child before the age of 7. Children with attentional deficit disorders who may be otherwise bright, with good language and perceptual abilities, may be unable to focus on school tasks because of an attentional deficit disorder.

While parents may refer to their child's learning and behavioral difficulties in school, upon questioning they answer that their child does not listen, is easily distracted, shows poor concentration with schoolwork, and has difficulty sticking to any type of activity. They also report that their child acts before thinking, is not able to stay on a task for any length of time, and shows excessive difficulty organizing homework. He is described as having difficulty sitting still or of fidgeting excessively. Parents sometimes describe a child like this as "driven by a motor." The onset, duration, and degree of this disorder can be obtained in an interview with the parents and in a report from the school. Manifestations of this disorder are evident upon observation of the child.

Borderline Intelligence and Mild Mental Retardation

Children with borderline intelligence (IQ 80–85) or with mild retardation (IQ 50–75) have deficits in cognitive ability and in adaptive behavior. Children who show more than mild retardation usually are identified by the school personnel as soon as they enter school, and they are placed in special classes according to their intellectual capabilities. Borderline or mildly retarded children tend to show relatively poor functioning in almost all areas. If these children are quiet and well-behaved and if they are personable and well-dressed, they can go unrecognized for years in school and may be misdiagnosed as underachieving, lazy, or unmotivated students. If they show inappropriate behavior, they are often thought to be emotionally disturbed. By interviewing the parents of such a child, the pediatrician almost always finds out that developmental milestones, especially in the area of language, were delayed. Usually, language milestones are more delayed than those pertaining to motor development. The child often is reported to play with younger children. The child displays a short attention span, poor memory, and difficulty expressing or understanding even simple concepts. He may need to have directions repeated. Parents report that he was late in learning letters and numbers. A school report may provide information that the child has difficulty in just about every aspect of school learning. Immature behavior may also be noted. Examination of the child reveals inappropriate behavior or behavior like that of a child much younger than is appropriate and skills and abilities uniformly well below average for age.

Primary Emotional Disturbance

This chapter cannot detail the many kinds of emotional difficulties that children may have. Often, children with primary emotional disturbance appear self-involved, unresponsive to a teacher, or inappropriate with other children. They may be extremely anxious, unduly depressed, or angry with little external explanation. They may show manneristic behavior and extreme withdrawal and rapidly changing moods. Behavior may range from their total withdrawal to acting out. Sometimes, it is hard to distinguish between a primary emotional disturbance and a reaction to frustration in learning because of a learning disability.

Parents may report a long-standing history of strange, inappropriate behavior. The school report corroborates inappropriate behavior. Examination of the child reveals strange affect, poor eye contact, inability to relate to the examiner, overfriendliness, or loose ideation, in the absence of specific perceptual, cognitive, or vocabulary deficits.

Developmental Expressive or Receptive Language Disorders

A developmental language disorder is the lack of development of appropriate vocal expression or comprehension of vocal expression despite relatively intact inner language. Children with this problem may be misdiagnosed as hearing impaired, mentally retarded, emotionally disturbed, or learning disabled. The child has extreme difficulties or delay in acquiring language. The school report notes that the child does not seem to understand what is being said or has little to say. Examination of the child reveals a paucity of language and poor verbal comprehension.

Other Conditions Impeding School Learning

The pediatrician must be sure to rule out visual and hearing problems, as undetected sensory impairments seriously impede learning. Extensive absence from school and frequent change in schools can account for a large gap in learning, lack of motivation, and poor school behavior. Extreme cultural deprivation is one of the most common causes of poor academic achievement in inner city children. Through understimulation during their preschool years, children with inherent abilities may be lacking in basic concepts, vocabulary, and a constructive attitude toward school. This can be detected in the interview with the parents by asking questions about home activities, family routine, and how children spend their waking hours. The pediatrician's impression of the parents' intelligence, concern for and understanding of their children, and availability can help in formulating this diagnosis. The school report may reflect poor motivation, inappropriate behavior, and poor skills on the part of the child and lack of contact and inappropriate interactions with parents. Examination of the child reveals whether there is adequate cognition, perception, or memory. In most cases, cultural deprivation alone does not account for a serious learning problem.

Follow-up Services

Even when the pediatrician has made the diagnosis, additional evaluations by specialists in psychology, special education, speech and language, and psychiatry may be needed in order to substantiate a disability and to help the child receive needed services. Usually, a school requires the documentation of a child's intellectual ability, academic achievement, language functioning, and emotional status in order to provide special services. Moreover, the specialists often can shed new light on the child's difficulties and can recommend specific strategies of intervention. Table 3 gives guidelines for follow-up services based on the differential diagnosis.

ONGOING ROLE OF PEDIATRICIAN

Despite referrals to various specialists, the pediatrician should continue to play a central role in the management of the child. Copies of all evaluations should be requested so that his records are complete. In subsequent vis-

TABLE 3. GUIDELINES FOR FOLLOW-UP SERVICES

Differential Diagnosis	Additional Evaluations	Treatment
Specific learning disability	Psychologic testing	Learning disabilities class or ancillary remedial services
Attentional deficit disorder		Behavioral modification program Trial of medication Child management strategies
Borderline mental retardation	Psychologic testing	Special education class
Primary emotional disturbance	Psychiatric evaluation	Psychotherapy
Developmental expressive or receptive language disorders	Speech and language evaluation	Special class placement Language therapy

its, the status of a child's achievement should be monitored to assess progress. This means that the pediatrician contacts the school personnel on an annual basis through a written form to the teacher or through telephone contacts, requesting information about academic achievement and behavior. Following a child with school learning difficulties requires a yearly reappraisal to see if current services continue to be appropriate and if new services should be added.

School learning difficulties often follow children into adulthood. Children with these problems need continuous support in coping with and adapting to their learning problems.

BIBLIOGRAPHY

Benton A, Pearl D (eds): Dyslexia, An Appraisal of Current Knowledge. New York, Oxford, 1978

Culbertson J, Ferry P: Learning disabilities. Pediatr Clin North Am 29:121, 1982

Denckla M: Minimal brain dysfunction and dyslexia: beyond diagnosis by exclusion. In Blaw M, Rapin I, Kinsbourne M (eds): Topics in Child Neurology. New York, Spectrum, 1977, pp 243–261

Duane D, Rome P: The Dyslexic Child. New York, Insight Publishing, 1981

Farnham-Diggory: Learning Disabilities, A Psychological Perspective. Cambridge, Mass, Harvard Univ Press, 1978

Kinsbourne M: School problems. Pediatrics 52:697, 1973

Knobloch H, Pasamanick B (eds): Gesell and Amatruda's Developmental Diagnosis, 3rd ed. New York, Harper & Row, 1974

Levine M, Brooks R, Shonkoff J: A Pediatric Approach to Learning Disorders. New York, Wiley, 1980

Levine M, Busch B, Aufseeser C: The dimension of inattention among children with school problems. Pediatrics 70:387, 1982

Lerer R, Lerer M: The effects of methylphenidate on the soft neurological signs of hyperactive children. Pediatrics 57:521, 1976

Louick D, Boland T: Psychologic tests: a guide for pediatricians. Pediatr Ann 7:12, 849, 1978

Rapin I: Children with Brain Dysfunction. New York, Raven, 1982

Smith S: No Easy Answers—The Learning Disabled Child. Superintendent of Documents, US Government Printing Office, Washington, DC 20402. DHEW Publication No (ADM) 79-825, June 1979

Wender EH: Learning disabilities in children. Pediatr Rev 3:91, 1981

Cross-Reference to *Pediatrics,* 17th ed.

TWENTY-SEVEN

Approach to the Child with Abnormal Stature

Paul Saenger

Abnormal statural growth is a subject pediatricians and endocrinologists alike confront with great frequency. Boys generally aspire to be taller, and girls frequently desire not to be too tall. Happily, in most instances, reassurance of the parent and the child is all that is necessary.

Before proceeding to a discussion of abnormal growth, a brief review of the physiologic mechanisms of normal growth is presented.

PHYSIOLOGIC MECHANISMS OF NORMAL GROWTH

Intrauterine Growth

Intrauterine growth is influenced by:

- Placental function
- Uterine crowding and/or constraints
- Maternal size
- Maternal ingestion of drugs (e.g., ethanol, nicotine, hydantoins)

Peak intrauterine growth velocity occurs at approximately 4 months of gestation. Size at birth appears to be dependent more on maternal than on genetic factors.

Several exogenous agents, such as ethanol, nicotine, hydantoins, and warfarin, may alter fetal growth. It is important to note that catch-up growth is usually not observed in the fetal hypoplastic syndromes due to these exogenous agents.

Hormonal regulators of *fetal growth* include insulin, thyroid hormones, and local tissue growth factors. The contribution of somatomedin to fetal growth is less clear, although to some extent somatomedin does correlate with fetal length and weight. The somatomedins, a family of polypeptides with structural homology to proinsulin, are all potent stimulators of cell proliferation. There is evidence that growth hormone stimulates somatomedin synthesis. Though predominantly synthesized in the liver, they are synthesized by multiple tissues in the fetus. However, children with hypopituitary dwarfism and children with Laron type dwarfism (a form of dwarfism probably caused by deficient somatomedin generation) have a nearly normal length and weight at birth, suggesting that growth hormone is relatively unimportant in utero. Thus, if somatomedins are important for fetal growth, their regulation in utero may depend less on growth hormone than on nutrition and insulin, two factors generally considered of paramount importance for fetal growth and development. The interrelationship between growth hormone and somatomedin is discussed under Hormonal Regulation of Normal Growth.

Postnatal Growth

The growth pattern of the infant shifts from a growth rate predominantly determined by maternal factors to one that is related to its own genetic background, as reflected by midparental size. Indeed, stature is one of the most heritable traits recognized in man; the coefficient of correlation for stature in monozygous twins is 0.95. The growth of the male infant for the first 6 months after birth is slightly faster than that of the female. Thereafter, there is no sex difference until the advent of adolescence. The early acceleration of male growth may be due to the transient increase in testosterone secretion in male newborn infants, which may last up to 200 days.

The shifting of the rate of linear growth from, say, the 75th percentile to the 10th percentile in some children or the reverse in others is a frequent and normal variant during the first 2 years of life. After age 2, there is a tendency for each child to follow the same percentile of the growth curve. Deviations may signal a pathologic process interfering with growth and should be investigated.

After rapid growth during infancy, both boys and girls grow between 6 and 8 cm/year (growth velocity) from 2–5 years of age. After 5 years of age and up to the beginning of rapid adolescent growth, both sexes grow at a rate of 4 to 8 cm per year.

Puberty is accompanied by a rapid increase in growth velocity. In the female, the growth spurt occurs relatively early in the sequence of pubertal events; in the male, it occurs about 2 years later. At the onset of the pubertal growth spurt, boys are on the average 10 cm taller than girls at the corresponding developmental stage. Thus, the difference in average stature between men and women is due both to the longer period of preadolescent growth in boys and their more intense and longer pubertal growth period (Fig. 1).

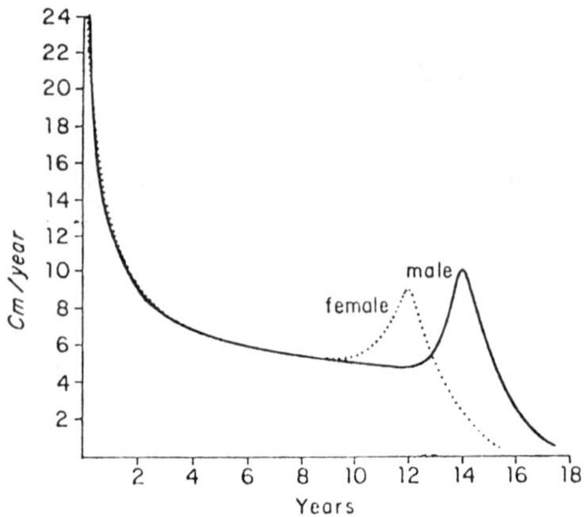

Figure 1. Individual velocity curves for length and height in males and females. Note the comparable deceleration in the rate of growth from infancy until the onset of adolescence. (*Adapted from Tanner JM, Whitehouse RH: Arch Dis Child 41:613, 1966.*)

Growth Curves and Body Proportions

The Iowa and Boston growth curves, still much in use, are 40 years old. The National Center for Health Statistics has published contemporary standard growth curves based on American children. Growth curves correcting for parental height have been developed by Tanner and have been reproduced by Smith. During periods of stable growth (2 to 9 years of age), these curves should be used in all children with abnormal stature.

Determination of body proportions provides additional information that is useful in classifying children with abnormal growth. Most widely used is the ratio of upper segment to lower segment (upper segment, crown to pubis; lower segment, pubis to heel). At birth, the upper/lower ratio is 1.7; it reaches 1.0 at 7–10 years and reaches 0.95 in adulthood. Blacks have relatively long limbs and reach an upper/lower ratio of 0.85. Another anthropometric index is arm span, which is usually within a few centimeters of total height. Short patients with primary disorders of the bone and cartilage or long-standing hypothyroidism have relatively disproportionately short extremities. Short children with nonendocrine disorders and children with growth hormone deficiency, constitutional delay in growth and adolescence, familial short stature, intrauterine growth retardation, and psychosocial dwarfism are normally proportioned. Patients with growth hormone excess and constitutional tall stature are also normally proportioned. Long extremities are seen in hypogonadal tall stature (e.g., Klinefelter's syndrome) and other rare disorders, such as Marfan's syndrome and homocystinuria.

Another useful reference point is the height age, the age at which the child's height corresponds to the 50th percentile.

Bone Age

Determination of the level of epiphyseal maturation or bone age is a most helpful aid in evaluating a child with abnormal stature, although a delayed bone age does not provide specific diagnostic information. Standards for both hand and wrist and knees are available. At minimal radiation dosage, this x-ray provides information on 30 bones or about 10% of those in the entire skeleton.

A number of methods have been derived to predict adult height based on height age and bone age. These predictions cannot take fully into account the pubertal growth spurt and are, therefore, at best an estimate. They are of great assistance, however, in reassuring normal, slowly maturing children. Estimate of adult height is also very important in the evaluation of a child with constitutional tall stature.

A delayed bone age (> 2 SD) is commonly seen in all of the endocrine disorders that cause short stature. The bone age is also retarded in constitutional delay, intrauterine growth retardation, and psychosocial dwarf-

ism. The bone age is usually normal in genetic or familial short stature.

HORMONAL REGULATION OF NORMAL GROWTH

Classic growth regulators include growth hormone, somatomedin, insulin, and thyroxin.

Growth hormone, insulin, and thyroxin have a major positive influence on growth rate, and corticosteroids have a major negative influence. Parathyroid hormone and vitamin D and its metabolites affect skeletal development and ossification. Gonadal and adrenal steroids are of particular importance in skeletal maturation and the pubertal growth spurt. Patients with isolated growth hormone deficiency undergo a blunted pubertal growth spurt and fuse their epiphyses eventually. Growth hormone and sex steroids probably act synergistically in normal puberty.

Growth Hormone

Pituitary growth hormone (GH) is the major stimulus for normal growth. Secretion of growth hormone is regulated by the interaction of two hypothalamic hormones, growth hormone releasing factor (GRF) and somatostatin. GRF has not been characterized in man. Somatostatin inhibits the secretion not only of growth hormone but of many pituitary, pancreatic, and parathyroid hormones.

Physiologic stimuli for growth hormone release are intake of food, strenuous exercise, and early sleep with a slow EEG pattern. The secretion of human growth hormone is enhanced by sex hormones. Ambulatory levels of growth hormone are higher in adult females than in males and may be increased by estrogen priming. Androgens also sensitize growth hormone releasing mechanisms.

Inhibition of growth hormone secretion occurs during hyperglycemia, in obesity, after prior stress-induced growth hormone secretion, with excessive glucocorticoids or inadequate levels of thyroid hormone, and in psychosocial deprivation. Growth hormone is secreted episodically. In infancy and childhood, growth hormone is secreted in bursts during sleep; this secretory pattern is established by 3 months of age.

Growth hormone has profound effects upon the metabolism of protein, fats, carbohydrates, and minerals. Growth hormone, however, does not directly affect skeletal growth but acts through production of somatomedins.

Somatomedin

The somatomedins are a group of peptides synthesized predominantly in the liver but also in muscle and kidney under the influence of growth hormone. Somatomedins (A,B,C) differ in their physiochemical properties. Somatomedin A (SmA) is a neutral protein with a MW of 2,000 daltons, SmB is an acidic peptide of 5,000 daltons, and SmC is a basic protein with a MW of 8,000 (20). Purified somatomedins resemble proinsulin in aminoacid sequence but have limited cross-reactivity with insulin in binding to receptors. An RIA assay for SmC is now commercially available. In serum, the somatomedins circulate bound to proteins.

Unlike those of growth hormones, somatomedin levels remain fairly constant throughout the day. Measurement of somatomedin in a single blood sample, therefore, provides an integrated estimate of the functional growth hormone status. Levels are age dependent and are much lower in children below 6 years of age. There is a distinct increase in somatomedins in boys and girls during adolescence at a time when the maximum growth spurt occurs. Changing levels of carrier protein or altering end-organ sensitivity may explain these age-dependent changes. For example, somatomedin receptor sites in newborns are markedly increased. Somatomedin production is decreased by a number of factors, including malnutrition, glucocorticoids, estrogens, systemic illness, and cirrhotic liver disease. Growth hormone, prolactin, insulin, and perhaps also thyroxin increase somatomedins.

Dietary protein appears to be particularly important for the generation of somatomedins and their action on growth cartilage. Evidence is now emerging that nutritional status is one of the most important determinants of somatomedin concentration in the serum. Serum levels are low in patients with protein-calorie malnutrition, despite extremely high levels of growth hormone. Even in well-nourished individuals, acute fasting causes a decline in serum concentrations within a few days. Suboptimal nutritional status may be an important mechanism whereby the SmC concentration is reduced in children with a wide variety of chronic illnesses.

The role of somatomedins in growth is indicated largely by correlations between somatomedin and growth velocity in children receiving growth hormone therapy. It seems likely, but not certain, that much of the postnatal growth is due to stimulation of cartilage growth by somatomedins. It should be stressed that, to date, only circumstantial evidence has accrued that somatomedin is truly the sole mediator of skeletal growth, since only in vivo assays with rather crude somatomedin preparations have been carried out.

Thyroid Hormones

Thyroid hormones do not appear to play a significant role in the early growth and development of the human fetus, since even those infants with congenital aplasia of the thyroid gland are of normal size at birth. Bone age and CNS development are retarded, however in the presence of decreased thyroid hormone. The importance of thyroid hormone for normal postnatal somatic growth is exemplified by the severe growth failure that regularly accompanies thyroid hormone deficiency. Severe hypothyroidism causes nearly absolute growth arrest and the most pronounced retardation in bone age development.

Insulin

Insulin is certainly a stimulator of fetal growth, as evidenced by the oversized infants born to diabetic mothers. Postnatally, the role of insulin as a growth promoting hormone is far from clear. In otherwise normal children with exogenous obesity and in hyperphagic children following surgery for craniopharyngioma, insulin levels may be markedly increased. In some of these children, acceleration of linear growth occurs.

Glucocorticoid Excess

Glucocorticoid excess appears to inhibit growth at the level of the chondrocyte. Growth hormone secretion is normal or depressed; serum somatomedin C concentrations may be normal or low. After prolonged exposure to daily high-dose glucocorticoids, catch-up growth is often insufficient to normalize the patient's height. Administration of glucocorticoids in growing rats resulted in permanent, profound biochemical and structural changes in the cartilage.

SHORT STATURE

A child is considered small if his standing height is 2 SD or more below the mean for age. Growth velocity (cm/year) is another important measurement in the evalution of a child who has abnormal growth. A growth rate of less than 4 cm/year at any time during the growth period is abnormal.

Since height measurements are obviously very important in the evaluation, these measurements (recumbent length up to 2 years of age, standing height in older children) should be obtained with the utmost accuracy.

Etiology and Differential Diagnosis

Normal Variants of Growth: Constitutional Delay in Growth and Adolescence and Familial Short Stature. The most frequent growth problem encountered by the pediatrician is that of an otherwise normal child with a steady, normal growth velocity who grows steadily below the 3rd percentile. Bone age is retarded but is consistent with height age. There is usually a strong family history of constitutional delay. Parent adjusted height may be abnormal. Final stature is within normal limits. These subjects are frequently delayed in growth at age 5 or 6. (See Table 1.)

By definition, puberty is delayed if there is a lack of testicular enlargement by age 14 or if there is no breast budding by the age of 13 years in girls (> 2.5 SD). By age 14, 1 of every 160 normal boys, and, by age 13, 1 of every 160 normal girls, do not exhibit any signs of puberty. Lack of progression through the stages of puberty, even if the onset is normal, may also require evaluation. A boy who has not completed secondary sexual maturation within 4–5 years after onset of puberty or a girl who does not menstruate within 5 years after onset of puberty may have a hypothalamic, pituitary, or gonadal disease.

A presumptive diagnosis of constitutional delay in growth may be made if the history and the pattern of growth reveal a long-standing history of short stature but consistent growth (growth velocity ≥ 4 cm/year). The family history typically includes parents or siblings with delayed puberty. Physical examination should reveal a normal sense of smell and visual fields. Skull films are normal, and the bone age is delayed proportionate to height age.

In children with constitutional delay, as in those with premature puberty, the skeletal age correlates far better with the onset of the pubertal growth spurt and other events in pubertal development than do either chronologic age or attained height. A decrease in growth velocity occurs in some patients just prior to the appearance of secondary sexual characteristics.

LH and FSH levels are normal for bone age. Elevation of gonadotropins and sex steroids precedes pubertal development by several months. Thus, LH, FSH, estradiol, or testosterone measurements will aid in predicting the course of development. Gonadotropin-releasing hormone (GnRH) stimulation tests can be used to differentiate hypogonadotropic states from pubertal delay. In the latter, GnRH will produce a rise in LH and FSH but not in hypogonadotropic hypogonadism.

Constitutional delay in growth has to be differentiated from familial short stature. Patients in the latter category are short but are normal for their family. Their growth velocity is normal. Parent adjusted height is normal and is, therefore, of great help in reassuring the parents and the patient alike. It is presumed that their short stature is due to genetic influence. These patients have a normal bone age and no family history of pubertal delay. Their final stature is short. There is no therapy to increase the final stature and the use of human growth hormone cannot be recommended at this time for patients with familial short stature even with normal hormonal findings and a normal growth velocity (Table 1).

Emotional Deprivation Syndrome and Other Environmental Causes. In a review of 185 cases of children hospitalized with a diagnosis of failure to thrive, 50 were found to have evidence of emotional deprivation. Children with emotional deprivation dwarfism have a reversible type of hypopituitarism. While exposed to the noxious environment in the disturbed home, children do not grow, but when removed to another environment, e.g., the hospital, they show rapid catch-up growth with restitution of pituitary function. These children do not respond to growth hormone therapy. Diagnosis of this condition can be established only by moving the child temporarily from his environment and documenting height and weight gain. This is best done in a hospital setting, where accurate measurements of food intake and eventual weight and height gain can be documented. A substitute mother from the nursing staff should be assigned to the patient throughout the hospital stay.

A stay of 3 weeks is often necessary to either prove or disprove the diagnosis of emotional deprivation syndrome. Short stature in this syndrome is presumably due to a defect in the release of the hypothalamic-releasing hormones secondary to emotional deprivation, although in some children hormonal data are entirely normal.

TABLE 1. NORMAL VARIANTS OF GROWTH

Features	Familial Short Stature	Familial Slow Maturation
Onset of growth deficiency	Postnatal	Postnatal (early childhood)
Rate of maturation	Normal	Slow and delayed
Bone age	Equals chronologic age	Retarded, equals height age
Family history	Short stature	Slow maturation
Final stature	Short	Normal
Therapy to increase eventual stature	None	None

(Adapted from Smith DW: Growth and Its Disorders, 1977, p. 64. Courtesy of W. B. Saunders Co.)

Intrauterine Growth Retardation. Intrauterine growth retardation may occur as an isolated condition or in the context of a recognizable syndrome, e.g., Bloom syndrome, Russell-Silver dwarfism, Cornelia de Lange syndrome.

A variety of intrauterine insults, such as rubella, syphilis, toxoplasmosis, and cytomegalic inclusion disease, and the maternal consumption of teratogens, such as ethanol, nicotine, hydantoins, and warfarin, may also severely reduce growth.

The unifying aspect probably is a defect in cellular proliferation. Postnatally, these patients usually do not show catch-up growth, and their hormonal profile (growth hormone, thyroid hormone, somatomedin) is normal. Skeletal maturation is normal or only moderately delayed. They reach puberty at a normal time and become short adults. The pubertal growth spurt is often blunted. Growth hormone therapy at stardard doses is not beneficial.

Chronic Diseases. Chronic disease of a nonendocrine organ system that may cause short stature include:

- Nutritional disorders (gastrointestinal disease, especially inflammatory bowel disease, but also, obstruction and malabsorption)
- Pulmonary disease
- Congenital heart disease with or without cyanosis
- Renal disease (acidosis, rickets, uremia)
- Liver disease (glycogen storage disease, cirrhosis)
- Hematologic disease (thalassemia, sickle cell disease)
- Central nervous system disease
- Bone and cartilage disease (skeletal dysplasia, often resulting in disproportionate short stature)
- Metabolic disorders
- Immunodeficiency states

Secondary growth deficiency is associated with many chronic diseases. Chronic liver disease may impair somatomedin generation. Chronic renal failure may give rise to somatomedin inhibitors that interfere with its action. Malabsorption in gastrointestinal disease can cause poor growth, as does the chronic catabolic state characteristic of many systemic chronic diseases. Puberty is usually delayed due to the underlying disease. Correction of the underlying disorder is often followed by catch-up growth.

Chromosomal Anomalies. Patients with abnormal or monosomic X chromosomes show continued slow growth and a lack of a pubertal growth spurt. The mean final height in patients with gonadal dysgenesis is 144 cm (range 133–161 cm). Patients with mosaicism are significantly taller than patients with 45/XO karyotype. The parent-child relation still holds true for 45/XO Turner syndrome: the taller parents have the taller children with this disorder. Growth hormone levels and somatomedin levels are normal in these children. In contrast, the XXY and XYY syndromes are associated with tall stature.

Growth Hormone Deficiency. Growth hormone deficiencies caused by intracranial lesions are listed below.

- Congenital
    Pituitary dysgenesis
    Septo-optic dysplasia
    Cleft palate
    Single central incisor syndrome
- Acquired
    Neoplasia
    Craniopharyngioma
    Glioma of the optic chiasm
    Ectopic pinealoma
    Adenoma of the pituitary
    Hand-Schüller-Christian disease
    Trauma (perinatal, postnatal)
    Infection (e.g., meningitis)
    Radiation therapy to the head and neck

Growth hormone deficiency may be idiopathic or organic (e.g., secondary to an intracranial lesion). Dysgenesis of the pituitary gland may occur as an isolated abnormality or in association with midline defects, such as cleft palate or the single central incisor syndrome.

Septo-optic dysplasia is a developmental defect characterized by an absent septum pellucidum and hypoplasia of the optic nerves and the optic chiasm. The optic foramen is often very small, and these patients may be blind. Gonadotropin secretion usually remains normal.

A number of tumors, listed above, may interfere with hypothalamic or pituitary function or both. In patients under 14 years of age, the most common intracranial tumor of nonglial origin is craniopharyngioma. Visual disturbances are more common presenting complaints than a fall in growth velocity. Removal of as much tumor as possible, with subsequent radiation therapy, is the treatment of choice. Total excision often cannot be achieved without putting the patient at risk for serious neurologic sequelae. Ten-year follow-up studies show that relapse is frequent. Careful endocrine follow-up studies are necessary following treatment to assess hypothalamic-pituitary function and to initiate appropriate hormonal replacement therapy. Although many children with carniopharyngioma grow poorly before surgery, normal or even catch-up growth has been observed following removal of the tumor. Postoperative growth is often associated with normal somatomedin, normal or increased insulin levels, hyperphagia, and progressive obesity. The patients should be carefully followed for temperature instability and essential hypernatremia with lack of an appropriate thirst mechanism.

Hand-Schüller-Christian disease is a chronic, disseminated reticuloendotheliosis that may involve the hypothalamus or the pituitary or both, leading to diabetes insipidus and growth hormone deficiency. On x-rays of the skull, lytic lesions of the bone are often present.

The increasing long-term survival of children who receive radiation therapy for tumors of the head and neck as well as for CNS sanctuary irradiation in leukemia has led to the recognition that such therapy may cause deficiency of growth hormone as well as other pituitary hormones. The effect on pituitary function may manifest itself only several years later.

In most children with hypopituitarism, no specific cause is immediately discernible. Review of the history reveals that in many cases perinatal insults (e.g. breech delivery) may precede hypopituitarism.

Battering in infancy may result in subdural hematomas, brain injury, and anterior hypopituitarism. The disorder may result from injury to the anterior pituitary itself, the pituitary stalk, or the hypothalamus. This suggests that all children with serious head injuries, regardless of cause, should have long-term observation for signs of impaired growth and hypopituitarism.

Idiopathic Growth Hormone Deficiency.

Autosomal recessive and X-linked recessive patterns of inheritance of GH deficiency have been described, although the great majority are sporadic. The prevalence of idiopathic growth hormone deficiency remains uncertain, since there is a considerable difference between the figures obtained, ranging from 1 in 30,000 to 1 in 5,000. It occurs more frequently in boys than in girls. The reasons for this discrepancy are not clear.

Idiopathic growth hormone deficiency may be isolated or may be associated with other hormone deficiencies. Hypopituitarism may thus become manifest in the newborn period. The infant is usually not small for age at this time. Hypoglycemia, seizures, micropenis, prolonged jaundice, and neonatal hepatitis may be presenting complaints. In older children, a progressive decrease in growth velocity is the most common finding, though hypoglycemia may also occur. Patients may have truncal obesity and a doll-like facial appearance, with marked frontal bossing and a depressed nasal bridge.

Growth hormone deficiency may be due to an abnormality at the level of the hypothalamus or the pituitary. There may be an abnormal neurotransmitter mechanism or impaired synthesis or secretion of growth hormone-releasing factors in the hypothalamus. At the pituitary level, there may be a receptor defect for growth hormone-releasing factors or deficient growth hormone synthesis (Table 2).

It appears now that release of an abnormal growth hormone molecule is a rare cause of dwarfism. In these patients, growth hormone is normal as measured by RIA, but it reacts weakly in the more discriminating radioreceptorassay (RRA). Somatomedin is low. Growth hormone therapy results in normal somatomedin generation. Some investigators have used the term "normal variant short stature" to describe this cohort of children. The term is, however, a misnomer, as the growth velocity of these patients is distinctly abnormal. These patients appear to secrete a biologically ineffective growth hormone and respond favorably to growth hormone therapy.

Another subgroup are patients with Laron type dwarfism, who have high circulating levels of growth hormone, and very low levels of somatomedin, that do not increase in response to exogenous growth hormone. Laron type dwarfism appears to involve a defect in somatomedin generation, and at present there is no therapy for this condition since somatomedin is not available for therapeutic use.

Recently, a defect in somatomedin unresponsiveness has been described. The patient had growth failure in the presence of normal growth hormone and elevated somatomedin, as assessed by bioassay, RRA, and RIA. This patient is different from pygmies who show peripheral unresponsiveness to human growth hormone levels (RIA) with *normal* somatomedin activity. (See Table 2.)

Hypothyroidism. Growth arrest and severe delay in bone age maturation are perhaps the most constant feature of primary hypothyroidism in infants and children. Congenital hypothyroidism is now readily detected by screening programs based on the measurement of thyroxin or TSH on filter-paper blood specimens.

In older children, acquired hypothyroidism is usually the result of Hashimoto's

TABLE 2. GROWTH HORMONE AND SOMATOMEDIN IN SHORT STATURE

	GH	SM		
		Basal	Stimulated with Exogenous GH	Growth Rate with GH Therapy
Normal	N	N	↑	N
Idiopathic GH deficiency	↓	↓	↑	↑
Pygmies	N	N	N	—
Laron dwarfism	↑ ↑	↓	↓	No therapy possible
Craniopharyngioma	↓	N	—	No therapy necessary
Biologically inactive GH	N (RIA)	↓	↑	↑
Peripheral unresponsiveness to SM	N (RIA)	(↑ RIA, RRA bioassay)	↑ ↑	↑

↓, decreased; ↑, increased; GH, growth hormone; N, normal; RIA, radioimmunoassay; RRA, radioreceptorassay; SM, somatomedin.

thyroiditis or decompensation of an ectopic, dysgenetic thyroid gland. Growth failure is a constant feature. Thyroid antibodies should be measured in the search for Hashimoto's thyroiditis.

Glucocorticoid Excess. Loss of diurnal variation in plasma cortisol and elevated urinary free cortisol excretion are present in Cushing's syndrome. Patients with Cushing's syndrome are obese and have striae, glucose intolerance, and poor growth. Conversely, review of growth charts of patients with exogenous obesity frequently reveals accelerated linear growth. Growth-retarding effects of glucocorticoid therapy can be reduced by giving single, large doses of the steroid on alternate days.

Differential Diagnosis

History. Approximately 2 million children in this country have statures falling more than 2 SD below the mean for their age, but most of these children have no disease and need not be evaluated. A normal child who suddenly stops growing may not fall more than 2 SD below the mean for a number of years, but this child should clearly be investigated long before the height percentile becomes subnormal. Thus, a child's current growth percentile on the growth curve must be contrasted against the genetic background (what is the height of parents and grandparents?), gestational and past medical history (what was the birth weight?), physical findings (were there any signs of nonendocrine systemic illness?), and, most important, the growth rate, i.e. the growth velocity, since birth and the current growth rate.

In any patient whose stature is more than 3 SD below the mean height for age, an immediate work-up is indicated. In children whose height is between 2 and 3 SD below the mean, a limited number of screening tests for common causes of growth failure are obtained on the initial clinic visit. If the growth rate on subsequent visits is found to be abnormal, more extensive testing, including mea-

surement of growth hormone, is advised. In any child in whom the growth velocity is less than normal for age, an evaluation is indicated, regardless of whether their absolute height is abnormal or not. These decisions are, of course, tempered by historical and physical findings.

The history should include a complete genetic pedigree, documenting achieved adult height and age at puberty (e.g., menarche or first shaving). The history should include a nutritional history, and the psychosocial environment should not be neglected. A history of intrauterine growth retardation often suggests some inherent deficiency in the cells to grow and divide.

Physical Examination. The physical examination is very useful in differentiating nonendocrine organ system malfunction from abnormalities of hormone secretion. If there is other organic disease or malabsorption, weight is often more severely affected than height. The physical examination may provide ready clues to skeletal disorders, dysmorphic syndromes, diseases of specific organ systems, and certain endocrine diseases, in particular, hypothyroidism and Cushing's syndrome.

Laboratory Examination. In the absence of diagnostic clues, the patient has to be screened for more silent causes of growth failure. This includes assessment of renal function to rule out unrecognized renal failure and tubular disorders (pH, specific gravity, BUN, creatinine, electrolytes), measurement of calcium and phosphorus and alkaline phosphatase to rule out subtle forms of rickets, and measurement of the serum somatomedin level to screen for growth hormone deficiency.

Thyroid function should be evaluated by measuring T4 and TSH. If the gland cannot be palpated, a thyroid scan is indicated to rule out an ectopic gland. Hypothyroidism must be corrected before growth hormone secretion can be evaluated. If the patient has secondary hypothyroidism, a thyroid-releasing hormone test to differentiate between hypothalamic and pituitary hypothyroidism is indicated.

An abnormality of the X chromosome should be sought in all short girls, regardless of the presence or absence of physical stigmata of Turner syndrome. The initial evaluation in girls with short stature includes, therefore, a karyotype of lymphocytes and measurements of FSH and LH. Gonadotropins are invariably elevated, even in the prepubertal child with gonadal dysgenesis.

An elevated erythrocyte sedimentation rate is often an early clue to a then mild asymptomatic malabsorption syndrome. Bone age aids little in the differential diagnosis; the bone age is useful in assessing the growth potential of the child. Lateral views of the skull are frequently helpful in disclosing an unsuspected, silent, intrasellar tumor.

After a disease of a major nonendocrine organ system has been ruled out, one has to decide which endocrine tests, if any, are indicated. Evaluation of the patient's growth velocity is very helpful in this assessment. The child who is growing at a normal rate is most unlikely to have an endocrinologic cause for short stature. Children with a history of constitutional or familial short stature and a normal growth rate do not require endocrinologic evaluation. Follow-up at 6-month intervals, however, is suggested. X-rays of the wrist for determination of the bone age as a predictor of mature height are indicated. Follow-up is mandatory in the child for whom growth data are not available so that a growth rate, based on at least 6-months observation period, can be determined over time.

When the growth velocity is consistently less than 4 cm per year and there is a significant delay of the bone age (> 2 SD), additional studies are indicated. Screening tests for growth hormone deficiency include strenuous exercise for 30 minutes with subsequent sampling for growth hormone, sleep studies where blood is obtained 60 minutes after sleep onset, and SmC measurements.

The incidence of a positive response in normal children after these screening procedures is approximately 70%. It follows, therefore, that a significant portion of normal children will not show a plasma growth hormone response. In these patients, definitive tests are needed.

Confirmation of the diagnosis of growth hormone deficiency depends on failure to respond to at least two of the following definitive stimuli, which may be used sequentially and on an ambulatory basis. The patient fasts overnight and is kept at rest before and during the test, since, as stated above, exercise can induce a growth hormone release and render the pituitary temporarily refractory to other stimuli. The four definitive tests used most widely are:

1. Insulin infusion to induce hypoglycemia
2. L-dopa administration
3. Arginine hydrochloride infusion
4. Glucagon given IM

Since growth hormone deficiency is often associated with abnormal secretion of other pituitary hormones, complete evaluation of pituitary function should be carried out by the endocrinologist.

Therapy of Short Stature

Specific therapy is indicated in children with treatable causes of short stature.

Hypothyroidism. L-thyroxin is the replacement drug of choice, given at a dose of 3–4 μg/kg/day (100 μg/m^2 surface area). Adequacy of treatment can be judged from the growth curve and normalization of TSH levels. Excessive L-thyroxin dosages may cause undue acceleration of the bone age.

Hypopituitarism.
Isolated Growth Hormone Deficiency. These patients should be treated with human growth hormone 0.1 U/kg up to 2 U per dose 3 times per week. Therapy is continued to a

height of 163 cm (5 feet 4 inches or 50th percentile) for girls and 168 cm (5 feet 6 inches or 10th percentile) for boys. Therapy is maintained as long as the patient responds adequately. The response to human growth hormone is greatest during the first year of treatment when most patients show catch-up growth (7–15 cm/year). Subsequently, the growth velocity usually declines to 4–7 cm/year.

After IM administration of growth hormone, hypopituitary patients demonstrate a peak response in immunoreactive somatomedin C between 16–24 hours and a fall to nearly basal levels by 48 hours. The delay in the somatomedin C response suggests that the hormone is not stored in a readily releasable form. There might be some rationale for conducting further studies to evaluate the daily administration of growth hormone in order to eliminate the troughs of somatomedin C levels seen using 3 times weekly regimens. Daily growth hormone injections are certainly indicated in the treatment of hypoglycemia-prone hypopituitary patients. Continuous subcutaneous infusion of growth hormone, as advocated by some groups, does not offer any therapeutic advantages.

Causes of poor response to human growth hormone therapy are listed:

- The patient is not growth hormone deficient.
- The patient developed unrecognized hypothyroidism during therapy.
- Inadequate dose was given.
- The patient does not comply.
- Hormone is not injected properly.
- The patient has emotional deprivation syndrome.
- The patient receives suboptimal caloric nutrition.

Since variations in nutritional status are as critical as growth hormone to the regulation of somatomedin C levels, particular attention has to be paid to caloric intake in those youngsters who are refractory to GH therapy.

At present, the only available source of human growth hormone is material extracted from human pituitary glands collected at autopsy. Human growth hormone is distributed free of charge by the National Pituitary Agency for approved projects to treatment centers but not for individual patients. There is presently enough material for all patients lacking growth hormone. Commercial sources charging $5,000–$6,000 per treatment-year are available in the United States. Bacterial synthesis of growth hormone using recombinant DNA techniques is not feasible. Recombinant DNA-derived human growth hormone expressed in *Escherichia coli* has an N-terminal methionine residue, i.e., one additional aminoacid. It is in its biologic activity indistinguishable from native pituitary growth hormone. Recombinant DNA-derived growth hormone is capable of producing insulin resistance and causes an elevation of somatomedin C. It is doubtful, however, whether growth hormone manufactured in this fashion will be in the foreseeable future any cheaper than the growth hormone offered through commercial sources.

Multiple Hormone Deficiencies. Appropriate replacement therapy should be given. The cortisol dose should be kept at a minimum, since larger doses interfere with somatomedin generation. Patients with multiple pituitary hormone deficiencies usually do not respond as well to human growth hormone therapy.

Constitutional Short Stature. Treatment of delayed puberty is dependent upon the diagnosis and nature of the disorder. Patients with constitutional delay in growth have spontaneous onset and eventually normal progression through puberty. Usually, sympathetic reassurance and continued observation are sufficient.

The developmental delay, which frequently causes impaired self-image, may lead to abnormal isolation and depression in teenagers, particularly in adolescent males. Some patients feel such intense pressure that only the appearance of signs of puberty will reassure them and enable them to participate in sports and social activities with their peers.

A brief course of testosterone enanthate (100–200 mg iM every 3–4 weeks for 3 months) in boys, or ethinyl estradiol (10µg per day for 3 months) or conjugated estrogen (0.3 mg per day for 3 months) in girls is an effective and safe means to induce the development of the first signs of maturation of the secondary sex characteristics. Longitudinal growth may also accelerate during this treatment. If puberty does not ensue, the treatment may be repeated. Usually only one to two courses of therapy are necessary. The skeletal age should be monitored carefully during this treatment. In addition to the obvious psychologic benefits, this treatment program helps also in the differential diagnosis of constitutional delay of puberty vs gonadotropin deficiency. When treatment is withdrawn after the bone age has been advanced to 14 years, patients with constitutional delay will continue further development on their own, while those with gonadotropin deficiency will not progress and may, in fact, regress. Current evidence suggests that anabolic agents (e.g., oxandrolone) do accelerate linear growth in the short run, i.e., the patient reaches his final height sooner. Final stature is unchanged, however. These androgens cause a significant transient depression of gonadotropins and testosterone. Cautious use of an anabolic agent is indicated when short stature creates physiologic problems that cannot be ameliorated in any other way. While the patient receives oxandrolone, the bone age should be monitored every 6 months to avoid missing undue acceleration of bone age maturation. Anabolic steroids, especially those substituted in the C_{17} position (e.g., methyltestosterone) are occasionally hepatotoxic

and may cause a cholestatis syndrome. Baseline tests of liver function and 6-monthly check-ups therefore are indicated. Hepatic tumors have been reported after high-dose androgen therapy, e.g., for aplastic anemia, but have not been observed in patients treated with low doses for developmental delay.

Treatment with a gonadotropin releasing hormone analog may also prove to be useful in the management of the rare patient with constitutional delay in growth and short stature who enters puberty early. If the predicted adult height in such a patient is less than 148 cm, therapy with a GnRH analog, thus prolonging the period of prepubertal growth, may increase final adult stature.

Intrauterine Growth Retardation. While regular doses of growth hormone are ineffective in intrauterine growth retardation, high-dose human growth hormone therapy using 5–10 times the physiologic dose may be beneficial in some patients. This question is currently being investigated.

Turner Syndrome. Girls with Turner syndrome may be treated with oxandrolone 0.15–0.2µg/kg in late childhood or adolescence, though the beneficial effect on final height is not proven. After age 15 or 16 years, secondary sex characteristics can be brought about by continuous estrogen therapy using conjugated estrogens or estradiol. Early estrogen therapy is contraindicated, since it will close the epiphyses prematurely. Prolonged unopposed estrogen therapy should be avoided. For continuing therapy, the patient may be maintained on cyclical therapy, e.g., estradiol (Estrace) and Provera. The patient should be maintained at the lowest possible therapeutic dose level (the level that will maintain regular cyclical bleeding). Further, patients receiving estrogen-progesterone therapy periodically should have an endometrial biopsy to determine if there is a silent endometrial abnormality.

A study is currently under way to evaluate the efficacy of high-dose human growth therapy in children with Turner syndrome.

TALL STATURE

Etiology
Causes of tall stature include:

ENDOCRINE DISORDERS	NONENDOCRINE CONDITIONS
Growth hormone excess	Constitutional tall stature
Abnormal sexual maturation	Cerebral gigantism
Precocious puberty	Marfan's syndrome
Virilization, feminization	Homocystinuria
Hypogonadism	

Compared to short stature, tall stature, i.e. height above the 97th percentile, is an infrequent complaint.

From a cultural standpoint, it affects girls to a far greater degree than boys. Contrary to the experience in Europe, it is extremely unusual for American families to be concerned that their sons are too tall.

Excessive growth hormone secretion in children and adolescents is caused by a functioning pituitary tumor, usually an eosinophilic adenoma. Neurofibromatosis can give rise to gliomas in the hypothalamus, which may lead to excessive growth hormone secretion.

Young patients with an excess of growth hormone are tall and grow at a rate more rapid than expected for their age. Their growth curve deviates more and more away from normal. Growth hormone excess in children will not lead to acromegalic features, as is seen in adults with growth hormone excess. Impaired vision and visual field abnormalities may be present.

Diagnosis
The diagnosis of growth hormone excess is confirmed by the failure to suppress plasma growth hormone by raising the blood sugar during a standard 5-hour oral glucose tolerance test. Normally, plasma growth hormone should fall to 5 ng/ml or less within 60–120 minutes after ingestion of the glucose load. Somatomedin C levels may be elevated as well. A CT scan of the head may help in localizing the tumor.

The treatment of growth hormone excess is directed at ablating the tumor, preferably through the transsphenoidal approach. Radiation therapy is not very effective and is only recommended when the tumor is inoperable because of its location.

Sexual precocity and virilizing disorders are the most common endocrine causes of increased statural growth. (For details, see Chapter 38.)

Two benign conditions that are not commonly associated with increased linear growth and must not be confused with sexual precocity are premature thelarche and adrenarche. (See Chapter 38.)

Constitutional tall stature is a normal variant that results in tall adult stature. Bone age and growth velocity are normal, and the growth curve is parallel to the 97th percentile.

Familial rapid maturation results only in a transient abnormality as the child goes through puberty sooner. Bone age may be advanced. Final adult height is normal or even short.

In this country, patients with constitutional tall stature seeking medical help are usually girls 2–4 SD above the mean height for age. The mean height in American girls is 64.5 inches. Usually one or both parents of these girls are also tall. Endocrine function is normal. Bone age determinations of the wrist and knee are necessary to estimate adult height. Some patients are well adjusted and happy. Others are withdrawn, depressed, and underachieving.

Therapy
Excessive growth can be prevented to a certain degree by the use of high-dose estrogen therapy. These estrogen doses are approx-

imately 10-fold larger than those used in contraceptive medications. The mechanism of action is acceleration of bone maturation and depression of somatomedin activity in the serum. The results of some published series are shown in Table 3. While the height reduction in some studies appears to be impressive, i.e., 6–7 cm, in other studies a reduction of only 3 cm was observed. It needs to be emphasized that this is a reduction of predicted mature height. It is still not clear whether the benefits of this therapy outweigh the risks of high-dose estrogen therapy and its delayed effects. Nausea at the onset of therapy is common, and obesity is a frequent side effect. One girl developed a thrombosis in a superficial vein of her calf. Ovarian cysts developed in two girls. Long-term potential hazards of high-dose estrogen therapy given over 2 years are not known. They include precipitation of diabetes mellitus or atherosclerosis, neoplasms of the genital tract, breast cancer, sterility, and hepatic adenoma.

Treatment of tall stature in girls remains a very controversial topic in pediatrics, and this author believes that the benefits of maybe 1–2 inches in reduction of a *predicted* adult height do not outweigh the risks of hormonal therapy.

CEREBRAL GIGANTISM

Cerebral gigantism (Soto's syndrome) is a nonendocrine disorder of unknown cause. The birth weight is often increased, and the bone age is increased. There is rapid growth in early infancy and childhood. Adult stature is normal in most instances. Mental retardation is common. Growth hormone and somatomedin levels are normal in these patients.

There is no treatment for cerebral gigantism. Management should be directed at maximizing intellectual development.

TABLE 3. RESULTS OF PUBLISHED SERIES USING ESTROGEN FOR TREATMENT FOR TALL GIRLS

Drug	Schoen et al. Conjugated Estrogens 10 mg/day	Wettenhall et al. Diethylstilbestrol 3 mg/day	Crawford Diethylstilbestrol 5 mg/day	Zachmann et al. Ethinyl Estradiol 0.3 mg/day	Puttkamer et al. Conjugated Estrogens 7.5 mg/day
Age at beginning of treatment (yr)	12.1	13.0	12.9	12.9	13.2
Skeletal age (yr)	12.0	13.2	13.2	13.4[†]	12.4
Premenarcheal:-postmenarcheal ratio	21:0	46:41	58:42	23:17	20:21
Height at start of treatment (cm)	169.7	172.7	174.0	—	174.8
Predicted mature height (cm)	182.9	182.1	182.6	181.9[†]	186.5
Actual mature height (cm)	179.1	178.6	176.5	177.4	179.2
Reduction due to treatment (cm)	3.8	3.5	6.1	4.6	7.3
Duration of treatment (mo)	24.7	25.2	17.2	20.4	22
Total no. of cases	21	87	100	40	41

*Intermittent: 21 days of treatment, 7 days of no treatment. All other estrogen treatment schedules were continuous.
[†]Bone age and growth prediction using TW-2 method; all others by Greulich and Pyle Atlas and Bayley and Pinneau tables. *(From Crawford JD: Pediatrics 62: (6) 1189, 1978.)*

BIBLIOGRAPHY

Bajorunas DR, Ghavimi F, Jereb E, et al.: Endocrine sequelae of antineoplastic therapy in childhood head and neck malignancies. J Clin Endocrinol Metab 50:329, 1980

Clemens RD, Van Wyk JJ, Ridgway EC, et al.: Evaluation of acromegaly of somatomedin C radioimmunoassay. N Engl J Med 301:1138, 1979

Comite F, Cutler GB Jr, Rivier J, et al.: Short-term treatment of idiopathic precocious puberty with a long-acting analogue of luteinizing hormone-releasing hormone. N Engl J Med 305:1546, 1981

Copeland KC, Underwood LE, Van Wyk JJ: Induction of immunoreactive somatomedin C in human serum by growth hormone: dose response relationships and effect on chromotographic profiles. J Clin Endocrinol Metab 50:690, 1980

Costin G, Fefferman RA, Kogut MD: Hypothalamic gigantism. J Pediatr 83:419, 1973

Craft HW, Underwood LE, Van Wyk JJ: High incidence of perinatal insult in children with idiopathic hypopituitarism. J Pediatr 96:397, 1980

Crawford JD: Treatment of tall girls with estrogen. Pediatrics suppl 1189: 62, 1978

———. Meat, potatoes and growth hormone. N Engl J Med 305:163, 1981

Daughaday WH, Laron Z, Pertzelan A, et al.: Defective sulfation factor generation: A possible etiologic link in dwarfism. Trans Assoc Am Physicians 82:129, 1969

D'Ercole JD: Use of the RIA for somatomedin C estimation. J Pediatr 99: 735, 1981

Finkelstein JW, Kream J, Ludan A, et al.: Sulfation factor (somatomedin): An explanation for continued growth in the absence of immunoassayable growth hormone in patients with hypothalamic tumors. J Clin Endocrinol Metab 35:13, 1972

Frasier SD: A review of growth hormone stimulation tests in children. Pediatrics 53:929, 1974

———. Growth disorders in children. Pediatr Clin North Am 26:3, 1979

Greulich WW, Pyle SI: Radiographic Atlas of Skeletal Development of the Hand and Wrist. Stanford Univ Press, 1959

Hopwood NJ, Kelch RP, Zipf WB, et al.: The effect of synthetic androgens on the hypothalamic-pituitary-gonadal axis in boys with constitutionally delayed growth. J Pediatr 94:657, 1979

Kowarski AA, Schneider J, Bel-Galim E, et al.: Growth failure with normal serum RIA-GH and low somatomedin activity: somatomedin restoration and growth acceleration after exogenous GH. J Clin Endocrinol Metab 47:461, 1978

Lanes R, Plotnick LP, Spencer EM, et al.: Dwarfism associated with normal serum growth hormone and increased bioassayable, receptorassayable, and immunoassayable somatomedin. J Clin Endocrinol Metab 59:485, 1980

Lovinger RD, Kaplan SL, Grumbach MM: Congenital hypopituitarism associated with neonatal hypoglycemia and microphallus: four cases secondary to hypothalamic hormone deficiencies. J Pediatr 87:1171, 1975

Lyen KR, Grant DB: Morbidity after surgery for craniopharyngeoma. Pediatr Res 15:1540, 1981 (abstr.)

Miller WL, Kaplan SL, Grumbach MM: Child abuse as a cause of post traumatic hypopituitarism. N Engl J Med 302:724, 1980

National Center for Health Statistics: NCHS Growth Charts. (Suppl HRA 76:1120), 1976, Vol 25

Phillips LS, Vassilopoulou-Sellin R: Somatomedins. I and II. N Engl J Med 302:371, 438, 1980

Puttkamer VK, Bierich JF, Schönberg D, et al.: Efficiency and mode of action of conjugated estrogens in the treatment of tall girls. Pediatr Res 9:685, 1975

Pyle SI, Hoerr NL: Radiographic Atlas of Skeletal Development of the Knee. Springfield, Il, Thomas, 1955

Raiti S (ed): Advances in Human Growth Hormone Research. DHEW Publication No (NIH) 74-612, 1974 p 321

Rimoin DL, Horton WA: Short stature. J Pediatr 92:523, 697, 1978

Rosenfeld RG, Northcraft GB, Hintz RL: A prospective randomized study of testosterone treatment of constitutional short stature in adolescent males. Pediatr Res 15:444, 1981 (abstr.)

Rosenfeld RG, Wilson DM, Bennett A, et al.: Recombinant DNA-derived human growth hormone is biologically active in humans. Pediatr Res 16:143A, 1982 (abstr.)

Rudman D, Davis GT, Priest JH, et al.: Prevalence of growth hormone deficiency in children with cleft lip or palate. J Pediatr 93:378, 1978

Rudman D, Kutner MH, Blackston RD, et al.: Children with normal variant short stature: treatment with human growth hormone for six months. N Engl J Med 305:123, 1981

Saenger P, Wiedemann E, Schwartz E, et al.: Somatomedin and growth after renal transplantation. Pediatr Res 8:163, 1974

Saenger P, Levine LS, Wiedemann E, et al.: Psychosocial dwarfism: normal somatomedin. Paediatr Paedol Suppl 5:1, 1977

________. Wiedemann E, et al.: Growth without radioimmunoassayable growth hormone. J Pediatr 88:137, 1976

________. Somatomedin in cerebral gigantism. J Pediatr 88:155, 1976

Sills RH: Failure to thrive. The role of clinical and laboratory evaluation. Am J Dis Child 132:967, 1978

Smith DW: Growth and Its Disorders—Major Problems in Clinical Pediatrics. Philadelphia, Saunders, 1977

________. Recognizable patterns of Human Malformation, 2nd ed. Philadelphia, Saunders, 1976

Underwood LE, Van Wyk JJ: Hormones in normal and abnormal growth. In Williams RH (ed): Textbook of Endocrinology, 6th ed. Philadelphia, Saunders, 1981, p 1149

Cross-Reference to *Pediatrics,* 17th ed.

TWENTY-EIGHT

Speech and Language Problems in Children

Marilyn B. Silver

A child has a communication disorder if one or more of the following problems are found: (1) impairment in the comprehension or expression of spoken or written language, and (2) abnormal production of speech sounds, abnormal voice patterns with regard to quality, pitch, duration, or loudness, and abnormal fluency affecting the rate and rhythm of speech.

Communication disorders are developmental or acquired, vary in degree of severity, and may be associated with physical, cognitive, or emotional problems.

Language and speech disorders may impact on various aspects of a child's development and the family's life. Parent-child interaction, sibling and peer relationships, school performance, and the child's development of self-esteem may all be affected. Early intervention, therefore, is desirable to minimize the problem and to maximize the child's performance.

It is usually the pediatrician to whom the parent first expresses concern about the child's hearing, language, or speech. It may be that the parent feels that the child's understanding or speaking is below expectation when compared to peers or siblings. They may report that the speech is not as clear as it should be, or they may be concerned that the child is stuttering.

However, it may be the pediatrician who first becomes aware that the child's hearing, language, or speech is not as it should be. Thus, the pediatrician is frequently in the position of screening for subtle as well as obvious communication problems within the context of the pediatric examination. In addition, being aware of the necessity for early intervention, the pediatrician must be able to help the parent understand the need for referral for diagnostic services and possibly for therapeutic intervention. Because of this role of case manager, the pediatrician must be able to support the family in coping with the child's special need with regard to therapy or schooling.

The thrust of this chapter is to provide the pediatrician with a method of screening and referring the child with a communication disorder.

LANGUAGE AND ITS RULES

Language is a structured system of arbitrary symbols. It enables us to communicate our ideas and feelings to others efficiently, to think abstractly, to process and store information for future use, to control our world to some extent, and to predict and anticipate future events. Speech is the mechanism for language. It involves the use of the speech sounds of the language, voice, and fluency.

Normal language and speech performance are dependent on an intact auditory system, neurologic maturation and integrity, intact vocal and articulatory structures, the ability to make adjustments in the vocal tract, cognitive maturation and integrity, and the ability to learn the rules of the language.

What are the rules that must be followed if the individual is to be a competent communicator? First, there is the grammar of a language. The phonologic, morphologic, and syntactic rules are subsumed under this heading.

Phonologic Rules

The phonologic rules provide the structure for putting speech sounds (phonemes) together for forming words. Thus, the child must learn the sounds of language and the acceptable sequences. Indeed, those of us who do crossword puzzles unconsciously utilize this linguistic knowledge. If one sees a sequence, such as "W, Q, N," the first response is that "something is wrong." We know that this is an unacceptable or incorrect combination of sounds in English.

Morphologic Rules

Morphologic rules deal with manipulating words to change meaning. For example, if we wish to indicate more than one, we add an *s* to a word. But we also learn that some words do not follow this rule, and they must be manipulated differently. It is not unusual to hear the maturing normal child go through a sequence, such as "I have a foot," then later, "I have two foots," then, with the awareness or irregularity, "I have two feets," and finally, "I have two feet."

Another example of a morphologic rule is that the addition of *ed* to a verb indicates past tense. One language-impaired child we saw could indicate tense only by adding a *time* word. He might say, "Me talk on the phone yesterday," or "Me talk on the phone today," or "Me talk on the phone tomorrow."

Syntactic Rules

Syntactic rules relate to the word order of the sentence. For example, in some languages, adjectives precede the noun. In others, adjectives follow the noun.

Semantic Rules

Semantic rules must be learned. While a sentence, such as "The wall put the dog on top of the sky" is gramatically correct, it is meaningless. Semantic rules enable us to make that decision.

There are also rules for the nonsegmental aspects of language. These deal with the utilization of *prosodic features*, such as intonation and stress. They convey meaning. A rising inflection at the end of an utterance indicates a question, a sharp drop, an imperative. Word boundaries or juncture also fall under this heading. For example, the difference between "I scream" and "ice cream" is that different boundaries are established between the speech sounds.

FUNCTIONAL USE OF LANGUAGE

Pragmatic rules govern the five functional uses of language: (1) to inform, (2) to control or persuade, (3) to express one's feelings, (4) to perform communicative rituals (e.g., a religious ceremony), and (5) to perform imaginary acts. The precursor to the actual use of verbal language to fulfill one of these uses can be seen in the first year, when the crying of the infant contains a directive function for the mother, as do pointing and words a little later on. There are also standards against which we make judgments about voice production and fluency. Thus, we decide if a person's voice is normal and if the individual is a fluent speaker or is so nonfluent as to be labelled a stutterer.

Thus, the language-developing child is not learning lists of words and phrases. Rather the child is learning the rules of language and acquiring a vocabulary that will fit within this framework. Knowing the rules of a language enables us to understand an utterance that was never before heard and generates an utterance that was never before spoken.

NORMAL LANGUAGE

The normal developmental sequence of auditory, vocal, and verbal behaviors is used to screen for language disorders. Key screening items are listed for different age groups, as well as possible etiologies that the pediatrician should consider in planning what action, if any, to take.

Three Months of Age
Normal Characteristics.

1. Responds to sound by becoming quiet or by changing behavior.
2. Responds to quiet sounds as well as loud sounds.
3. Discriminates between angry and friendly, familiar and unfamiliar, male and female voices.
4. Is soothed by a pleasant adult voice. Often looks at speaker and responds by smiling.
5. Coos, producing long vowel and vowel-like sounds.
6. Babbles. One syllable is repeated over and over again. May start using the consonants /b/, /d/, and /m/.

At Risk Features.

1. Fails to consistently respond to auditory stimuli.
2. There is a reduced amount of babbling, and/or very few different speech sounds are heard.

Possible Working Hypothesis.

1. Decreased hearing acuity.

Action.

1. Refer the child for otologic examination and hearing evaluation. Decreased hearing acuity has a marked impact on the development of language and speech, regardless of type and degree of loss. Therefore, every child who has suspicious auditory behavior or whose vocalizations are different from that of a normal child must have a hearing evaluation. Current instrumentation and techniques can provide information about a child's hearing, regardless of age. Thus, for this and the following age groups, this recommendation applies to every case.
2. If there is decreased hearing that cannot be ameliorated by medical or surgical intervention, a referral is made for the audiologist to perform a hearing aid evaluation to determine if the child will benefit from amplification.
3. A referral should be made for an infant auditory training program. The emphasis is on development of language and speech, utilizing various techniques. The parents, as well as other family members, become active participants in the program and are taught how to carry it out at home.

Nine Months to Twelve Months of Age
Normal Characteristics.

1. Understands simple verbal requests accompanied by gesture.
2. Recognizes objects by name.
3. Has at least one or two individual words other than "ma-ma" or "da-da." (Words may also be "sentences.")
4. Repeats sounds made by self and others.
5. Gestures. Plays "pat-a-cake," waves "bye-bye."

6. Uses jargon. "Talks" to play objects or to people in inflected utterances but without true words. (It is different from babbling in that one utterance will contain many different syllables.)

At Risk Features.

1. Comprehension is poor.
2. There is very little vocal play ("quiet child").
3. Has not acquired first words yet.

Possible Working Hypothesis.

1. Decreased hearing acuity.

Action.

1. Refer for otologic examination and hearing evaluation and follow-up if indicated.
2. If there is no hearing loss, the child's development of language and speech should be closely monitored.

Twelve to Eighteen Months of Age
Normal Characteristics.

1. Responds to simple commands accompanied by gestures at first and then without gestures (15 months).
2. Demonstrates some echolalia.
3. Uses speech intentionally. Has a vocabulary of 7–20 words.
4. Consistently uses a greater variety of consonants: /b/, /d/, /t/, /g/, /h/, /m/, /n/.
5. Starts to ask for objects by name.

At Risk Features.

1. Does not respond to commands without accompanying gestures.
2. Shows no growth in acquisition of vocabulary, or no more than one or two words.
3. Uses only a few consonants during vocalizations.
4. Shows no naming skills.

Possible Working Hypothesis.

1. Decreased hearing acuity.
2. Language impairment.

Action.

1. Refer for otologic examination and hearing evaluation and follow up if indicated.
2. Refer for evaluation of speech and language. If indicated, a structured language stimulation program will be set up for the parents to carry out with the child at home. The speech and language pathologist will meet with the parents and see the child on a regular basis to chart the child's progress and to modify the program as needed.

Eighteen Months to Two Years of Age
Normal Characteristics.

1. Recognizes pictures by pointing.
2. Recognizes 1 body part (18 months), 3 body parts (21 months) and then 5 body parts (23 months).
3. Says name on request.
4. Has a vocabulary of approximately 100–200 words.
5. Has first 2-word sentences or 2-word phrases. Occasional 3- and 4-word sentences (24 months).
6. Asks questions by rising intonation at the end of a phrase.
7. Begins to use pronouns.
8. Uses speech that is 65% intelligible.

At Risk Features.

1. Does not understand names of objects or pictures of objects or names of body parts.
2. Has very limited vocabulary.
3. Has not started putting words together.
4. Uses speech that is unintelligible to people other than family members.

Possible Working Hypothesis.

1. Decreased hearing acuity.
2. Language impairment.
3. Cognitive deficit.

Action.

1. Refer for otologic examination and evaluation of hearing.
2. Refer for evaluation of language and speech.

Two and One-half Years of Age
Normal Characteristics.

1. Responds to simple, related, two-part commands.
2. Understands prepositions "in" and "on."
3. Is beginning to use verbs.
4. Asks questions, e.g., "What dat?" "Go bye-bye?" "Where ball?"

At Risk Features.

1. Seems not to understand without gesture and demonstration.
2. Does not ask questions. This is a key screening question for this age and older. Questions are a primary means of learning about ourselves and our environment. In order to ask questions, at this age, the child must have age-level language, cognitive and socialization skills, curiosity, and a view of the adult (or older child) as a partner in this exploration. Children with language problems tend to use questions less frequently than do normal children.

Possible Working Hypothesis.

1. Decrease in hearing acuity.
2. Language impairment.
3. Mental retardation.
4. Emotional problems.

Action.

1. Refer for otologic examination and audiologic evaluation.
2. Refer for evaluation of language and speech. At this age and older, if therapy is indicated, the speech and language pathologist will work directly with the child and utilize the parents as co-therapists to carry out the program at home.
3. Referral for a psychologic evaluation.

Three Years of Age
Normal Characteristics.

1. Has a vocabulary of approximately 900 words.
2. Has 3–4 word sentences.
3. Is able to name 4–5 pictures of common objects.
4. Can tell own name.
5. Uses plural suffix(es).
6. Uses past tense.
7. Uses "Who" question.
8. Uses speech that is 90% intelligible.

At Risk Features.

1. Verbal comprehension is significantly below age level.
2. Vocabulary is small.
3. Sentences are absent.
4. Speech is not understood by people outside immediate family and frequently not by family members.
5. Utterances are simple and always in the present tense.
6. "Who" questions are not used.

Possible Working Hypothesis.

1. Decrease in hearing acuity.
2. Language impairment.
3. Mental retardation.
4. Emotional problems.
5. Very little language stimulation at home.

Action.

1. Refer for otologic examination and audiologic evaluation.
2. Refer for evaluation of language and speech.
3. Refer for a psychologic evaluation.
4. Recommend nursery school.

Four Years of Age
Normal Characteristics.

1. Follows three-part unrelated commands.
2. Understands all spatial prepositions.
3. Has a vocabulary of approximately 1,500 words
4. Has 4–8 word sentences.
5. Uses complex sentences.
6. Uses "why" "how" "when" and "where" questions.
7. Uses irregular plurals consistently.
8. Has intelligible speech.
9. Holds conversation.

At Risk Features.

1. Comprehension of verbal language is below age level.
2. Small vocabulary.
3. Is unable to adequately express himself verbally.
4. Is unable to converse with people.

Possible Working Hypothesis.

1. Decrease in hearing acuity.
2. Language impairment.
3. Mental retardation.
4. Emotional problems.

Action.

1. Refer for otologic examination and audiologic evaluation.
2. Refer for an evaluation of language and speech.

3. Refer for a psychologic evaluation.
4. Consider evaluation for special preschool program.

Five to Six and One-half Years of Age
Normal Characteristics.

1. Understands almost all that is said to him/her.
2. Has mastered all grammatical rules.
3. Has vocabulary that continues to grow.

At Risk Features.

1. Comprehension of verbal language is below age level.
2. Small vocabulary.
3. Is unable to adequately express himself verbally.
4. Is unable to converse with people.

Possible Working Hypothesis.

1. Decrease in hearing acuity.
2. Language impairment.
3. Mental retardation.
4. Emotional problems.

Action.

1. Refer for otologic examination and audiologic evaluation.
2. Refer for evaluation of language and speech.
3. Referral for a psychologic evaluation.
4. Referral for evaluation for special school placement.

TYPES OF COMMUNICATION PROBLEMS

In this section, profiles of children with different types of communication problems are presented, as well as a methodology for screening for these deficits.

The Language-impaired Child

The language-impaired child has not internalized all the rules of language. The child either has not been able to learn them or has learned them atypically. This results in deviant language performance. In addition, some children have such a pervasive symbolic disorder that other nonverbal behaviors are depressed. Thus, the child may demonstrate one or more of the following:

1. Difficulty understanding what is said, either verbally or in writing, depending on age.
2. Difficulty expressing ideas and feelings verbally or in writing, depending on age, because of depressed vocabulary or atypical organization of language.
3. Difficulty understanding or using vocal nuances and gestures.
4. Difficulty with symbolic play.

It is not unusual for language-impaired children to have temper tantrums. John was 2 years 8 months old when he was brought for an evaluation. He was found to have both comprehension and expressive language difficulties. It was after he was started in language therapy that his mother shared with us that he had several tantrums a day. They occurred whenever there was to be a change in what he was doing. These were not necessarily unpleasant changes. For example, when she would start to put on his outdoor clothes to go to MacDonald's (which he loved) or to see his grandmother (whom he loved and with whom he always had a nice time), he would throw himself on the floor and scream. An analysis of the situations that provoked the tantrums led to the hypothesis that he did not understand what his mother was teling him and did not know what was going to happen to him. Therefore, photographs were taken of the rooms in the house, of places where they might go, and of people he would visit or who would visit him. His mother would tell him what he was going to do. If he was going to be visiting his grandmother, his mother would show him the grandmother's photograph.

There was a dramatic decrease in tantrums during the first week of this procedure.

The Child with an Articulation Disorder

The child with an articulation disorder has not measured the production of speech sounds appropriate to the child's chronologic age. The child omits, substitutes, or distorts the sounds in the initial, medial, or final positions in words. The disorder may be mild and not impair intelligibility as, for example, with an interdental lisp in which a /th/ is substituted for /s/. At the other end of the spectrum, the disorder may be severe enough to render speech almost completely unintelligible to people outside the immediate family and sometimes to family members as well.

Frequently, these children are reported to have been "late talkers." There is a developmental sequence for the acquisition of speech sounds (phonemes). Vowels and consonants requiring comparatively gross movements of the articulators are acquired first. Consonants and consonant clusters, e.g., sp, str, ks, requiring finer movements are mastered later.

Some children with impaired articulation have poor auditory monitoring skills.

Jessica was 5 years 5 months of age and had a moderate to severe articulation problem. (She pronounced her name as "dedikuh.") She was unintelligible more than 50% of the time. During the evaluation, she was asked the name of her dog. She replied. "Peh-buh." After repeating it several times, she was still not understood. Finally, the listener said "Oh" in a way to imply understanding, but Jessica was not falling for that one. She told the individual, "You say it." What could the response be other than "Peh-buh?" "Yes," she replied. The dog's name was Pebbles.

Not only was Jessica unable to monitor her own poor productions, she was unable to perceive any difference between what was said in imitation of her and the correct production that she always heard at other times.

TABLE 1. PHONEMIC DEVELOPMENT

CA	Phonemes and Phoneme-Blends	CA	Phonemes and Phoneme-Blends
3 years	Vowels: ē, ĭ, ĕ, ă, ŏ, ŭ, o͝o, o͞o, ō, ô, à, ûr Diphthongs: u̇, ā, ī, ou, oi Consonants: m-, -m-, -m, n-, -n-, -n, -ng-, -ng, p-, -p-, -p, t-, -t-, -t, k-, -k-, b-, -b-, d-, -d-, g-, -g-, f-, -f-, -f, h-, -h-, w-, -w- Double-consonant blends: -ngk	5 years	Consonants: -j- Double-consonant blends: fl-, -rp, -lb, -rd, -rf, -rn, -shr Triple-consonant blends: str-, -mbr
3.5	Consonants: -s-, -z-, -r, y-, -y- Double-consonant blends: -rk, -ks, -mp, -pt, -rm, -mr, -nr, -pr, -kr, -br, -dr, -gr, -sm	6 years	Consonants: -t-, th-, -th-, -th-, v-, -v, -th-, -l Double-consonant blends: -lk, -rb, -rg, -rth, -nt, -nd, -thr, -pl, -kl, -bl, -gl, -fl, -sl Triple-consonant blends: skw-, -str, -rst, -ngkl, -nggl, -rj, -ntth, -rch
4 years	Consonants: -k, -b, -d, -g, s-, sh-, -sh, -v-, j-, r-, -r-, l-, -l- Double-consonant blends: pl-, pr-, tr-, tw-, kl-, kr-, kw-, bl-, br-, dr-, gl-, sk-, sm-, sn-, sp-, st-, -lp, -rt, -ft, -lt, -fr Triple-consonant blends: -mpt, -mps	7 years	Consonants: th-, th-, z-, -z, -zh-, -zh, -j Double-consonant blends: thr-, shr, sl-, sw-, -lz, -zm, -lth, -sk, -st Triple-consonant blends: skr-, spl-, spr-, -skr, -kst, -jd
4.5	Consonants: -s, -sh-, ch-, -ch-, -ch Double-consonant blends: gr-, fr-, -lf	8 years	Double-consonant blends: -kt, -tr, -sp

(From Templin, MC: Certain language skills in children. Child Welfare Monograph No. 26. University of Minnesota Press, Minneapolis, © Copyright 1957 by the University of Minnesota. p. 51.)

The normal stages of speech-sound mastery are used to screen for articulation disorders, as with Templin's Table of Phonemic Development (Table 1).

At Risk Features.

1. Phoneme mastery is below age level.
2. Speech is not understood or difficult to understand.
3. Phonemes at the ends of words are omitted.
4. Sibilant phonemes, such as /s/, /z/, /zh/, /sh/, and the affricate phonemes, /ch/ and /j/, sound blunted. For example, the sentence, "My teacher told me to tie my shoe" sounds something like "My teacder told me to tie my toos."
5. Double or triple consonant blends are reduced to one phoneme.
6. There are many distortion errors.

Possible Working Hypothesis.

1. Hearing loss.
2. Structural anomalies, e.g., cleft palate.
3. Perceptual deficits.
4. Malocclusion.
5. A congenitally short lingual frenulum attached close to the tip of the tongue. This occurs in very rare cases. In most cases where there is a shortened frenulum, there is adequate tongue mobility for speech.
6. Poor neuromuscular control of the articulators.

Action.

1. Refer for otolaryngologic examination.
2. Refer for evaluation of hearing.
3. Refer to speech and language pathologist.

In addition to testing perceptual skills, the speech and language pathologist will analyze the errors and determine if they are related, for example, to a malocclusion or to poor neuromotor functioning of the articulators. A recommendation for referral to a dentist or orthodontist might be an outcome of this evaluation.

The Hearing-impaired Child

Since hearing loss is a significant cause of depressed language and speech functioning, the following is a profile of the hearing-impaired child.

The speech and language patterns of the hearing-impaired child are dependent on the type and extent of hearing loss, the age at which it was acquired, and the length of time the child has had it.

Characteristics.

1. The earlier the hearing loss is acquired, the poorer will be speech and language performance.

2. Generally, the deaf child (who will have a sensory-neural loss) will demonstrate:
   a. Distortion of voice in terms of loudness, pitch and quality.
   b. Abnormal inflections and phrasing.
   c. Marked distortion of speech sounds and, thus, poor intelligibility.
   d. Marked language problems, primarily of vocabulary, morphology, and syntax.
3. The hard-of-hearing child may have a sensory-neural, conductive, or mixed hearing loss. Vocal quality will generally be normal for all types.
   a. The child with a sensory-neural hearing loss *will tend* to demonstrate distortions of high-frequency consonants, e.g., s, z, sh, zh, ch, j, th, omission of final consonants, and, if all of the frequencies are involved, impaired language performance.
   b. The child with a conductive hearing loss *tends* to demonstrate a soft voice, some degree of retracted vocal quality, and possibly, if all the frequencies are involved, impaired language performance.

There is evidence that children who have had a number of incidents of middle ear effusion during the preschool years are more likely to have communication deficits than children without this history. It is hypothesized that the auditory deprivation that occurs during the episodes has a significant impact on language and speech development.

Michael was first seen for a speech and language evaluation at 24 months of age. He had had a myringotomy and the insertion of tubes 11 days before this visit. The parents reported that there had been a dramatic change in listening behavior and vocabulary acquisition in this very short time.

A formal evaluation revealed that his language skills ranged from 12 to 8 months. He was combining words, he had a sparse repertoire of speech sounds, and only about 20% of his utterances were intelligible. He was put on a home language stimulation program.

He was seen again at 26 months of age. Language skills were now at the 24-month level. Vocabulary had increased. He was using bisyllabic words, 2-word phrases, and verbs. However, speech was still generally unintelligible, although he now had 3 times more consonants. The home program was modified and continued. He was evaluated a third time when he was 28 months old. Now language skills ranged from 30 months to 36 months. (He was also able to read all the letters of the alphabet.) He was using 3- to 4-word phrases and sentences. However, many were syntactically incorrect. He asked simple questions and answered "where" questions. Speech was still markedly unintelligible. He was referred for formal language and speech therapy.

The Mentally Retarded Child

Language and speech problems are frequently associated with mental retardation. The following is a profile of the mentally retarded child.

The term "mental retardation" refers to significantly subaverage general intellectual functioning (e.g., more than 2 SD from the mean on formal tests). Deficits in adaptive behavior manifested during the developmental period exist concurrently. Adaptive behavior deficits vary according to age. The developmental period is from 0–18 years.

Communication disorders are a frequent concomitant of mental retardation. These deficits show a heterogeneity of type and degree. They may be associated with:

1. Language-learning problems.
2. Depressed hearing levels.
3. Structural anomalies.
4. Motoric problems.

The mentally retarded child may demonstrate one or more of the following:

1. Impaired language.
2. Abnormal articulation.
3. Stuttering.
4. Voice disorder.
5. Concrete, nonelaborative language performance.

The Bilingual Child

One is frequently asked if a bilingual environment is responsible for a child having a language impairment. First what is meant by the term? "Bilingualism" is defined as the practice of alternately using two languages. There are two types.

Infant Bilingualism or Simultaneous Acquisition of Language. The child receives input from two languages from infancy, so that both are being learned together. There is parallel development of phonology, morphology, and syntax. Between the ages of 2½ and 3 years, the normal child is aware of his own bilingualism and is able to translate messages from one language into the other.

Childhood Bilingualism or Sequential Acquisition. This term refers to the establishment of a second language during the early school years after the first language has been learned in the family.

Bilingualism, unto itself, does not cause a communication disorder. The proportion of bilingual children with genuine communication disorders is the same as that found with monolingual children. A language-impaired child from a bilingual environment has impaired functioning in *both* languages, although they may do better in one than the other.

The Child with a Voice Disorder

A voice disorder exists when one or more of the following conditions are present:

1. A defective structure or organic disorder of the vocal organs produces patterns of pitch, loudness, or quality that are sufficiently atypical to interfere with communication.
2. Voice production *results* in organic disorders of the vocal organs.
3. The habitual manner of voice production results in atypical patterns not appropriate to the sex and chronologic age of the speaker.

Most of the voice problems children have tend to fall into one of two categories: disorders of *quality* or of *resonance*. In the former, the major manifestation is chronic hoarseness, generally caused by excessive tension of the vocal folds or the appearance of vocal nodules. Both are frequently the result of vocal abuse, i.e., excessive shouting and yelling for a significant time.

Resonance problems are manifested in excessive or too little nasality. There are three phonemes in English that are nasal by definition: m, n, ng (si*ng*). When they are produced, the oral cavity is closed off, and the breath stream is directed through the nose. Other phonemes have a nasal coloring due to their proximity to the nasals. For example, the "a" in the word "man" will normally be somewhat nasal. However, there is no nasal component for the word "cat."

Findings of Excessive Nasality.

1. Cleft palate.
2. Submucosal cleft of the palate (which may also cause nasal snorting during speech).
3. Inadequate velopharyngeal closure, which may be secondary to structural problems (too short palate), poor neuromotor control, or paralysis.

Findings in Denasality. Denasality occurs with lack of nasal resonance when the /m/, /n/, and /ng/ are produced.

1. Structural problems of the nose.
2. An obstruction in the nasal passages, such as enlarged adenoids.

Action.

1. Refer to a otolaryngologist. A speech and language pathologist will not work with someone with a voice problem until the individual has had a thorough examination by a pediatrician or otolaryngologist and it is their opinion that referral is appropriate.
2. If there is evidence of a structural problem, such as cleft palate or submucosal cleft, the referral should be to a cleft palate center.

The Stuttering Child

Stuttering is defined as consisting ". . . of brief periods of interruptions in speech that have abnormal duration or frequency."[1]

Vocal performance that is labeled as stuttering may also be seen, to a lesser degree, in the speech of normal children. Many children between the ages of 3 and 5 years go through a period of "normal nonfluency." This disappears after a while. They demonstrate:

1. Repetitions (as opposed to prolongations, hard contacts, and silent intervals) that tend *not* to be associated with specific speech sounds, words, or speaking situations.
2. No secondary symptoms (facial, vocal, and/or body mannerisms).
3. No inhibitions in speaking freely.

The stuttering child tends to demonstrate the first two characteristics to a greater extent and has more periods of acute frustration to which he responds by no longer speaking freely.

---

[1]Bloodstein O: Speech Pathology: An Introduction. Boston, Houghton Mifflin, 1979.

Some children stutter for a while, and then it disappears. For some children, the stuttering comes and goes. It either disappears or becomes firmly established. In addition to repetitions, the child may now demonstrate prolongations, hard contacts, or silent intervals. Frequently, secondary symptoms are incorporated into the stuttering pattern.

At Risk Features.

1. History of stuttering in the family.
2. Parents anxiety about child's nonfluency.
3. Child has been told to "slow down, take a deep breath," and so on and/or has been teased about his speech.
4. Child is avoiding speaking, and/or secondary characteristics are observed.

Action.

1. For the young child, the pediatrician may counsel parents regarding "normal nonfluency" and make suggestions that they take pressure off the child "to speak better." However, to say "Don't worry, he'll outgrow it" is to imply that this "it" is not "normal," and the covert message may be that they do indeed have something to be concerned about.
2. Refer for a speech and language evaluation if:
   a. It is believed that the parents have a need to have a specialist evaluate the child.
   b. The amount of nonfluency is considered beyond acceptable boundaries.
   c. The child exhibits secondary characteristics.

THE SCREENING PROCESS

Screening may take the form of questioning the parent or direct observation of the child. The pediatrician need not have an armamentarium of tests for the latter. A box of com-

mon objects may be all that is necessary to provide language and speech samples. For example:

Activity. Depending on child's age, give commands using the objects, such as, "Put the key on your chair" or "Put the key on your chair and the pencil on the floor."

Product. (Refer back to normal language, and speech information.) Sample auditory verbal comprehension, auditory memory skills, understanding of spatial prepositions.

Activity. Child chooses one object at a time and tells something about it.

Product. Sample of connected discourse, naming skills, articulation, voice, and fluency.

THE REFERRAL PROCESS

If the child "fails" the screening, the referral letter, in addition to a statement about the findings and the medical and social history, should also request that the results of the evaluation be sent to the pediatrician, including recommendations, plans for implementation, and the parents' response when they were informed of them.

THE CASE MANAGING PROCESS

If the child is to be seen for some type of intervention program, the pediatrician should request that the agency or individual have periodic reports sent about the child's progress and of any change in the program.

SUMMARY

Early intervention for children with speech and language disorders is imperative. The pediatrician, both by design and because the parents place him in the role, must screen for these problems during the routine examination of the child. It is mandatory to appropriately refer the child who fails the screening and to then monitor his progress.

It is intended that this chapter serve as a guide for such a systematic approach.

BIBLIOGRAPHY

Bloodstein O: Speech Pathology: An Introduction. Boston, Houghton Mifflin, 1979

Hopper R, Naremore R: Children's Speech: A Practical Introduction to Communication Development, 2nd ed. New York, Harper & Row, 1978

Irwin J: Disorders of Articulation. Indianapolis, Bobbs-Merrill, 1972

Kleffner F: Language Disorders in Children. Indianapolis, Bobbs-Merrill, 1976

Menyuk P: The Development of Speech. Indianapolis, Bobbs-Merrill, 1972

Moskowitz B: The acquisition of language. Sci. Am Nov 1978, pp 92–108

Reilly A (ed): The Communication Game: Perspectives in Development: Speech, Language and Non-Verbal Communication Skills. Pediatric Round Table: 4, New York, Johnson & Johnson Baby Products Company, 1980

Sak R, Ruben R: Recurrent middle ear effusion in childhood: implications of temporary auditory deprivation for language and learning. Am Otol Rhinol Laryngol 90:546, 1981

Schwartz AH, Murphy MW: Cues for screening language disorders in preschool children. Pediatrics 55: 717, 1975

Cross-Reference to *Pediatrics,* 17th ed.

Development	p 1577	Mental Retardation	p 399–402
Hearing Loss	p 65, 888, 897, 1578, 1615	Speech	p 80, 899, 1613
Language	p 25, 45, 63–64	Stuttering	p 63–64

Acute and Chronic Illness of Various Body Systems

TWENTY-NINE

Cardiac Signs and Symptoms

Bernard Fish

All pediatric practitioners are faced daily with the evaluation of infants and children with symptoms and signs suggestive of cardiac malfunction. Since the vast majority of these children do not have heart disease, the major task is to differentiate the normal from the abnormal. The intent of this chapter is to present information that will be helpful to practitioners in sorting out signs and symptoms possibly referable to the heart. This chapter focuses on the asymptomatic child with a murmur. Evaluation of the neonate with possible congestive heart failure or with cyanosis is also discussed.

THE CHILD WITH A HEART MURMUR

This section is intended as a guide for the differentiation of innocent murmurs from organic murmurs in children beyond infancy. Clinical features of the most common defects that produce organic murmurs are described, along with criteria for assessment of their severity. Children with overt cardiac signs and symptoms are not discussed in detail.

Innocent Murmur vs Organic Murmur

Innocent murmurs are the most common ones found in children. Tables 1 and 2 list their characteristics and the noncardiac factors that influence their intensity. Organic murmurs are those that are considered to be associated with anatomic cardiac defects (Table 3). If a murmur can be identified with certainty as innocent, no further evaluation is necessary. The child and family should be advised as to what an innocent murmur is, since many families believe that the term "heart murmur" is synonymous with the term "heart defect." It is important to stress that no abnormality is present and that no special precautions should be taken. Activity should not be restricted. Lifestyle and career planning should not be affected. The practitioner should be prepared to respond to requests from schools, health care agencies, employers, and insurance companies to certify that there is no increased risk of morbidity or mortality associated with an innocent murmur.

Special Note Regarding Murmurs in Neonates

We believe that a murmur detected in the newborn period should never be diagnosed as innocent. All of these infants need to be monitored closely for cyanosis or for signs of CHF. Frequent evaluation of color, breathing, feeding habits, and growth will allow identification of infants in difficulty.

TABLE 1. DIFFERENTIATION OF INNOCENT VS ORGANIC MURMUR

Parameter	Findings with *Innocent* Murmur and Normal Cardiac Function	Findings with *Organic* Murmur and/or Cardiac Overload	Differential Diagnosis of Abnormal Findings
Position on chest where murmur is heard	Precordium (may be widely transmitted)	Precordium	
	Neck (venous hum)	Neck	AS, PS, PDA, Coarct
		Lung fields	PPS
		Back	PDA, PPS, fistula
Timing	Systolic ejection	Systolic Ejection	PS, AS
		Pansystolic	VSD
	Diastolic (venous hum)	Diastolic decrescendo	AI, PI
		Middiastolic flow rumble	ASD if tricuspid flow rumble
			VSD, MI, PDA if mitral flow rumble
	Continuous (mammary souffle)	Continuous	PDA
Intensity	I–III	I–VI	
Quality	Vibratory, musical	Harsh	AS, PS, VSD
		High-pitched, blowing	MI, tiny VSD
Thrill	Absent	May be present over precordium, suprasternal notch, or carotid arteries	Indicates grade IV–VI intensity
S_1	May be split	S_1 may be inaudible	LV dysfunction
Ejection sounds	None	Ejection click (pulmonic area, Ao area)	PS, AS
		Midsystolic click	Mitral valve prolapse
S_2	Physiologically split	Fixed split	ASD, RBBB, PS, or PPS
	P_2 may be $>$ A_2 in children	Loud A_2	*d*-transposition, *l*-transposition (anterior aorta)
			Systemic hypertension
		Loud P_2	Pulmonary hypertension, PPS
		A_2 or P_2 inaudible (single S_2)	AS, PS, tetralogy of Fallot
Early diastole		Opening snap	MS
Mid diastole	Physiologic S_3 may be present in older children and adolescents	S_3 gallop	LV dysfunction, volume overload
Late diastole		S_4	Decreased compliance, cardiomyopathy

(*continued*)

TABLE 1 (*Continued*)

Parameter	Findings with *Innocent* Murmur and Normal Cardiac Function	Findings with *Organic* Murmur and/or Cardiac Overload	Differential Diagnosis of Abnormal Findings
Response to change in position	May change intensity	May change intensity	Mitral valve prolapse, pedunculated intra-cardiac mass
Response to exercise	Intensity may increase	Intensity may increase	
	S_3 may become audible	Diastolic flow rumble may become audible	
Response to Valsalva maneuver	Intensity should decrease	Intensity may increase	IHSS, occasionally mitral valve prolapse
		Intensity may decrease	All other defects
Response to isometric load	Variable	Intensity may increase	AI, mitral valve prolapse, VSD, MI
		Intensity may decrease	IHSS, AS
Cardiac impulse	Normal	RV heave	ADS, PS, tetralogy of Fallot
		LV heave	LV volume or pressure load
		Apex may be deviated laterally (LV)	LV dysfunction (cardiomyopathy), LV volume load (AI, MI, VSD, PDA, and soon)
Pulses, BP	Normal and equal in arms and legs	May be absent in legs	Coarctation of the aorta

AI, aortic insufficiency; AS, aortic stenosis; ASD, atrial septal defect; Coarct, coarctation of aorta; IHSS, idiopathic hypertrophic subaortic stenosis; LBBB, left bundle branch block; LV, left ventricle; MI, mitral insufficiency; MS, mitral stenosis; PDA, patent ductus arteriosus; PI, pulmonic insufficiency; PPS, peripheral pulmonic stenosis; PS, pulmonic stenosis; RBBB, right bundle branch block; RV, right ventricle; VSD, ventricular septal defect.

EVALUATION OF MURMURS IN OLDER CHILDREN

History

Most children with heart murmurs are asymptomatic, and the relevant history is negative. It is important to ask about symptoms of cardiac decompensation in the neonatal period or symptoms of acute rheumatic fever during childhood. Records should be obtained from other practitioners and from prior hospitalizations to determine when the murmur was first detected. A history of symptoms, such as dyspnea on exercise, orthopnea, weight loss, or chronic fever, should be sought.

Chest pain is usually not a cardiac symptom. The types of heart disease that produce

TABLE 2. CAUSES OF INCREASED CARDIAC OUTPUT THAT MAY INCREASE INTENSITY OF HEART MURMURS

Fever
Activity
Anemia
Medications
A-V malformations
Hyperthyroidism
Beri-beri (may be induced during recovery
  from severe malnutrition)
Hyperkinetic heart syndrome

chronic chest pain include severe forms of aortic stenosis or subaortic stenosis, congestive cardiomyopathy, Eisenmenger's syndrome, pericarditis, and myocarditis. These usually are recognized immediately on physical examination and EKG. If there are no overt cardiac findings, the physician should look elsewhere for the source of chest pain.

Physical Examination

Evidence of a systemic or an inherited disorder that could predispose to a cardiac defect should be sought, such as fetal alcohol syndrome and Turner's syndrome. Respiratory rate and heart rate should be counted. Tachypnea at rest is a sign of cardiac decompensation in both infants and children. Blood pressure is measured in the right arm. If elevated, it should be measured in all four limbs.

On examination of the chest, a precordial bulge indicates chronic cardiac enlargement. A parasternal (right ventricular) or apical (left ventricular) heave is significant. Lateral displacement of the left border of the heart or of the apical impulse indicates cardiac enlargement. A thrill indicates that the murmur associated with it is at least grade IV/VI in intensity. (See Table 4 for grading of the intensity of murmurs.)

The significance of abnormal findings on auscultation is presented in Table 1. The murmur is evaluated for timing, quality, in-

TABLE 3. ETIOLOGY OF ORGANIC MURMURS

Some Rather Frequent Causes of Organic Murmurs in Asymptomatic Children

Aortic valve disease
  Congenital (bicuspid aortic valve is the most
    common)
  Rheumatic (usually presents with AI, not AS,
    in childhood)
Atrial septal defect (ostium secundum)
Mitral insufficiency
  Rheumatic
  Nonrheumatic (prolapse is the most common)
Patent ductus arteriosus
Pulmonic stenosis
Ventricular septal defect

Cardiac Problems Found Less Frequently in Asymptomatic Children

Mitral stenosis
  Rheumatic
  Nonrheumatic

Ostium primum ASD (with cleft mitral valve)
Peripheral pulmonic stenosis
Tetralogy of Fallot (rarely asymptomatic)
Hypertrophic obstructive cardiomyopathy
  (HOCM), also referred to as IHSS

Significant Cardiac Problems that May Present without a Heart Murmur

Acute myocarditis
Coarctation of the aorta
Congestive cardiomyopathy
Pericarditis

TABLE 4. GUIDE FOR GRADING OF INTENSITY OF SYSTOLIC HEART MURMURS

Grade	Intensity
I	Faint, heard only with special effort
II	Faint, easily heard
III	Prominent, not loud
IV	Loud, usually associated with palpable shrill
V	Very loud, heard with the edge of the stethoscope on chest
VI	Exceptionally loud, heard even with stethoscope off chest

tensity, location, and transmission. The neck and back are auscultated in order to define distant transmission of the murmur. Ejection or nonejection (late systolic) clicks (an extra sound occurring during systole) should be looked for. The second sound is examined for physiologic splitting and intensity of the pulmonary component. Diastole should be scanned for gallops and diastolic murmurs.

Enlargement of the liver may be a sign of venous engorgement. Enlargement of the spleen occurs with venous engorgement and with generalized disease, such as bacterial endocarditis. The extremities are examined for the character of the pulses, color, and perfusion. Absence of a pulse in the legs indicates obstruction to arterial flow, which occurs with coarctation of the aorta. Bounding pulses indicate patent ductus arteriosus or aortic insufficiency. Generalized weak pulses and poor perfusion may indicate congestive cardiomyopathy or severe aortic stenosis. Peripheral edema is a late sign of cardiac decompensation. If edema is present without signs of severe cardiac dysfunction, the possibility of renal disease or hypoalbuminemia should be considered.

Laboratory Procedures

The noninvasive laboratory procedures used for evaluation of children with cardiac problems include hematocrit determination, electrocardiogram, chest x-ray, echocardiogram, Holter monitor, and stress test. Occasionally, a radionuclide scan is helpful.

MANAGEMENT

Indications for Subspecialty Referral

Cardiology consultation for evaluation of a heart murmur is indicated in children who are symptomatic or who are suspected of having organic disease. The chest x-ray, electrocardiogram, and hematocrit can be requested by the pediatric practitioner. If these are normal, but there is still some question of the possibility of organic cardiac disease, referral to a cardiologist is indicated. Children with the recent onset of congestive heart failure or progression of signs of cardiac overload should be admitted to the cardiac center without delay to rule out such illnesses as acute rheumatic fever, myocarditis, pericarditis, or bacterial endocarditis.

Management of Asymptomatic Children with Organic Murmurs

Once the diagnosis of an organic murmur has been confirmed or established by the pediatric cardiologist, decisions need to be made regarding everyday management of the child. Areas of concern include the need for restriction of physical activity and the institution of antibiotic therapy in special situations, in addition to long-term prognosis and what benefits might occur with treatment. The consultant must communicate this information to the child and the family as well as to the pediatric practitioner. The practitioner then needs to reinforce the information in a follow-up visit with the family. In this way, errors in interpretation of the advice given will be minimized.

Physical Exertion. Exercise is not restricted unless there are specific indications, such as in the child with severe aortic stenosis or severe cardiomyopathy. Children with mild aortic or pulmonic stenosis or with a ventricular septal defect and a small left-to-right shunt are allowed normal activity, including strenuous exertion.

Antibiotic Prophylaxis. In general, all cardiac defects predispose to the development of bacterial endocarditis. The goal of prophylaxis is to administer appropriate antibiotics so that therapeutic concentrations will be present in the bloodstream before bacteria are released (Table 5). Colonization of any rough edges inside the heart or major blood vessels thus may be prevented. Prophylaxis is against gram-positive organisms before dental, skin, and ear-nose-and-throat procedures and before any procedure during which endotracheal intubation is necessary. Uncomplicated herniorrhaphy, testicular operations, and similar genital and perineal procedures should be included in this group. Prophylaxis against both gram-positive and gram-negative organisms is given for intra-abdominal procedures and urologic procedures involving instrumentation of the urinary tract. There is controversy regarding the necessity for prophylaxis prior to a clean abortion by dilatation and curettage. Minor trauma and common childhood infections are handled in the usual fashion.

Children who have had rheumatic fever must be protected against further infection with the group A streptococcus. This requires giving daily oral penicillin in small doses or monthly injections of long-acting penicillin. Children allergic to penicillin may be protected with a sulfonamide or erythromycin. Children whose heart valves have been damaged by rheumatic fever need prophylaxis against bacterial endocarditis as well.

THE NEONATE WITH CONGESTIVE HEART FAILURE

Rapid identification of the neonate in congestive heart failure (CHF) is essential in order to provide appropriate diagnostic and therapeutic intervention. The initial signs and symptoms of disease often are subtle. Identification and emergency treatment of the infant with cardiac disease is emphasized in this section, since definitive diagnosis, treatment, and long-term management are in the domain of the pediatric cardiologist.

Etiology

Though the most important conditions causing cardiac failure in the neonate are congenital anatomic defects of the heart and great vessels, other conditions must be considered as well. The various etiologies can be considered under five headings:

1. Anatomic obstruction and hypoplasia of the left heart
2. Myocardial dysfunction, with or without cardiac defect
3. Arrhythmia
4. Left-to-right shunt
5. Fluid overload

The age of the infant serves as a clue to the etiology. Left heart obstruction becomes symptomatic as soon as the ductus begins to close (i.e., during the first days of life), leaving the lower body with no source of blood flow. Ventricular dysfunction also may appear within the first days of life, often in the setting of gestational diabetes or perinatal stress.

In contrast, the appearance of CHF in an infant with a left-to-right shunt is usually delayed for weeks to months in full-term babies with well-developed pulmonary arterioles. In premature infants, left-to-right shunts may cause failure much earlier, since their pulmonary arterioles are less well developed. Arrhythmias may cause heart failure in utero or at any time after birth. Fluid overload may become a factor any time intravenous fluids are used in neonates but may occur also in utero or at birth with severe anemia (as in erythroblastosis fetalis).

TABLE 5. RECOMMENDED ANTIBIOTIC PROPHYLAXIS FOR INFECTIVE ENDOCARDITIS

	No Contraindication to Penicillin	Penicillin Allergy or Resistance
Dental and upper respiratory tract procedures*		
Usual patient	1. 30 minutes to 1 hour before procedure, give aqueous penicillin G 30,000 IU/kg mixed with 600,000 IU of procaine penicillin G intramuscularly, then oral penicillin V at 250 mg every 6 hours for four to eight doses (500 mg if child weighs more than 30 kg) OR 2. Oral penicillin V (1 g), followed by 250 mg every 6 hours for four to eight doses (double these doses if weight is more than 30 kg)	1 to 1.5 hours before procedure give oral erythromycin at 20 mg/kg, then 10 mg/kg every 6 hours for four to eight doses
Patient with prosthetic valve	Intramuscular penicillin as above, plus intramuscular streptomycin 20 mg/kg; repeat these once daily for 2 days	30 minutes to 1 hour before procedure, give intravenous infusion of vancomycin at 20 mg/kg, then erythromycin at 10 mg/kg every 6 hours for eight doses by mouth
Gastrointestinal and genitourinary procedures†		
Usual patient	30 minutes to 1 hour before procedure, give intramuscular aqueous penicillin G at 30,000 IU/kg plus streptomycin at 20 mg/kg; repeat every 12 hours for two doses	30 minutes to 1 hour before procedure, give intravenous infusion of vancomycin at 20 mg/kg plus intramuscular streptomycin at 20 mg/kg; can repeat once 12 hours later
Patient with prosthetic valve	As above; some use intramuscular or intravenous ampicillin at 50 mg/kg instead of penicillin, and intramuscular or intravenous gentamicin at 2 mg/kg instead of streptomycin; repeat every 8 hours for 2 hours	As above

*Bacteremia is usually due to streptococci, although diphtheroids and occasional staphylococci have been reported. Almost all the invading organisms are penicillin-sensitive.

†Bacteremia usually with enterococci (*Streptococcus faecalis*) or gram-negative bacilli, but only the former are likely to cause bacterial endocarditis. *(From: Rudolph AM (ed): Pediatrics, 17th ed, Appleton-Century-Crofts 1982.)*

Differential Diagnosis

History. The important points relate to family history, difficulties with gestation, and the stress of delivery. A history of another infant with cardiac disease is important, since some forms of heart disease are more likely to be familial (e.g., endocardial fibroelastosis). Maternal illness during pregnancy, especially rubella, may lead to congenital heart defects. Diabetes mellitus, even if only gestational, is a predisposing factor in left ventricular dysfunction, transient hypertrophic obstructive cardiomyopathy, persistence of fetal circulatory pathway, and cyanotic congenital heart disease. Perinatal stress and asphyxia also may lead to persistence of fetal circulatory pathway or left ventricular dysfunction.

Parental concerns over noisy or rapid breathing and sweating or irritability with feeding must not be dismissed. Questions concerning changes in color (pallor, cyanosis) and cyanosis or mottling with crying should be asked.

Physical Examination. Two axioms are useful in examining neonates suspected of having a cardiac defect:

1. A murmur detected in a neonate should never be diagnosed as innocent.

2. Absence of a heart murmur should not dissuade one from cardiac evaluation if other findings point in that direction.

Table 6 summarizes the important points to be looked for in the assessment of an infant.

Though tachypnea is an important early sign of elevated pulmonary venous pressure, other systems must be investigated when tachypnea is found (Table 7). Since tachypnea associated with mild to moderate pulmonary venous hypertension is not accompanied by respiratory distress, one must count the respiratory rate in order to recognize this sign in a baby. Other characteristic physical findings with CHF are pallor, precordial heave, and accentuated (or distant) heart sounds. A gallop rhythm may be present. Hepatomegaly, abnormal pulses, and decreased peripheral perfusion (cool extremities) are all relatively late signs. Peripheral edema is not commonly seen in infants with CHF.

Laboratory Procedures.
Blood Studies. Anemia, hypoglycemia, and hypocalcemia must be ruled out in any baby with cardiac decompensation, since these may be the cause of a baby's difficulty or may

---

TABLE 6. SIGNS OF CARDIAC DECOMPENSATION

Observation and/or History	Physical Examination
Decreased growth	Tachypnea
Poor feeding	Cardiac heave and/or enlargement by palpation
Irritability	Gallop rhythm
Abnormal respirations	Enlargement of liver and/or spleen
Tachypnea at rest	Weak pulses
Dyspnea on exertion	Differential BP (arms > legs)
Orthopnea (babies may become irritable when lying flat)	Murmur (may be absent)
Decreased perfusion (cool extremities)	
Color change (pallor, cyanosis, mottling)	
Sweating (diaphoresis)	

**TABLE 7. CONDITIONS OTHER THAN
CARDIAC THAT MAY PRODUCE TACHYPNEA
OR CYANOSIS IN THE NEONATE**

Large and small airway disease
Pleural effusion or empyema
Pneumonitis
Central nervous system infections
Metabolic acidosis
Fluid retention with or without edema
Intestinal obstruction or paralytic ileus
Diaphragmatic hernia
Methemoglobinemia, hemoglobin M disease
Persistence of fetal circulatory pathway (PFCP)

be contributing factors. Acidosis, especially a metabolic base deficit, may indicate inadequate systemic blood flow.

Electrocardiogram. In neonates, the electrocardiogram reflects fetal physiology (Table 8). For this reason, interpretation of the EKG in the neonate requires an appreciation of the differences from the older child because of the special conditions during fetal life.

In neonates with CHF, the EKG findings for LV hypoplasia are the same as those with severe RVH. With LV dysfunction or obstruction, the EKG shows only ST-T wave changes, since there has not been time for changes in QRS to develop. In severely stressed neonates, patterns associated with acute myocardial infarction may evolve. Left axis deviation or indeterminate axis may indicate a complex defect, such as complete atrioventricular canal, double outlet right ventricle, or tricuspid atresia. In babies with VSD or PDA, the most common defects, the EKG may be normal, reflecting normal development of LV and RV muscle mass prior to birth. Thus, in most infants, the EKG is not very useful in assessing the severity of a defect. Nevertheless, it may help to identify those with complex defects, and it is obviously helpful in evaluating arrhythmias.

Chest X-ray. The chest x-ray is useful for the evaluation of increased or decreased pulmonary blood flow, cardiac enlargement and configuration, and pulmonary venous hypertension (Table 9). Occasionally, the shape of the heart on chest x-ray may provide a clue to the specific diagnosis.

Echocardiography. Echocardiography (Table 10) can aid in differentiating babies with left ventricular dysfunction from those with left-to-right shunts and from those with severe left ventricular outflow tract obstruction or hypoplastic left heart syndrome, since all of these conditions may present in similar fashion. Complex defects, such as A-V canal, single ventricle, and double outlet right ventricle, are recognized. It is important to understand, however, that uncomplicated ventricular septal defect is not necessarily differentiated from ductus arteriosus, since neither defect can be reliably visualized in neonates. Both defects appear as left-to-right shunts, with large left atrium and hyperkinetic left ventricle.

Management

Once a diagnosis of congestive heart failure is suspected, consultation with a pediatric cardiologist is essential. There are, however, some basic guidelines that should be followed even prior to or coincident with the request for assistance.

Initial and Immediate Management. The clinical state of the infant dictates how aggressive the management of congestive heart failure should be. The child in mild CHF presents with poor feeding, tachypnea, tachycardia, and possibly poor growth. Most often, these simple measures indicated below will be all that is required to stabilize this infant prior to consultation with a cardiologist or neonatologist on site or in preparation for transfer. Occasionally, heroic measures may be necessary in the baby who appears shocky, perhaps unconscious, gray in color, with poor

TABLE 8. EKG FINDINGS IN NEONATES

	Criteria	Significance
Normal	RV dominance, RAD in term babies LV dominance in premature babies Use normative tables	Seen in neonates with normal development of both ventricles; VSD, PDA, mild valvular deformities; *d*-transposition and tetralogy of Fallot do not interfere with fetal development of ventricular mass and therefore may present with normal EKG
RVH	Increase in RV forces for age R in V_3R, V_1, V_2; S in V_5, V_6 Use normative table *Or* relatively inconspicuous LV forces (greater than normal RV dominance for age)	Seen with mild to moderate PS but not with severe PS where RV is relatively hypoplastic; also seen with total anomalous pulmonary venous drainage where all veins drain to the right side during fetal life so that the RV carries more than normal flow
	Or upright T in lead V_1 after 48–72 h	Severe LV outflow obstruction may cause the RV to take over more of the fetal cardiac output and produce fetal RVH and relatively hypoplastic LV; defects include coarctation of the aorta, severe AS, mitral abnormalities, and hypoplastic left heart syndrome
LVH	Increase in LV forces for age S in V_3R, V_1, V_2; R in V_5, V_6 *Or* relatively inconspicuous RV forces	Seen with LV outflow obstruction that is relatively mild so as not to produce LV hypoplasia; also seen with cardiomyopathies such as that seen in infants of diabetic mothers; also seen with RV hypoplasia as in severe PS, pulmonary atresia, tricuspid atresia
Atrial hypertrophy	It is often difficult to be certain in neonates which atrium is involved; large RA sometimes produces posterior forces (negative deflection in V_1) and LAE sometimes produces a large P wave in lead II	If seen in the first few days of life this indicates fetal heart failure as seen in hydrops, severe arrhythmia, or fetal valvular insufficiency (e.g., Ebstein's anomaly) or atresia (e.g., tricuspid atresia)

pulses, poor peripheral perfusion, i.e., cool extremities, poor filling of the nailbeds, and poor heart sounds. Table 11 indicates a sequence of measures to take during initial management of CHF. The following discussion deals with the acutely ill infant in congestive heart failure.

Initial laboratory assessment includes determination of arterial blood gas (pH, PaO_2, $PaCO_2$), complete blood count (hematocrit), serum electrolytes (sodium, potassium, bicarbonate, calcium), and a serum glucose. Maintenance of a flow sheet with all the laboratory determinations, times of their

TABLE 9. FEATURES SEEN ON X-RAY THAT MAY BE HELPFUL

Heart size and shape
Pulmonary vascular markings
  Arteries
    Pulmonary overcirculation (L-R shunt)
    Pulmonary undercirculation (RV obstruc-
      tion)
  Veins
    Pulmonary venous hypertension (heart
      failure, left heart obstruction)
  Capillaries
    Edema
Position of vital structures (relative to abnor-
    malities of situs)
  Aortic arch
  Cardiac apex
  Stomach bubble
  Liver
  Thoracic situs
Skeleton
  (Syndromes)

TABLE 10. HEART DEFECTS THAT CAN BE DIAGNOSED BY ECHOCARDIOGRAM IN CYANOTIC NEWBORNS

d-Transposition (great vessel position)
Ebstein's anomaly of the tricuspid valve (tri-
    cuspid position)
Endocardial cushion defect (A-V valve motion)
Hypoplastic left heart syndrome
Severe aortic stenosis (fibrotic aortic valve)
Severe mitral stenosis (motion of mitral valve)
Tetralogy, pulmonary atresia, truncus ar-
    teriosus (overriding aorta)
Total anomalous pulmonary venous return,
    cor triatriatum (pulmonary venous chamber
    behind heart)
Tricuspid atresia, single ventricle (presence of
    only one ventricle)

measurement, and therapy given for repair of abnormalities, is very helpful in organizing therapy.

One begins with maintenance of an adequate airway. Treatment of hypoxemia is begun immediately. We strive to raise the PaO_2 to 100 torr or greater; in the absence of a right-to-left shunt, this usually can be achieved by giving oxygen with an FiO_2 of 0.4 (40% oxygen concentration). The method of delivery varies according to the infant's condition. For the infant breathing on his own and not requiring ventilatory support, a head box is adequate.

Temperature is maintained using an open warmer controlled by a thermistor attached to the baby's skin and set at 35C (95F). This allows access to the infant so that other procedures may be performed. Electrodes are attached to the baby's chest so that heart and respiratory rates can be monitored continuously.

An occasional infant will require mechanical support of ventilation. Trans-laryngeal intubation (orotracheal or nasotracheal) is established, the infant is paralyzed with pancuronium (0.1 mg/kg intravenously as needed), and oxygen is given to keep the PaO_2 above 100 torr, as mentioned above.

Simultaneous with the establishment of adequate oxygenation, an assessment of the need for glucose, calcium, and bicarbonate is made. The blood glucose should be maintained above 100 mg/dl, but not high enough to overcome the renal threshhold (usually 160–180 mg/dl). This can be achieved by using 5–10% glucose in the intravenous solution. If the infant has severe hypoglycemia (less than 50 mg/dl at full term), rapid correction is essential (Table 11), using 25% glucose in water. If no metabolic acidosis exists, extra bicarbonate does not have to be given. If the pH is below 7.1, 1–2 mEq/kg of $NaHCO_3$ should be given intravenously along with the oxygen. If the pH is 7.1 or higher, one can wait to see what improvement is obtained after oxygen therapy ventilatory support (if indicated) and improvement in cardiac output.

Hypocalcemia can be managed by infusing calcium gluconate 300–500 mg/kg/24 h

TABLE 11. MANAGEMENT OF ACUTE CIRCULATORY FAILURE

Condition	Medication	Dose	Method of Administration	Aim of Therapy
Hypoxemia	Oxygen	40%	Head box, CPAP, or intubation	↑ paO_2 >100 mm Hg
Hypoventilation	Ventilatory support		CPAP or Mechanical	↑ paO_2 >100 mm Hg ↓ $paCO_2$ <40 mm Hg
Metabolic acidosis	Sodium Bicarbonate	1–2 mEq/kg	Intravenous bolus diluted 1:3	↑ pH to 7.2
Pulmonary edema	Furosemide	1 mg/Kg	Intravenous bolus	↓ work of breathing ↑ $pa\ O_2$ ↓ $pa\ CO_2$
Inadequate contractility	Dopamine	10 mcg/kg/min (5–20 mcg/kg/min)	Continuous Infusion*	↑ Cardiac output ↓ Metabolic acidosis
Hypoglycemia	Glucose 25%	2–4 cc/kg	Intravenous Bolus	Glucose between 100 and 150
Hypocalcemia (STAT)	Calcium gluconate 10%=100/mg/cc	100 mg/kg 1 cc/kg	Slow intra-venous bolus	Ion Ca 3–4 mEq/ml Total Ca 7.5–8 mg/dl
Hypocalcemia (Continuous)	same	500 mg/kg 5 cc/kg	Continuous in-fusion over 24 hours	same
Anemia	Blood	10 cc/kg	Packed red cells	↑ Hematocrit to 35–40%
Hyponatremia severe (Na <120 mEq/L)	NaCl 3%	5–6 cc/kg	Intravenous bolus	Na >120 mEq/l

*The stock concentration of dopamine is 40 mg/cc. A dilution of 60 mg/100 cc given at a rate of 1cc/Kg/Hr provides 10 mcg/Kg/min.

by constant IV infusion, following calcium levels frequently intravenously, with adjustment of the dose as needed.

Hyperkalemia (serum K above 6.5 mEq/L) will improve as the acidosis is treated and urine flow is established. Severe hyponatremia (less than 120 mEq/L) should be managed by infusing 3% NaCl 5–6 ml/kg rapidly, along with a diuretic.

As all these measures are being carried out, furosemide should be given intravenously in a dose of 1 mg/kg. If the infant is judged to be extremely ill, the bladder is catheterized so that urine flow can be monitored continuously. In the less ill infant, a urine collecting bag, externally applied, is sufficient. Vital signs (temperature, heart rate, respiratory rate, and blood pressure) are followed. Accurate weights before and during therapy are essential.

In the seriously ill child, cardiac inotropes are administered by continuous intravenous infusion. We have used dopamine as our initial inotrope, beginning with a dose of 10 µg/kg/min by constant infusion. No loading dose is necessary.

Marked improvement in the infant's condition should be noted within 10–15 minutes after the onset of dopamine if the dose is adequate. The dopamine drip rate can be adjusted down or up as needed to maintain the circulation. Color, quality of pulses, heart sounds, level of consciousness, and perfusion of the extremities will all look, feel, and sound much more normal. Arterial blood gas determinations will show a return of the pH to near normal and an increase in PaO_2 and a decrease in $PaCO_2$. Improvement with these measures may be very temporary in these infants. Diagnosis and definitive treatment must proceed on an urgent basis.

We do not believe that digoxin plays a part in the immediate stabilization of a child in acute or impending cardiopulmonary collapse. We still believe that digoxin is useful in the treatment of chronic congestive heart failure but that the decision to begin using it, the method of its administration, and the dose to be used can await the cardiologist. (See Table 12 for doses.) The decision to use prostaglandin inhibitors (indomethacin, aspirin) to induce closure of the ductus arteriosus likewise is a decision left to the cardiologist or neonatologist, as is the use of prostaglandin E_2 in order to keep a ductus arteriosus open.

In the great majority of instances, the correction of metabolic disturbances and the use of a diuretic, oxygen, and digoxin will stabilize the infant's condition. If the baby needs to be transferred to a distant facility or if the pediatric cardiologist is not immediately available, these measures should be initiated by the pediatric practitioner, since the stabilization of the infant in congestive heart failure is essential prior to transportation.

Indication for Cardiac Catheterization and Surgery. A discussion of these aspects of care is beyond the scope of this chapter. The timing of these decisions is complex, based on the accumulation of diagnostic data and the response of the infant to medical management, and requires the expertise of both the cardiologist and the cardiac surgeon. For a discussion of how these decisions are made and of chronic medical management, follow-up, and prognosis, page references to the 17th edition of *Pediatrics* are given at the end of this chapter.

Chronic Medical Management of CHF

If surgery is to be delayed, CHF is treated chronically by continuation of oral digoxin and diuretics, with careful observation of

TABLE 12. DIGITALIZING THE NEWBORN INFANT

Age	Total Loading Dose Divided over 18–36 HR	Usual Daily Maintenance Dose
Premature	20–40 mcg/kg	7–12 mcg/kg/day
Term–1 mo	40–50 mcg/kg	10–15 mcg/kg/day
1 mo–2 years	60–75 mcg/kg	15–20 mcg/kg/day

1. Correct metabolic disturbances; especially, Na, K, pH.
2. Baseline 12 lead EKG.
3. Divide Loading dose into 3–4 doses at intervals of 4–8 hours. (e.g., ½; ¼; ¼ or ¼; ¼; ¼; ¼)
4. Observe by auscultation and rhythm strips for 2° heart block; ventricular ectopic beats and other arrhythmias.
5. 12 Lead EKG after digitalization for changes in P-R interval and T waves (digitalis effect).
6. The maintenance dose is determined by improvement achieved, side effects experienced, and renal status. Maintenance is usually divided B.I.D. in babies.

Doses are reduced if myocarditis or electrolyte disturbance is suspected.

mineral balance (sodium, potassium, calcium) and acid-base balance. Some babies will need spironolactone or potassium supplements. Oral vasodilators are reported to be beneficial in LV dysfunction but have not been used in babies with left-to-right shunts. Additional supportive measures include high-calorie feedings, protection from thermal stress, and careful observation for and treatment of intercurrent infections. Respiratory rate, feeding pattern, response to infection, and growth are carefully monitored during ambulatory follow-up. Medications are increased to keep up with growth. The timing of elective repair varies from institution to institution.

THE NEONATE WITH CYANOSIS

The cyanotic infant requires rapid establishment of the underlying cause and institution of therapeutic measures. Though a right-to-left shunt can produce cyanosis, other conditions need to be considered (Table 7), including diseases of red cells, upper and lower airways, pneumonia, infection, and persistence of the fetal circulatory pathway. Initial consultation with a neonatologist is suggested, especially when a cardiac cause for the cyanosis is not obvious, in order to aid in proper diagnosis and management. The discussion that follows focuses on cardiac conditions that can produce cyanosis.

Etiology

The two groups of heart defects that produce cyanosis in the neonate are those with severe obstruction to pulmonary blood flow (e.g., tricuspid atresia and severe Tetralogy of Fallot) and those that produce parallel pulmonary and systemic circulations with inadequate mixing of blood (e.g., transposition of the great vessels). Another condition, persistence of the fetal circulatory pathway (PFCP), though not associated with an anatomic defect, is also a cardiac cause of cyanosis. PFCP may be seen in normal newborns predisposed to it by such factors as diabetes mellitus in the mother, acidosis, hypoglycemia, hypocalcemia, polycythemia, infection, or any perinatal stress.

Differential Diagnosis

History. Attention to the details of the prenatal course, delivery, and immediate postnatal period is very important. Prolonged ruptured membranes and fever in the mother point to infection as a cause for the cyanosis. A low Apgar score, associated with a difficult delivery, suggests the possibility of central nervous system insult, meconium aspiration, or sepsis. An infant who had been doing well, with no history of risk factors, who suddenly deteriorates and becomes cyanotic, may have sepsis or a cerebral hemorrhage.

Physical Examination. Physical examination, with attention to the degree of cyanosis and respiratory distress, may be helpful. As a general rule, infants with cyanosis related to the respiratory tract have significant difficulty in breathing, while cardiac and metabolic defects produce tachypnea with much less distress. Sepsis or cerebral insult may produce cyanosis on the basis of hypoventilation. Presence or absence of a murmur does not establish or exclude cardiac disease. Conditions, such as tricuspid atresia, often are not associated with a murmur, whereas in cyanosis due to metabolic causes, especially if associated with cardiac failure, a systolic murmur of mitral or tricuspid insufficiency may be heard.

Laboratory Procedures. A complete blood count, arterial blood gases, glucose, calcium, serum electrolytes, blood and urine cultures, chest x-ray, and electrocardiogram are all necessary. Polycythemia as a cause of cyanosis can be ruled out with a normal hematocrit. A normal PaO_2 in the presence of cyanosis suggests the diagnosis of methemoglobinemia. Hypoglycemia and hypocalcemia must be corrected, whatever the etiology, as should any abnormalities of serum electrolytes.

The electrocardiogram may or may not be helpful. As in babies with congestive heart failure, the EKG generally reflects intrauterine physiology. (See Table 8.)

Chest X-ray (Table 9). Assessment of pulmonary blood flow is useful because it leads immediately to a decision regarding therapy. Decreased pulmonary blood flow indicates severe obstruction. Babies with this pattern may depend on a patent ductus for adequate pulmonary blood flow, and they may benefit from infusion of prostaglandin. Increased pulmonary blood flow in a severely cyanotic baby suggests transposition of the great vessels. Occasionally, however, transposition presents with severe pulmonary vasoconstriction, and the x-ray will be misleading.

The heart size or configuration may be helpful. A markedly enlarged heart with large right atrium is seen with Ebstein's anomaly of the tricuspid valve and with pulmonary atresia associated with tricuspid insufficiency. Some x-rays of babies with pulmonary atresia will show the characteristic absence of the main pulmonary arterial segment on the frontal film.

The position of other structures, such as aortic knob, cardiac apex, bronchi, stomach bubble, and liver, may be indicative of abnormalities of the aortic arch or abnormalities of situs that are associated with congenital heart defects.

Echocardiography can identify babies without cardiac defects and can separate those with defects into various categories. Echocardiography does not often replace cardiac catheterization in babies with cyanotic heart defects but may allow a diagnosis to be made with fewer angiograms and, therefore, less morbidity.

Management of the Cyanotic Neonate

Consultation with a neonatologist or cardiologist is necessary in infants with cyanosis. However, the stabilization of all such infants, using principles described in the section on congestive heart failure, applies to these infants as well.

Management of Patients with Cyanotic Heart Defects Once Diagnosis Is Established and Palliation Completed

Oxygen Delivery. Babies with adequate balloon septostomies will maintain arterial Po_2 anywhere above 29–30. Typical Po_2 in infants with aorta-to-pulmonary artery shunts will be about 40–45 mm Hg. As long as there is enough oxygen to maintain aerobic metabolism and neurologic development, growth will progress. Thus, *careful observation for metabolic acidosis* in addition to arterial Po_2 is essential during recovery from surgery and during intercurrent illness.

Blood oxygen-carrying capacity (red cell volume) must be maintained during acute phases of management.

During chronic ambulatory monitoring, hematocrit and hemoglobin or RBC morphology are followed as guides to:

1. Bone marrow response to hypoxia
2. Relative iron deficiency

A rising hematocrit indicates worsening of hypoxia. Therefore, a rising hematocrit should prompt referral to the cardiac center for consideration of further surgery. Above a hematocrit of about 65% there are often symptoms of headache and tiredness as well as a risk of stroke. If surgery is not immediately feasible, hematophoresis should be carried out, using saline, albumin, or plasma to replace red cells removed.

Cyanotic spells are characterized by episodes of sudden onset of dyspnea and cyanosis. Sometimes the spells are apparently spontaneous. Sometimes they are preceded by feeding, defecating, or exertion. Once each episode begins, it seems to be self-perpetuating even though the individual rests or squats. Sometimes the dyspnea and cyanosis go on to stupor or syncope. There is usually gradual resolution over a variable period of time. On the other hand, an episode may lead to prolonged hypoxia, acidosis, and brain damage.

If cyanotic spells are identified by history, one would refer the baby back to the cardiac center for further testing and, perhaps, further palliative or corrective surgery.

Intravenous Infusions. It must be stressed that at any time during which intravenous infusions are necessary, care must be taken *not* to infuse bubbles or particles, as either may embolize directly to the brain.

Prophylaxis Against Bacterial Endocarditis. See Table 5. For a discussion of the management of neonates with specific cyanotic conditions, see references to *Pediatrics,* 17th ed., at the end of this chapter.

BIBLIOGRAPHY

Barlow JB, Pocock WA: The problem of non-ejection systolic clicks and associated mitral systolic murmurs: Emphasis on the billowing mitral leaflet syndrome. Am Heart J 90:636, 1975

Benzing G III, Schubert W, Hug G, Kaplan S: Simultaneous hypoglycemia and acute congestive heart failure. Circulation 40:209, 1969

Bleifer S, Dorioso E, Grishman A: The auscultatory and phonocardiographic signs of ventricular septal defects. Am J Cardiol 5:191, 1960

Bristow JD, Metcalf J: Physical signs in congestive heart failure. Progr Cardiovasc Dis 10:236, 1967

Cutler JG, Ongley PA, Schwachman H, Massell FB, Nadas AS: Bacterial endocarditis in children with heart disease. Pediatrics 22:706, 1958

Minhas K, Gasul BM: Systolic clicks: A clinical, phonocardiographic and hemodynamic evaluation. Am Heart J 57:49, 1959

Shah P, Sinch WSA, Rose V, Keith JD: Incidence of bacterial endocarditis in ventricular septal defects. Circulation 34:127, 1966

Tavel ME: Clinical Phonocardiography and External Pulse Recording, 3rd ed. Chicago, Year Book, 1978

Talner NS: Congestive heart failure in the infant: A functional approach. Pediatr Clin North Am 18:1011, 1971

Talner NS, et al.: Guidelines for insurability of the patient with congenital heart disease. Circulation 62:1419A, 1980

Whitmer JT, James FW, Kaplan S, Schwartz DC, Knight MJS: Exercise testing in children before and after surgical treatment of aortic stenosis. Circulation 63:254, 1981

Cross-Reference to *Pediatrics,* 17th ed.

THIRTY

Dental Development and Common Dental Problems

Harold Diner

Parental concerns about a wide variety of common dental conditions in young children are frequently directed initially to the pediatric practitioner and other pediatric health workers. Conversely, the dentist may seek pediatric advice about dental care for a child with chronic medical disease.

Some of these concerns may derive from normal dental growth and development and require only reassurance. However, other conditions may require therapeutic intervention or the initiation of a pediatrically directed preventive dental health regimen.

Many of the common dental problems of childhood are directly related to various stages of dental development. The clinical features of the most common dental disorders and their management are presented, therefore, in a temporal sequence. Major consideration has been given to dental conditions that are associated with local causative factors rather than to the oral manifestations of systemic diseases. A summary of the subjects discussed is given in Table 1.

THE NEWBORN INFANT

Minor structural variations of the mouth and face are difficult to assess in the newborn infant, since they may represent either the normal oral-facial development for a particular child or manifestations of significant developmental abnormalities.

Detailed oral examination of the newborn child requires good lighting and the use of a dental mouth mirror for retraction and better visibility. It is desirable to do the examination after a feeding when the child is less readily disturbed. A surgical scrub technique is obligatory. Palpation is a necessary part of the examination and particular attention should be paid to the following:

1. Palate: abnormal length and depth, clefting, abnormalities of the uvula
2. Pharynx: oropharyngeal dimension, lymphoid tissue aggregates, tonsillar crypts
3. Alveolar ridges: abnormal consistency,

413

TABLE 1. DENTAL DEVELOPMENT AND COMMON DENTAL PROBLEMS

Newborn Period
Oral facial relationship—cranial-facial ratio
Intraoral findings
  Epstein's pearls
  Dental lamina cysts
  Bohn's nodules
  Epithelial tags
  Eruption cysts
  Mucoceles
  Congenital epulis
  Natal teeth
  Capillary hemangioma, fibroma, papilloma, lipoma

Teething Period (Primary Dentition—4 Months–3 Years)
Constitutional symptoms—nonspecific, controversial
  Fever
  Loss of appetite
  Sleeplessness
  Increased salivation
  Gastrointestinal upset
Local features
  Gingival and mucosal inflammation and ulceration
  Cheek rash and angular cheilitis (commissural irritation)
  Eruption cyst
  Eruptive gingival inflammation—most common during period of mixed dentition with exfoliation of primary teeth and eruption of permanent successors

Dental Variations
Spacing and facial asymmetry
Eruption delay or acceleration
Differences in tooth number
Tooth discolorations
  Extrinsic stains
  Intrinsic (ineradicable) discolorations

Oral Soft Tissue Lesions
Viral infections—relatively common
  Acute herpetic gingivostomatitis (primary herpes)
  Herpangina
  Herpes labialis (cold sores)

Bacterial infections—relatively rare, more commonly secondarily imposed on primary diseases from other causes
  Chronic marginal gingivitis—common, generally innocuous in childhood, may lead to periodontitis
  Acute necrotizing ulcerative gingivostomatitis
Common oral findings (nonspecific etiology)
  Aphthous stomatitis (canker sores)
  Benign migratory glossitis
Factitial (self-induced, traumatic) lesions
  Cheek, tongue, and lip biting and chewing
Physically and chemically induced lesions
  Electrical burns
  Topical chemical burns
  Systemically administered drugs

Oral Habits
Bruxism (tooth grinding)
Thumb or digit sucking
Tongue thrust swallow
Obstructive mouth breathing
Articulatory defects
  Oral structural variations
  Malaligned or missing teeth
  Abnormal frenular attachments
Selection of orthodontic nipples and pacifiers

Dental Trauma
Crown and root fracture
Abscess formation
Subluxation, intrusion, and avulsion of teeth
Reimplantation of teeth
Injuries related to child abuse

Infections of Dental Origin and Dental Pain
Localized abscess formation
Cellulitis
Antibiotic usage
Incision and drainage

Role of Pediatrician in Prevention of Dental Caries
Fluoride utilization
Feeding and dietary measures
Undesirable feeding supplements
General dental management

Requests by Dentists for Consultation with Pediatrician

enlargement, clefting, asymmetry, exostoses

4. Gingivae: elevations, cysts, discoloration, ulcerations
5. Vestibules and the floor of the mouth: abnormal frenular attachments, salivary duct patency, elevations
6. Tongue: abnormal mobility, size, deviation, lobulation, fissures
7. Lips: clefts, pits, commisural inflammation

In the normal neonate, facial asymmetry is not uncommon. Although the mandible may appear to be micrognathic, actually it is usually retrognathic due to the large cranium: face ratio. The tongue also may appear enlarged due to retropositioning of the mandible and the absence of teeth. The shallowness of facial depth, which is approximately 35% of the adult depth, may account for the appearance of midface hypoplasia. The palate is generally flat in infants, and maxillary ridges, supplemented by palatal fat pads, appear broad. Frenular attachments, particularly in the anterior upper dental arch, are broadly attached to the crest of the alveolar ridge, producing a transitional notching which may simulate minor clefting. In general, the period from birth to 3 years is an active period for oral-facial growth and development, and during the eruption of the primary dentition, considerable alteration in palatal and alveolar architecture may occur.

By far the most common oral findings in the newborn are many small cysts that have been classified on the basis of their location and embryologic origin. They occur almost universally and generally disappear spontaneously within a few months. *Epstein's pearls* are remnants of epithelial tissue trapped along the midline palatal raphe. They occur only in the midline at or near the junction of the hard and soft palates. They are raised, keratin-filled cysts, which appear singly, in grapelike clusters, or extend beadlike along the midline. *Dental lamina cysts* are remnants

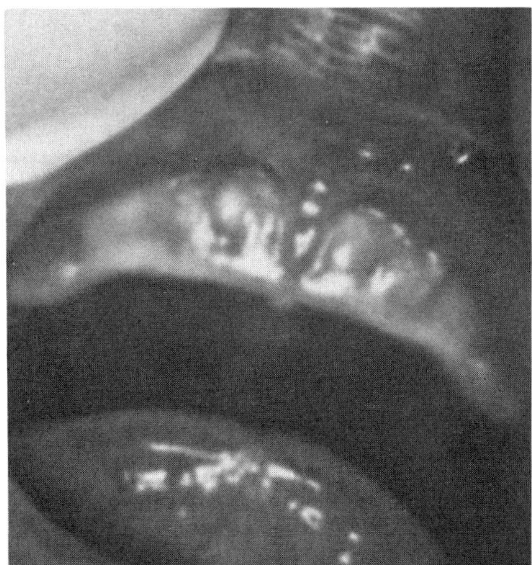

Figure 1. Bohn's nodules on the labial gingival surface.

of the epithelial anlage of actual tooth structure; they usually have a translucent appearance and occur invariably on the crest of the alveolar process. *Bohn's nodules* (Fig. 1) are remnants of mucous gland tissue entrapped by oral epithelium. Dental lamina cysts and Bohn's nodules are small, firm masses and almost always resolve before any appreciable

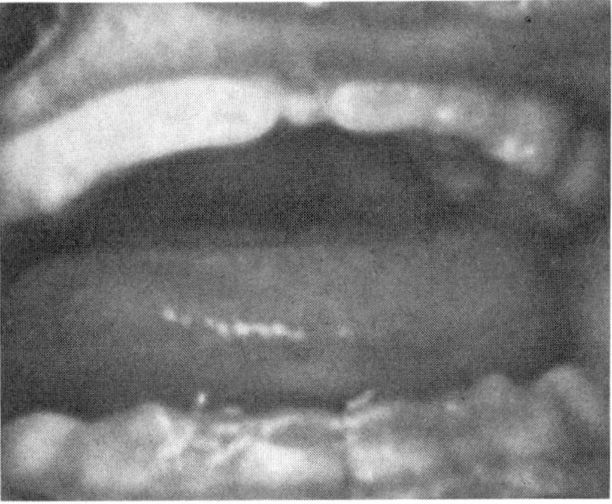

Figure 2. Epithelial tags are common, innocuous soft tissue elevations on the crestal ridge.

cystic enlargement occurs. *Epithelial tags* are nonsessile, noncystic tissue elevations on the crest of the alveolar process (Fig. 2). *Eruption cysts* result from expansion of the dental follicle of an erupting tooth. In young children, they appear most frequently in the region of the first primary molar on the crest of the alveolar ridge. Occasionally, particularly in erupting permanent teeth, an *eruption hematoma* may form (Fig. 3). Eruption cysts usually extravasate spontaneously, but if they persist, referral for dental radiographs to confirm their follicular association with erupting teeth should be made. Simple needle aspiration usually results in total resolution. *Mucoceles,* although sometimes developmental, usually occur after occlusion of minor salivary gland ducts traumatized after dental eruption. They are usually a deeper blue than eruption cysts and are more firmly based. They are generally single lesions and

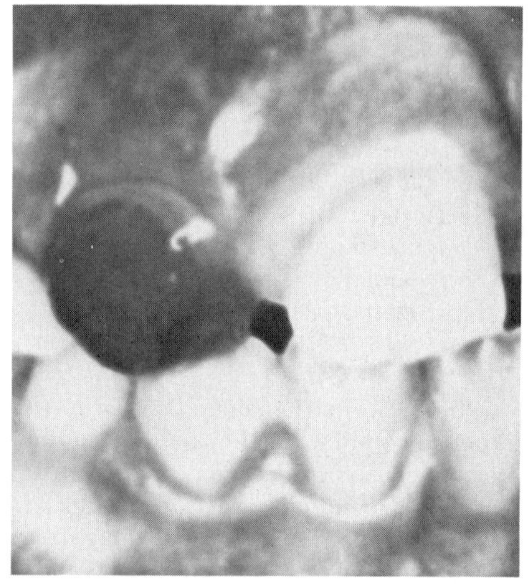

Figure 3. Eruption hematoma is a superficial, blood-filled follicular cyst.

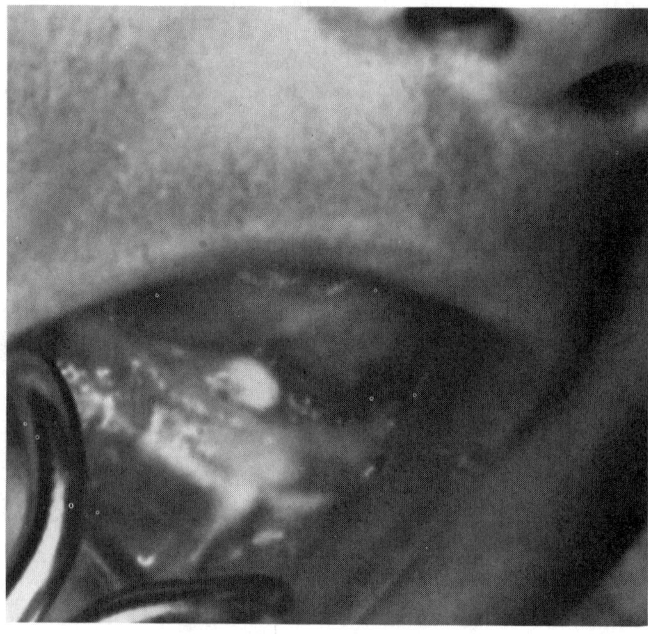

Figure 4. Transitory occlusion of the submaxillary salivary gland duct.

are most frequently found on the mucocutaneous border of the lips or on the mucous membranes of the lips and cheeks. Spontaneous extravasation or needle aspiration offers only temporary remission. They should be treated by surgical excision to the base of the lesion to prevent recurrence. Occasionally, *temporary occlusion of the orifice of the main submaxillary salivary gland duct* may produce a small, whitish, firm elevation under the base of the tongue (Fig. 4). Spontaneous opening of the duct usually occurs, but, if not, simple needle puncture is usually sufficient. *Congenital epulis* is a benign, sometimes stalked, soft tissue tumor attached directly to the crest of the alveolar ridge (Fig. 5). It occurs most frequently in the maxilla and is found most often in females. It can assume considerable dimension and interfere with normal feeding. Surgical removal is easily performed, and recurrence is unusual. *Natal teeth* occur in 1 in 4,000 births; they are poorly calcified, and their tenuous attachment invites the possibility of spontaneous loosening and aspiration. Natal teeth also are capable of producing traumatic ulceration of the tongue in association with suckling (Riga-Fede dis-

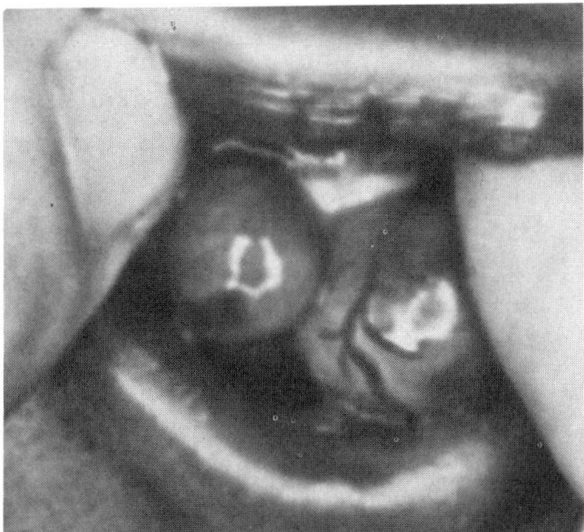

Figure 5. Congenital epulis of the newborn on the anterior mandibular ridge.

ease). They should be removed after explanation to the parent that their retention is potentially more detrimental than their absence in the primary dentition. Removal of natal teeth is easily accomplished with a hemostat without local anesthesia. Bleeding is controlled simply by local application of gauze packs (Fig. 6). A gauze apron should be held behind the teeth to prevent the necessity for intraoral retrieval of the extracted teeth.

A variety of common benign oral tumors occur in older infants and young children. They include fibroma, papilloma, lipoma, and hemangioma. Therapy for capillary hemangiomata should be deferred, since these tumors frequently involute spontaneously with age. Oral tumors should be referred routinely for biopsy, excision, and histologic review.

Dental consultation should be requested for all instances of major and minor clefting, enlargements or masses and other pronounced variations of oral and facial structures, and intraoral ulcerations and inflammation. Early orthodontic support may help to achieve improved surgical results in cleft lip and palate repair. Prosthetic appliances for palatal coverage may reduce early feeding problems. Minor oral surgical procedures may ameliorate the problem of glossoptosis and obstruction in severe micrognathia.

TEETHING PERIOD

The relationship of teething to constitutional disturbances, such as fever, loss of appetite, sleeplessness, gastrointestinal upset, and jaw grinding, remains controversial. Mucosal and gingival inflammation or ulceration in the edentulous infant may be due to the use of hard teething objects. Irritation of the lips and rashes on the cheeks may be due to increased salivary flow during teething and limited capacity to swallow the increased flow. Local tissue changes are relatively unre-

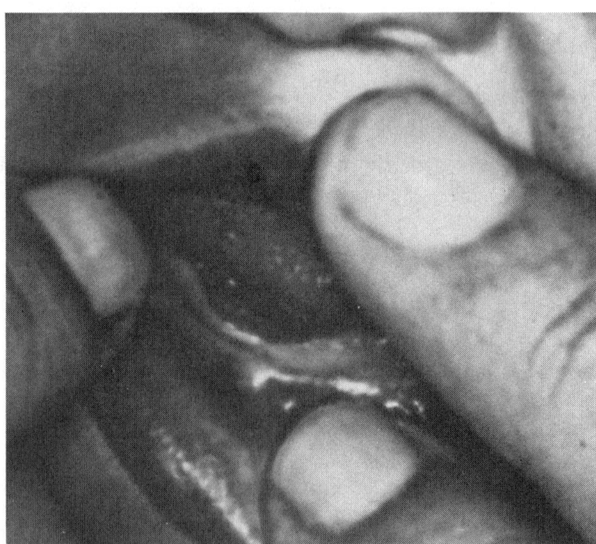

Figure 6. Postoperative response to extraction of natal teeth.

markable during the eruption period of the primary teeth. These include a mild and usually transitory inflammatory response, generally with little discomfort, even in association with an eruption cyst (expanded dental follicle). During the period of mixed dentition, mild discomfort and inflammation may be associated with loosening and exfoliation of primary teeth and eruption of permanent dentition. Constitutional responses during permanent tooth eruption are reported less frequently than during primary teething in spite of a decidedly more complicated eruption sequence and the greater potential for local inflammatory and irritative responses. Hence, it is difficult to reconcile the high percentage (95%) of reported constitutional responses to teething before 18 months and the very low percentage reported thereafter. The attribution of symptoms and signs of potentially serious organic disease to teething can create critical diagnostic errors. In addition, the risk of iatrogenic disease is always present when drugs are prescribed for nonspecific complaints. On balance, teething can hardly be considered the primary etiologic factor in the constitutional disturbances de-

scribed. For the management of mild local discomfort, a topically applied salve of 2.5% Xylocaine ointment and Orabase (oral adhesive), applied several times a day, is an effective palliative measure.

DENTITIONAL VARIATIONS

Spacing and Facial Asymmetry

Problems of eruption due to local causative factors, i.e., discrepancies in jaw-tooth size relationships, supernumerary teeth, ectopic eruption patterns, and abnormal resorptions of teeth are relatively uncommon in the primary dentition. It is unusual to see dental crowding of primary teeth, since primary teeth are usually spaced to accommodate wider permanent tooth dimensions. The absence of such developmental spacing in the primary dental arch causes lack of available space for the permanent teeth and subsequently may create malocclusion. Crowding of primary teeth may be a better indicator of a truly small jaw than visual comparison with other facial features (Fig. 7). Variations in the order of tooth eruption and/or certain oral habits,

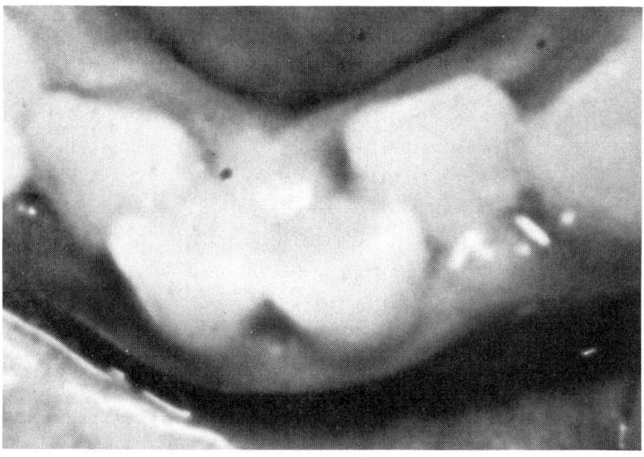

Figure 7. Crowding of lower primary anterior teeth in micrognathia.

such as thumbsucking, may create a dental crossbite which is characterized by abnormal tooth contacts when the jaws are closed (Fig. 8). This pattern of eccentric jaw closure may create the illusion of true facial asymmetry that may be mistakenly attributed to neuromuscular impairment, such as facial paralysis, cranial nerve abnormality, or facial skeletal abnormalities, such as hemiatrophy or hypertrophy or hemifacial microsomia. If the dental midlines of the upper and lower jaws approximate exactly during jaw closure before tooth contact, and mandibular deviation occurs after complete jaw closure, it can be assumed that premature dental contact is forcing the mandible to shift laterally. Dental consultation can determine the dental contribution to any facial asymmetry and provide corrective measures if indicated.

Eruption Delay

Eruptive delay or acceleration is most frequently familial. The comparison of dental to chronologic age, unless remarkably deviant, is basically unreliable in the mixed dentition because of a variety of local factors that may impede eruption. Early loss of primary teeth may accelerate or delay eruption of the permanent successors depending on the degree of root formation of the secondary teeth. With the exception of certain disease entities, such as endocrinopathies, Down syndrome,

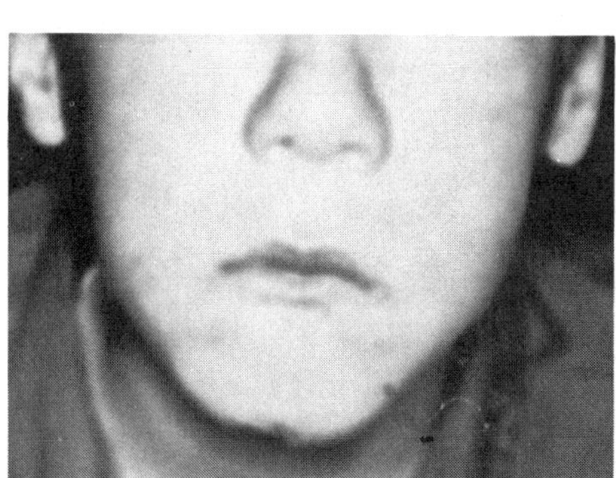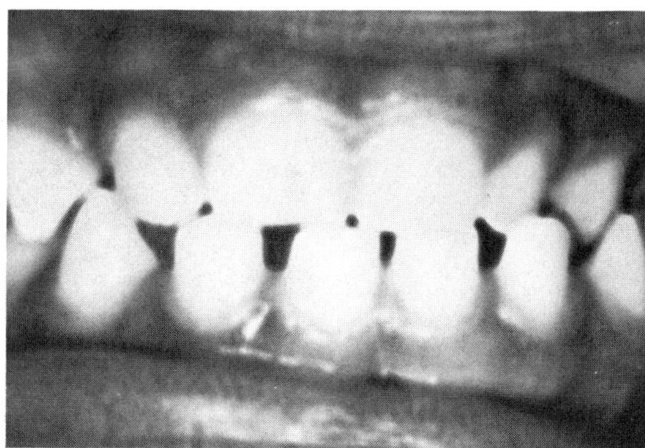

Figure 8. Dental crossbite causing facial asymmetry.

craniostenosis, and benign osteopetrosis, the relationship of dental age to bone age may have little clinical significance. Rates of calcification of teeth estimated from dental radiographs generally provide a more reliable assessment of dental development and maturation in primary and permanent dentitions. Markedly delayed eruption should be viewed with greater suspicion than early appearance of teeth. Unless a definitive family history of delayed eruption can be elicited, referral for dental radiographs should be made if no teeth have appeared by *1 year of age*.

Differences in Tooth Number and Enamel Dysplasias

The incidence of missing or extra primary teeth in normal populations is remarkably low. Congenital absence is much higher in the permanent dentition, particularly when third molars are included in the comparative survey. Hypodontia or hyperdontia are inherent features of certain diseases (Down syndrome, ectodermal dysplasia, chondroectodermal dysplasia, cleidocranial dysplasia, and cleft palate) or may be transmitted as single gene traits. While minimal discrepancies in tooth number and minor variations in tooth morphology may defy ready recognition by the pediatrician, enamel dysplasias are more easily identifiable. Developmental enamel defects may be imposed by systemic disease during tooth development and may represent a characteristic feature in some syndromes or may occur as a primary genetic defect with no other structures involved. Enamel dysplasias (hypoplasia, hypocalcification, hypomaturation) may be temporally related to serious constitutional disease during several stages of dental formation (Fig. 9). Formation of dental matrix and varying degrees of calcification of all primary teeth occur during gestation. Calcification of the permanent dentition occurs postnatally, with the first permanent molar (6-year molar) beginning to calcify at birth. Enamel dysplasias in the primary teeth represent indelible markers of abnormal gestational events and, thus, provide diagnostically useful information. Chronologic enamel lesions derive from the death of enamel-forming cells (ameloblasts) or incomplete calcification and maturation of

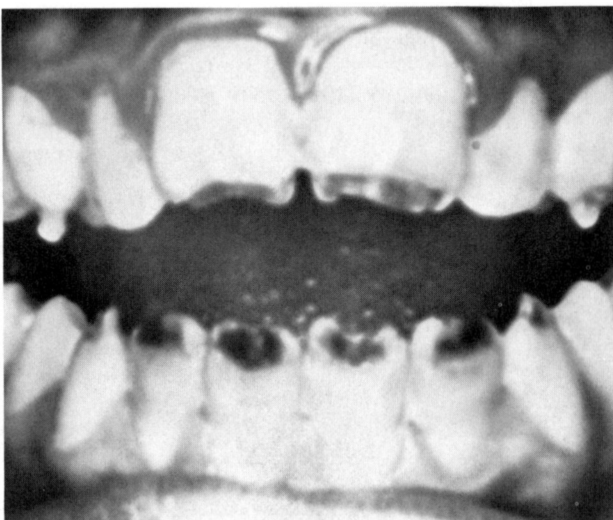

Figure 9. Chronologic enamel hypoplasia in the permanent dentition.

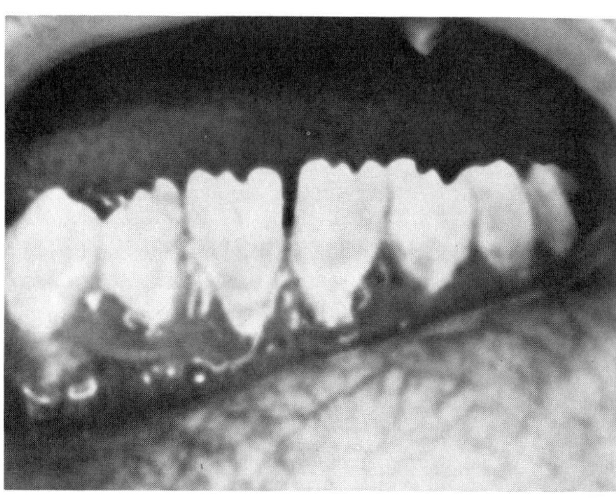

Figure 10. Intrinsic tooth staining in dentinogenesis imperfecta in association with osteogenesis imperfecta.

dental enamel during formation in response to a variety of physiologic insults. They have a distinct linearity and symmetry and differ from the primary enamel disorders of genetic origin, amelogenesis imperfecta. These genetically imposed dysplasias are divided into 12 distinct types on the basis of structural defect and mode of transmission. They usually occur in both the primary and permanent dentitions and demonstrate global tooth surface involvement rather than having a linear distribution.

Tooth Discolorations

Most discolorations of teeth are of exogenous origin and may appear as orange, green, brown-black, or yellow and green stains. They are usually related to oral chromogenic bacteria, inadequate oral cleansing, food and beverage stains, or chemical stains (e.g., oral iron solutions). They usually can be distinguished easily from intrinsically (permanently) stained teeth by vigorous scrubbing with a mild abrasive on a moistened gauze pad. Ineradicable discolorations may be related to dental caries, blood and bacterial pigments associated with pulpal necrosis, endemic fluorosis, tetracycline incorporation

(brown, gray, black), greenish blue teeth in neonatal jaundice, or the burgundy colored teeth of erythropoietic porphyria; these are all examples of intrinsic staining. The brown-blue of dentinogenesis imperfecta, as a primary disorder of dentin, or in association with osteogenesis imperfecta, is quite characteristic (Fig. 10). The denudation of enamel in some forms of amelogenesis imperfecta may impart a yellow-brown discoloration to the teeth.

ORAL SOFT TISSUE LESIONS

Oral soft tissue lesions, during the first year of life, are generally benign and, for the most part, related to minor trauma. *Bednar's aphthae* (pterygoid ulcers) are benign, superficial ulcers of the hard palate that are related to nipple pressure during nursing. Serious primary oral lesions, such as ulcerations, areas of necrosis, and focal inflammatory infiltrates, occurring prior to or after dental eruptions are usually related to systemic diseases. These may include blood dyscrasias, autoimmune and deficiency diseases, metabolic disturbances, histiocytoses (especially Letterer-Siwe disease), and nutritional deficiencies.

Viral Infections

The most common viral infections in childhood are herpes simplex type 1 infections and herpangina. *Acute primary herpetic gingivostomatitis* occurs from contact with herpes simplex virus following loss of maternal antibodies. Oral features include marked erythema, edema of the gingiva, and the appearance of vesicles and ulcers distributed throughout the mouth. Fever, malaise, generalized discomfort, and oral pain are common symptoms, which usually subside in approximately 7 days. Acute primary herpes is clinically differentiated from *herpangina* due to group A Coxsackie virus, which affects the oropharynx and posterior oral regions without gingival enlargement. Symptoms are generally mild with few complications, and the disease runs it course in 7–10 days.

These viral infections are treated with soft, bland diets, increased fluid intake, and Xylocaine oral rinses. Antibiotic therapy has little effect and is indicated only if, in the clinician's estimation, there is a secondarily imposed bacterial infection. Recurrence is extremely rare and is generally indicative of altered immunologic status or related to prolonged corticosteroid therapy.

Recurrence is a common feature of *herpes labialis* (cold sore), which is also caused by herpes simplex virus. These lesions are vesicular, with subsequent ulceration, and occur along the mucocutaneous border of the lips without intraoral involvement. Crusting, along the cutaneous border, may extend the normal healing period beyond the usual 7–10 days. Factors inducing viral activation include exposure to the sun, febrile diseases, colds, mechanical trauma, and emotional stress. Treatment is essentially limited to the application of protective creams and topical analgesics.

Bacterial Infections

Primary oral soft tissue bacterial infections are rare but may be secondarily imposed on active viral lesions or occur in association with bacterial pharyngeal infections. In children, mild inflammation of the borders of the gingiva (chronic marginal gingivitis) is common but ordinarily innocuous. The inflammation is generally attributable to mouth breathing and drying of the gingiva, malposed teeth which encourage food impaction, poor oral hygiene, or dental appliances which contribute to food retention. Salivary calculus (tartar), an additional irritant of the gingival margin, does form on children's teeth but usually not to the same extent as in adults. More marked degrees of gingival inflammation and hypertrophy are more typical of adolescents, in whom irritative factors are seemingly enhanced by nonspecific hormonal changes (Fig. 11). Inattention to regular oral hygiene measures and frequent snacking are additional contributing factors in gingival disease. *Acute necrotizing ulcerative gingivostomatitis* (Vincent's infection), although relatively uncommon in young children, is the most frequent bacterial infection of the oral tissues (Fig. 12). It is characterized by necrosis and ulceration of the interdental gingival papillae, oral fetor, pain, elevated temperature, lymphadenopathy, and general malaise. It is not contagious but left untre-

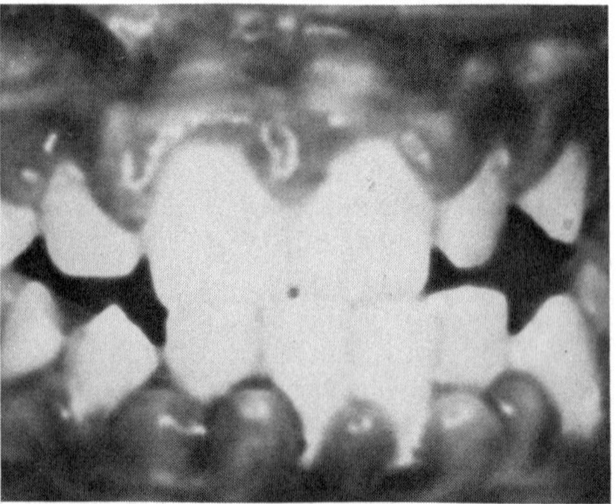

Figure 11. Postpubertal chronic marginal gingivitis.

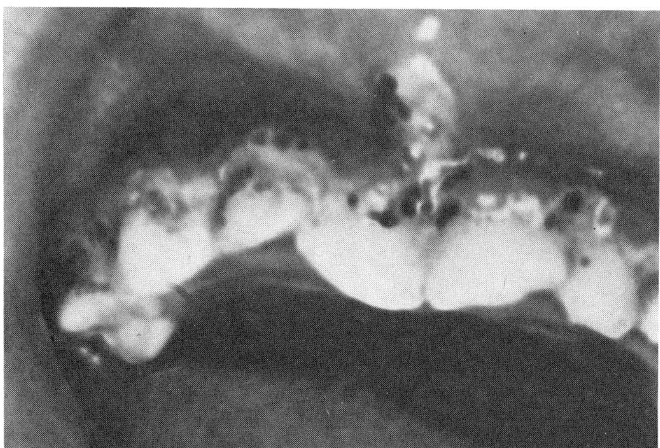

Figure 12. Acute necrotizing ulcerative gingivostomatitis in a 4 year old.

ated, can result in severe periodontal breakdown. It is a fusospirochetal infection and may respond dramatically to systemic penicillin within a few days. However, antibiotic treatment must be accompanied by vigorous periodontal scaling and curettage to prevent recurrence.

Common Oral Findings

Oral aphthae (canker sores) have been attributed to viral or bacterial agents, food allergy, hormonal disturbances, trauma, abnormal immune response, and emotional stress (Fig. 13). These aphthae are single or multiple, painful ulcerations, which may oc-

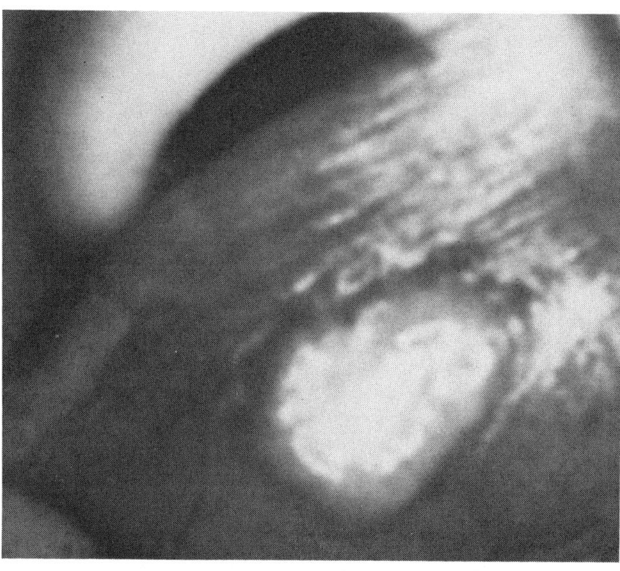

Figure 13. Aphthous ulcer on the upper lip.

cur on the lip, cheek, tongue, palate, gingiva, floor of the mouth, or pharynx. They are sometimes difficult to visualize, particularly in the posterior mucobuccal folds. The acute discomfort they cause is frequently misinterpreted as being of dental origin. They usually last from 7 to 14 days. Bland mouth rinses have been suggested to reduce discomfort and to shorten the duration of the lesions. Frequently, complete cessation of pain can be achieved by cauterization of noncoalescent lesions by a single topical application of Negatan (negatol solution 45%—netacresol sulfonic acid with formaldehyde).

Benign migratory glossitis (geographic tongue) is a common, mild, wandering, innocuous inflammation of the tongue. The lesions are not fixed and are characterized by a smooth, atrophic red center surrounded by a white keratotic border, most frequently on the dorsum of the tongue. Emotional stress and a possible genetic predisposition are considered the major etiologic factors.

Factitial

Self-induced oral lesions occur most frequently in children with developmental disabilities, such as mental retardation or serious emotional disorders (Fig. 14). They may become so destructive that an oral protective device, hand binding, and even dental extractions may be warranted. Lip biting or chewing, in association with local anesthetic usage, is a common occurrence in young and handicapped children (Fig. 15).

Physically and Chemically Induced Lesions

Electric burns of the mouth usually occur at the lip commissures and are usually more deep-seated than is apparent clinically. Surgical lip revision is deferred until after initial healing. Severe retraction can be reduced by the use of a prosthetic commissural expander under mild and sustained tension (Fig. 16).

Severe caustics, such as lye, can produce grave local and systemic damage. The common practice of placing aspirin tablets on the oral tissues for toothache or nonspecific oral complaints can produce local sloughing and ulceration.

Untoward responses to systemically administered drugs can produce manifestations in the oral soft tissues in a variety of ways, including oral discomfort, erythema vesicles, bullae and vesiculobullous lesions, ulcers,

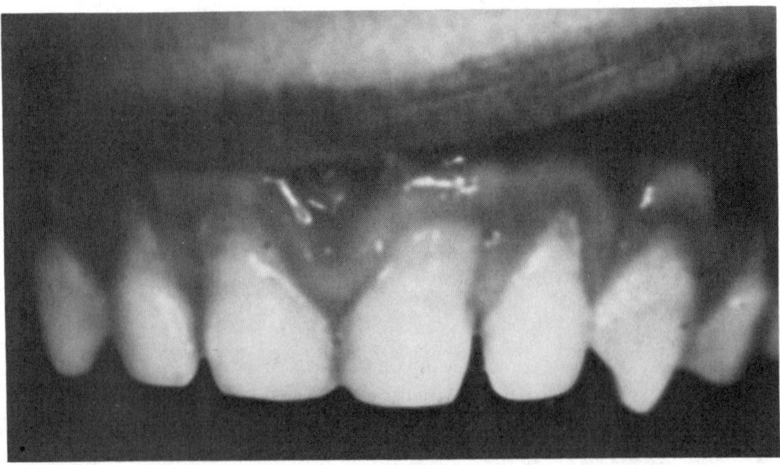

Figure 14. Self-induced oral lesions.

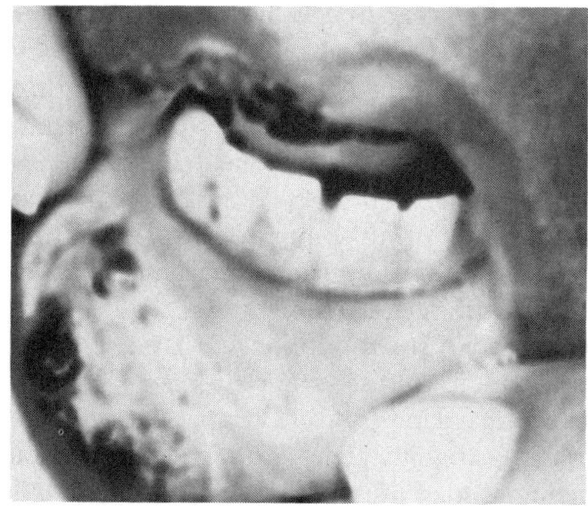

Figure 15. Post local anesthetic lip trauma.

and erosions. Most of these drug reactions appear to be allergic in nature, and they may be particularly idiosyncratic, such as gingival hyperplasia in chronic Dilantin usage. Drug-related oral reactions in children are due most frequently to alterations in the oral flora from antibiotics. With broad-spectrum antibiotics, a shift in the bacterial-mycotic flora may permit the depression of some organisms and allow overgrowth of others. Candidiasis and black, hairy tongue may occur as a result of such a shift. In some instances, denudation of the tongue papillae and generalized erythema of the oral tissues may occur in response to antibiotics (antibiotic stomatitis). Vesiculobullous eruption, probably the most common oral lesion related to drug allergy, may occur as an allergic response to barbiturates, salicylates, and antibiotics. The oral mucosa may be involved also in general drug-induced disturbances, such as petechial hemorrhages in oral tissues resulting from platelet deficiency in drug-induced marrow suppression.

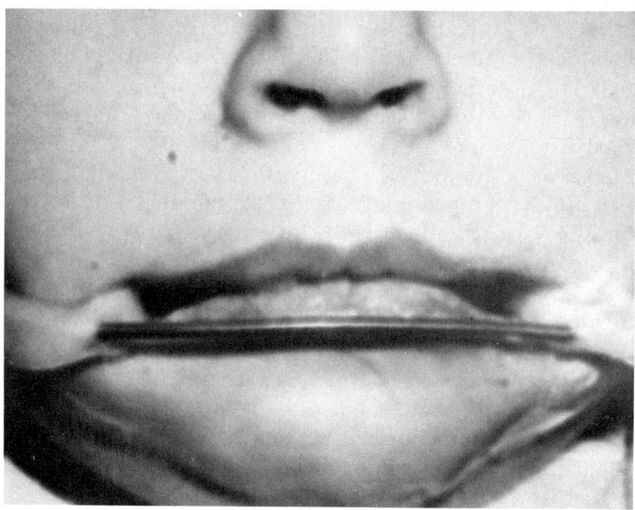

Figure 16. Commissural extender for presurgical management of electric burns.

ORAL HABITS

Bruxism

Bruxism (tooth gnashing and grinding) is a relatively common childhood habit and appears to have little psychologic significance. There is inadequate evidence to support some of the systemic etiologic factors that have been suggested, such as intestinal parasites, subclinical nutritional deficiencies, and allergic and endocrine disorders. The habit may be quite audible, particularly at night, or it may go entirely unnoticed by the parent. Other than the obvious and extensive wear facets that it may produce on the teeth, it infrequently causes any clinical detriment to young dentitions. A simple prosthetic mouth guard can be fabricated should the grinding be disquieting to other household members, cause lip and cheek biting, create soreness of teeth, or result in actual periodontal breakdown. Experience suggests that the habit decreases with age. It should be noted, however, that in neuromuscular impairment, such as spastic and athetotic cerebral palsy, tooth attrition may be so marked as to completely obliterate the usual occlusal anatomic features.

Thumbsucking

Thumbsucking, one of the so-called compulsive habits, may provoke considerable parental concern. Chronic thumbsucking was commonly considered to be an emotional disturbance. However, it is now interpreted as a simple habit or learned response, which usually can be effectively and safely extinguished in older children. Children who persist in sucking their thumb are no more likely to exhibit neurotic symptoms or abnormal behavior than other children.

Restrictive measures to control the habit should not be attempted in the preschool years. The habit frequently lessens spontaneously by age 6 or disappears completely at about 11 years, possibly as a result of peer disapproval. Dental changes created by thumbsucking in the primary dentition are usually correctable when therapy is initiated during the period of the early mixed dentition. Mechanically, a properly constructed palatal crib or rake provides an extinction process that permits thumb placement but removes the reinforcement associated with sucking. This orthodontic appliance is fixed to the teeth to discourage thumb placement in the usual position it occupies during the sucking habit. The appliance may be pronged so as to irritate the thumb when it is placed in the sucking position. For most children, this approach to the elimination of digit sucking habits is tolerated well. Coercion, threats, appeals to reason, and rewards are still dependent on patient cooperation and are, thus, generally less effective. It is reported that such minor symptoms as increased fingernail biting, chewing of clothing, and handling of the genitals may develop after correction of the habit. These habits usually are transitory and can be disregarded.

Tongue Thrusting

In the normal adult swallowing pattern, the teeth are brought together, the lips close, and the tongue is held against the palate behind the upper incisor teeth. In abnormal tongue thrust swallow (reverse swallow, perverted and deviant swallow), the tongue is positioned forward in association with abnormal functioning of the lips, mentalis, and other circumoral muscles. Persistent tongue thrusters are reported to have larger tonsils and higher and narrower palates and to demonstrate more digit sucking and mouth breathing. Tongue thrusting is said to create anterior open bite (failure of the anterior teeth to contact in jaw closure), lisping, posterior or lateral open bite, and increased labial prominence of the upper anterior teeth (bucking). However, it has never been proven satisfactorily that tongue thrusting is a primary etiologic factor in dental malocclusion.

Tongue thrust swallow occurs almost universally in infancy and diminishes at 2½–3 years with the advent of the adult swallowing pattern. Since 50% of 6 year olds and only 2% of 11 year olds demonstrate the habit, it is generally considered a transitional stage of development for most children. However, differences of opinion exist concerning treatment of children with persistent tongue thrust swallow and dental malocclusion. Orthodontic therapy is the most usual mode of treatment for cases of dental malocclusion with tongue thrusting. Proponents of myofunctional therapy (retraining for correct tongue placement and normal perioral muscle activity) propose that there is a strong causal and reciprocal relationship among tongue thrusting, lisping, and dental malocclusion. They advise that in many instances myofunctional therapy is an essential adjunct to orthodontic treatment. Myofunctional measures require patience and forebearance and are time consuming. Their value in dental therapy is currently in question, and consensus suggests that while tongue thrusting and lisping may occur simultaneously, no causal relationship between them has been established.

Obstructive Mouth Breathing

Nasal airway obstruction necessitating compensatory mouth breathing may be caused by congenitally large or allergically hypertrophied turbinates, choanal atresia, narrow maxillary nasal passages, deviated nasal septa, allergic rhinitis, extensive nasopharyngeal lymphoid tissue, polyp formation, and neoplasm. Children with genetically narrow faces and small nasopharynx are more inclined to demonstrate airway obstruction when the adenoids are swollen and edematous. Chronic mouth breathing may be accompanied by vigorous and persistent tongue thrusting and cause improper facial muscle pressures that can affect dentofacial morphology during periods of oral-facial growth. This deviant muscle activity may interfere with the acceptable alignment of teeth and achievement of a pleasing facial balance. There are optimal maxillary-mandibular growth periods for achieving maximal orthodontic results. However, in individual children, these growth periods may not coincide with physiologic regression of pharyngeal tonsillar tissue. From the orthodontic point of view, removal of tonsils and adenoids may be critical to the success and stability of complicated orthodontic therapy for some children. Since other medical indications for tonsillectomy and adenoidectomy are quite strict, controversy concerning its advisability arises.

The pediatrician is frequently drawn into this arena, and his assessment of potential gain or detriment may be critical in making the final decision. He should be aware that orthodontic therapy is not purely cosmetic. The achievement of optimal tooth-to-tooth relationships and favorable occlusal harmony is significant in limiting dental caries susceptibility and the progress of periodontal disease.

Articulatory Defects

Articulatory defects are not significantly related to dental malocclusions, malaligned or missing teeth, or oral structural variations, such as highly arched and constricted palatal vaults. The replacement of missing primary teeth is of greater important in the maintenance of adequate space for permanent tooth eruption and the prevention of dental crowding and malocclusion. There is, as well, little evidence to support the belief that lisping or other speech defects result from a tight lingual frenum (tongue-tie). The eruption of teeth, which is accompanied by growth of supporting bone and gingiva, usually results

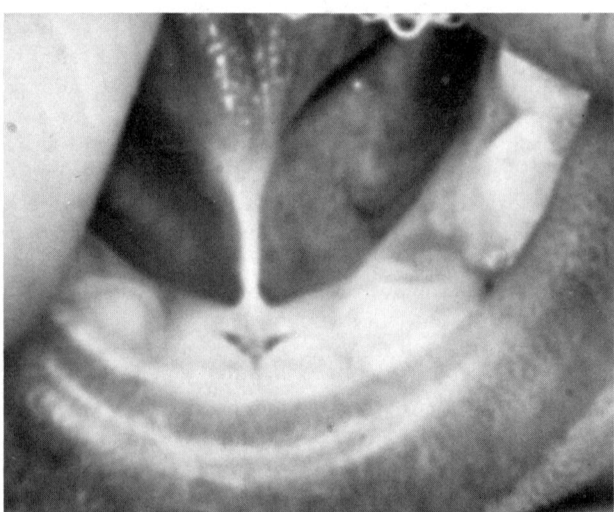

Figure 17. Indication for lingual frenectomy.

in a more appropriate repositioning of the frenum. Tightness of the frenum rarely if ever interferes with tongue function, nor is tongue function ever significantly improved by frenectomy. Cutting the frenum is not entirely an innocuous procedure and may, on occasion, promote bacterial invasion with possible infection of the submaxillary salivary glands. Surgical release of a frenum which inserts into the crest of the lingual attached gingivae is indicated only if tongue movements cause clinical retraction of the tooth-gingival attachment and predispose that area to periodontal breakdown (Fig. 17). Resection may also be indicated in those instances where the frenum may interfere with the placement of a dental prosthesis or where a frenum is so broad and fibrous so as to interfere with approximation of adjacent teeth.

Selection of Orthodontic Nipples and Pacifiers

It has been proposed that properly designed feeding nipples and pacifiers reduce mouth breathing, strengthen lip activity, reduce deforming tongue thrust activity, and provide sensory gratification. Since it is estimated that the work of the muscles of mastication in the breastfed infant is about 50 times greater than that of infants fed by bottles, any feeding modifications that simulate maternal nursing may provide a strong deterrent to excessive thumb and finger sucking. It is claimed that the initial use of the orthodontic nipple, in contrast to the conventional easy-flow nipple provides these benefits and, when followed by a secondary physiologic exerciser, the orthodontic pacifier, facilitates the transition from the infantile to the mature swallowing pattern. Several reports have confirmed the preventive orthodontic value of these suggested regimens. However, some parental reports indicate that the nipple is frustrating to use and that feeding time is prolonged unduly. Decisions for the use of pacifiers should, therefore, be individualized. There is no reason to use them if there are no existing oral habits, such as blanket chewing or finger sucking. If the thumbsucking habit is already deeply entrenched, it is likely that the pacifier will be rejected. Pacifiers are probably most useful when there are beginning indications of habit formation.

Dental Trauma

Trauma to the primary teeth occurs most frequently between ages 1½ and 2½ years. The maxillary incisors are the teeth most frequently traumatized, although other teeth may be affected in unusual and severe accidents. The primary teeth can be subject to crown fracture, discoloration, root fracture, abscess formation, subluxation, intrusion, and avulsion. Many intruded teeth will reerupt spontaneously within a relatively short period of time; prolonged delay requires dental consultation. Trauma and infection of primary teeth, or both, can affect the perma-

nent successors during their early formative stages by producing pulpal damage, displacement of the tooth germ, or delayed eruption or enamel defects (Turner teeth) (Fig. 18). Turner teeth are permanent teeth that may demonstrate enamel defects due to trauma or infection of the primary teeth they are replacing. Total luxation (avulsion) of primary teeth warrants referral for dental radiography for possible retention of root fragments. If the normal exchange time is not imminent, decisions for prosthetic replacement may be important for esthetics, mastication, and, for some children, the avoidance of deleterious habits. Reimplantation or replacement of avulsed teeth should be considered for permanent teeth only. The long-term prognosis depends on the time lapse; optimally, this is within 30 minutes after traumatic exfoliation. The pediatrician's intervention may be crit-

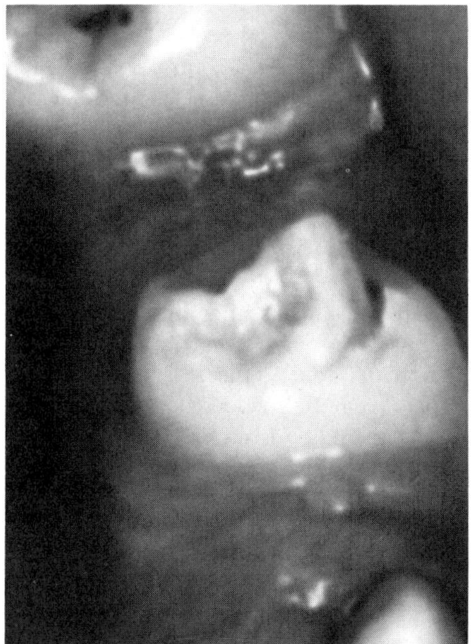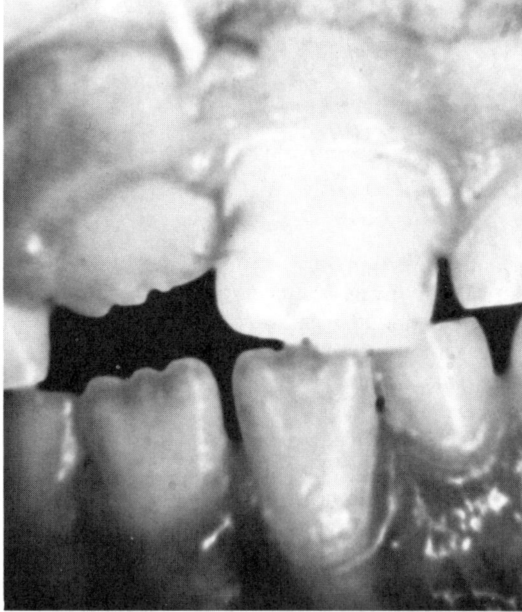

Figure 18. Turner teeth.

ical if dental help is not immediately available. Simply washing the tooth in warm water, replacing it in the tooth socket in its proper relationship, and stabilizing the tooth with gentle finger pressure for 5–10 minutes is the first and most critical aspect of treatment. Dental referral, as soon as possible, is essential for firmer stabilization, pulpal therapy, and continued observation.

As a general rule, particularly where trauma to teeth is accompanied by lacerations of the lips and gums, dental consultation is recommended. Opposing and adjacent teeth, although seemingly unaffected, may have sustained root fracture or pulpal injury that may not become clinically apparent until some later time.

The relationship between dental trauma and child abuse is forensically important to the pediatrician. A recent survey indicated that oral-facial trauma is present in nearly 50% of reported cases. The most common features included fractures of the teeth (32%), oral bruises (24%), oral lacerations (14%), fractures of the maxilla and mandible (11%), and oral burns (5%).

INFECTIONS OF DENTAL ORIGIN AND DENTAL PAIN

Dental infections are common in children and almost invariably related to pulpal necrosis due to dental decay or traumatic injury of sufficient intensity to cause pulp death. The teeth may remain totally asymptomatic or may be locally painful, or, in some instances, the pain may be referred to other areas on the same side of the dental arch. Clinical manifestations of odontogenic infections may include localized abscess formation with chronic fistulas, localized erythema and inflammation of the gingiva, swelling (cellulitis), and fever and general malaise. In many instances, after the acute phase, root canal therapy can restore these teeth to a healthy functional state. However, acute dental infections accompanied by facial swelling require immediate attention. Antibiotics, incision and drainage, and debridement of infected tissues (where fluctuance is evident) are the usual emergency measures. Initial recommendations for antibiotic control of odontogenic infections may frequently be a responsibility of the pediatrician. Penicillin V is the most widely used drug in such infections. It is effective against aerobic Gram-positive organisms, such as alpha-hemolytic streptococci, and against anaerobic bacteria and fusospirochetal infections. For young children, on an outpatient basis, penicillin V 250 mg qid for 5 days is recommended initially, with immediate referral to the dentist. Local dental measures can effect more rapid resolution of the infection, and decisions for increased or continued dosage can be made by the dentist. For older children, and depending on the severity of the infection, starting doses may be elevated to 500 mg qid. For a child allergic to penicillin, erythromycin, although not as effective against obligate anaerobic bacteria as penicillin, is an adequate substitute against the various forms of alpha-hemolytic streptococci. The recommended dosage of erythromycin, initially, is 30–50 mg/kg/day. Nausea and abdominal pain are not uncommon with erythromycin, but it has the advantage of being absorbed easily when taken after a meal. Other antibiotic drugs, oral cephalosporins (Keflex) and amoxicillin, are useful in odontogenic infections, but they may be allergenic in penicillin-sensitive patients. Doxycycline is an effective substitute for penicillin for fusospirochetal infections in sensitive patients, but it may cause staining of the teeth, as does its counterpart, tetracycline. On balance, penicillin V and erythromycin are almost invariably the antibiotic drugs of choice in the outpatient management of infections of odontogenic origin in children.

Prophylaxis for Subacute Bacterial Endocarditis

Children with congenital or acquired heart defects are at risk for infective endocarditis during dental treatment. In the dental office, penicillin V, orally, is most frequently used for chemoprophylaxis.

Children. *Penicillin V* 2.0 g is given orally 30 minutes–1 hour prior to procedure, then 500 mg orally every 6 hours for 8 doses in children over 60 pounds. For children less than 60 pounds, 1.0 g orally 30 minutes–1 hour prior to the procedure is given, then 250 mg orally every 6 hours for 8 doses.

Erythromycin (penicillin allergy) 20 mg/kg is given orally 1½–2 hours prior to the procedure, then 10 mg/kg every 6 hours for 8 doses.

For children with increased susceptibility to infective endocarditis, intramuscular aqueous penicillin mixed with procaine penicillin plus streptomycin are suggested. For penicillin-sensitive children, vancomycin IV plus oral erythromycin are recommended.

For a more complete review of recommendations, the pediatrician is referred to a brochure "Prevention of Bacterial Endocarditis," American Heart Association, or *Circulation* 56:139A, 1977.

Oral Pain

By far the most frequent cause of oral pain is related to the teeth themselves. Inflammation of the pulp can be transitory as well as chronic. Transitory dental pain can be related to dental trauma, pulpal hyperemia sometimes related to cavity preparation, and thermal conductivity with metallic dental restoration. Chronic inflammation of the dental pulp may exist for long periods of time without symptoms, but acute flare-ups can occur if the patient's resistance is lowered by sys-

temic disease or an infection. Referred pain simulating pain of dental origin can occur with otitis media, allergic rhinitis, upper respiratory infection, and maxillary sinusitis.

THE ROLE OF THE PEDIATRICIAN IN PREVENTION OF DENTAL CARIES

Accumulation of data concerning dental caries in the primary dentition strongly supports the need for the initiation of preventive oral hygiene starting practically at birth. Prefluoridation surveys indicate that at 1 year of age about 5% of children exhibit dental decay, about 10% at age 2, 40–55% by ages 3–4, and about 75% at age 5.

There are several major contributions to preventive dental health that are related to primary pediatric care; these include fluoride utilization and both desirable and undesirable feeding and dietary measures.

Fluoride Utilization

Systemic fluoride utilization during the formative stages of dental development has effected a 60–70% overall reduction in caries attack rates in children. Supplementation with fluoride dentifrices and topical fluoride application has provided an additional 10–15% reduction in caries susceptibility. However, constant review of fluoride utilization is an ongoing process. Since the pediatrician is frequently involved initially in supervising ingested fluoride supplementation he should be familiar with current principles of its use.

1. At present, there is insufficient evidence that prenatal fluoride supplementation is effective in preventing caries in either primary and secondary dentitions to warrant its routine use.
2. Adequate fluoride intake should be de-

rived principally from water and ordinary foods. When fluoride ingestion from dietary sources and water is deficient, as determined by consulting the local Department of Health, special supplements, such as tablets or drops, may be used. Earlier recommendations for supplementary fluoride regimens based on age or the arbitrary use of combined vitamin-fluoride preparations may, in some cases, have caused temporary overdosage. Optimal systemic intake of fluoride is 1 ppm in drinking water. Although high concentrations (4–9 ppm) over long periods of time may infrequently cause increased bone density, there has been no indication of functional impairment or any relationship to clinical disease. However, these higher fluoride doses can cause fluorosis of teeth (white opacities, surface pitting, and brown opaque areas). While mild fluorosis is too slight to impair the appearance of the teeth, moderate fluorosis (above 1.8 ppm) is decidedly undesirable. Although there need be no concern for fluoride toxicity in controlled fluoridation systems, concentrated fluoride preparations for home use should be kept out of reach of children. The lethal dose of sodium fluoride for adults ranges from 2–5 g taken orally; in children, smaller amounts may cause symptoms of poisoning or even death.

3. Human and cow's milk have much lower fluoride content than previously reported, generally far below 0.1 mg/L. Absorption of fluoride from milk is less complete than from water.

4. Current fluoride dosage recommendation for systemic use is given in Table 2).

Commercial formulas (ready-to-use) contain 0.2 mg of fluoride per quart, which is adequate for children from 0–2 years. Concentrated liquid and powdered formulas contain similar or lower fluoride levels when diluted with nonfluoridated water. However,

TABLE 2. CURRENT FLUORIDE DOSAGE RECOMMENDATIONS FOR SYSTEMIC USE

Fluoride Content of Drinking Water (ppm)	Fluoride Supplementation (m/24 hr)		
	Birth to 2 yr	2–3 yr	3–4 yr
Less than 0.3	0.25	0.50	1.00
0.3–0.7	0	0.25	0.50
Over 0.7	Fluoride dietary supplements unnecessary		

when concentrated liquid formulas are mixed with fluoridated water, the content of fluoride equals 0.5–0.6 mg/quart. Powdered formula, diluted with fluoridated water, usually contains about 0.8 mg fluoride per quart. Hence, concentrated liquid or powdered formulas require no supplemental fluoride when mixed with fluoridated water.

In general, water exceeding the optimal fluoride content for caries prevention should not be used for dilution of infant formulas. Even though the use of distilled water in formula feeding is admittedly impractical, it is the only approach that avoids excessive fluoride intake. It appears that fluoride supplementation is indicated only when human or unmodified cow's milk is being fed, and then only if the fluoride content of the individual water supply is remarkably low. Breastfed infants in communities with nonfluoridated water supplies should have fluoride supplementation as outlined above.

Feeding and Dietary Measures

Rampant caries in association with prolonged use of the nursing bottle is not an uncommon finding. Prolonged nocturnal bottle feeding is a well-documented etiologic factor in this type of dental decay (nursing bottle caries). Increased caries activity associated with prolonged bottle feeding with milk formulas, refined sugar, or fruit juices before going to sleep has been well established. There are indications as well that human milk alone or with supplemental carbohydrates can also be cariogenic. The cariogenicity of both human and bovine milk, because of their lactose content, is enhanced if the milk is permitted to stagnate on the teeth.

Several basic feeding guidelines can diminish appreciably these causes of early onset caries:

1. From birth, the infant should be held while feeding, and the bottle should be removed after the child falls asleep to prevent pooling of milk.
2. Frequent short feeding periods are preferable to long, sustained ones which encourage cariogenic activity.
3. After eruption, the teeth should be cleansed regularly, particularly after feeding. Wiping with gauze pads or cotton balls is adequate. The use of dentifrices for young children can be started at about 2 years, but brushing must be either performed or supervised by the parent. A soft bristle brush with a small head is essential to prevent gingival injury.
4. Nursing should be discontinued as soon as cup drinking is achieved, usually at about 12–15 months.

Undesirable Feeding Supplements

Many young parents, particularly organic food enthusiasts, are substituting foods that contain natural sugar for refined sugar products in the belief that they are more nutritious. As an example, it is frequently assumed that honey is less cariogenic than other sweet products, such as jams, jellies, or syrups that contain high concentrations of refined sugar. It should be recognized that the foremost adulterant of honey is sucrose, added directly or fed to bees. Additionally, the sticky consistency of honey is even more likely to cause caries than its action as a substrate for caries-producing organisms. Honey, applied to the nipple to enhance bottle feeding, is unquestionably an undesirable feeding practice. It has been demonstrated that even low concentrations of sucrose combined with starchy foods render the food highly cariogenic. Honey is probably at least as cariogenic as sucrose and, when ingested with natural foods, probably retains its highly cariogenic character even at very low concentration.

General Dental Management

Children generally respond well in the dental office, even at ages of 2½–3 years, the time of the traditional first visit. Children with earlier signs of caries, usually nursing bottle caries, should be referred immediately after recognition of the caries. Current techniques of dental management are, for the most part, not resisted by most children. On occasion, mild verbal and physical coercive measures are required. Local anesthesia and nitrous oxide inhalational analgesia have become fairly routine components of standard practice in children's dentistry. Nitrous oxide and oxygen, at analgesic levels, is an excellent psychosedative for relieving anxiety. In this range, it is physiologically safe and effective, with remarkably few medical contraindications. (It is nonaddictive, and there is certainly no evidence to indicate that its use in dentistry predisposes susceptible children to experiment with other drugs.)

Dental examinations should be done twice yearly, particularly in children who demonstrate active caries activity. The mixed dentition period is developmentally dynamic, and opportunities for preventive and interceptive orthodontic measures may be lost if dental monitoring is irregular and widely spaced.

Dental radiography is an essential element of comprehensive dental health care. However, the concern about exposure to radiation in the dental office is reasonable and justified. At present, periodic examination of dental radiology units is obligatory in many states. Improved radiologic techniques, utilizing fast speed film and shielding devices (lead aprons), are common practices in most dental offices. It is difficult however, to establish criteria for optimal radiation safety. Dental radiographs are important in dental trauma, marked developmental lag, pulpal therapy, caries susceptibility, and in children with developing malocclusions. The pediatrician asked about the need for dental radiography should assure parents that the dental profession is aware of the hazards of radiation and has become considerably more circumspect in the clinical application of this absolutely necessary adjunct to good dental care. However, parents should not be discouraged from discussing their concerns with the child's dentist.

REQUESTS BY DENTISTS FOR CONSULTATION WITH THE PEDIATRICIAN

The dentist will frequently request pediatric consultation for children with chronic medical disorders or developmental disability and for children who exhibit marked situational reactivity toward dental treatment. Consultation may be requested particularly about drugs to be used in dental management. There are many aspects of dental and oral surgical treatment that may affect the child's medical status. It is difficult for the pediatrician to suggest methods of handling children who are overanxious about dental procedures. Dental procedures are mechanically exacting and time consuming. Premedication dosage, especially with oral administration of drugs with dosages predicted on age and weight, is notoriously unreliable. Inhalational methods, such as nitrous oxide in anal-

gesic ranges, rectal placements, intramuscular injections, and intravenous routes are more dependable for achieving sedation for outpatients. In some instances, hospital admission and the use of operating room facilities may be required for children with severe behavioral resistance. The common premedication drugs used in dental practice include chloral hydrate, Vistaril, Demerol, Phenergan, Valium, and barbiturate preparations. Their sedative action is enhanced if accompanied by nitrous-oxide-oxygen analgesic levels. Most dentists are familiar with these drugs, but decisions for their use may require consultation. In most communities, the oral surgeon and the pedodontist can provide this therapeutic support. In any case, suggestions for the use of drugs should not be given casually, and both undersedation and oversedation should be avoided.

Any meaningful control over the common dental disorders, such as dental caries, periodontal disease, and malocclusion, must be based on prevention. Thus, the future of good dental health in this country must begin in childhood, and this can never be adequately accomplished without the knowledgeable assistance and support of the practicing pediatrician.

BIBLIOGRAPHY

David JM, Law DB, Lewis TM: An Atlas of Pedodontics, 2nd ed. Philadelphia, Saunders, 1981

Fromm A: Epstein's pearls, Bohn's nodules and inclusion-cysts of the oral cavity. J Dent Child 34:275, 1967

Snawder KD: Handbook of Clinical Pedodontics. St. Louis, Mosby, 1980

White GE: Clinical Oral Pediatrics. Chicago, Quintessence Publishing Co., 1981

Cross-Reference to *Pediatrics,* 17th ed.

THIRTY-ONE

The Abnormal Urine and Urinary Tract Disease

David Goldsmith

Proteinuria, hematuria, and leukocyturia, either alone or in combination, are common findings in pediatric patients.[1-3] Interpretation of the urinalysis may be difficult, since well-established, age-related standards for the amount of protein, red blood cells, and white blood cells considered normal in healthy children are lacking. Moreover, each of these abnormalities is nonspecific; any disease of the urinary tract may cause proteinuria or an abnormal urinary sediment. In addition, nonrenal disease, such as appendicitis or other febrile illnesses, can result in similar abnormalities.

Urinary findings sufficient to establish the diagnosis of hematuria or proteinuria are set forth in Table 1. Urinary and other findings that help to establish various categories of renal disease, such as urinary tract infection, nephritis, and renal failure, are included in Table 1 also. It should be clear that the entities listed in Table 1 represent broad diagnostic categories and not specific diseases. They are useful designations, however, since they are easily established by history, physical examination, and simple laboratory testing.[4] The various sections of this chapter describe the differential diagnosis of these conditions and the management of commonly encountered disorders. Entities not encountered frequently in pediatric practice, such as renal tubular disorders, and the management of conditions for which consultation with a pediatric nephrologist is required, such as chronic glomerulonephritis or renal failure, are not included. The reader is referred elsewhere for a more complete discussion.[4,5]

ASYMPTOMATIC HEMATURIA AND PROTEINURIA

Definition

The definition of significant hematuria and proteinuria is somewhat arbitrary because no systematic studies of red cell and protein excretion rates in a large number of children have been reported. More importantly, in large surveys of the epidemiology of hematuria and proteinuria in school-age children, Dodge et al.[3] found only 8 of 6,070 children screened to have renal disease, as judged by their primary care physician. Vehaskari et

TABLE 1. CATEGORIES OF PRESENTATION OF RENAL AND URINARY TRACT DISEASE

Entity	Diagnostic Characteristics
Asymptomatic urinary abnormalities	
Hematuria	(1) 3 analyses demonstrating more than trace on strip test *or* (2) more than 6 RBC/mm^3 in unspun urine *or* (3) more than 3 RBC/hpf in sediment from centrifuged random urine *or* (4) more than 15,000 RBC/hr/m^2 in an Addis count
Proteinuria	(1) 3 analyses of $\geq$ 1+ in random specimens *or* (2) > 40 mg/m^2/hr in urine made and collected in the recumbent position
Asymptomatic bacteriuria	Bacteriuria, > 100,000 organisms/ml in clean-catch urine
Urinary tract infection	(1) Bacteriuria > 100,000 organisms/ml in clean-catch or catheterized urine or any bacteria in a sample obtained by suprapubic aspiration in combination with (2) dysuria, frequency, fever, flank pain, or previous UTI
Nephritis	(1) Red blood cell casts or hematuria *and* (2) oliguria, edema hypertension, or elevated serum creatinine
Nephrotic syndrome	(1) Heavy proteinuria > 40 mg/m^2/hr *and* (2) serum albumin < 0.25 g/dl
Abdominal mass	Palpable lesion in the perinephric or suprapubic region
Hypertension	Blood pressure, 95th percentile for age and sex
Renal failure	(1) Creatine clearance* < 20 ml/min/1.73 m^2 *or* (2) anuria *or* (3) oliguria and rapidly rising serum creatinine

*Creatinine clearance can be estimated using the following formula: Clearance (ml/min/1.73/m^2) = 0.55 × body length (cm)/plasma creatinine (mg/dl)

al.[1,2] found only 2 of 8,954 children to have specific abnormalities. None of the 10 patients in these two studies considered to have renal disease had isolated hematuria; 6 of the 10 had isolated proteinuria. It should be appreciated that these 10 patients with recognizable renal or genitourinary abnormalities accounted for less than 5% of the children with a persistently abnormal urinalysis.

These findings suggest that evaluation of patients with asymptomatic urinary abnormalities will uncover significant pathology infrequently. On the other hand, in unpublished studies of the International Study of Kidney Disease in Children, histologic abnormalities of the kidney were found in nearly 40% of children with isolated hematuria of more than 6 months duration. The natural history and, thus, the prognosis for these children are unknown.

Until well-defined age-adjusted rates of red cell and protein excretion are established and more precise information about the clinical significance of asymptomatic hematuria or proteinuria is available, no precise definition can be made for asymptomatic urinary abnormalities. Nevertheless, most authors would agree that the criteria shown in Table 1 do provide reasonable guidelines for the diagnosis.[1–9]

Differential Diagnosis

Most of the diseases that are included in the differential diagnosis of hematuria and proteinuria (Table 2) belong to categories of presentation other than an asymptomatic child with an abnormal urine. However, should the disease be mild or at an early stage, other findings often are absent and even minimal diagnostic criteria cannot be met. For exam-

TABLE 2. CAUSES OF ASYMPTOMATIC URINARY ABNORMALITIES

	Other Modes of Presentation	Proteinuria	Hematuria Microscopic	Macroscopic	Casts
Glomerular diseases					
Acute glomerulonephritis	Renal failure, nephritis	+ +	+ +	+ +	+
Chronic glomerulonephritis	Renal failure, nephritis	+ +	+ +	+	+
Benign recurrent hematuria (familial or nonfamilial)	Nephritis	−	+ +	+ +	+
Familial nephritis or nephropathy	Renal failure, nephritis	+ +	+ +	+ +	+
Berger's disease (IgA nephropathy)	Nephritis	+ +	+ +	+ +	+
Exercise hematuria	—	+	+ +	−	−
Drugs and nephrotoxins	Nephritis, renal failure, nephrotic syndrome	+ +	+ +	+	−
Orthostatic proteinuria	—	+ +	−	−	−
Subclinical minimal change nephrotic syndrome	Nephrotic syndrome	+ +	+	−	−
Nonglomerular diseases					
Infection of urinary tract	—	+	+ +	+	−
Congenital anomalies (hydronephrosis, polycystic kidney)	Abdominal mass	+	+ +	+	−
Trauma	—	−	+	+ +	−
Tumors	Abdominal mass	−	+	+ +	−
Foreign bodies	UTI	−	+ +	+	−
Stones	—	+	+ +	+	−
Sickle cell trait or disease	—	+	+ +	+ +	−
Bleeding diatheses	—	−	−	+ +	−
Renal venous thrombosis	Renal failure, abdominal mass	+	−	+ +	−
AV malformation	—	−	+	+ +	−

ple, Sagel and her co-workers[10] demonstrated significant renal histologic abnormalities in children with asymptomatic hematuria known to have had a group A beta-hemolytic streptococcal infection during the previous month. These children clearly had mild poststreptococcal acute glomerulonephritis, although none had edema, hypertension, oliguria, or abnormal renal function.

In Table 2, diagnostic entities are separated according to the location of the lesion. Clues to the diagnosis are provided by the nature of the associated urinary abnormalities. For example, the presence of red cell casts indicates that the lesion is most likely to be found at the level of the glomerulus, and work-up for the more common forms of glomerulonephritis should be undertaken. Grossly bloody urine, in contrast to tea-colored or smokey urine, is not characteristic of glomerular lesions, and other causes, such as trauma, arteriovenous malformations, or sickle cell trait or disease, should be sought. The three-glass test also helps to distinguish bleeding from the kidney and ureter from that due to lesions in the bladder and urethra. Most nonglomerular diseases are associated with minimal or absent proteinuria except when the hematuria is massive. The presence of clots usually indicates lower tract bleeding, although clots may form in the renal pelvis following local trauma. The history and renal colic suggest the correct diagnosis.

History and Physical Examination. A history of renal disease in family members is found frequently in familial nephritis, benign recurrent hematuria, polycystic kidney disease, metabolic disorders associated with renal stones (such as cystinuria or oxalosis), sickle cell disease or trait, and bleeding diatheses. Nerve deafness and ocular abnormalities in family members suggests familial nephritis (Alport's disease). A history of recent or concurrent illness suggests the possibilities of acute nephritis (poststreptococcal or other postinfectious etiology), an acute exacerbation of minimal change nephrotic syndrome, and benign recurrent hematuria. Dysuria is often found in urinary tract infections and in instances of intravesicular foreign body.

The physical examination can help to determine the etiology of the urinary abnormalities. Perineal irritation and meatal ulceration are obvious causes of microscopic hematuria. Attention should be paid to detecting the presence of hypertension, edema, rashes, arthritis, fever, pallor, ocular and auditory abnormalities, abnormal growth, and abdominal masses.

Laboratory Evaluation. The first step in the evaluation of hematuria or proteinuria is to confirm their presence and persistence. These abnormalities often resolve spontaneously, and no further work-up is required. Microscopic hematuria was found by Dodge et al. in 4–6% of schoolchildren, but it persisted for more than 6 months in fewer than 0.5%. More than two thirds of children found to have proteinuria had at least one normal urinalysis when the test was repeated on two other occasions.[3] These findings, taken together with the low incidence of renal or GU abnormalities in children with isolated urinary abnormalitites,[1-3] support the argument favoring a limited work-up of these patients. In all instances, however, a urine culture should be performed early in the evaluation because the test is noninvasive and inexpensive. Quantitative determination of urinary protein excretion is also carried out as part of the initial work-up (Figs. 1 and 2).

Isolated Microscopic Hematuria. Patients with isolated hematuria are evaluated according to the algorithm shown in Figure 1. It is advisable to examine the urine of other family members and to obtain audiograms even in the absence of a family history of nephritis or renal disease, because there is a high degree of variability in the expression and penetrance of the gene,[11,12] and nearly 20% of the cases may represent spontaneous new mutations.[13] Tests for sickle hemoglobin should be done in black patients. Since hematuria may be an early sign of hypercalciuria and stone formation, urinary calcium is measured quantitatively.[14,15] This can be done on the same sample of urine collected for the measurement of excretion of protein.

The role of excretory urography in the evaluation of patients with isolated microscopic hematuria is not clear. Few children found to have hematuria have renal disease, but half of those with disease have abnormal excretory urograms.[3] Therefore, many pediatric nephrologists recommend radiographic evaluation if the isolated microscopic hematuria persists for 6 months or more.

Renal biopsy is not indicated in the ma-

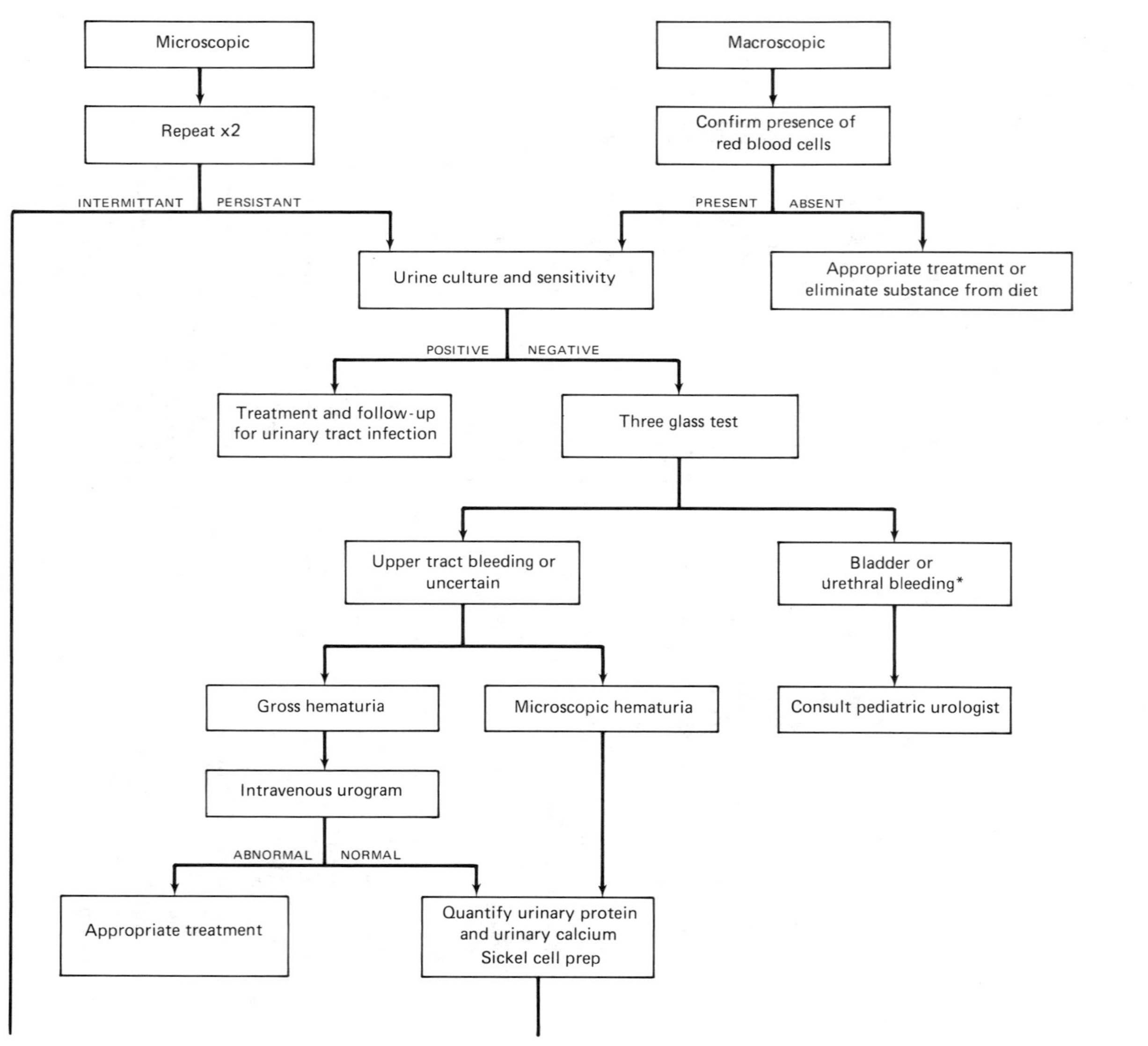

Microscopic
Macroscopic
Repeat x2
Confirm presence of red blood cells
INTERMITTANT
PERSISTANT
PRESENT
ABSENT
Urine culture and sensitivity
Appropriate treatment or eliminate substance from diet
POSITIVE
NEGATIVE
Treatment and follow-up for urinary tract infection
Three glass test
Upper tract bleeding or uncertain
Bladder or urethral bleeding*
Gross hematuria
Microscopic hematuria
Consult pediatric urologist
Intravenous urogram
ABNORMAL
NORMAL
Appropriate treatment
Quantify urinary protein and urinary calcium Sickel cell prep

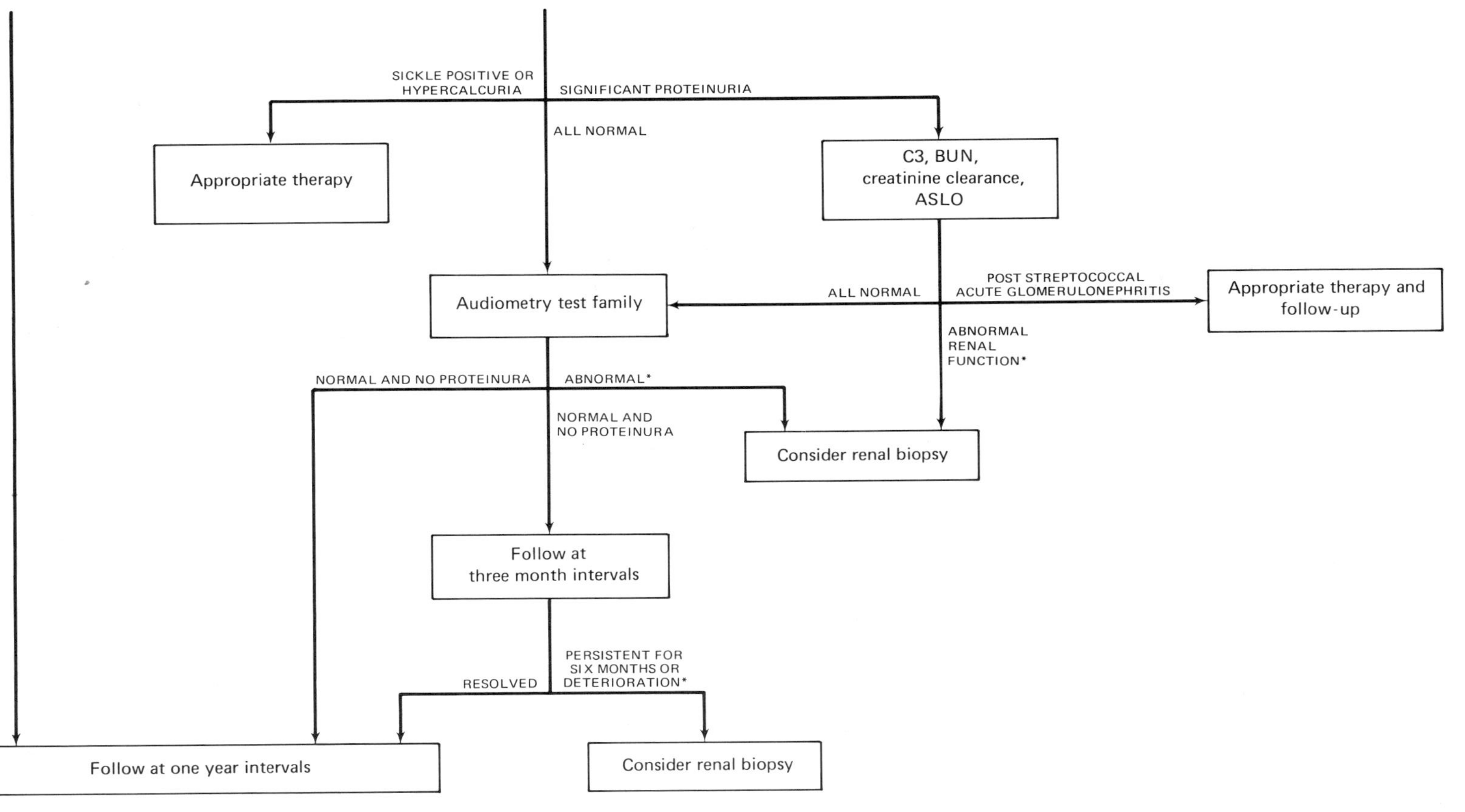

Figure 1. Evaluation of Hematuria.

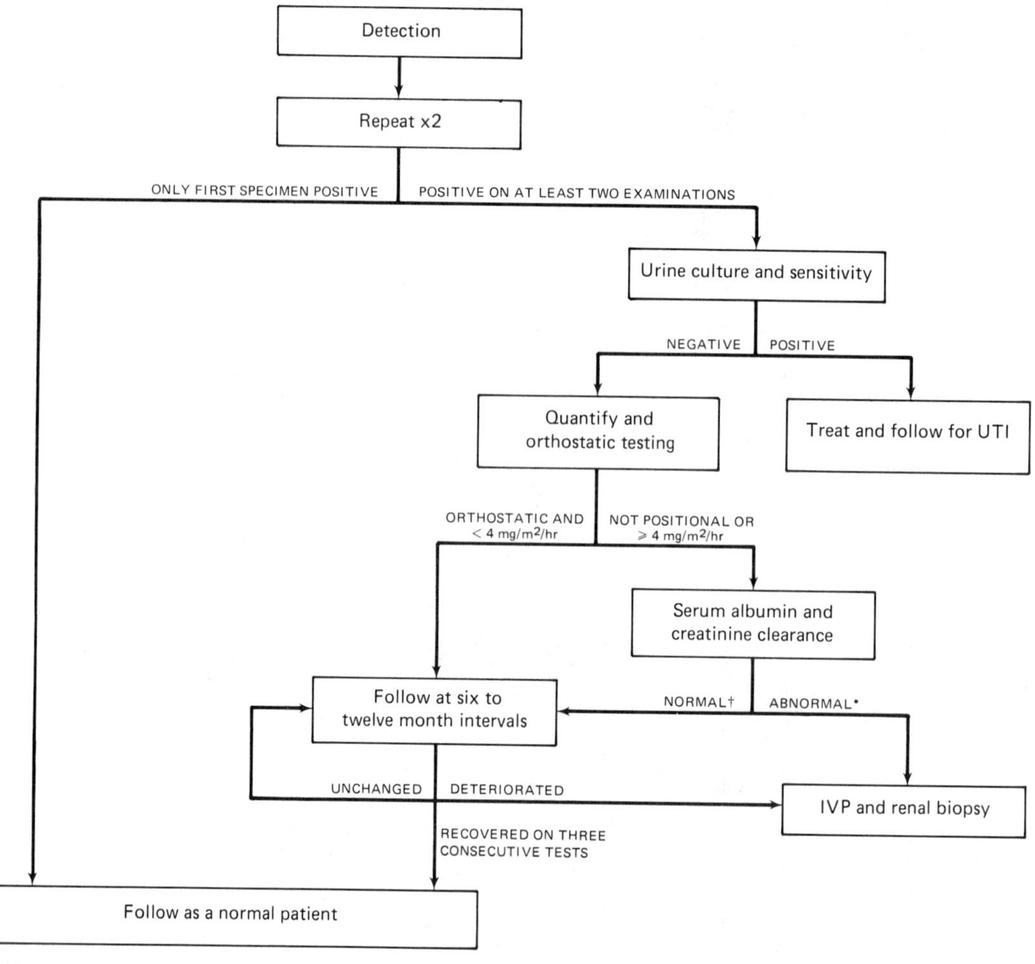

Figure 2. Evaluation of Proteinura.

jority of patients with isolated hematuria because, in almost all instances, specific therapy of the conditions likely to be diagnosed is not available. Moreover, the prognostic significance of many of the histologic lesions remains unknown.[16] One exception is to consider renal biopsy in children whose hematuria persists into their teens because genetic counseling may be advisable.

Microscopic Hematuria and Proteinuria. If hematuria can be demonstrated to be of glomerular origin by the presence of casts or by the association with proteinuria, measurements of the serum creatinine and blood urea nitrogen and an estimate of the glomerular filtration rate[17] are obtained (Fig. 1). Serologic tests for streptococcal infection are done and serum complement of C3 is measured early in the evaluation to identify children with asymptomatic, acute, poststreptococcal glomerulonephritis. In the patients with abnormal renal function and for whom no cause has been established, consultation with a pediatric nephrologist is indicated.

Gross Hematuria. It is not necessary to await confirmation of gross hematuria in multiple specimens prior to initiating a work-up. Suffice it to say that care must be taken to assure the absence of factitious hematuria and pigments that may give the urine a red color in the absence of blood. Examples of the latter are urate crystals on the diaper, hemoglobinuria and myoglobinuria, and red dyes found in certain foods (such as beets) or added as food coloring.

The disease entities that may be responsible for gross hematuria are quite similar to those causing microscopic hematuria (Table 2), but their frequency is different. Urinary tract infection was diagnosed in half of 144 children who presented with gross hematuria in a general pediatric setting, but only 6 children were shown to have acute nephritis.[18]

In most instances the cause of gross hematuria is readily identifiable from the history and physical examination. In those cases where the diagnosis is more elusive, a work-up similar to that described for microscopic hematuria is followed, with several important differences, included in Figure 1. It is usually unrewarding to obtain quantitative assessment of urinary protein excretion, because some protein is likely to be found in all children with gross hematuria. Nevertheless, if 4+ proteinuria is documented, the underlying lesion is likely to be glomerular. Patients with gross hematuria should be evaluated for bleeding diatheses, although that diagnosis is usually established before the occurrence of an episode of gross hematuria. Unless a simple diagnosis can be made, such as bleeding from meatal ulceration, consultation with a pediatric nephrologist or urologist and the performance of an intravenous urogram (especially in infants) are recommended.

Isolated Proteinuria. Isolated proteinuria is generally considered to be a more ominous sign than hematuria, although most children do not have a serious underlying disease. The first two diagnoses to be considered are urinary tract infection and orthostatic proteinuria. The former can be confirmed by obtaining a urine culture, and the latter is established by demonstrating the absence of proteinuria during recumbency.

Although patients with all forms of renal disease have greater rates of excretion of protein during activity than at bed rest, orthostatic proteinuria is diagnosed when protein-free urine is obtained while the patient is recumbent and significant amounts of proteinuria are detected while the patient is upright or ambulatory. Since orthostatic proteinuria appears to be of little clinical significance,[19,20] patients with this condition require no further evaluation; the status of proteinuria is reassessed at 6–12 month intervals.

In most children with isolated proteinuria, it is transient or orthostatic. Patients with persistent proteinuria that is not orthostatic nearly always have flomerular disease. For this reason, measurement of the glomerular filtration rate and consultation with a nephrologist are recommended. Some authors have suggested performance of an intravenous urogram,[6,21] but there is little information currently available on which to base this recommendation.

URINARY TRACT INFECTION

Definition

Urinary tract infection (UTI) is a common nephrologic problem in pediatric practice, second only to nocturnal enuresis in its frequency. It is defined as the presence of bacteria in the urinary tract, diagnosed usually by the finding of greater than 100,000 bacteria per ml of urine in a clean-catch specimen.

Differential Diagnosis

In contrast to the other presentations of renal disease, urinary tract infection usually does not pose any problem of differential diagnosis. However, a careful search must be made for underlying conditions that predispose to or may lead to complications of infection. The history should focus on evidence of previous episodes of undiagnosed infections. Examples are recurrent febrile illnesses in the absence of a diagnosis, recurrent episodes of abdominal pain, feeding difficulties in infancy, and poor growth. In addition, the history should elicit the voiding pattern of the patient, particular attention being paid to the quality of the stream in males, the frequency of urination, and indications of dysuria, such as hesitancy or crying during micturition.

On physical examination, attention should be paid to whether the bladder is palpable and, if so, its size. Meticulous examination of the abdomen is done to determine if the kidneys are palpable or if there are abdominal masses. The external genitalia are examined for any abnormality. The back is examined for evidence of spinal abnormality, such as a hairy nevus or dimple in the sacral area. A neurologic examination is performed to look for evidence of a neurogenic bladder.

There is a vast literature regarding clinical and laboratory signs that help the physician to distinguish between urinary tract infections that involve the kidney and those localized to the bladder and urethra.[22–26] The importance of making this distinction lies in the relative likelihood of an underlying abnormality of the urinary tract. Infections that are confined to the bladder do not cause renal damage and are associated less frequently with urinary tract malformations. High fever, flank pain, and costovertebral angle tenderness suggest the diagnosis of pyelonephritis. Unfortunately, the various enzymatic tests, the presence or absence of clumps of white cells or glitter cells in the urine, and the urinary concentrating capacity are not consistently reliable indicators of upper or lower tract disease.

Diagnosis

The diagnosis of UTI is suggested by the symptoms of frequency, dysuria, urgency, and abdominal or suprapubic pain. The urine may have a strong ammoniacal or putrid smell. Urinalysis reveals increased numbers of leukocytes and often a small amount of protein. The diagnosis of UTI is established by demonstration of bacteria in the urine. Although urine normally is sterile, most techniques of collection permit the introduction of small numbers of bacteria. Therefore, it is important to quantify the numbers of organisms, in order to differentiate true bacteriuria from contamination.

Laboratories will perform a bacterial count on urine specimens received for culture. A count of 10^5 per ml or greater is indicative of bacteriuria. In most healthy subjects in the absence of infection, bacterial counts on urines obtained by a clean voiding technique or by catheterization of the bladder are less than 10^4, and usually less than 10^3 organisms per ml. Counts between 10^3 or 10^4 and 10^5 are considered equivocal.

Since results from the bacteriology laboratory are not immediately available, it is useful to examine the urinary sediment for bacteria. Microscopic identification of a single organism in a noncentrifuged specimen of urine indicates a bacterial count of 10^5 per ml or more. On a centrifuged specimen, numerous organisms will be seen in every field if the count is 10^5. Finding a few organisms in most fields is an equivocal result. In noninfected individuals, rare or no organisms will be seen.

In infants, the urine is examined usually with a specimen obtained by application of a sterile plastic bag to the previously cleansed perineum. Negative results with this procedure are reliable. If the urine is positive for bacteria, there is a strong possibility that the urine has been contaminated, even if the count exceeds 10^5. In such instances, urine should be obtained by suprapubic aspiration of the bladder, and the presence of any number of organisms is indicative of UTI. Although an occasional urine specimen obtained by suprapubic puncture from a child presumed to be free of infection will be found to have a bacterial count in excess of 10^3 per ml,[27] bacteria found in urine obtained with this technique from an ill patient should be regarded as proof of infection.

Treatment

Treatment is almost always begun prior to identification of the organism and antibiotic sensitivity testing. In most instances, organisms encountered in uncomplicated infections are sensitive to ampicillin, a sulfonamide, or nitrofurantoin. Any of these can be used as intial treatment. If the patient does not have a prompt response to treatment, with improvement or loss of all symptoms in 24 to 48 hours, choice of another antibiotic is based on sensitivity testing.

It is generally recommended that children receive 7–10 days of treatment even though they may be entirely well clinically in hours. Recent studies suggest that in patients with uncomplicated lower urinary tract infection, 3 days of treatment or even a large single dose of antibiotic is sufficient.

In severely ill patients, children thought to have pyelonephritis, or those who fail to respond to therapy despite administration of an appropriate antibiotic, consultation with a pediatric nephrologist is recommended.

Evaluation and Follow-up

In addition to the bacterial investigations necessary to identify the organism and determine its sensitivity to antibiotics, the evaluation and follow-up of a child with a urinary tract infection must make provisions for identifying malformations, renal scars, and recurrent infections. It is usually recommended that all children with a urinary tract

infection undergo radiographic evaluation, consisting of IVP and voiding cystourethrography. These studies usually are obtained 6 or 8 weeks after the infection has been eradicated, in order to allow for resolution of any inflammation of the ureteral orifices.

The recommendation that all children be evaluated radiographically after the first urinary tract infection is controversial, since the incidence of abnormalities in girls can be as low as 1–2%.[28] Nevertheless, it is generally agreed that only females with symptoms specifically and clearly localized to the lower urinary tract be exempt from radiographic evaluation. It is important to note that the incidence of renal scars is substantially higher in girls with asymptomatic bacteriuria than in those with symptoms localized to the bladder.[28] Thus, the recommendation regarding radiographic evaluation applies to children with asymptomatic bacteriuria as well.

Consultation with a pediatric urologist is indicated for children with an abnormal intravenous urogram or vesicoureteral reflux into a dilated renal pelvis. Low-grade reflux limited to the ureter or into a normally appearing pelvis seems to be of little clinical importance. These children can be followed by the pediatrician. Consultation is recommended if there are morphologic or functional abnormalities of the kidney, if the reflux persists, or if other complications develop. Since reflux has been recently shown to be associated with the development of severe and progressive renal disease,[29–31] follow-up should provide for the detection of proteinuria, hypertension, or altered glomerular filtration rate, in addition to performance of cystourethrography at yearly intervals.

In order to assure eradication of the initial infection and to identify recurrences, urinalysis and culture should be repeated 48 hours after initiation of treatment, 2–3 days and 2–3 weeks after discontinuing therapy, and at 3-monthly intervals for the first year.

Recurrent urinary tract infections often present difficult problems of management, and consultation with a pediatric nephrologist or urologist is advisable.

NEPHRITIS

Definition

The clincial syndrome of nephritis comprises the combination of hematuria or red cell casts with altered renal function (elevation in the serum creatinine), oliguria, edema, or hypertension. It most instances, proteinuria is also present. It may be the result of either acute or chronic injury, and it follows a variable clinical course, dependent upon the underlying disease. The acute forms are characterized by a sudden onset and, in severe cases, may be complicated by congestive heart failure, pulmonary edema, hypertensive encephalopathy, and renal failure. Mild forms are usually self-limited and are managed adequately by a conservative approach.

It is to be noted that the term "nephritis," as used here, does not imply any particular histopathologic change. Some conditions, such as the nephritis associated with EB virus, involve primarily the renal interstitium but are included in the differential diagnosis, whereas some histologic forms of glomerulonephritis, such as those associated with dermatomyositis, rheumatoid arthritis, and scleroderma, are not included in this section because heavy proteinuria and the nephrotic syndrome are the predominant clinical findings. Since there is substantial overlap between nephrotic syndrome and nephritis, a list of conditions that are often associated with either is provided (Table 3).

The term "chronic glomerulonephritis" implies persistence of urinary abnormalities and progressive loss of renal function. Children with chronic progressive renal disease should be managed in consultation with a pediatric nephrologist, and their treatment is not discussed in this chapter.

Differential Diagnosis of Acute Nephritis

A wide variety of conditions may present as acute nephritis (Table 4), but most are encountered rarely in pediatrics. Even so, the diagnosis of uncommon conditions is often apparent, such as in cases of shunt nephritis, subacute bacterial endocarditis, or radiation nephritis.

In practice, the differential diagnosis of acute nephritis is limited mainly to poststreptococcal glomerulonephritis, anaphylactoid purpura, hemolytic-uremic syndrome, systemic lupus erythematosus, and hereditary

TABLE 3. DISEASES COMMONLY PRESENTING AS NEPHRITIS AND/OR THE NEPHROTIC SYNDROME

Associated with Infection	Associated with Systemic Illness
Malaria	Systemic lupus erythematosus
Syphilis	Anaphylactoid purpura
Inherited	Polyarteritis
Hereditary onycho-osteodysplasia (nail-patella syndrome)	Dermatomyositis
Sickle cell disease	Rheumatoid arthritis
	Scleroderma
	Idiopathic
	Membranoproliferative glomerulonephritis
	Focal segmental glomerulosclerosis

TABLE 4. DIFFERENTIAL DIAGNOSIS OF NEPHRITIS

Disease	Findings		
	Historical	Physical	Laboratory
I. Infectious			
Poststeptococcal	Pharyngitis or impetigo	Impetigo	Low C3, C4, elevated ASLO
Viral (varicella, mumps, Ebstein-Barr)	Exposure and lack of immunization	Concurrent illness	Viral studies
Bacterial endocarditis	—	Cardiac murmur	Positive blood culture
Shunt nephritis	Hydrocephalus	Shunt in place	Low C3, positive blood culture
Malaria (acute)	Exposure	Hepatosplenomegaly	Low C3, parasites on blood smear
II. Associated with Systemic Illness			
Anaphylactoid purpura	Joint pain, abdominal pain, previous episode	Characteristic rash, arthritis	Normal C3
SLE	Weight loss, antecedent signs of other organ involvement	Female: fever, malar rash, arthritis	Elevated ESR, low C3, C4 Coombs positive anemia, anti DNA titers, FANA
Hemolytic-uremic syndrome	Mild gastroenteritis	Pallor	Schistocytes, severe hemolytic anemia
Polyarteritis	Antecedent signs of other organ involvement	Male: fever, characteristic rash, arthritis, lung involvement	Elevated ESR, leukocytosis eosinophilia, normal C3
Goodpasture's syndrome	—	Pulmonary hemorrhage	Circulating antibasement membrane antibodies
Mixed connective tissue disease	—	Combined characteristics of SLE, scleroderma, dermatomyositis, rheumatoid arthritis	Circulating immune complexes
Cryoglobulinemia	Disease associated with cryoglobulinemia	—	Cold-precipitable proteins
III. Other			
Membranoproliferative glomerulonephritis	Nonspecific	Nonspecific	Low serum C3
Focal glomerulonephritis	Nonspecific	Nonspecific	Nonspecific
Interstitial nephritis	Exposure to toxin (e.g., phenacetin)	Nonspecific	Nonspecific
Proliferative glomerulonephritis	Nonspecific	Nonspecific	Nonspecific

nephritis. Anaphylactoid purpura and systemic lupus erythematosus are recognized by the involvement of other organ systems, characteristic rashes, and laboratory studies. The diagnosis of hemolytic-uremic syndrome is made on the basis of the history of an antecedent gastrointestinal disturbance, acute renal failure, anemia, and the presence of schistocytes in the peripheral smear. Hereditary nephritis is suggested by the family history and the presence of auditory or ocular abnormalities. The single most common form of nephritis, namely, poststreptococcal acute glomerulonephritis, is suggested in most instances by a history of antecedent pharyngitis or the presence of impetiginous lesions.

In addition to providing clues to the appropriate diagnosis, the history and physical examination should also be directed toward uncovering the severity of the episode. The presence of headaches or irritability suggests impending hypertensive encephalopathy. A marked decrease in urinary volume or frank anuria suggests the diagnosis of acute renal failure. Alterations in respiratory rate or the presence of pulmonary rales implies that a congestive heart failure and pulmonary edema have supervened.

Treatment

Treatment of mild cases of acute glomerulonephritis, either poststreptococcal or associated with anaphylactoid purpura, can be undertaken by the primary physician. Severe cases and those associated with other diagnoses should be managed in consultation with a pediatric nephrologist because renal biopsy often is necessary to establish the diagnosis and/or prognosis.

Treatment is mainly expectant, with the child being observed closely for the development of complications; this may require hospitalization. Bed rest often is recommended during the early stages, but there are no data to support its value. Limitation of intake of salt and fluid restriction are instituted in order to avoid volume overload. The blood pressure is measured frequently to detect the onset of hypertension. If the blood pressure tends to rise, antihypertensive medication should be instituted promptly. (See Chapter 32.) If the patient develops renal failure, consultation with a pediatric nephrologist should be sought. Complete recovery is anticipated in over 95% of children.

NEPHROTIC SYNDROME

Definition

The nephrotic syndrome is characterized by edema, proteinuria, hypoalbuminemia, and hyperlipidemia (hypercholesterolemia). However, as indicated in Table 1, the presence of heavy proteinuria ($> 40mg/m^2/hr$) and a reduction in the serum albumin to less than 2.5 g/dl are the most important features.[32] It is common, therefore, to apply the term to all patients having these two characteristics even if the others are absent.

Differential Diagnosis and Evaluation

The nephrotic syndrome can be divided into two groups: (1) primary idiopathic conditions that involve only the kidney and (2) secondary forms associated with systemic diseases or those due to known toxins or allergic phenomena. The diseases are listed in Table 5 according to their relative frequency within the group.[33–35] It can be seen that the majority of patients with idiopathic nephrotic syndrome in childhood have minimal change nephrotic syndrome (MCNS), an entity that is usually responsive to steroid therapy and does not lead to progressive renal insufficiency. The high rate of response in MCNS contrasts markedly with that of other forms of primary nephrotic syndrome. Because of this, a therapeutic trial of prednisone can be used as a diagnostic tool.[36] The exception to the general rule of a therapeutic trial of prednisone lies in the patient with a low serum

TABLE 5. CAUSES OF NEPHROTIC SYNDROME

Primary	Frequency
Minimal change nephrotic syndrome	Very common (75–80%)
Focal segmental glomerulosclerosis	Uncommon (5–10%)
Membranoproliferative glomerulonephritis	Uncommon (5–10%)
Membranous nephropathy	Rare
Mesangioproliferative nephrotic syndrome	Rare
Proliferative glomerulonephritis	Rare
Secondary	
Infectious	
Syphilis	Uncommon (5–10%)
Malaria (chronic)	Rare
Associated with systemic disease	
Anaphylactoid purpura	Common (20%)
Systemic lupus erythematosus	Common (20%)
Sickle cell disease	Unusual (10–15%)
Amyloidosis	Rare
Hemolytic-uremic syndrome	Rare
Dermatomyositis	Rare
Scleroderma	Rare
Inherited	
Hereditary onycho-osteodystrophy	Uncommon (5–10%)
Congenital nephrotic syndrome	Rare
Toxic	
Heavy metal (gold, mercury)	Rare
Bee sting	Uncommon (5–10%)
Poison oak	Rare
Drugs	
Pencillamine	Rare
Trimethedione	Rare

complement, since this laboratory finding is very common in patients with membranoproliferative glomerulonephritis,[33] a disease in which severe hypertension may develop with daily steroid administration.[37]

The use of clinical characteristics at the time of onset, such as age, presence or absence of hematuria, hypertension, and edema, fails to distinguish patients with MCNS from those with more severe diseases. Renal biopsy is the sole method for establishing the diagnosis in steroid-nonresponsive patients.

The secondary nephrotic syndrome occurs far less frequently than does the primary nephrotic syndrome; it is usually due to anaphylactoid purpura, systemic lupus erythematosus, sickle cell nephropathy, or hereditary nephritis. The other causes listed in Table 5 are seen rarely. The historical and physical findings of anaphylactoid purpura, systemic lupus erythematosus, and hereditary nephritis are included in the section dealing with nephritis and Table 4 because these entities usually present as such rather than as the nephrotic syndrome.

Treatment

Patients with nephrotic syndrome who fail to respond to prednisone therapy should be referred to a pediatric nephrologist for evaluation and treatment. Many children with MCNS can be managed by the primary physician without need for consultation.

Treatment is begun with prednisone, 60 mg/m²/day divided into 3–4 doses, and is given for 28 days. During this period, almost all children with MCNS will lose their proteinuria. At the end of the 28-day period of treatment, the dosage is reduced to 40 mg/m²/day and is given as a single dose either every other day or 3 consecutive days of each week. This alternate day or intermittent therapy is continued for another 28 days.

Most children with MCNS will have a recurrence of proteinuria within the subsequent months. With such a relapse, prednisone is started at the intitial dosage but kept at this level only until the urine is protein free for 3 days. Four weeks of alternate day or intermittent therapy is then given, as with treatment of the initial episode.

Many children with MCNS have frequent relapses,[38,39] requiring repeated courses of treatment with steroids, thus making them prone to the development of steroid toxicity. Such children should be referred to a pediatric nephrologist for consideration for other forms of treatment.

Children suspected of having MCNS who fail to respond to the initial 4 weeks of therapy should be referred for consultation. Similarly, the previously steroid-responsive child who becomes nonresponsive should be referred.

The fluid retention of children with MCNS is usually not severe enough to warrant diuretic therapy and can be expected to abate as the patient responds to steroid therapy. Severe edema associated with compromise of circulatory or respiratory status can be treated with a combination of intravenous albumin and furosemide. This should be done in consultation with a pediatric nephrologist.

Although children with the nephrotic syndrome are prone to infection, antibiotic prophylaxis is not indicated. These children should be observed closely and treated promptly if infectious complications develop.

REFERENCES

1. Vehaskari VM, Rapola J: Isolated proteinuria: Analysis of a school-age population. J Pediatr 101:66, 1982

2. Vehaskari VM, Rapola J, Koskimie O, et al.: Microscopic hematuria in schoolchildren: Epidemiology and clincopathologic evaluation. J Pediatr 95:676, 1979

3. Dodge WF, West EF, Smith EH, et al.: Proteinuria and hematuria in school children: Epidemiology and early natural history. J Pediatr 88:327, 1976

4. Goldsmith DI, Spitzer A: Evaluation of infants and children for kidney disease. Pediatrician 8:246, 1979

5. Edelmann CM Jr (ed): Pediatric Kidney Disease. Boston, Little Brown, 1978

6. West CA: Asymptomatic hematuria and proteinuria in children. J Pediatr 89:173, 1976.

7. Silverberg DS, Allard MJ, Ulan RA, et al.: City-wide screening for urinary abnormalities in schoolgirls. Can Med Assoc J 109:981, 1973

8. Silverberg DS: City-wide screening for urinary abnormalities in school boys. Can Med Assoc J 111:410, 1974

9. Northway JD: Hematuria in children. J Pediatr 78:381, 1971

10. Sagel D, Treser G, Ty A, et al.: Occurrence and nature of glomerular lesions after group A streptococcal infections in children. Ann Intern Med 79:492, 1973

11. Hallberg A: Alport's syndrome: A report of three Swedish families. Acta Paediatr Scand 65:49, 1976

12. Shaw RF, Glover RA: Abnormal segregation in hereditary renal disease with

deafness. Am J Human Genet 13:89, 1961

13. Shaw RF, Kallen RJ: Population genetics of Alport's syndrome: Hypothesis of abnormal segregation and the necessary existence of mutation. Nephron 16:427, 1976

14. Kalia A, Travis LB, Browhard BH: The association of idiopathic hypercalciuric and asymptomatic gross hematuria in children. J Pediatr 99:716, 1981

15. Roy S III, Stapleton FB, Doe HN, et al.: Hematuria preceding renal calculus formation in children with hypercalciuria. J Pediatr 99:712, 1981

16. Trachtman H, Weiss, R, Greifer I: Hematuria in children: Indications for renal biopsy. Kidney Int 23:138, 1983 (Abstract)

17. Schwartz GJ, Haycock GB, Edelmann CM Jr, et al.: A simple estimate of glomerular filtration rate in children derived from body length and plasma creatinine. Pediatrics 58:259, 1976

18. Ingelfinger JR, Davis AE, Grupe WE: Frequency and etiology of gross hematuria in a general pediatric setting. Pediatrics 59:57, 1977

19. Levitt JI: The prognostic significance of proteinuria in young college students. Ann Intern Med 66:685, 1967

20. Robinson RR: Idiopathic proteinuria. Ann Intern Med 71:1019, 1975

21. Robson AM, Manley CB: Proteinuria: Physiologic and clinical considerations. Curr Probl Pediatr 1:27, 1970

22. Donatas AS, Marketos SG, Papanayiotou PC, et al.: Simplified water-loading test in bacteriuria. Nephron 12:121, 1974

23. Bank N, Bailine SH: Urinary beta-glucuronidase activity in patients with urinary tract infection. N Engl J Med 272:70, 1965

24. Carvajal HF, Passey RB, Berger M, et al.: Urinary tract dehydrogenase isoenzyme 5 in the differential diagnosis of kidney and bladder infections. Kidney Int 8:176, 1975

25. Anderson HJ, Berstrom T, Lincoln K, et al.: Studies of urinary tract infections in infancy and children. VI. Determination of *E. coli* antibody titers in the diagnosis of acute urinary tract infections lacking the usual urinary findings. J Pediatr 67:1080, 1965

26. Hewstone AS, Whitaker J: The correlation of ureteric urine bacteriology and homologous antibody titer in children with urinary infection. J Pediat 74:540, 1969

27. Pryles CV, Atkin MD, Morse TS, et al.: A comparative bacteriologic study of urine obtained by percutaneous suprapubic aspiration of the bladder and by catheter in children. Pediatrics 24:983, 1959

28. Winberg, J, Anderson HJ, Bergstrom T, et al.: Epidemiology of symptomatic urinary tract infection in childhood. Acta Paediatr Scand [Suppl 252] 63:1, 1974

29. Aladjem M, Schoeneman MJ, Bennett B, et al.: Focal segmental glomerulosclerosis with proteinuria and chronic interstitial nephritis. NY State J Med March 1978, p 579

30. Cotran RS: Glomerulosclerosis in reflux nephropathy. Kidney Int 21:528, 1982

31. Arant BS Jr, Sotelo-Avila C, Bernstein J, et al.: "Segmental hypoplasia" of the kidney (Ask-Upmark). J Pediatr 95:931, 1979

32. Abramowitz M, Arneil GC, Barnett HL, et al.: Controlled trial of azathiaprine in children with nephrotic syndrome. A report for the International Study of Kidney Disease in Children. Lancet 1:959, 1970

33. International Study of Kidney Disease in Children. The nephrotic syndrome in children. Prediction of histopathology from clinical and laboratory characteristics at the time of diagnosis. Kidney Int 13:43, 1978

34. White RHR, Glasgow EF, Mills RJ: Clinicopathologic study of nephrotic syndrome in childhood. Lancet 1:1353, 1970

35. Habib R, Kleinknect C: The primary nephrotic syndrome of childhood. Classification and clinicopathologic study of 406 cases. In Sommers SC (ed): Pathology Annual, New York, Appleton-Century-Crofts, 1971, p 165

36. A report of the International Study of Kidney Disease in Children. The primary nephrotic syndrome in children: Identification of patients with minimal change nephrotic syndrome from initial response to prednisone. J Pediatr 98:561, 1981

37. White RHR, Cameron JS, Trounce JR: Immuno-suppressive therapy in steroid-resistant proliferative glomerulonephritis accompanied by the nephrotic syndrome. Biol Med J 2:853, 1966

38. A report of the International Study of Kidney Disease in Children. Primary nephrotic syndrome in children: Clinical significance of histopathologic variants of minimal change and of diffuse mesangial hypercellularity. Kidney Int 20:765, 1981

39. A report of the International Study of Kidney Disease in Children. Identification of frequent relapses among children with minimal change nephrotic syndrome. J Pediatr 101:514, 1982

Cross-Reference to *Pediatrics,* 17th ed.

THIRTY-TWO

Hypertension

Chester M. Edelmann, Jr.

Hypertension in adults is a common condition and, in most instances, a primary disease (i.e., without known etiology), thus termed *essential* hypertension. In contrast, hypertension in children is commonly viewed as a rare disorder, usually secondary to an identifiable disease. It is now well established, however, that hypertension in children is *not* uncommon and that in the majority of cases the diagnosis is essential. What seems to have led to this confusion is that in prior years most children diagnosed as hypertensive had *severe* disease. Severe hypertension in this age group indeed is usually secondary to an identifiable disorder. However, it is now clear that the majority of children with hypertension in fact have mild disease, either overlooked or discounted in previous decades. In most of these children the diagnosis is essential hypertension.

It behooves the pediatric practitioner to be aware of hypertension as a relatively common disorder, to know how to determine blood pressure accurately and reliably, and to understand the initial approach to diagnosis and management.

DEFINITION

Hypertension is defined as a level of blood pressure, systolic or diastolic, that exceeds the 95th percentile for blood pressure levels in healthy children of the same age and sex. With this definition, 5% of all children will be found to have levels of blood pressure that are in the hypertensive range. The minority have levels that *greatly* exceed the 95th percentile; these children can be diagnosed as truly hypertensive when first detected. Most children with blood pressure levels just above the 95th percentile do not have an abnormality in blood pressure control. Rather, it would appear that they simply represent the upper end of the normal range. However, some of these children ultimately will have levels that are unequivocably abnormal and, therefore, of concern. Presently, it is not possible to identify them prospectively.

Another problem is that the 95th percentile for blood pressure levels in adolescents exceeds 140 torr systolic and 90 torr diastolic, values taken as the upper limit of normal in adults. The significance of this observation is unknown. As a practical matter, however, the upper limits applied to adults are considered valid at any age, even though for a particular adolescent the blood pressure reading may not exceed the 95th percentile for age.

The ranges of blood pressure found in children from 2 to 18 years of age are shown in Figures 1 and 2. Fewer data are available for children below the age of 2. The 95th percentiles are somewhat lower, approximately 100 systolic and 45 diastolic from 6

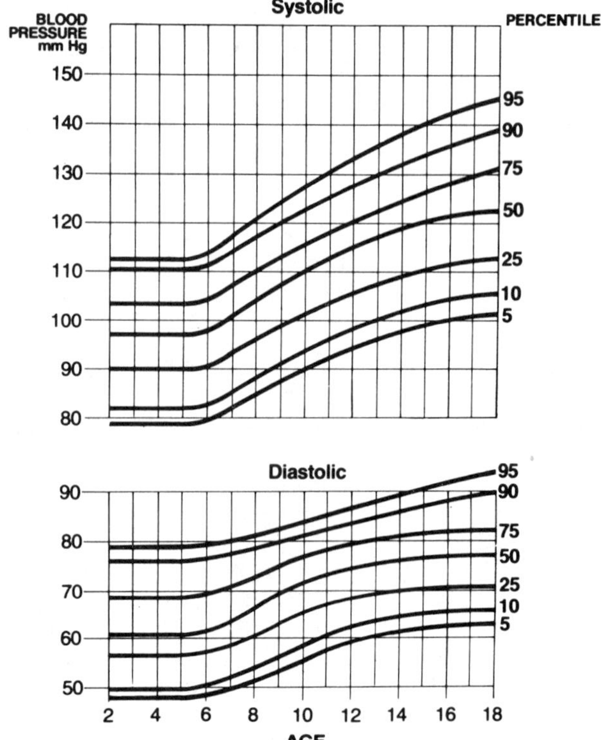

Figure 1. Fifth to ninety-fifth percentiles for blood pressure in normal girls, according to age. (Based on data from the Report of the National Heart, Lung and Blood Institute's Task Force on Blood Pressure Control in Children Pediatrics 59 (Suppl.): 797, 1977.)

months to 2 years of age, and 5–10 torr lower in younger infants. Even fewer studies have been done of blood pressure levels in newborn infants.

Blood pressure levels up to 10 torr above the 95th percentile are considered indicative of mild hypertension. Levels 10–20 torr above the 95th percentile represent moderate hypertension. Levels above this are considered severe hypertension.

DETERMINATION OF BLOOD PRESSURE

The most common method of measuring the blood pressure is auscultation. It is essential that a cuff of proper width be utilized and that it completely encircle the circumference of the arm. Blood pressure is determined with the child in the sitting position, with the arm at the level of the heart. The bladder should cover two thirds of the length of the arm; usually the largest cuff that will fit the child is used. After inflating the cuff well above systolic, the pressure is allowed to decrease 2–3 torr per second. The first sounds heard are taken to indicate the systolic pressure. The level at which the sounds become muffled is the best indicator of the diastolic pressure, rather than the level at which the sounds disappear. Both of these levels should be recorded, along with the systolic reading, for example 105/75/70. In some children, there is no clear level at which the sounds become muffled. In such a case, the recording would be 105/70/70.

If elevated levels of blood pressure are

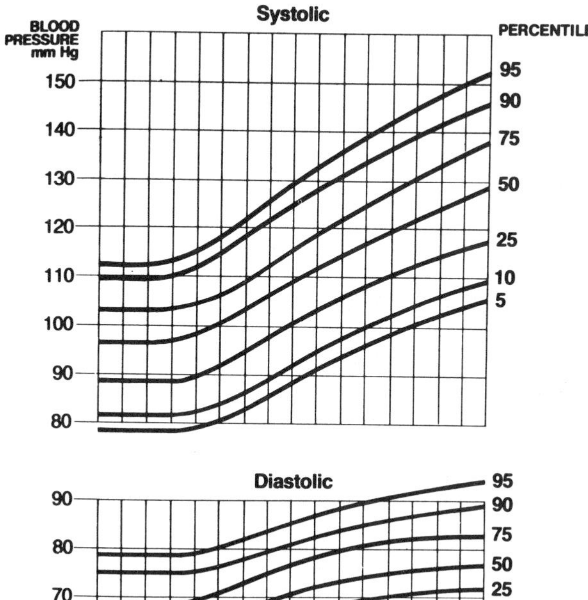

Figure 2. Fifth to ninety-fifth percentiles for blood pressure in normal boys, according to age. (Based on data from the Report of the National Heart, Lung, and Blood Institute's Task Force on Blood Pressure Control in Children Pediatrics 59 (Suppl.): 797, 1977.)

found, the blood pressure should be measured again after an interval of a few minutes. Often, lower values are found as the child relaxes. The pulse rate should be recorded, since tachycardia, which is a reliable indicator of anxiety, may increase cardiac output and thus elevate the blood pressure.

Blood pressure in infants is determined most accurately using ultrasonic devices that utilize the Doppler effect. An electronic transducer converts pressure waves into sound. When systolic pressure is reached, the change in the frequency of the reflected waves is identified by a change in sound. At the diastolic level, the sounds become muffled. Blood pressure in infants can be determined also by the *flush method*. With a blood pressure cuff in place, elastic material (such as a rubber glove) is wrapped tightly around the hand to squeeze blood out of the arterial vessels and capillaries. The pressure in the cuff is then raised above systolic, and the elastic wrapping is removed. While one observer watches the sphygmomanometer, another watches the hand to determine the point of flushing as the cuff pressure is slowly reduced. The point of flushing correlates well with the mean blood pressure.

ETIOLOGY

Essential Hypertension

Essential hypertension by definition is a condition in which no underlying cause for the hypertension can be found. Essential hypertension is considered to be a disorder of blood pressure control mechanisms, be it at the level of the kidney or related to some other system. It may account for as many as 95% of children with hypertension, although, as mentioned above, most instances are mild.

Renal Disease

The most common cause other than essential hypertension is renal disease. Hypertension is encountered in most forms of acute and chronic renal disease, particularly when there is renal insufficiency. The cause of hypertension in patients with parenchymal renal disease is unknown. Presumably, the disease process interferes in some way with the kidney's normal role in blood pressure control. In chronic renal insufficiency, this is often associated with sodium retention and expansion of the vascular volume. In other patients, there appears to be a disturbance in the renal renin-angiotensin system. In still other patients, the abnormality in blood pressure control cannot be defined.

Renovascular Disease

A special form of renal disease, renovascular disease, is an important cause of hypertension. It is rare in children but important, since it often can be cured by surgical intervention. Its pathogenesis is still controversial but seems to relate to impaired blood flow to the kidney or to one segment of the kidney. Renal ischemia results in overproduction of renin, stimulating the excessive production of angiotensin II. Angiotensin II is a potent vasoconstrictor. It stimulates the release of norepinephrine from certain sympathetic nerve endings, it has a central action (raising blood pressure through neural mechanisms), and it stimulates the production of aldosterone, leading to retention of sodium and volume expansion.

Pheochromocytoma

Pheochromocytoma is a tumor of chromaffin cells, most commonly of the adrenal medulla but occurring at any site in which chromaffin cells are found. Production by these tumors of catecholamines, which are potent vasocon-strictors, results in hypertension. The other clinical manifestations of pheochromocytoma are related also to catecholamine excess. These include excessive sweating, tachycardia, polydipsia, polyuria, anorexia, and body wasting. Hypertension in adults is often paroxysmal. This is much less common in children, in whom sustained, marked elevation in blood pressure is usual.

Hyperaldosteronism

Primary hyperaldosteronism, caused by adrenal hyperplasia or neoplasia, is rare in children. Excessive production of aldosterone results in retention of sodium, volume expansion, and hypertension. Hyperaldosteronism also causes excessive urinary loss of potassium, resulting in polyuria, hypokalemia, and metabolic alkalosis, which may serve as clues to the diagnosis.

Other Causes

Elevated levels of blood pressure are encountered in children with dysautonomia, thyrotoxicosis, Cushing disease, coarctation of the aorta, neuroblastoma and other neural crest tumors, and renin-secreting tumors. Congenital adrenal hyperplasia due to deficiency of 11-beta-hydroxylase or 17-alpha-hydroxylase may be associated with hypertension. A number of drugs and other substances may result in hypertension, including oral contraceptives, adrenocortical steroids, sympathomimetic amines, and licorice.

DIFFERENTIAL DIAGNOSIS

History

Since there is a strong familial prevalence of essential hypertension, the status of other family members, particularly first-order relatives, should be determined. Another infant in the family with congenital adrenal hyperplasia is an obvious clue to etiology. Information should be sought about family members with renal disease, since conditions such as polycystic kidney disease are genetically transmitted.

Questions should be asked to determine the duration of hypertension and associated abnormalities. A history of headaches, shortness of breath, and fatigue may be indicative of long-standing hypertension. Hematuria or edema suggests the diagnosis of renal disease. Weight loss, sweating, and tremulousness point to the diagnosis of pheochromocytoma. Other characteristic symptoms may suggest thyrotoxicosis. Weakness and polyuria suggest hyperaldosteronism. Ingestion of drugs that may cause hypertension should be investigated.

Physical Examination

Accurate measurement of the blood pressure and confirmation of the presence of hypertension is, of course, essential. Examination of the fundi is useful in assessing the duration and severity of hypertension. Physical features that might suggest a particular etiology should be sought. Pallor might reflect the anemia of chronic renal insufficiency. Café au lait spots suggest neurofibromatosis. Examination should include a search for the classic features of thyrotoxicosis, in addition to examination for thyroid hypertrophy. Body wasting, tremor, and sweating suggest pheochromocytoma. An abdominal mass may represent an enlarged kidney (hydronephrosis, polycystic kidney disease) or a tumor (Wilms, adrenal, or other). Auscultation of the abdomen for a bruit is useful in the diagnosis of renovascular hypertension. The diagnosis of coarctation of the aorta should be readily made on the basis of the characteristic murmur and the blood pressure differential between the upper and lower extremities. Features of the Cushing syndrome suggest pituitary or adrenal disease or ingestion of adrenocortical steroid drugs.

Laboratory Examination

The most important laboratory test is the urinalysis (Fig. 3). A normal urine examination makes the diagnosis of renal disease unlikely. Conversely, the presence of marked hematuria and proteinuria may result in the prompt exclusion of other etiologies. It must be understood, however, that hypertension of any cause can result in renal damage, resulting in urinary abnormalities. In the absence of intrinsic renal disease or very severe hypertension, however, these abnormalities are usually minimal.

Measurement of serum urea, creatinine, electrolytes, and pH may lead directly to the diagnosis of renal disease. Hypokalemic alkalosis suggests hyperaldosteronism, which, however, may be either primary or secondary. Patients suspected of having thyrotoxicosis should, of course, have thyroid function tests. Similarly, in the infant with suspected congenital adrenal hyperplasia, specific blood and urine studies are done to identify the abnormality. Pheochromocytoma is diagnosed by finding increased excretion of catecholamines in the urine. Provocative tests, such as the intravenous injection of histamine or the manual application of pressure to a tumor, are dangerous and should never be done. The administration of phentolamine has been used as a diagnostic test for pheochromocytoma, a postive response being a significant fall in blood pressure. The frequency of false positive and false negative results with this test renders it unreliable, and its use is not recommended.

When renal disease is suspected as the etiology, a variety of studies utilizing radiographic, sonographic, or radionuclide techniques may be useful. Renal arteriography and measurement of renal venous renin concentrations may be needed to establish the diagnosis of renovascular hypertension.

SCHEMA FOR EVALUATION OF A CHILD WITH HYPERTENSION

Infants

During the first month of life, hypertension is usually caused by vascular or cardiac disease. From 1 to 12 months, hypertension most commonly is secondary to renal disease (including renovascular disease), and the work-

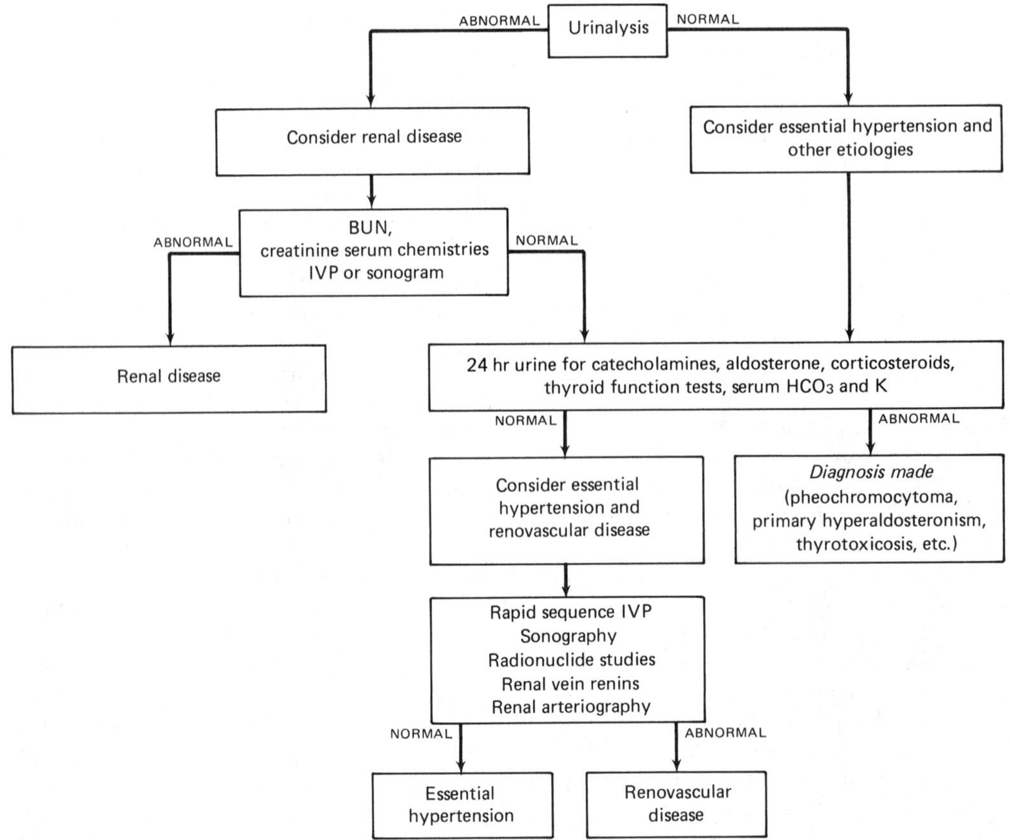

Figure 3. Differential diagnosis of hypertension.

up should proceed accordingly. Other diagnoses to be considered include Wilms tumor, coarctation of the aorta, congenital adrenal hyperplasia, and dysautonomia. Essential hypertension and other forms of secondary hypertension are either rare or nonexistent.

Children Beyond Infancy

Features of thyrotoxicosis, Cushing syndrome, pheochromocytoma, or coarctation of the aorta may lead to a prompt diagnosis, with performance of specific tests to confirm the original impression. Work-up of such patients should be done in consultation with the appropriate consultant. With a history of ingestion of licorice, oral contraceptives, or other drugs that produce hypertension, the potentially offending agent should be discontinued to see if the hypertension ameliorates.

In most children, the diagnosis will prove to be essential hypertension, and there are no immediate clues as to etiology. The approach is somewhat different for children with moderate or severe hypertension and for those with minimal elevations in blood pressure, which may prove to be transient or inconsequential. The child with minimal elevation of blood pressure and no other clinical findings should be examined on several occasions to confirm its persistence. There is no urgency to proceed rapidly with complicated, expensive, and anxiety-producing laboratory tests.

If the child is persistently but minimally hypertensive or demonstrates labile hypertension (hypertensive at times, normotensive at other times), a urinalysis and blood chemistries should be done. Abnormalities suggesting renal disease or hyperaldosteronism should lead to consultation with the pediatric nephrologist or endocrinologist and, at times, referral for further evaluation.

With mild hypertension, normal urinalysis, and normal blood chemistries, the diagnosis of essential hypertension is most likely, and it is recommended that no further laboratory examinations be done. An intravenous urogram may be indicated in the child in whom essential hypertension seems unlikely, based on a negative family history, the absence of obesity, the age of the child (essential hypertension is seen mostly in adolescents), and blood pressure readings that are at times more than minimally elevated.

The child with moderate or severe degrees of hypertension requires prompt attention. In most instances, the child with severe hypertension should receive serious consideration for hospitalization for observation, diagnosis, and treatment.

As discussed above under mild hypertension, the initial urinalysis and blood chemistries may suggest a specific diagnosis. If these examinations are negative, other tests for renal disease are performed, such as intravenous urography. Urine collections are made for measurement of catecholamines and aldosterone. Further work-up should proceed in consultation with a pediatric nephrologist. If an endocrine disorder or parenchymal renal disease has not been diagnosed, evaluation is done for renovascular disease, including renal arteriography and measurement of renin levels in the left and right renal veins. If these studies are negative, the diagnosis of essential hypertension is made.

TREATMENT

Management of secondary hypertension is the management of the underlying condition. This may be treatment of thyrotoxicosis, extirpation of a pheochromocytoma, surgical correction of a coarctation of the aorta or a strictured renal artery, or discontinuation of oral contraceptives. In these instances, treatment of the primary disease usually results in return of blood pressure levels to normal.

Management of essential hypertension or hypertension secondary to parenchymal renal disease is symptomatic, i.e., specifically directed toward measures that will lower the blood pressure. Since the cause of essential hypertension is not known, no other approach is possible. Unfortunately, treatment is available for very few renal diseases, and hypertension per se must be treated, even though it is secondary.

Mild Hypertension

It has been well established that treatment of moderate or severe hypertension in adults results in decreased morbidity and mortality. This would seem to apply to children as well. Treatment of mild hypertension in adults remains controversial. Outcome data are not available concerning treatment of mild hypertension in children. Our recommendation, therefore, is that they be followed closely, evaluated at 6-monthly or yearly intervals, and counseled with regard to the minimal nature of their hypertension and the possibility that it may be self-limited or may become more severe with time. Reduction of extreme degrees of obesity is recommended, as well as limitation of salt intake in the child whose intake clearly is excessive. Pharmacologic therapy is not recommended.

Moderate or Severe Hypertension

Specific efforts should be made to lower the blood pressure to normal in children with moderate or severe degrees of hypertension.

Nonpharmacologic Management. Salt intake should be limited to 2–4 g a day, depending on the age and size of the child. This requires considerable cooperation from other family members, who must agree to have foods prepared without added salt and be willing not to add salt at the table and thus tempt the hypertensive child. Salted pretzels and potato chips and processed foods high in salt content should not be in the home.

In the obese child, efforts at weight reduction, if successful, may be all that is required to return the blood pressure to normal.

The role of exercise in management of the hypertensive child is unknown. It seems reasonable to recommend a moderate level of physical exercise. Strenuous competitive sports should be permitted only after the patient has had an exercise test. Isometric exercises, which lead to elevation of blood pressure and do little to contribute to physical fitness, cannot be recommended, but there are insufficient data to know whether or not they are contraindicated.

Drug Therapy. If restriction of salt intake or weight reduction does not result in normalization of the blood pressure, pharmacologic treatment is indicated. The lowest effective dose of each agent should be the guide to initiating therapy. If blood pressure control is not achieved, the dosage can be increased gradually over a period of weeks. Exceeding recommended maximum dosages does not add to the efficacy of antihypertensive agents but does make side effects more likely.

Since all forms of hypertension may respond to reduction in the vascular volume, diuretics are the first drugs to be administered. They are often effective by themselves in rendering the blood pressure normal, cause little in the way of side effects, and are relatively inexpensive (Table 1). Diuretics often cause hypokalemia in adults, but this is uncommon in children. Blood levels of potassium should be checked every few months, however, and a potassium supplement provided if hypokalemia is detected.

If diuretic therapy alone is not successful in bringing the blood pressure to normal, an antihypertensive drug is added. We prefer initially to use a beta blocker in combination with the diuretic agent. If the blood pressure becomes normal, an attempt is made to discontinue the diuretic. If hypertension returns, the diuretic is reintroduced.

If a beta blocker plus the diuretic is not successful, hydralazine or prazosin is added as a third drug. If this regimen is not successful, the patient can be switched to more potent agents. At this point, however, therapeutic decisions should be made in consultation with a pediatric nephrologist.

There are no data to guide the duration of treatment of essential hypertension in children. It seems reasonable to attempt to discontinue therapy if the blood pressure has remained normal for a period of 2 years. This should be done gradually and with close observation of the child for return of hypertension.

Emergency Treatment of Severe Hypertension

Hypertension of extreme degrees, particularly when associated with heart failure, hypertensive retinopathy, or encephalopathy, is a medical emergency. The goal is to lower the blood pressure quickly to moderate levels and then to continue treatment to bring the blood pressure to a normal level over the subsequent days and weeks.

Diazoxide is an extremely effective drug in the treatment of severe hypertension. It is given intravenously in a dosage of 5 mg per kg body weight. If the desired response is not achieved, the dose can be repeated every 30–60 minutes. If the patient is volume expanded, intravenous administration of a potent diuretic, such as furosemide, may help to control hypertension. This is given slowly, in a dosage of 1–2 mg per kg.

Sodium nitroprusside is a potent anti-

TABLE 1. DOSAGES AND CHARACTERISTIC OF COMMONLY USED ANTIHYPERTENSIVE AGENTS

Drug	Useful Dosage Range (mg/kg/day)	Frequency of Administration (per day)	Frequency of Dose Adjustment (days)	Mode of Action	Major Side Effects
Chlorothiazide*	10–20	1–2	14	↓ ECF (short term); ↓ PVR (long term)	Hypokalemia, hyperglycemia, hyperuricemia, hyperlipidemia
Hydrochlorothiazide*	1–2	1–2	14	Same as for chlorothiazide	Same as for chlorothiazide
Chlorthalidone*	0.5–1	1	14	Same as for chlorothiazide	Same as for chlorothiazide
Metolazone*	Adult dose 2.5–5 mg/day[†]	1	14	Same as for chlorothiazide	Same as for chlorothiazide
Propranolol	1–6[‡]	2–3	3–6	β-adrenergic blockade CNS action	Congestive heart failure, bronchospasm, fatigue
Nadolol[§]	Adult dose 40–640 mg/day[†]	1	3–6	Same as for propranolol	Same as for propranolol
Metoprolol	Adult dose 100–450 mg/day[†]	2	3–6	Same as for propranolol	Same as for propranolol
Pindolol	Adult dose 10–40 mg/day[†]	3–4	3–6	Same as for propranolol	Same as for propranolol
Methyldopa[§]	10–40	3	3–6	CNS effect leading to ↓ PVR	Postural hypotension, sedation, lassitude, drowsiness
Hydralazine	1–7	3	3–6	Vasodilatation leading to ↓ PVR	Tachycardia, flushing, headaches, dizziness, palpitations
Prazosin	0.04–0.3	3	2–3	Vasodilatation leading to ↓ PVR	Dizziness, headache, drowsiness, lack of energy, weakness, palpitations, nausea, syncope

*Not effective with renal failure. Use furosemide.

[†]Pediatric dosage not established.

[‡]Maximum dose not established. Doses much greater than 6 mg/kg/day have been used safely.

[§]Adjust dosage for renal failure.

CNS, central nervous system; ECF, extracellular fluid; PVR, peripheral vascular resistance. *(From Gauthier B, Edelmann CM Jr, Barnett HL (eds): Nephrology and Urology for the Pediatrician. Little, Brown and Co., 1982.)*

hypertensive agent that may be used instead of diazoxide or when that drug fails to lower the blood pressure. It is given as an intravenous infusion, starting at a dosage of 1 μg per minute per kg body weight. In contrast to diazoxide, which rarely produces hypotension, nitroprusside consistently causes hypotension if given in excessive dosage. Therefore, the blood pressure must be monitored continuously, with change in the rate of administration of nitroprusside being based on the blood pressure response.

Once the blood pressure has been controlled with these emergency measures, other antihypertensive agents should be started to maintain the effect (Table 1).

REFERENCES

General

Adams FH, Landaw EM: What are healthy blood pressures for children? Pediatrics 68:268, 1981

Giovanelli G, New MI, Gorini S (eds): Hypertension in Children and Adolescents. New York, Raven Press, 1981

Goldring D, Hernandez A: Hypertension in children. Pediatr Rev 3:235, 1982

Ingelfinger JR: Pediatric Hypertension. Philadelphia, Saunders, 1982

Essential Hypertension

Bailie MD, Mattiol LF: Hypertension relationships between pathophysiology and therapy. J Pediatr 96:789, 1980

Jesse MJ: Essential hypertension in children. Hosp Practice 22:81, 1982

Lieberman E: Essential hypertension in children and youth: a pediatric perspective. J Pediatr 85:1, 1974

Loggie JMH, New MI, Robson AM: Hyper-tension in the pediatric patient: a reappraisal. J Pediatr 94:685, 1979

Renal Disease

Gauthier B, Edelmann CM Jr, Barnett HL: Hypertension. In Nephrology and Urology for the Pediatrician. Boston, Little, Brown, 1982, p 21

Ingelfinger JR: Renal parenchymal and structural causes of hypertension in childhood. In Pediatric Hypertension. Philadelphia, Saunders, 1982, p 168

Mulrow PJ, Siegel NJ: Mechanisms in hypertension. In Edelmann CM Jr (ed): Pediatric Kidney Disease. Boston, Little, Brown, 1978, p 325

Renovascular Disease

Stickler G: Renal arterial disease and renovascular hypertension. In Edelmann CM Jr (ed): Pediatric Kidney Disease. Boston, Little, Brown, 1978, p 1093.

Endocrine Causes of Hypertension

Bryan TB, Brouhard BH: Hypertension in children: endocrine aspects. Nephron 23:106, 1979

Gitlow SE, Mendlowitz M, Wilk EK, et al.: Excretion of catecholamine catabolites by normal children. J Lab Clin Med 72:612, 1968

New MI, Levine LS: Adrenocortical hypertension. Pediatr Clin North Am 25:67, 1978

New MI, Baum CJ, Levine LS: Nomograms relating aldosterone excretion to urinary sodium and potassium in the pediatric population: their application to the study of childhood hypertension. Am J Cardiol 37:658, 1976

Scott HW, Oates JA, Nies AS, et al.: Pheochromocytoma: present diagnosis and management. Ann Surg 183:587, 1976

Cross-Reference to *Pediatrics,* 17th ed.

THIRTY-THREE

Approach to the Pediatric Patient with Inflammatory Skin Disease

Marcos Sastre

DIFFERENTIAL DIAGNOSIS

The clinical diagnosis in the pediatric patient with skin disease requires the usual, systematic approach to the history, physical examination, and laboratory testing.

History

It is usually counterproductive to yield to the temptation of making an instantaneous clinical diagnosis on the basis of the appearance of the rash without eliciting pertinent historical data. A careful inquiry of the onset and progression of the rash should be made, including the temporal relationship between the appearance of the rash or its recurrence and exposure to drugs, sunlight, or possible allergic contactants, such as metals or plants. The presence of pruritus or pain is the most important subjective symptom. Fever or prodomal symptoms usually indicate an infectious etiology.

Physical Examination

The three essential elements of a physical examination are (1) the type of lesion, (2) its configuration, and (3) its distribution on the body.

Type of Lesion. The association of certain lesions permits the classification of inflammatory skin diseases into certain reaction patterns that are helpful in the process of differential diagnosis. The following are the most important lesions:

Macule	Atrophy
Papule	Sclerosis
Plaque	Fissure
Nodule	Erosion
Wheal	Ulcer
Vesicle	Scar
Bulla	Scale
Pustule	Crust
Abscess	Telangiectasia
Sinus	Lichenification
Cyst	Gangrene

Macule. A macule is a circumscribed area of change in normal skin color. Erythematous macules are caused by dilatation of dermal capillaries and are blanchable by pressing with a glass slide (diascopy). Purpura and petechiae are defined as extravasation of red blood cells in the dermis; the lesions are not blanchable on diascopy. They are called petechiae or ecchymosis according to size. Alteration in the quantity of distribution of melanin pigment leads to hyperpigmented or hypopigmented macules.

Papule. A papule is a circumscribed elevation of the skin. It may result from thickening of the epidermis, as in the common wart, or by accumulation in the dermis of cells, edema fluid, or metabolic products. Papules sometimes involve the pilar apparatus and are called follicular papules (e.g., keratosis pilaris), or involve the sweat duct (e.g., miliaria).

The shape of the papule may be flat (e.g., lichen planus), conical or acuminate (e.g., keratosis pilaris), dome-shaped (e.g., melanocytic nervus), or umbilicated (e.g., molluscum contagiosum). The color is also important and can be erythematous (e.g., insect bite), violaceous (e.g., lichen planus), pearly (e.g., molluscum), copper-colored (e.g., lues), white (e.g., lichen sclerosis et atrophicus), or yellow (e.g., xanthomas).

The topography of the surface is usually helpful in the diagnosis. It may be smooth, keratotic (with scale), as in Darier's disease, or verrucous (with minute projections), as in warts.

Plaque. A plaque is an elevation above the skin surface that is large in proportion to its thickness. It sometimes results from coalescence of papules. The lesion of psoriasis is the typical example.

Nodule. A nodule is a palpable, elevated lesion, usually 1 cm or larger in diameter. It may be located in the epidermis (e.g., squamous cell carcinoma), the dermis (e.g., tuberculosis), or in the subcutaneous tissue (e.g., panniculitis).

Wheal. A wheal is a papule or plaque that results from dermal vasodilatation and edema. It is usually evanescent, disappearing in a few hours.

Vesicle and Bulla. A vesicle is a fluid-containing, circumscribed elevation of the skin. Bullae are larger lesions. They result from cleavage of the skin at two essential levels, intraepidermal and subepidermal. Epidermal vesicles tend to be flaccid and rupture relatively easily, whereas subepidermal vesicles tend to be tense and remain intact longer. When a blister ruptures, the circumscribed denuded area that results is called an "erosion."

Pustule. A pustule is a circumscribed elevation of the skin that contains pus. It may arise de novo or evolve from preexisting vesicles. It is located in the epidermis, the pilar apparatus (follicular pustule), or the eccrine sweat duct.

Abscess. An abscess is a localized accumulation of pus, usually deep in the dermis or in the subcutaneous tissue, so that the pus is not visible on the surface. A sinus is a tract connecting a suppurative cavity with the skin surface.

Cyst. A cyst is a sac, lined by epithelium, that contains liquid or semisolid material. It is resilient on palpation.

Atrophy. Atrophy is thinning or loss of substance of the epidermis, dermis, or subcutaneous tissue. Epidermal atrophy results in fine wrinkling or in a transparent, ironed-out appearance. Dermal atrophy is related to a decrease in elastic or collagen tissue or both and appears as a depression on the skin. An atrophic panniculus also results in a depression but of less defined outlines.

Sclerosis. Sclerosis is a circumscribed or diffuse hardening of the skin resulting from a relative or absolute increase in fibrous tissue.

Fissure. A fissure is a linear cleavage of the skin surface, which may be painful.

Ulcer. An ulcer is a circumscribed defect in the continuity of the skin with loss of the epidermis and the superficial dermis. It usually heals with scarring.

Scar. A scar results from the laying down of fibrous connective tissue as a repair mechanism of lacerations, ulcerations, or surgical wounds. Scars may be atrophic or hypertrophic.

Scale. A scale is the result of visible desquamation of the stratum corneum. It may result from accelerated epidermal proliferation or abnormal cohesion of desquamated horny cells.

Crust. A crust is the result of drying of a serous, purulent, or hemorrhagic exudate on the skin surface.

Lichenification. Lichenification is the result of repeated rubbing of the skin and resembles a tree bark. There is thickening of the epidermis, increased skin markings, and hyperpigmentation.

Gangrene. Gangrene is necrosis of the dermis, epidermis, or subcutaneous tissue due to compromise in the blood supply. It may be of infectious origin or result from inherent pathology of the blood vessels.

Configuration of the Lesions. Certain groupings of the lesions are helpful in diagnosis. Lesions are described as linear, annular, herpetiform, zosteriform, segmental, and reticular.

A linear configuration suggests an exogenous cause, as in poison ivy (*Rhus radicans*) dermatitis. An annular or ring-shaped configuration occurs when the process spreads peripherally and tends to clear in the center, as in tinea corporis.

In herpes simplex the vesicles are arranged in groups, described by the term "herpetiform." A zosteriform configuration occurs when grouped lesions follow a dermatome, as in herpes zoster. A bandlike arrangement that does not exactly follow the distribution of a nerve is called segmental, as in segmental vitiligo. The term "reticulate" indicates a netlike arrangement as seen in certain vascular responses, such as livedo reticularis, or pigmentary alterations, as seen in radiodermatitis.

Distribution of the Lesions. Skin diseases can be localized, regional, generalized, or universal, including hair and nails. A bilateral, symmetrical eruption suggests an endogenous cause. Lesions present in areas exposed to sunlight or trauma suggest the etiologic factor. Many skin diseases have characteristic patterns of distribution that help in the diagnosis, as described under the specific entities discussed later.

Laboratory Examination

Among the many tests that can aid in the diagnosis of skin diseases, the following are most useful:

- Gram stain
- KOH mount (examination of scales for fungi)
- Tzank smear (skin scraping stained with Giemsa)
- Wood's light (black ultraviolet light)
- Patch tests (to different chemicals)
- Darkfield (i.e., primary lues)
- Biopsy
- Immunofluorescence
- Blood chemistry

REACTION PATTERNS

Reaction patterns of the skin in inflammatory dermatoses include the following:

- Eczematous
- Papulosquamous
- Vesiculobullous and pustular
- Vascular
- Dermal
- Subcutaneous nodules, Panniculitis
- Sclerosis and atrophy

Eczematous Reaction Pattern

The term "dermatitis" or "eczema" refers to an inflammatory reaction of the skin to a variety of exogenous or endogenous factors. Dermatitis can be classified as acute, subacute, or chronic. In acute dermatitis there is erythema, edema, erosions, oozing, and crusting. In subacute dermatitis, which can be confused with a papulosquamous reaction, there is erythema and scales. In chronic dermatitis there is lichenification, fissuring, and pigmentary changes.

The most important types of eczematous dermatitis are atopic dermatitis, contact dermatitis, nummular dermatitis, lichen simplex chronicus, seborrheic dermatitis, superficial fungal infections (also papulosquamous), dyshidrosis, autoeczematization or id reaction, infectious eczematoid dermatitis, and exfoliative dermatitis.

The key clinical characteristics and laboratory tests that are helpful in differential diagnosis are described in Table 1.

Atopic Dermatitis. Atopic dermatitis is a genetically determined, chronic, pruritic, inflammatory reaction of the skin, frequently associated with personal or familial history of asthma or hay fever. The skin is hyperirritable, with a lowered threshold for pruritis. Rather than a "rash that itches," it is an "itch that rashes." The increased irritability of the skin triggers an itch sensation leading to scratching by the patient, with subsequent ex-

coriation, lichenification, and pruriginous lesions. Many of these patients have increased IgE blood levels, abnormal vascular responses, such as white dermographism (blanching upon stroking with a blunt instrument, possibly due to accumulation of edema fluid), and increased susceptibility to certain infections, especially *Staphylococcus* and *Candida*.

In infancy, the dermatitis usually begins 2–3 weeks after birth, with involvement of the face, the scalp, and the extensor surface of the extremities. The reaction is acute or subacute with erythema, edema, vesicles, oozing, and crusting.

In childhood the characteristic lesions are excoriated, hypertrophic (pruriginous) papules and lichenification, located in the neck and flexural folds of the extremities.

In adolescence the disease resembles the childhood form but can also involve the face, chest, and scalp. Frequently, the disease involves only the palms or soles or both.

Like many allergic processes, the dermatitis becomes less severe as the patient grows older. Frequently associated findings are xerosis (dry skin), cataracts, ichthyosis vulgaris, and keratosis pilaris.

Contact Dermatitis. Contact dermatitis is caused by contact with a chemical agent that acts as an allergic sensitizer or as a primary irritant. The distribution in areas of exposure is characteristic. Linear configuration of the lesions (erythema, papules, vesicles, and scale) is frequently found. The diagnosis is confirmed by patch tests with the specific allergen.

Nummular Dermatitis. Nummular dermatitis is characterized by coin-shaped, eczematous patches. The elementary lesions appear as pinhead-size papules or vesicles, followed by oozing, crusting, and scaling, with lichenification appearing later. The lesions are usually quite pruritic. The most

TABLE 1. DIFFERENTIAL DIAGNOSIS OF THE ECZEMATOUS REACTION PATTERN

Disease	Key Clinical Findings	Helpful Laboratory Tests
Atopic dermatitis	Personal or family history of atopy; in infants, subacute, with erythema, edema, oozing, and crusting on scalp, face, and extensor aspects of extremities; in childhood, presents with lichenification and pruriginous papules in flexural creases	Serum IgE frequently elevated
Contact dermatitis	Acute, subacute, or chronic eczema with linear or irregular configuration and with distribution in exposed areas, suggesting an exogenous cause	Patch test to suspected allergen(s)
Nummular dermatitis	Coin-shaped lesions	Biopsy helpful, negative KOH
Lichen simplex chronicus	Well-delineated plaque of lichenification, location helpful	Biopsy suggestive
Seborrheic dermatitis	Greasy scale, location in seborrheic areas	—
Tinea corporis	Often annular lesions with peripheral active margin; on scalp, hairs broken at different levels with scaling on the surface	Wood's light fluorescence sometimes positive on scalp, fungal culture, KOH
Dyshidrosis	Location on volar surface of hands and feet. "Sago grain" vesicles	
Autoeczematization, id reaction	Initial focus of eczema or infection followed by bilateral and symmetrical eczematous rash	KOH, culture at primary focus negative on id lesions
Exfoliative dermatitis	Generalized erythroderm, sometimes lesions or history of previous dermatosis pinpoints etiology	Biopsy usually not helpful

common location is the extensor surface of the extremities and trunk. The etiology is unknown.

Lichen Simplex Chronicus. Lichen simplex chronicus is a circumscribed neurodermatitis, characterized by a well-defined plaque of lichenification, most frequently located on the ankles, neck, or pretibial areas. The disorder results from chronic rubbing and scratching by the patient.

Seborrheic Dermatitis. Seborrheic dermatitis is an eczematous dermatitis localized in the seborrheic areas of the face (eyebrows, eyelids, and nasolabial folds), the neck, presternal and interscapular areas, the scalp, axillas, and groins. It is characterized by an orange-brown erythema with a greasy scale.

In the infant, seborrheic dermatitis involves predominantly the scalp. Sometimes it is generalized, presenting as an exfoliative erythroderma (Leiner's disease).

Dyshidrosis. Dyshidrosis is a vesicular eruption of the volar surface of the fingers, palms, and soles. The elementary lesion is a small (*sago grain*) vesicle. Intense pruritus is usually the rule. The disease is characterized by exacerbations and remissions. In some patients there is a history of atopic dermatitis or hypersensitivity to nickel. Despite its name, there is no abnormality of sweating.

Autoeczematization, Id Reaction. Autoeczematization is a symmetrical generalized eruption appearing in patients with severe localized eczematous dermatitis. It is probably mediated by antibodies to epidermal antigens.

An id reaction is a generalized, symmetrical, eczematous dermatitis distant to foci of infection (bacterial, fungal, or tuberculous). The lesions are characteristically bilateral and symmetrical and do not contain the infectious organism, but they do respond to specific antimicrobial therapy.

Infectious Eczematoid Dermatitis. Infectious eczematoid dermatitis is an eczematous dermatitis present in areas of draining purulent exudates, such as an abcess or a chronic middle ear infection. It is characterized by erythema, edema, oozing, and crusting and probably represents a reaction to the products of the infectious process.

Exfoliative Dermatitis. Exfoliative dermatitis affects the entire integument, with diffuse erythema and scale. It may be the progression of (1) a preexisting dermatitis, such as psoriasis, atopic dermatitis, lichen planus, seborrheic dermatitis, pityriasis rubra pilaris, (2) a result of a contact dermatitis, or (3) associated with malignancies, such as lymphoma or leukemia. However, a large proportion of cases are idiopathic.

Papulosquamous Diseases

The papulosquamous reaction pattern includes a heterogeneous group of disorders characterized clinically by the presence of erythema and scale. They are as follows:

- Pityriasis rosea
- Secondary lues
- Psoriasis
- Seborrheic dermatitis (also eczematous)
- Tinea versicolor
- Lichen planus
- Parapsoriasis
- Superficial fungal infections
- Pityriasis rubra pilaris
- Lupus erythematosus

The key clinical characteristics and laboratory tests helpful in the diagnosis are shown in Table 2.

Pityriasis Rosea. Pityriasis rosea is an acute exanthematous eruption distributed symmetrically on the trunk and proximal extremities. It is usually preceded by a single, scaly lesion called a "herald patch." The lesions are oval, erythematous patches with a collarette of scale and their axes parallel to Langer's lines. The eruption usually lasts from 4 to 6 weeks. It can be indistinguishable from secondary lues, and serologic tests should always be done for differential diagnosis.

Secondary Lues. Secondary lues is a bilaterally symmetrical eruption of erythematous (ham- or copper-colored) macules and papules with varying amounts of scale, located mainly on the trunk, with prominent involvement of palms and soles. The mucous membranes characteristically are involved (mucous patches). Other lesions of secondary disease are sometimes found, such as split papules on the corners of the mouth, annular syphilides, and condylomata lata. Associated manifestations include fever, pharyngitis, lymphadenitis, hepatosplenomegaly, uveitis, and orchitis.

The diagnosis is made by the characteristic distribution and is confirmed by specific serologic tests.

Psoriasis. Psoriasis is a chronic proliferative epidermal disease of polygenic inheritance.

It usually starts in adult life but is not

TABLE 2. DIFFERENTIAL DIAGNOSIS OF PAPULOSQUAMOUS DISEASES

Disease	Key Clinical Findings	Helpful Laboratory Tests
Pityriasis rosea	Symmetrical, with involvement of trunk, proximal extremities; oval lesions with collarette of scale; herald patch; usually does not involve palms and soles	Serology to rule out secondary lues
Secondary lues	Generalized and symmetrical but with involvement of palms, soles, and mucous membranes; frequent systemic manifestations	Serology
Psoriasis	Well-defined plaques of erythema with silvery scale; usually scalp and extensor surface of the extremities; nail changes	Biopsy
Seborrheic dermatitis	Greasy scale, in seborrheic areas	
Tinea corporis	Often annular lesions with peripheral active margin; on scalp, hair broken at different levels, with scaling on the surface	Wood's light fluorescence sometimes positive, KOH, fungal culture
Tinea versicolor	Mainly trunk; erythematous or hypopigmented; sometimes confluent	KOH shows hyphae and spores, Wood's light fluorescence occasionally
Lichen planus	Symmetrical; violaceous flat-topped pruritic polygonal papules; Wickham's striae; mucous membrane involvement	Mineral oil, biopsy
Parapsoriasis	Chronic, asymptomatic, and resistant to treatment	Biopsy sometimes helpful
Pityriasis rubra pilaris	Triad of salmon orange follicular scaly papules, palmar and plantar hyperkeratosis, and islands of sparing; symmetrical distribution	Biopsy suggestive but not diagnostic
Lupus erythematosus	Atrophy, telangiectasia, follicular plugging, scarring, pigmentary change	Biopsy usually diagnostic; immunofluorescence shows immunoglobulins at dermoepidermal junction; serum antinuclear antibody

rare in children. The characteristic lesion is a well-defined plaque of erythema and silvery scale. Removal of the scale may show multiple bleeding points (Auspitz sign).

Psoriasis characteristically involves the extensor surface of the extremities, scalp, nails, and presacral areas. The nails show pitting, onycholysis (separation of the nail), and subungual debris. Occasionally, the disease occurs as an eruptive process, most frequently associated with streptococcal infections.

Tinea Versicolor. Tinea versicolor is a papulosquamous symmetrical eruption located centrally on the trunk. It is due to overgrowth of saprophytic yeasts (*Pityrosporon* species). The lesions are salmon-colored macules or papules with fine scale. They become confluent into large patches with irregular geographic (maplike) outlines. In the dark races, hypopigmentation is fairly common.

The diagnosis is made by scraping and KOH mount of the scales. Short hyphae and round spores are characteristic (spaghetti and meatballs). Occasionally the lesions show a yellow fluorescence under Wood's light.

Lichen Planus. Lichen planus is a generalized pruritic symmetrical eruption of unknown etiology. The elementary lesions are flat-topped, polygonal, violaceous papules that sometimes coalesce to form plaques. A reticulate white appearance can be observed on the surface of the lesions by applying mineral oil (Wickham's striae). Involvement of the mucous membranes is common. In the buccal mucosa, reticulated (netlike) white patches are characteristic.

Parapsoriasis. Parapsoriasis is a heterogeneous group of disorders of unknown origin. It can be present with small or large plaques of erythema with fine scale, with or without atrophy. The lesions are usually long lasting, resistant to treatment, and often nonpruritic. Poikiloderma (reticulated pigmentation, atrophy, and telangiectasia) is sometimes found. Large plaques, with atrophy and poikiloderma, are sometimes the early manifestation of mycosis fungoides (cutaneous T cell lymphoma).

Tinea Corporis. Tinea corporis is a superficial fungal infection of the glabrous (hairless) skin, usually present with asymmetrical, solitary, or annular plaques with fine scale. These lesions are due to infection by dermatophytes (fungi belonging to the genera *trichophyton*, *Epidermophyton*, or *Microsporum*).

The diagnosis is made by scraping the scales and mounting them with KOH on a glass slide. Hyphae can be seen, parasitizing the superficial corneal cells. Fungal cultures are needed to identify the organism. Nail involvement (tinea unguium) is common.

In children, involvement of the scalp is much more common than that of glabrous skin or nails. The characteristic lesions are patches of erythema and scale with broken-off hairs. Infections with some fungal species (*Trichophyton tonsurans*, *Trichophyton schoenleinii*) result in permanent alopecia. Occasionally, the lesions become purulent (kerion). Certain species fluoresce readily with Wood's light. By examining the parasitized hairs under the microscope, spores can be found inside or outside the hair shaft, depending on the infecting species.

Pityriasis Rubra Pilaris. Pityriasis rubra pilaris occurs as a generalized, erythematous, orangy eruption consisting of acuminate (cone-shaped), keratotic, folliculate papules. The most common locations are the dorsal surface of the fingers, elbows, and knees, side of neck, and extensor surface of the extremities. When the eruption is confluent, small islands of uninvolved skin are characteristic. A frequent finding is hyperkeratosis of palms and soles. The eruption is usually long lasting and responds poorly to treatment.

Lupus Erythematosus. The chronic form of lupus erythematosus presents with atrophic erythematous scaly patches, with telangiectasia and hyperpigmentation or hypopigmentation. It usually heals with scarring. It is more common in areas exposed to sun, especially the face. When it affects the scalp, it leaves permanent, scarring alopecia.

In the systemic form, patches of erythema, edema, and telangiectasia are common. A malar (butterfly) rash on the face is characteristic. Periungual erythema and telangiectasia with hypertrophy of the nail cuticle are helpful diagnostic signs. Vasculitic lesions, presenting as palpable purpura with or without ulcerations and scarring, are not uncommon.

Vesiculobullous and Pustular Reaction Pattern

This group of skin diseases, characterized by blisters, bullae, or pustules with erosions and crusts, includes the following:

- Viral diseases
- Acute eczematous diseases (see eczematous reaction pattern)
- Erythema multiforme (toxic epidermal necrolysis)
- Dermatitis herpetiformis
- Chronic bullous disease of childhood
- Epidermolysis bullosa
- Impetigo
- Hailey-Hailey disease
- Pemphigus vulgaris

Clinical features and laboratory tests helpful in diagnosis are shown in Table 3.

Viral Blisters. In recurrent herpes simplex infections the lesions are grouped, umbilicated vesicles on an erythematous base, located most frequently near the mouth, nose, genitalia, or sacral area. The diagnosis is confirmed by scraping the base of the blisters and staining the smear with Giemsa or Wright stain and finding multinucleate giant cells and edematous (balloon) cells (Tzank smear).

In herpes zoster similar lesions are found, following the distribution of a nerve. In chickenpox superficial vesicles on an erythematous base occur in several crops. As a result, the exanthem is polymorphous, with lesions in different stages: papules, vesicles, pustules, or crusted erosions, with increased density of lesions on the trunk (centripetal distribution). The Tzank smear shows findings similar to those in herpes simplex. The viruses are easily differentiated by culture.

In smallpox, the blisters are larger and more deeply seated. The patient is usually very sick, and the lesions heal with scarring. There is a prodrome of high fever, headache, and backache. The blisters are more numerous in the acral portions of the body (centrifugal distribution). The Tzank smear

sometimes shows eosinophillic inclusions in the cytoplasm of the epidermal cells (Guarnieri bodies).

Erythema Multiforme. Erythema multiforme or toxic epidermal necrolysis is a syndrome characterized by generalized erythema, edema, and exfoliation in large sheets, which gives the skin the appearance of a scalded burn. In infants and children the disease is due to a soluble toxin produced by *Staphylcoccus aureus*, phage group 2, type 71.

In adults toxic epidermal necrolysis is more often due to hypersensitivity to certain drugs (penicillin, phenolphthalein, phenylbutazone). It involves the mucous membranes, with erosions and crusting, and it is considered a form of erythema multiforme. Both types can be distinguished histologically by the level of the epidermal separation, which is high (at the granular layer) in the infantile form and low (at the level of the basal layer) in the adult form. Immunofluorescence studies fail to demonstrate immunoglobulins in either form.

Dermatitis Herpetiformis. Dermatitis herpetiformis presents as a bilaterally symmetrical eruption, which is usually exquisitely pruritic. The lesions are edematous papules or papulovesicles, present in groups on the extensor surface of the extremities, buttocks, and back.

The histology of early lesions shows accumulation of neutrophils in the dermal papillae (microabscesses). Immunofluorescent studies of frozen sections of involved or uninvolved skin show granular deposits of IgA at the dermoepidermal junction. Circulating antibodies usually are not present in the blood. A gluten-sensitive enteropathy frequently is associated.

Chronic Bullous Disease. Chronic bullous disease of childhood is usually a disease of the first decade of life. The lesions are tense bullae sitting in erythematous or normal-appearing skin. The most commonly involved

**TABLE 3. DIFFERENTIAL DIAGNOSIS OF THE VESICULOBULLOUS AND PUSTULAR
REACTION PATTERN**

Disease	Key Clinical Findings	Helpful Laboratory Tests
Viral blisters	Herpetiform or zosteriform configuration of grouped, umbilicated vesicles; in chickenpox, lesions in different stages, centripetal; in smallpox, lesions in same stage, centrifugal	Tzank smear, viral culture
Acute eczematous dermatitis	Distribution and configuration helpful in distinguishing contact dermatitis, id, and others	KOH, patch test
Toxic epidermal necrolysis	Infant form is staphylococcal; adult form is drug-induced	Culture for *Staphylococcus* in primary focus, histologic level of split helpful
Dermatitis herpetiformis	Bilateral, symmetrical eruption on extensor surfaces; grouped papulovesicles	Biopsy, immunofluorescence: granular IgA in basement membrane
Chronic bullous disease of childhood	Extremities, lower trunk, and genitalia	Immunofluorescence: linear IgA deposits in basement membrane
Epidermolysis bullosa	Increased skin fragility with blistering, with or without scarring and milia	Biopsy, electron microscopy
Impetigo contagiosa	Preschool children; exposed areas; erosions with honey-colored crusts	Gram stain, culture
Bullous impetigo	Infants; blisters and varnishlike crusts	Gram stain, culture
Hailey-Hailey disease	Familial history; flexural areas	Biopsy
Pemphigus vulgaris	Superficial blisters on a noninflammatory base that rupture easily; crusted erosions; mucous membrane involvement	Biopsy, epidermal intercellular IgA by immunofluorescence

sites are the lower extremities, lower part of
the trunk, and genitalia. Linear IgA deposits
at the dermoepidermal junction can be demonstrated in some patients.

Epidermolysis Bullosa. Epidermolysis bullosa is a group of hereditary diseases that
have in common an increased fragility of the
skin with a tendency to blistering as a result of
mechanical trauma.

Epidermolysis bullosa simplex is inherited as an autosomal trait. Blisters are produced on the sites of trauma, usually without
associated erythema. The histology shows
that the separation is due to degeneration of
the basal cells.

Epidermolysis bullosa of the hands and
feet (Weber-Cokayne) is inherited as an autosomal dominant trait. The onset is in childhood or later, with blisters on the palms and

soles. Histologically, the separation occurs above the basal layer. The lesions heal without scarring.

Junctional bullous epidermatosis (Herlitz disease) is inherited as an autosomal recessive disorder and usually presents at birth with blisters and erosions. Mucous membrane involvement and dystrophic changes of the nails are common. Few patients survive to adulthood. Electron microscopy shows that the separation occurs between the plasma membrane of the basal cells and the basal lamina.

Epidermolysis bullosa dystrophica occurs in two forms, autosomal dominant and autosomal recessive. Both are characterized by extensive blistering, with scarring, dystrophy of the nails, and contractures and later fusion of the digits. Secondary infection of the lesions is common. Early death may occur from infection, amyloidosis, or general debilitation. Squamous cell carcinoma occasionally develops in scarred lesions.

Acquired epidermolysis bullosa is a mild dystrophic form occurring in patients without a family history. The diagnosis is made by exclusion of other blistering disorders.

Impetigo. There are two forms of impetigo. Impetigo contagiosa is due to hemolytic streptococci. It usually affects preschool age children in exposed areas of the body. The lesions start with erythema and blisters, followed by pustules that rupture rapidly to form the characteristic honey-colored crusts.

Bullous impetigo is usually a disease of infants and is caused by *Staphylococcus aureus*. The lesions are superficial blisters that rupture, leaving erosions covered with varnishlike crusts.

Hailey-Hailey Disease. Hailey-Hailey disease is a benign familial pemphigoid disease, characterized by erythema, vesicles, scale, and vegetations, usually affecting the flexural folds: neck, axillae, and groins. It is inherited as an autosomal dominant trait.

Acantholysis and dyskeratosis are the most prominent histologic findings.

Pemphigus Vulgaris. Pemphigus vulgaris is a blistering process that results from the presence of autoantibodies against the intercellular substance of the epidermis. Initially, it involves the mucous membranes. On the skin it presents with superficial blisters, with a noninflammatory base, that rupture easily, leaving crusted erosions.

The histology shows destruction of desmosomes (acantholysis) above the basal layer, which usually remains intact. The diagnosis is confirmed by immunofluorescence, which shows immunoglobulins and complement in the intercellular spaces of the epidermis.

Vascular Reaction Pattern

The basic process in the vascular reaction pattern is an alteration of the dermal blood vessels. The most important entities of this group are:

- Urticaria
- Toxic erythema
- Erythema multiforme
- Vasculitis

Clinical features and laboratory tests useful in differential diagnosis are shown in Table 4.

Urticaria. The lesions of urticaria are wheals, elevated edematous lesions that are quite pruritic and last only a few hours. The lesions are the result of mast cell degranulation with release of vasoactive substances, such as histamine and bradykinins.

The etiologic factors can be immunologic (antigens) or nonimmunologic (drugs or physical agents).

Toxic Erythema. Erythematous macular and papular eruptions are classified as toxic erythema, including viral exanthems (measles, rubella, roseola, erythema infectiosum),

TABLE 4. DIFFERENTIAL DIAGNOSIS OF THE VASCULAR REACTION PATTERN

Disease	Key Clinical Findings	Helpful Laboratory Tests
Urticaria	Evanescent wheals	Laboratory test sometimes helpful in pinpointing etiology
Toxic erythema	Distribution often helpful; drug history; fever and prodrome in viral rashes	Viral cultures, serologic studies
Erythema multiforme	Target lesions; bilateral symmetrical polymorphous eruption with involvement of mucous membranes	Biopsy helpful, negative immunofluorescence
Vasculitis	Palpable purpura; symmetrical: allergic; acral asymmetrical: septic	Biopsy, gram stain, culture

bacterial toxemias (such as scarlet fever), and allergic drug eruptions (such as penicillin hypersensitivity).

Erythema Multiforme. Erythema multiforme is a bilaterally symmetrical, generalized eruption consisting of macules, papules, urticarial lesions, blisters, and, sometimes, purpura. There is prominent involvement of mucous membranes of the mouth, nose, conjuctivae, and genitalia, with edema, erosions, and crusting. The lesion is thought to be a hypersensitivity reaction, and it has been associated with a variety of infectious agents and drugs. In many cases the etiology is obscure. The biopsy usually shows dermal edema, perivascular mononuclear infiltrates, and various degrees of epidermal necrosis. The immunofluorescence usually is negative.

Vasculitis. Vasculitis is the presence of palpable purpura denoting extravasation of blood and inflammation of the vessel wall. Two broad categories are distinguished. *Allergic vasculitis* frequently presents with numerous lesions distributed bilaterally and symmetrically. The histologic picture is usually that of a leukocytoblastic venulitis with infiltration of neutrophils, nuclear dust, and fibrinoid necrosis of the vessel wall. In *septic vasculitis* the lesions are most frequently asymmetrical, few in numbers, and located in the acral portions of the body. The lesions usually are due to bacterial embolization associated with meningococcemia, gonococcemia, and bacterial endocarditis and present as purpuric macules, papules, or pustules. The histologic picture in septic vasculitis is that of capillary thrombosis. Sometimes, bacterial antigens can be demonstrated by immunofluorescence. Occasionally, the diagnosis can be made by gram stain or culture of the lesions.

Dermal Reaction Pattern: Granulomatous Disease

In the dermal reaction pattern there are usually no changes in the epidermis, but there is infiltration of the dermis by cells, edema fluid, metabolic products, and degenerated collagen. The granulomatous diseases are the most prominent members of this group. The most important granulomatous diseases are:

- Lupus vulgaris
- Swimming pool granuloma
- Deep fungal disease
- Granuloma annulare
- Sarcoidosis

The clinical features and laboratory findings are summarized in Table 5.

**TABLE 5. DERMAL REACTION PATTERN:
DIFFERENTIAL DIAGNOSIS OF THE GRANULOMATOUS DISEASES**

Disease	Key Clinical Findings	Helpful Laboratory Tests
Tuberculosis (lupus vulgaris)	Apple-jelly nodules with scarring and ulceration, diascopy	Acid-fast stain and culture
Swimming pool granuloma	History of trauma; verrucous infiltrated plaques	Acid-fast stain and culture
Deep fungal disease	Dermal nodules or plaques, vegetations, ulceration	Biopsy (with fungal stains), culture
Granuloma annulare	Annular lesions	Biopsy: palisading granuloma with mucin stain
Sarcoidosis	Skin-colored nodules, other organ involvement	Biopsy: sarcoidal granulomas, not diagnostic

Lupus Vulgaris. Lupus vulgaris is the typical example of secondary tuberculosis of the skin. The characteristic lesions are apple-jelly-colored infiltrated papules, nodules, and plaques, located most frequently on the face. Scarring and ulceration can lead to significant disfigurement. By pressing the lesions with a glass slide (diascopy), the characteristic color can be better appreciated. The biopsy shows tuberculous granulomas, usually with few acid-fast bacilli. Proper cultures should be obtained.

Swimming Pool Granuloma. Swimming pool granulomas are verrucous, infiltrated plaques affecting exposed areas as a result of trauma and inoculation with *Mycobacterium balnei.* The diagnosis is made by histologic examination, acid-fast staining, and culture.

Deep Fungal Disease. Cutaneous involvement is common in blastomycosis, coccidioidomycosis, and cryptococcosis. Dermal nodules and plaques, with or without vegetations, and ulceration are the usual findings. The diagnosis is made by demonstrating organisms in the lesions with PAS or silver stains and by obtaining proper cultures.

Granuloma Annulare. The typical lesions of granuloma annulare are annular erythematous plaques, usually present on the extensor surface of the extremities. The condition is relatively common in children and generally is self-limited. The biopsy shows a palisading granuloma, accumulations of mucins surrounded by histiocytes in a palisade arrangement.

Sarcoidosis. The cutaneous lesions of sarcoidosis are skin-colored papules and nodules that on diascopy disclose an apple-jelly color. They are commonly located on the face, around the mouth, nose, and eyes.

The biopsy shows epithelioid cell tubercles with a paucity of mononuclear cells. The involvement of other organs, such as hilar adenopathy, uveitis, osteitis cystica, and hepatosplenomegaly, is necessary for a positive diagnosis.

Subcutaneous Nodules, Panniculitis

Panniculitis is a reaction pattern characterized by deep, ill-defined subcutaneous nodules. The diagnosis is made mainly on histologic grounds. The most important types of panniculitis are:

- Erythema nodosum,
- Erythema induratum
- Weber-Christian disease
- Subcutaneous fat necrosis of the newborn

Clinical features and laboratory findings are shown in Table 6.

Erythema Nodosum. Erythema nodosum presents as crops of tender, warm, erythematous, deep-seated nodules, most commonly located on the anterior surface of the legs.

The surface of the lesions changes in color from shades of erythema to blue and brown, resembling the evolution of a hematoma. The condition may be idiopathic or a manifestation of drug hypersensitivity, sarcoidosis, tuberculosis, or deep fungal infection. The biopsy shows an inflammation of the connective tissue septa separating the fat lobules (septal panniculitis).

Erythema Induratum. Erythema induratum is a nodular vasculitis that previously was thought to be tuberculous but currently is considered a hypersensitivity reaction. The lesions present as tender, indurated, deep-seated nodules found usually on the calfs. They have a tendency to ulcerate, drain, and heal with scarring. The biopsy shows a granulomatous vasculitis with a conspicuous amount of fat necrosis.

Weber-Christian Disease. Weber-Christian disease is characterized by subcutaneous nodules appearing in crops, with associated fever, arthralgia, and leukocytosis. The histology shows three different stages: neutrophilic infiltrates, fat necrosis with foamy macrophages, and fibrosis.

Subcutaneous Fat Necrosis of the Newborn. Subcutaneous fat necrosis of the newborn presents as nodules or plaques in an otherwise healthy infant. The lesions have a tendency to ulcerate. Histologically, there is fat necrosis and granulomas with histiocytes showing cholesterol crystals in the cytoplasm.

Atrophy and Sclerosis

Diseases with atrophy and sclerosis include:

- Striae distensae
- Anetoderma
- Atrophoderma of Pasini and Pierini
- Morphea
- Necrobiosis lipoidica
- Lichen sclerosus et atrophicus

Atrophy is a loss of tissue substance and may involve the epidermis, dermis, or both. Sclerosis or fibrosis is a relative increase in connective tissue fibers and may be associated with atrophy. Clinical features and laboratory findings are shown in Table 7.

TABLE 6. DIFFERENTIAL DIAGNOSIS OF THE SUBCUTANEOUS NODULES, PANNICULITIS REACTION PATTERN

Disease	Key Clinical Findings	Helpful Laboratory Tests
Erythema nodosum	Painful nodules; changes color like hematoma; no ulceration	Biopsy
Erythema induratum	Nodules usually show ulceration and scarring	Biopsy; vasculitis
Weber-Christian disease	Fever and crops of lesions	Leukocytosis, biopsy
Subcutaneous fat necrosis of the newborn	Indolent nodules	Biopsy: fat necrosis, cholesterol crystals in histiocytes

TABLE 7. DIFFERENTIAL DIAGNOSIS OF DISEASES WITH SCLEROSIS AND ATROPHY

Disease	Key Clinical Findings	Helpful Laboratory Tests
Striae distensae	Linear lesions	—
Anetoderma	Palpating finger pushes through	Compare biopsy of the lesions with that of normal skin
Atrophoderma of Pasini and Pierini	Slate color; cliff-drop sign	Biopsy
Necrobiosis lipoidica	Orange-brown plaques with atrophy and telangiectasia, often in diabetic	Biopsy: palisading granuloma
Lichen sclerosis et atrophicus	White atrophic papules; frequently atrophy and sclerosis of genitalia	Biopsy
Morphea	Indurated bound down plaques; initially edematous with violaceus border, later sclerotic	Biopsy

Striae Distensae. The lesions of striae distensae are longitudinal bands of thinned and wrinkled skin over the abdomen, breasts, and thighs. Obesity and pregnancy are predisposing factors.

Anetoderma. Anetoderma, also called "macular atrophy," usually presents with localized areas of dermal atrophy. The palpating finger pushes through a bladderlike area of decreased tissue resistance. The epidermis over the lesions appears finely wrinkled. Occasionally, some lesions are preceded by an inflammatory phase. The biopsy shows a decreased amount of collagen and elastic tissue in the dermis. The etiology is obscure.

Atrophoderma of Pasini and Pierini. The lesions of atrophoderma of Pasini and Pierini are slate colored, depressed, and located mainly on the trunk. The border is well defined to the palpating finger (cliff-drop sign). The condition is thought by some to be a variant of morphea.

Morphea. Morphea is a localized induration of the skin that initially shows a violaceous border. Eventually the inflammation subsides, and varying amounts of atrophy can be observed. The histologic picture shows an increased layering of collagen at the dermal-subcutaneous interphase, indistinguishable from the lesions of systemic scleroderma.

Necrobiosis Lipoidica. Necrobiosis lipoidica occurs as atrophic, yellow-brown plaques, with prominent induration and telangiactasia, located mainly in the pretibial areas. The biopsy shows areas of degenerated collagen with palisading granulomas and thickening of the vessels. Many patients have abnormal glucose tolerance tests or overt diabetes.

Lichen Sclerosus et Atrophicus. The main changes of lichen sclerosus et atrophicus are localized areas of epidermal atrophy and edematous induration of the connective tissue, followed by scarring. The initial elementary lesions are flat-topped, whitish papules with central depression. These lesions coalesce into plaques, sometimes with prominent follicular plugging. Involvement of the genitalia and perineal areas is common.

GENERAL PRINCIPLES OF MANAGEMENT OF INFLAMMATORY SKIN DISEASES

The skin and mucous membranes are unique in their easy access to a therapeutic preparation that can be administered directly by topical application. Two essential elements take part in a topical formulation: the active ingredient(s) and the vehicle. Both have to be appropriate for the condition being treated. An old principle of dermatologic therapeutics is that an acutely inflamed, oozing process should be dried and that a chronic dry condition should be moisturized. Here the vehicle plays a key role in the therapeutic benefit.

Basic Dermatologic Vehicles

The Open Wet Dressing. Wet dressings help in drying inflammatory exudates by enhancing evaporation. Their primary indication is in treatment of processes with blisters, pustules, erosions, oozing, crusting, and maceration. Water is the essential ingredient, but the addition of mild antiseptics, such as aluminum acetate (Burow's solution) or potassium permanganate, sometimes is helpful.

Powders, Lotions, and Aerosols. These substances act as absorbents by their large particulate surface. In flexural intertriginous areas they reduce maceration and friction. Powders can be applied as such or as medically active or inert ingredients in lotions where the particles are suspended in a liquid vehicle. In aerosols the solid or liquid particulates are suspended in a gaseous vehicle under pressure.

Creams and Gels. Creams are emulsions of oil in water. Since the aqueous solvent is the largest component, they have some drying action. Gels are greaseless, colloidal, usually hydroalcoholic vehicles especially suitable for application in hairy areas.

Ointments. Ointments are emulsions of water in oil. They form a protective barrier that prevents evaporation and enhances water retention in the lesion. Their most useful indication is in the treatment of chronic, dry, or lichenified dermatoses.

Pastes. Pastes are mixtures of powders and ointments. They also have a moisturizing action.

Topical Steroids

Which ones should be used? This is one of the most confusing topics for a nondermatologist because of the large number of drugs and preparations available. The best way to approach this dilemma is to learn the relative efficacy of these agents in steroid-responsive dermatoses. The use of the most potent pharmacologic agents should be restricted to conditions that are relatively steroid resistant, since the frequency and severity of side effects are usually proportional to potency.

It is also important to know that certain areas of the body, such as the face and the intertriginous folds, are prone to develop untoward reactions associated with topical steroids, including folliculitis, atrophy, telangiectasia, striae, and secondary infection. Therefore, in those areas compounds of low potency should be used to minimize the secondary effects. The potency of the preparation also correlates with the greater or lesser occlusive properties of the vehicle. Ointments are the most occlusive, followed by creams and lotions. Sometimes, for a relatively unresponsive dermatosis or for certain areas of the body with thick skin, such as the hands and feet, this occlusion can be enhanced by using a plastic film, such as a polyethylene wrap. The steroid compound is applied generously to the affected area and the plastic dressing is then used, commonly overnight, to promote sweating, skin hydration, and steroid penetration.

Topical steroids can be classified as of

TABLE 8. CLASSIFICATION OF TOPICAL STEROIDS

High Potency
Fluocinonide (Lidex)
Halcinonide (Halog)
Betamethasone dipropionate (Diprosone)

Intermediate Potency
Triamcinolone acetonide (Kenalog) (Aristocort)
Betamethasone valerate (Valisone)
Betamethasone benzoate (Uticort)
Desonide (Tridesilon)
Fluocinolone acetonide (Synalar)

Low Potency
Hydrocortisone (Hytone)

high, intermediate, or low potency, as shown in Table 8. From a practical point of view, it is best to become experienced with the use of a few preparations in each category.

Antibiotics

When they are needed, antibiotics should not be used topically! To treat local, bacterial, skin infection, such as impetigo, it is important to use a proper systemic antibiotic. Studies have shown that topical antibiotic preparations do not decrease the local bacterial count of common pathogens. Mild local antiseptics, such as providone-iodine, hexachlorophene, or chlorhexidine, are usually preferable to topical antibiotics but do not substitute for proper systemic antibiotic therapy.

Therapeutic Hints for Treatment of the Most Common Dermatoses

Eczematous Diseases. The acute, exudative, eczematous dermatitides, such as dyshidrosis and acute contact dermatitis, should be treated initially with cool, wet dressings, followed by topical steroid lotions. Chronic eczematous processes, such as atopic dermatitis, lichen sclerosus et atrophicus, and seborrheic dermatitis, should be treated with steroid creams or ointments. Sick patients with extensive involvement of atopic derma-

titis, autoeczematization, acute contact dermatitis, or exfoliative erythroderm can be treated with systemic corticosteroids.

Papulosquamous Diseases. Papulosquamous diseases usually are less steroid-responsive than the eczematous processes. Pityriasis rosea is usually self-limiting and does not require treatment. Tinea versicolor, superficial fungal infections, and secondary lues all have specific etiologic treatment with topical or systemic antifungals or systemic antibiotics, respectively.

Psoriasis and lichen planus are usually responsive to topical steroids and sometimes to ultraviolet radiation, with or without chemotherapy with psoralens (photochemotherapy). Pityriasis rubra pilaris is difficult to control. The new oral retinoids (vitamin A-related compounds) offer some promise.

Lupus erythematosus is a systemic disease that can be treated with systemic steroids and immunosuppressants when there is multiple organ involvement. Localized lesions can be infiltrated with steroids, or if the cutaneous lesions are extensive, antimalarials can be used, provided that adequate ophthalmologic follow-up is secured to prevent retinal damage.

Vesiculobullous Diseases. The best local treatment of vesicobullous lesions, as stated before, is open wet dressings to enhance drying and healing. Certain bullous diseases, such as pemphigus vulgaris are steroid-responsive. Dermatitis herpetiformis responds to dapsone and a gluten-free diet. Chronic bullous disease of childhood usually responds to a combination of dapsone and systemic steroids. The treatment of Hailey-Hailey disease and epidermolysis bullosa is not very effective. Impetigo, as noted before, should be treated with systemic antibiotics.

Vascular Diseases. The treatment of vascular diseases usually is symptomatic, with antihistamines in urticaria and erythema multiforme. If the etiologic agent is known (drug allergen), steps should be taken to eliminate the exposure to it. Systemic steroids are used in severe reactions, but their efficacy is questionable.

Granulomatous Diseases. The treatment of lupus vulgaris is with systemic antituberculous drugs. Swimming pool granuloma responds poorly to these agents, but excision of the lesion or local application of heat sometimes is helpful.

Sarcoidosis and granuloma annulare sometimes respond to local steroid injections. The treatment of deep fungal infections generally is the administration of systemic antifungal agents, such as amphotericin B, miconazole, and ketoconazole.

Panniculitis. Systemic steroids are sometimes used in erythema nodosum, erythema induratum, and Weber-Christian disease. Subcutaneous fat necrosis of the newborn generally is self-limiting.

Sclerotic and Atrophic Diseases. The response of the sclerotic and atrophic diseases to treatment usually is disappointing. However, many of them tend to improve with time.

PRIMARY CARE BY THE PEDIATRICIAN VS CONSULTATION WITH THE DERMATOLOGIST

Eczematous Diseases
By the Pediatrician. Atopic dermatitis, nummular dermatitis, lichen simplex chronicus, seborrheic dermatitis, dyshidrosis, id reactions, and infectious eczemas can be managed directly by the clinician.

By the Dermatologist. Contact dermatitis usually requires patch testing, which is available in the dermatologist's office and is of difficult interpretation in children. Exfoliative dermatitis is of difficult etiologic diagnosis,

and its management can be beset by complications.

Papulosquamous Diseases
By the Pediatrician. Pityriasis rosea, secondary lues, psoriasis, seborrheic dermatitis, tinea versicolor, and lichen planus can be treated by the clinician.

By the Dermatologist. Parapsoriasis is difficult to diagnosis and manage. Fungal infections require skill in interpretation of KOH scrapings and cultures. Pityriasis rubra pilaris is relatively rare and responds poorly to treatment. Lupus erythematosus is best managed by cooperation between both specialists.

Vesiculobullous Diseases
By the Pediatrician. Viral exanthems, erythema multiforme, and impetigo can be managed by the pediatrician.

By the Dermatologist. Generalized bullous diseases, such as dermatitis herpetiformis, chronic bullous disease of childhood, epidermolysis bullosa, Hailey-Hailey disease, pemphigus vulgaris, and toxic epidermal necrolysis, are sometimes difficult to diagnose and manage. Complications of steroid therapy, due to the large doses required, are common. In most instances, a dermatologic consultation is advisable.

Vascular Reaction Pattern
By the Pediatrician. Urticarias and toxic erythemas can be handled by the pediatrician.

By the Dermatologist. A consultation for the differential diagnosis of the numerous entities presenting with vasculitis is usually required.

Dermal Diseases
Most of these diseases require biopsy and/or culture. A dermatologic consultation is usually helpful.

Panniculitides

The differential diagnosis is commonly difficult, and a biopsy is necessary. Therefore,
consultation is advised.

Diseases with Sclerosis and Atrophy

Since response to therapy is slow or poor, a
dermatologic consultation is required.

Cross-reference to *Pediatrics,* 17th ed.

THIRTY-FOUR

Gait Disturbances

Paul Harris

One of the most frequent concerns of parents consulting pediatricians involves questions regarding gait. At the time the toddler is beginning to walk, attention focuses on the lower extremities and feet. The pediatrician must be familiar with the normal growth and development of the lower extremities, the variations of normal, and the natural history of pathologic conditions.

Since most of the conditions discussed in this chapter have their origin in utero, an attempt is made to show how these positional deformities differ from acquired diseases and to consider them over a longitudinal time frame. The pediatrician can be effective in (1) reassuring parents about normal conditions, (2) following variations until such time as intervention is warranted, and (3) instituting prompt preventive measures where indicated. In some instances, such as congenital dislocation of the hip, early recognition is essential to proper management.

The pediatrician must be able to institute practical, simple, and inexpensive intervention where warranted and to discourage the use of unnecessary, useless measures or overly aggressive surgical procedures. Only by working closely with a competent pediatric orthopedist can the full benefit of preventive and interventive treatment be realized.

DEFINITION OF PROBLEM

Chapter 15 considered acute conditions affecting gait in the young or older child. This symptom has generally been described in terms of an active or dynamic process affecting joints of the lower extremity: hips, knees, ankle. In this chapter we will consider some of the static deformities or malformations of the lower extremities that manifest themselves as *perceived* disturbances of gait.

Since gait is a complex function, comprised of both static or structural components as well as active or dynamic movements at different levels, it is necessary to understand normal patterns of development and variations of normal in order to advise parents on their child's ultimate outcome. In addition, gait represents a summation of many factors occurring at several different levels—hip, femora, tibiae, foot—which may result in a single observation by the parent or pediatrician that the child's gait is abnormal.

At birth, the infant is observed by the practitioner for the influence of two major factors—congenital malformations that are usually genetic in origin vs congenital deformations secondary to intrauterine position and forces. Specific commonly occurring conditions in this latter category will be considered. In addition, as the child grows, develops, and learns to walk, certain changes take place normally as fetal, positional effects diminish and other familial patterns become more important in the ultimate achievement of a normal, neutral gait.

The major problems that pediatric practitioners face are in separating the extreme variations of normal from abnormal development and in determining when therapeutic intervention is warranted. There are many trends in thinking that have attributed undue benefit to preventive measures, which may have little or no effect on the natural development of the lower extremities, e.g., the choice of various types of shoes and arch supports for flatfoot. Overzealous surgical intervention at an early age for a condition, such as genu varum (which may correct spontaneously), is just as serious an error as non-aggressive early treatment for metatarsus adductus or congenital hip dislocations. Therefore, the pediatrician must work together with the family and orthopedist, on the one hand to reassure and to bide time when appropriate, and on the other hand, to recommend and facilitate surgical or other intervention when it is indicated.

ETIOLOGY

The causes of the common disturbances of gait are summarized in Table 1.

Congenital Dislocation of the Hip

Congenital hip dislocation (CHD) is included here because it is an important developmental neonatal condition that will ultimately result in gait disturbance if not recognized and treated during the first few months of life. Since it involves the hip joint and is thus not a static deformity, it is necessary to administer a screening or diagnostic manuever to detect its presence. Like most of the other conditions considered in this chapter, there is a definite relationship between intrauterine

TABLE 1. ETIOLOGY OF DISTURBANCE IN GAIT

Level	Condition
Hip	Congenital hip dislocation
	Excessive femoral anteversion
Knee	Genu varus
	Genu valgum
	Blount's disease
	Rickets
	Hyperextension, genu recurvatum
Tibia	External tibial torsion
	Internal tibial torsion
Foot	Metatarsus adductus
	Talipes equinovarus
	Pes planus, pes cavus
	Calcaneovalgus

position of the infant and subsequent development of the deformity.

Congenital hip dislocation is more often a congenital deformation, i.e., something acquired shortly before or after birth, than a congenital malformation of embryologic maldevelopment. Between 30 and 50% of children with CHD are delivered by breech. Therefore, it has been recommended that all infants delivered by breech should be fully evaluated for the possibility of CHD.

In most instances, newborn infants have dislocatable hips, with otherwise normal structural anatomy except for loose or stretched joint ligaments. In about 20% of cases the deformity is more severe and long standing, with resultant in utero deformity of the femoral head and acetabulum. The former cases respond to positional treatment, whereas the latter may require more aggressive intervention.

CHD is 6 times more common in females than males, and the left hip is 4 times more likely to be the involved joint, although bilateral hip dislocation occurs in 25% of cases.

Excessive Femoral Anteversion

Excessive femoral anteversion is a torsional deformity that occurs at the level of the hip and might better be termed "femoral tortion." Actually, all infants have femoral anteversion at birth, and it is not until 1–2 years of age that the femur begins to rotate externally in relation to the neck of the femur. Femoral anteversion represents a failure of progression and a persistence into childhood and adult life of the normally anteverted position.

A familial pattern may be partially responsible for failure to respond to the normal weightbearing forces in shaping the neck and head of the femur. There is still some debate as to whether abnormal sitting position (reverse tailor position) (Fig. 1) is primary or secondary in this condition. Some authors believe that the condition arises because children sit incorrectly, while others believe that they are able to sit in this position only because of the deformity. We subscribe to the latter but do not encourage children to sit in the W position as it may exacerbate or prolong an already existing deformity.

Genu Varus (Bowlegs) and Genu Valgus (Knock-knee)

Most normal infants are born with mildly to moderately bowed legs, physiologic bowing. The bowing is clearly related to the intra-uterine position, where the lower extremities

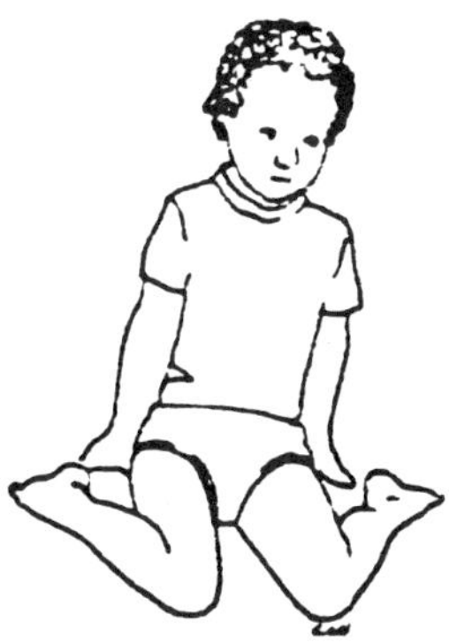

Figure 1. Reverse tailor or W position. *(From Staheli LT: Pediatr Clin North Am 24:810, 1977.)*

are folded up cross-legged on one another. The natural history of physiologic bowing is such that there is a gradual disappearance of the bowing during the first 2 years of life, by which time the tibiofemoral angle approaches 0° (Fig. 2). The process does not stop here, since most normal children then go to a phase of physiologic valgus. This peaks at age 3, after which it returns to about 5° of valgus by age 7.

The etiology of excessive physiologic bowing or excessive valgus deformity is unknown, but it is thought that hereditary factors play more of a role than environmental factors, such as walking habits. As long as the development is symmetrical and not excessive, bowleg under the age of 2½ and knock-knees between 2½ and 7 years of age should be considered variants of normal.

Blount's Disease

Blount's disease, or tibia vara, is a growth disturbance resulting in severe genu varum deformity. It is often associated with internal tibial torsion, which tends to exacerbate the condition.

The etiology of this progressive disease, which represents a growth disturbance of the epiphyseal and metaphyseal region of the posterior-medial aspect of the proximal tibia, is disputed. One school of thought suggests that there is a disturbance in growth and ossification (dysplasia of bone) of the medial part of the proximal tibial epiphysis-metaphysis. The other school attributes the problem to abnormal lines of force transmitted across the medial tibiofemoral compartment secondary to early walking patterns.

The condition is most common among blacks, with many cases reported from the West Indies and West Africa. Blount's disease has also been reported in Scandinavia. Initially, it may be impossible to differentiate excessive physiologic genu varum from early Blount's disease, even with radiologic criteria. We suggest that the spectrum of genu varum may include Blount's disease at the ex-

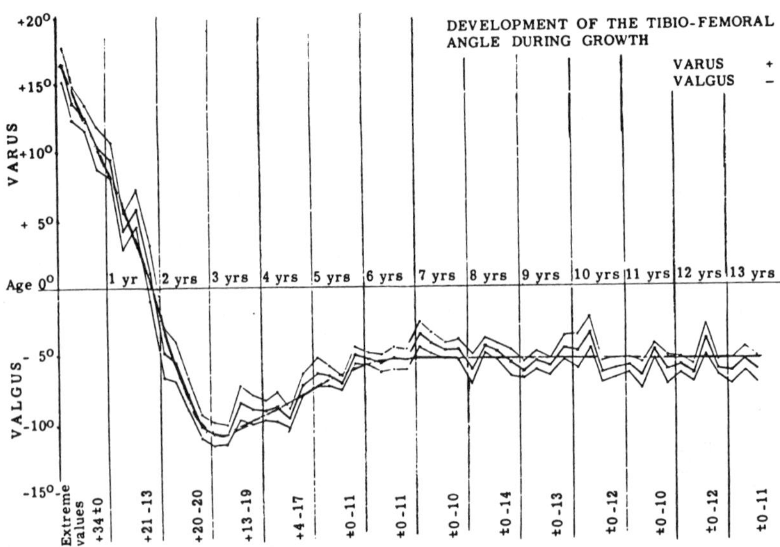

Figure 2. Development of the tibiofemoral angle during growth based on 1480 measurements of the tibiofemoral angle of children at different ages. *(From Salenius P, Vankka E: J Bone Joint Surg 57A:259, 1975.)*

treme and that familial or genetic predisposition probably accounts for its occurrence in some families and not in others.

Tibial Torsion

Whether or not an infant presents with tibial torsion is largely due to three factors: heredity, intrauterine position, and sleeping position. Probably the most significant of these is intrauterine position, which determines the basic deformity. Sleeping position is never causative but may further exacerbate the condition or prevent spontaneous resolution by maintaining the abnormal position for many hours during the day and night. Although there may be familial trends in gait patterns and torsional deformities, there are no specific hereditary patterns that have been documented.

The more common deformity is internal tibial torsion, frequently associated with metatarsus adductus. Although this condi-

tion may resolve spontaneously with weight-bearing, progression without resolution prior to 18 months of age results in lifelong gait disturbance.

External tibial torsion is usually of little significance unless extreme or asymmetric with greater than 20° variance between extremities.

Foot Deformities

By far the most common cause of foot deformities resulting in a gait disturbance is intrauterine fetal position with subsequent molding. Metatarsus adductus, which is often associated with internal tibial torsion, is usually a flexible forefoot deformity that can be corrected passively by manual manipulation. On the other hand, rigid metatarsus and talipes equinovarus (clubfoot) probably represents deformity of longer intrauterine positioning and is not spontaneously correctable with surgical intervention.

Calcaneovalgus deformity is another positional condition, usually of minor significance, which corrects spontaneously. Pes planus of the flexible or hypermobile type is so common as to be hardly considered a deformity. It probably derives from ligamentous laxity and hereditary predisposition rather than intrauterine fetal positioning.

Rigid pes planus, or flatfoot, secondary to tight heel cords may indicate another etiology, either skeletal or neuromuscular. All of the above conditions are relatively common etiologies for gait disturbance secondary to static conditions.

DIFFERENTIAL DIAGNOSIS

History

In contrast to limp (see Chapter 15), where the history is stressed as being the most important aspect of clinical evaluation, the history in the various gait disturbances considered here is not particularly helpful. In most of these conditions, symptoms are few or absent, and the diagnosis is based upon physical findings or maneuvers performed on a routine basis during newborn and health care maintenance visits. Additionally, stasic or structural deformity may not interfere significantly enough with function to elicit significant symptoms.

However, the natural history of each condition producing gait disturbance is important in determining in the individual child whether or not a particular condition is abnormal. For example, mild to moderate bowing is not abnormal in an 8-month-old infant but may be a sign of progressive disease in a 3 year old. Similarly, genu valgum in a 4 year old is not as bothersome to the pediatrician as this same finding in a 1 year old. Flatfoot in a toddler does not warrant great concern nor require therapeutic intervention.

Family history is often of help in evaluating gait disturbances, as tendencies towards torsional deformities, genu varum or valgus, and foot deformities often have repetitive familial patterns. This may help to reassure the anxious parent, on the one hand, or serve to alert the physician to a predisposition toward physiologic excess.

Any information on intrauterine position and observations made by parents or staff soon after birth are useful, as ultimately most conditions have their onset at that time. Thus, a history of breech delivery should help in evaluating the presence of congenital hip dislocation. Age of onset or when first observed helps to place the condition within its natural historical background.

Often, the pediatrician's role is simply to determine whether or not the condition is resolving or progressive. This may be accomplished both by accurate historical data and by sequential evaluations. Many of the conditions discussed may be bilateral, and most of the physiologic or minor positional variations tend to be symmetric, whereas more severe deformities are often unilateral or asymmetric. Therefore, the parents' perception of which side is worse or abnormal is important. Ethnic considerations provide only a few clues, such as the increased incidence of congenital hip dislocation in Lapps, Southern Tyrolean Italians, and certain Navajo Indian peoples, or the significant preponderance of excessive bowing and Blount's disease in West Indian blacks.

Historical data should include information on the child's preferred sleeping position. We do not believe that orthopedic gait disturbances are caused by aberrant sleeping positions, but they may well be prevented from spontaneous resolution or be exacerbated by continued fixation of an existing deformity. Most torsional deformities are exacerbated by the infant's sleeping in the prone position, whereas supine slumbering will allow natural resolution to occur more rapidly. Many parents are afraid to allow young infants to sleep on their backs for fear of regurgitation and aspiration. However, it has not been shown that the supine sleeping position for infants is safer than the prone. Can the older child sit cross-legged Indian style, or does he prefer to sit in the reverse tailor position? Does he run with a flailing or eggbeater pattern? These characteristics are all compatible with the diagnosis of excessive femoral anteversion.

Many concerns of parents are focused on the gait of the toddler who is just beginning to stand or walk. Feet and legs turning in or out, bowing, stumbling, falling, and waddling may all be normal stages of development in the newly ambulatory child, but excessive clumsiness and frequent falling over his own feet in a toddler may imply internal tibial torsion with metatarsus adductus.

Physical Examination

Physical examination is the most important procedure in evaluating a child with gait disturbance. The child must be observed with shoes on but otherwise fully undressed. If old enough to walk, gait should be evaluated by having the child walk and run, first with clothes on and subsequently undressed. Examination on the examining table should be performed in several positions, and the various manuevers described below must be performed.

Since gait is the summation of many factors at different levels affecting the lower extremities, physical examination will help to answer the following questions.

1. At what level (hips, femur, knees, tibia, foot) does the condition(s) exist?
2. Is the condition within range of normal for a developing infant or child, or does it represent an aberration of severe degree?
3. Is the condition bilateral or asymmetric?
4. Is the gait disturbance made up of several components, compensatory or cumulative?
5. What is the specific pathognomonic or diagnostic sign present to confirm or rule out the diagnosis being considered?

Examination of Hip of the Newborn. Physical examination of the hip joints is performed at birth, at the time of discharge from the nursery, at 2–3 weeks of age, and again at 4–6 weeks. Frequent and complete range of motion tests are necessary to screen for the presence of hip dislocation and to confirm the absence of pathology in infants noted to have ligamentous laxity or ligamentous clicks. With the infant lying comfortable supine on a firm surface, a reduction maneuver (Ortoloni maneuver) is performed by grasping the lower limb with the fingers extended over the greater trochanter and simultaneously lifting and abducting (Fig. 3). The maneuver should be performed gently but firmly. If dislocation is present, a palpable clunk will be appreciated as the head of the femur pops back into the acetabulum.

The reverse maneuver or dislocation test, known as the Barlow test, is performed by grasping the leg in the same manner but pressing down and simultaneously adducting. If the femur pops out, it will be felt and can be confirmed by the Ortolani maneuver. Small degrees of crepitance or slight sensations of clicking are usually due to ligaments, cartilage, or other soft tissue structures and do not indicate dislocation.

Shortening of one extremity or asymmetric skin folds may be suggestive of a problem but are difficult to assess and may be unreliable in arriving at a diagnosis, especially since the condition may be bilateral and thus appear symmetric.

Although it is desirable to make the diagnosis on physical grounds alone within the first month of life, examination of the hip joints should be repeated at all routine examinations during the first year (Fig. 4). In the older infant (2–4 months) the tests described above no longer yield positive results, as the dislocated hip is not easily reduced by a simple manual manuever. The most prominent and pathognomonic finding is severe limitation of abduction of the hip joint. Shortening and asymmetry with telescoping become

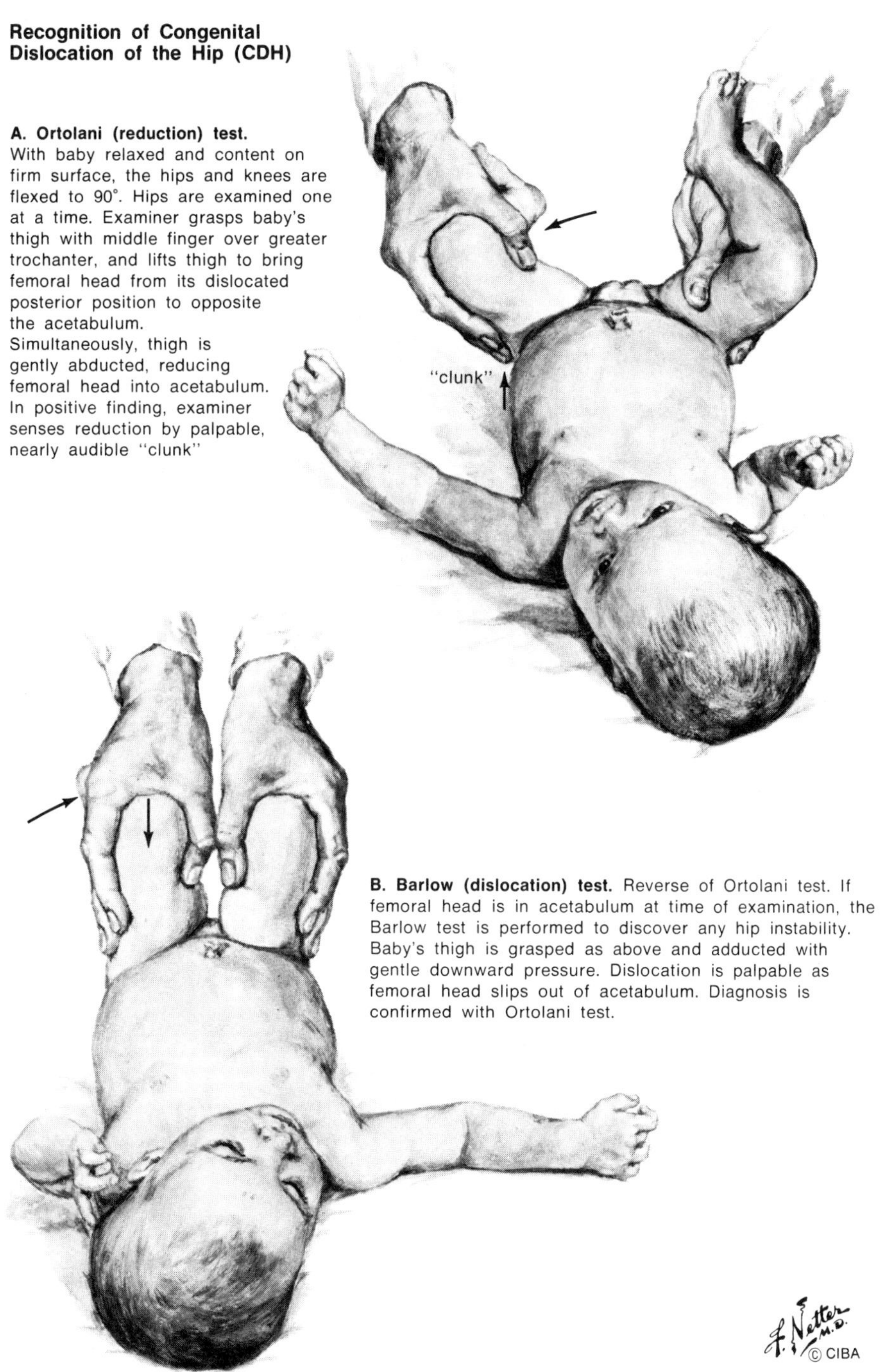

Figure 3. Recognition of congenital dislocation of the hip (CDH). *(From Hensiger RN: Ciba Clin Symp 31:1, 1979 © Copyright 1979, CIBA Pharmaceutical Company. Division of CIBA-GEIGY Corporation. Reprinted with permission from* Clinical Symposia, *illustrated by Frank H. Netter, M.D. All rights reserved.)*

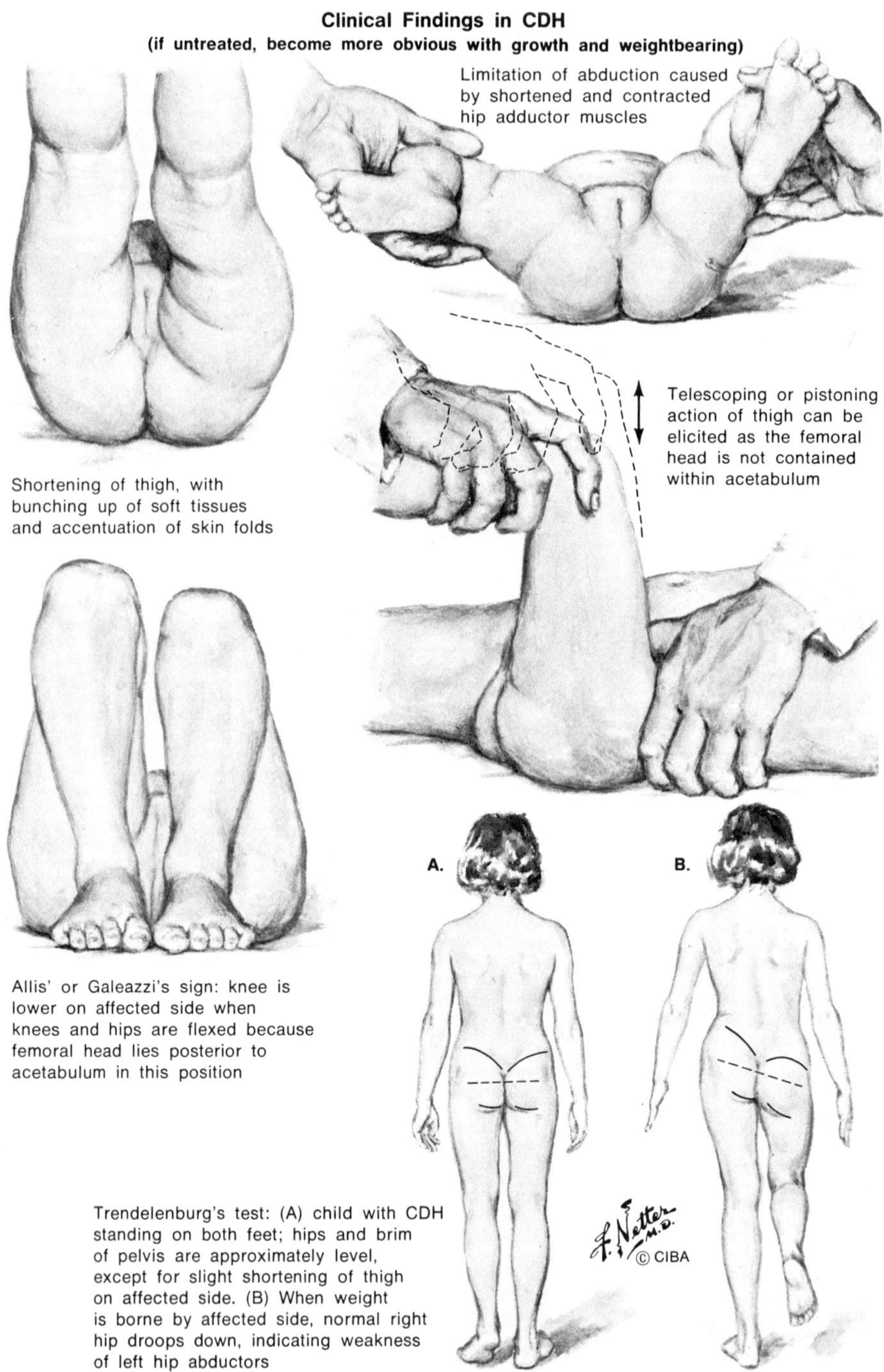

Figure 4. Clinical findings in CDH. If untreated, symptoms become more obvious with growth and weightbearing. *(From Hensiger RN: Ciba Clin Symp 31:1, 1979 © Copyright 1979, CIBA Pharmaceutical Company. Division of CIBA-GEIGY Corporation. Reprinted with permission from* **Clinical Symposia,** *illustrated by Frank H. Netter, M.D. All rights reserved.)*

more prominent and recognizable in unilateral disease. In the older child who has begun to walk, the development of Trendelenburg gait or sign or both should be considered to be indicative of congenital hip dislocation until proven otherwise. However, the natural history of this condition is such that patients may learn to walk, run, and compensate without symptoms or obvious signs of gait disturbance (such as waddling) until their teens or even young adulthood, at which time severe deformity of the acetabulum, femoral head, and false acetabulum have occurred.

Assessment of Level of Involvement. The three components that must be evaluated are hip rotation, thigh-foot angle, and foot axis or shape. All three of these are most easily measured with the infant lying comfortably on his belly with someone playing with him at the head of the examining table. With the knee flexed, the thigh/leg is allowed to fall laterally from the vertical position as far as it will naturally go from the midline. This rotates the thigh internally; the number of degrees of internal rotation is the angle made by the lower leg and the vertical midline position. Similarly, the leg is now folded inward to and across the midline, and the angle of external rotation of the femur is recorded on the other side of the midline. Normally, the sum of external and internal rotation is 100° or more. The limits of internal and external rotation vary with age. Infants have up to 90° of external rotation, and they can easily bring the leg all the way down on the table, but they may only have 10–20° internal rotation. As the child becomes older, the external rotation diminishes and the ability to internally rotate increases. Evaluation of rotational components should be performed separately on each leg (Fig. 5A, B, C).

Physical examination of the child who is being evaluated for a torsional deformity is performed in order to determine the level and the degree of deformity. The resultant components of femoral, tibial, and pedal contributions will produce a neutral gait, outtoeing, or intoeing. The term "angle of gait," refers to the angle that the foot makes with an imaginary line on the floor in the direction the child is walking (line of progression) (Fig. 5E). Most toddlers learn to walk outtoe about 20° from this line and gradually approach 5–10° by age 2. Outtoeing is common in the general population and is not abnormal. Intoeing gait is expressed in negative degrees from the straight line and may represent components of internal tibial torsion, femoral torsion, or metatarus adductus.

Angle of Gait. The angle of gait in a child who is not yet walking obviously is not obtainable, and even the child who is able to strut around the office is often self-conscious and will vary his gait tremendously. Therefore, casual observations and parental observations of gait are most helpful. Symmetric gait angles will also help the pediatrician to concentrate on which side is most affected.

Thigh–Foot Axis. The next measurement is the thigh–foot axis, which defines the degree of tibial torsion. The foot is dorsiflexed passively to 90° while the child continues to lie prone and while the examiner grasps the toes and distal foot. The angle observed between the axis of the thigh and the axis of the foot is approximated by observation and expressed positively for the outtoeing foot and negatively for the foot which points inward (Fig. 5C). Although it is also possible to evaluate the degree of torsion with the child sitting and flexing the knee and ankle joints to determine the relative axis of joint movements, we find that this requires more interpretation by the examiner and more infantile cooperation than the prone thigh–foot axis measurement described above.

Examination of the Foot. With the infant still prone, the shape of the bottom of the foot is observed, and the axis of the hindfoot is

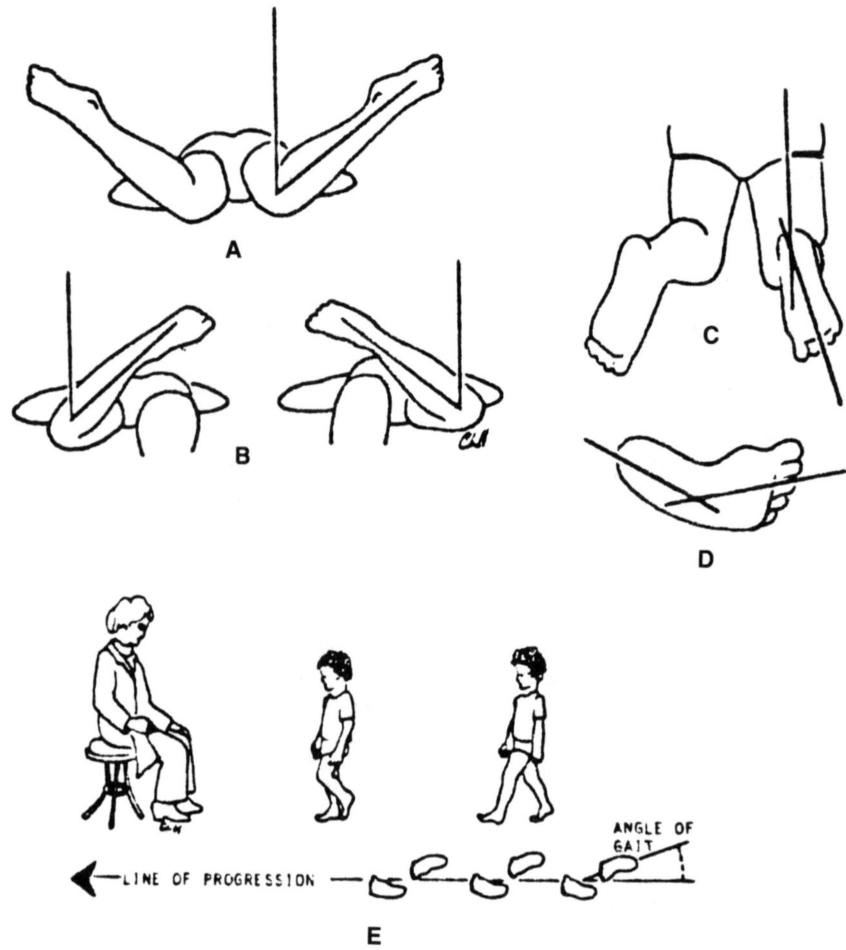

Figure 5. Evaluation for torsional deformity. A, B. Assessment of hip rotation. C, D. Assessment of thigh-foot axis. E. Assessment of angle of gait is made by estimating the average angle of each step while watching the child walk. *(From Staheli LT: Pediatr Clin North Am 24:810, 1977.)*

compared with the axis of the forefoot. Normally the two should make a straight line. In forefoot deformity, such as metatarsus adductus, the forefoot axis makes an obtuse angle, toward the midline with the hindfoot axis (Fig. 5D). At this point, it is essential to palpate the foot and determine its rigidity or suppleness. The degree to which the forefoot can be brought passively to the midline axis of the hindfoot will largely determine the severity of the deformity and the treatment indicated. Other physical findings compatible with the diagnosis of metatarsus adductus or varus are convexity on the lateral side of the foot and concavity with a crease on the medial side. Prominence or bulging at the base of the fifth metatarsal and a wide space between the first and second toes may also be noted but are not in themselves diagnostic. In metatarsus adductus, the deformity is limited to the forefoot, which is adducted and often supinated, whereas in clubfoot there is an additional heel varus and ankle equinas that is rigid.

Calcaneovalgus deformity may also be noted; this merely denotes a foot held naturally in dorsiflexion and eversion but which is usually supple and may be passively brought into normal position.

Another measure which we like to perform for the sake of both the pediatrician and the parents is to fold the baby back up into the most naturally occurring fetal position, which usually involves crossing the legs and folding in the feet. In this manner, it is easy to demonstrate the contribution of fetal intrauterine position to the various torsional components.

Physical examination of the lower extremities to evaluate bowleg (genu varus) and knock-knees (genu valgus) is largely a matter of observation. One should inspect the child visually both walking, if of age, and while lying in the supine position. The degree of varus or valgus deformity will usually be apparent as mild, moderate, or severe and is subject to interpretation as physiologic or pathologic depending upon the degree of deformity, the age of the child, and the presence or absence of symmetry. It is important to feel the knee and other joints for ligamentous laxity, and it may be helpful to measure the distance between the knees and the ankles in the standing older child. However, these methods are only clinical approximations of the tibiofemoral angle, which must be determined radiographically if pathology is suspected.

Pes planus or flatfoot is only mentioned here because of its association with external tibial torsion and as a cause of outtoeing. The

TABLE 2. PHYSICAL FINDINGS IN GAIT DISTURBANCES

Conditions	Physical Findings
Congenital hip dysplasia	Positive Ortoloni maneuver and/or Barlow test
	Shortening of leg
	Asymmetry of skin folds
	Limitation of abduction
	Trendelenburg gait
Excessive femoral anteversion	Characteristic sitting position
	Increased internal rotation
	Decreased external rotation
	Compensatory external tibial torsion
	Intoeing—negative angle of gait
Genu varus	Increased tibiofemoral angle 25°
Genu valgum	Negative tibiofemoral angle 15°
Blount's disease	Severe progressive bowing—bilateral with radiographic findings
Internal tibial torsion	Intoeing gait
	Negative thigh–foot axis—10 to 15°
External tibial torsion	Positive thigh–foot axis
	Outtoeing gait
Metatarsus adductus	Wide space between first and second toes
	Prominence at base of fifth metatarsal convexity of lateral border of foot
	Concave crease on medial aspect of foot
Talipes equinovarsus (club foot)	Forefoot adduction
	Supination heel varus
	Ankle equinus
Pes planus or cavus	Rigidity of arch or foot

hypermobile or everted foot may cause excessive positive angle of gait but rarely causes pain. Physical examination is synonymous with determining the relative degree of suppleness or rigidity. A supple foot may be considered to be normal in the infant and toddler. One should ask the older child to stand on tiptoes to demonstrate the functioning presence of an arch and ligaments. If the foot is rigid, whether flat or deeply arched (pes cavus), the examination is considered abnormal. Excessive eversion with bulging of the astragalus and concomitant outtoeing is the only significant criterion for abnormality.

A summary of the common physical findings found in infants or children with gait disturbances is found in Table 2.

Laboratory Examination

There are no laboratory tests other than radiologic that are useful, with the exception of genu varus 2° to rickets. Even radiographs are not uniformly indicated unless extreme variations of physiologic processes or pathology is suspected. Furthermore, many orthopedists and pediatricians caution on the interpretation of roentgenograms in congenital hip dislocation taken under 2 months of age, which may be inconclusive and misleading (Fig. 6).

Radiographic findings in various conditions that result in disturbances of gait are shown in Table 3.

MANAGEMENT

In general, the management of the conditions affecting gait described in this chapter require neither acute nor aggressive intervention (Table 4). With the exception of congenital hip dislocation, which does require early identification and prompt intervention to prevent further disability, the approach to management should be longitudinal. More often than not, the pediatric management of

TABLE 3. RADIOGRAPHIC FINDINGS IN GAIT DISTURBANCES

Condition	Radiographic Finding
Congenital hip dislocation	Increase in acetabular angle Lateral displacement of femoral neck Discontinuous Shenton's line (Fig. 6)
Excessive femoral anteversion	Anteversion of femoral neck >50°
Genu varus	Tibiofemoral angle >25° of varus Tibiofemoral angle >15° of valgus Asymmetry Short stature
Blount's disease	Abrupt medial angulation and fragmentation of proximal tibia Stages I–V
Rickets	Osteoporosis Bowing Widening of epiphyseal plate Fraying of metaphysis and cortical thinning
Tibial torsion	Not helpful
Metatarsus adductus	Usually normal
Equinovarus	Complex
Pes planus	Normal

torsional deformities, genu varus and valgus, and nonrigid foot deformities requires patience, observation, reassurance, and close long-term evaluation. Frequently, it may be necessary to advise parents and orthopedic consultants to avoid seeking and implementing aggressive surgical techniques for conditions that will resolve spontaneously if allowed to follow their predicted natural course. The pediatrician must be able to assess the degree of deformity, the direction in which it is proceeding over time (improving or be-

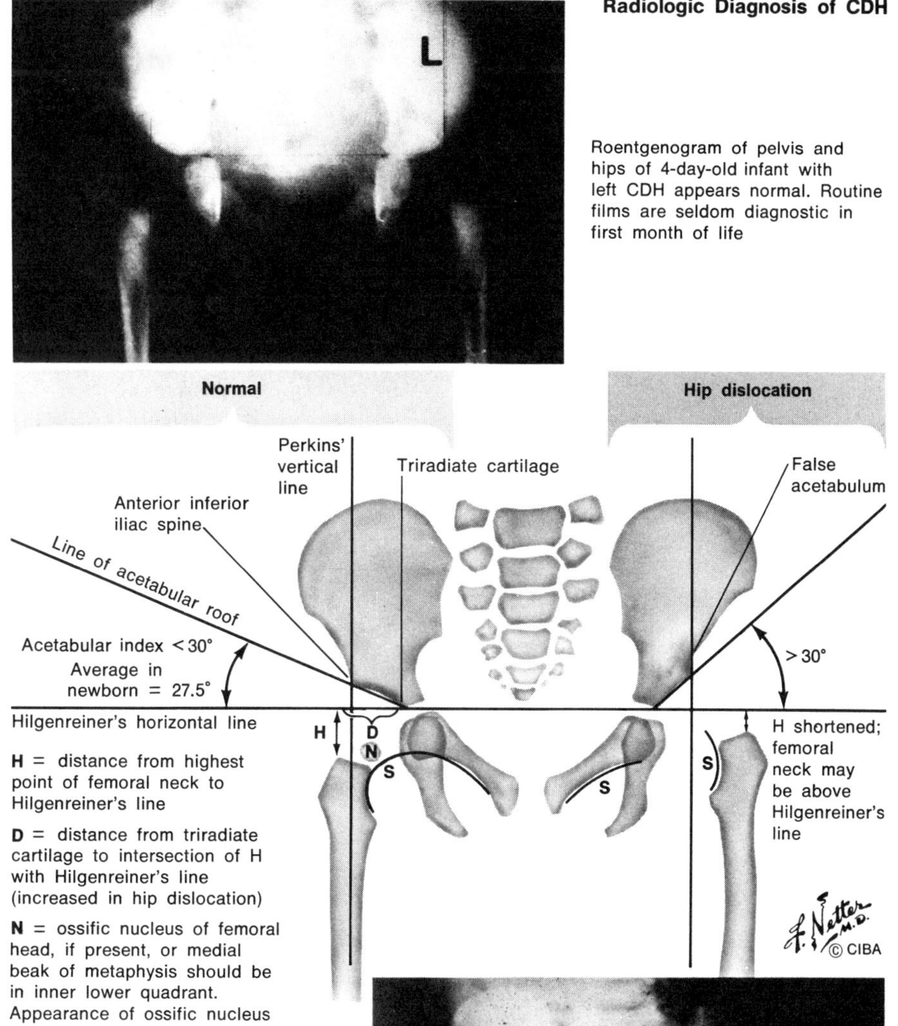

Figure 6. Radiologic diagnosis of CHD. *(From Hensiger RN: Ciba Clin Symp 31:5, 1979 © Copyright 1979, CIBA Pharmaceutical Company. Division of CIBA-GEIGY Corporation. Reprinted with permission from* **Clinical Symposia,** *illustrated by Frank H. Netter, M.D. All rights reserved.)*

TABLE 4. MANAGEMENT OF GAIT DISTURBANCES

Conditions	Pediatric Treatment	Joint Orthopedist Treatment with Pediatrician
Congenital hip dysplasia	Infant with reducible hip under 6 months: triple diapers or Frejka pillow or Ravelik harness	Child older than 6 months nonreducible hip: casting surgical procedures
Excessive femoral anteversion	No treatment, advise against reverse tailor squat	Over 18 years of age with severe disability, chondromalacia patella: derotational femoral osteotomy
Genu varus	Physiologic to age 2 years	Bracing 25°
Genu vargum	Physiologic to age 7 years	Surgrey 15° or asymmetric
Blount's disease	Diagnose	Bracing and surgery prn
Internal tibial torsion	Up to 18 months: sleeping position, Denis Browne bar up to 3 years	Severe over 3 years or 18 months to 3 years
External tibial torsion	Usually no treatment	Severe or asymmetric
Metatarsus adductus	Flexible: passive, stretching exercises	Rigid: casting
Clubfoot	Diagnose	Casting and surgery
Pes planus	Flexible	Rigid or painful: surgery
Pes cavus	No treatment	Rigid or painful: surgery

(From Gross RH: Pediatr Clinic N Amer 24:4, 1977, p 815.)

coming worse), and whether or not intervention at a particular state of development will ultimately produce desirable results.

Anecdotally, we have seen cases of rather severe genu varus in 2 year olds for whom tibial osteotomy was considered. These children were shown to resolve spontaneously over the next few years without surgery, avoiding the significant risk of neurovascular complications. On the other hand, it is much simpler to correct a severe rigid forefoot deformity by the application of corrective casts in the first few months of life than to allow the condition to persist until the child is of walking age, when surgical intervention would be required, and the results are less satisfactory.

Congenital Hip Dislocation

Pediatric management of the child with congenital hip dislocation should be restricted to the young infant recognized early to have clinically reducible hip dislocation. There are various simple positioning devices and regimens available to maintain the hip in the flexed and abducted position long enough to allow for normal acetabular development. In these most common and simple cases, it is not necessary to obtain x-rays, which are usually inconclusive at an early age. It is important, however, to evaluate these infants after 2 weeks and at subsequent intervals to be certain that the goal of continued reduction and loss of subluxation is accomplished.

Although the infant under 6 months of age with a clinically reducible dislocation of the hip can successfully be managed by an experienced pediatrician without the benefit of orthopedic consultations and many older pediatricians have avoided calling in an orthopedist, there may indeed be some significant value in consulting early, even in apparently simple cases. Experienced pediatric orthopedists are more readily available now and can establish rapport and direct knowledge of the patient's condition early should complications arise later. They can also lend a second opinion and reassurance, to both the family and the referring pediatrician, that the condition has been correctly identified and that adequate treatment is in progress.

The simplest method of management for the mildly affected infant is the use of triple diapers. However, the method is reliable only (1) if the parent knows how to perform the Ortaloni maneuver in order to be certain that the hip is in correct position and (2) if the parent is shown how to diaper the child correctly. It is not sufficient just to put on three layers of diapers. At least one diaper must be folded under two others to provide sufficient bulk to keep the hips abducted. Cloth diapers are superior to disposable diapers for this method.

Another simple method for the child with a sublxated or dislocated hip is the Frejka pillow, which is merely a large bulky device to keep the hips positioned correctly.

Other devices that are more effective and reliable are the Craig or Iufeld splint, the Von Rosen splint, and the Plavelik harness. Of these, we prefer the Pavelik harness for the child with significant dislocation that must be brought back into the acetabulum and held in place but that must be allowed to rotate within the socket. These methods can be used for children under 6 months of age on an outpatient basis. The duration of treatment (usually several months) will be determined by the progress of the individual infant.

Children over 6 months of age with frank dislocation that will not spontaneously reduce with the Ortonloni maneuver must be referred to a pediatric orthopedist for evaluation and treatment. During the first year of life, the developing acetabulum will respond by molding to the shape of a femoral head

that is in place, and the goal of management is to maintain position of the head of the femur within the acetabulum without compromising the vascular supply. At no time should forceful maneuvers or devices be applied that will damage these delicate structures. In the child between 1 and 5 years of age, various methods of treatment (molding, traction, casting, and surgical reduction) may be necessary and warranted, but in the child over 5 years of age, the end result of attempting to bring the femur down into the acetabulum may be unsatisfactory. In these cases, where there is no chance of having a normally functioning hip joint, many orthopedists recommend leaving the dislocated femur in its false acetabulum rather than attempting complex heroic surgical procedures.

The management of the child becomes a joint venture, and the pediatrician should not abandon the patient nor defer to all orthopedic opinion. Continued support, interpretation, evaluation of compliance, and advice to the family will make the orthopedist's intervention more effective and sensitive to the family's needs and, in the long run, will lead to a successful outcome.

Torsional Deformities

The management of torsional deformities in children is largely pediatric, as very few surgical interventions are warranted, and the pediatrician should be knowledgeable in determining which conditions need treatment and how to use the few effective splints or devices available.

There is no known preventive treatment for excessive femoral anteversion other than cautioning the parents not to allow the child to sit in the reverse tailor position. Sitting cross-legged (Indian style) will prevent further progression of this deformity, but the ultimate outcome must await young adulthood. If the disability at that time is judged to be severe, with a very abnormal gait, patellofemoral malalignment syndrome, and attendant chondromalacia patellae, femoral osteotomy may be indicated. However, there is no evidence that continued femoral anteversion leads to hip joint disease (arthritis) in later life, and, therefore, if signs and symptoms are tolerable, surgery should be avoided. Many patients are shown to have compensatory external tibial torsion that corrects the angle of gait when walking and provides good cosmetic appearance. In these instances, only athletic activities (including running) will be significantly altered, and the decision regarding surgery is elective.

Metatarsus Adductus

Mild to moderate forefoot deformities that are flexible are handled by the pediatrician and the parent without orthopedic intervention. Since this condition most often resolves spontaneously, it is not clear whether or not passive stretching exercises with each diaper change and handling of the infant are really contributory or more for peace of mind. We believe, however, that sleeping position is important in internal tibial torsion. If the infant can be encouraged to sleep in the supine position, the continuous pressure on the lateral aspect of the foot is removed, allowing the forefoot to develop normally.

In severe, asymmetric, or rigid forefoot abnormalities the application of casts changed every 2 weeks is recommended. This may be followed with outflare shoes to maintain position in combination with a Denis Browne splint if associated with internal tibial torsion.

Flatfoot or Pes Planus

There is still some controversy over the management of flexible flatfoot. While many podiatrists and orthopedists still recommend high-topped shoes with a Thomas heel and scaphoid pad, we do not recommend any special treatment for asymptomatic pes planus. It is quite possible that special shoes or arches may make the pronation and eversion less noticeable, but there is no evidence that any nonsurgical treatment alters the natural configuration of the foot.

On the other hand, if there is any degree of rigidity, pes cavus, or pain associated with foot deformity, orthopedic intervention is warranted and may involve surgical procedures.

Reassurance that all infants appear flatfooted until chubbiness has resolved and that arch function develops with walking is helpful, as is the observation that up to 50% of the population has some degree of flatfoot without disability.

Internal Tibial Torsion

The most common form of intoeing is internal tibial tortion, which is often associated with varying degrees of metatarsus adductus. The two together result in an abnormal gait, often noticed when the child begins to walk. In most mild to moderate situations, the condition will resolve spontaneously without treatment before 18 months. However, since the condition is positional in nature, sleeping posture may exacerbate or prevent spontaneous resolution. The parent should be advised as early as possible to encourage sleeping in the supine position. One helpful hint is to hang a mobile above the child's crib to attract attention and allow him to fall asleep on his back.

After 18 months of age spontaneous correction is unlikely, and night splints are necessary. The most successful method is to use a Denis Browne splint, which is a bar with adjustably mounted high-topped shoes. The shoes are adjusted 6–8 inches apart and externally rotated 35–40°. Children often do not tolerate this well at first, and parents must receive firm encouragement. Another method for milder deformities is to tie the heels of an old pair of shoes together after cutting off the toes. The child sleeps with these shoes on. Straight last or reverse last shoes or even shoes put on the opposite foot will help in mild flexible metatarsus adductus, but care must be exercised to be sure that pressure necrosis does not occur on the medial aspect on the foot or great toe.

All the above methods must result in

complete correction by age 3 years, after which only surgery is effective. The goal is to avoid tibial rotational osteotomy by early effective bracing and positioning, as this type of surgery is often fraught with complications.

External tibial tortion is rarely a problem, as a slight outtoeing gait is quite normal and tolerable. Very severe asymmetric conditions may also be managed by splinting as above.

Genu Varum and Genu Valgum

The management of physiologic symmetric genu valgum and genu varus requires no intervention whatever. No special shoes, exercises, or braces are indicated, and the use of a Denis Browne splint will actually exacerbate bowed legs. Reassurance that the bowing noted in toddlers under the age of 2 and the knock-knees commonly observed between 2 and 7 years are within the normal range is the most important aspect of pediatric assessment and counseling.

On the other hand, the pediatrician must be able to recognize when either of these conditions is asymmetric or of extreme variation with a poor prognosis. Severe varus deformity with a tibiofemoral angle of greater than 25°, which has not resolved by age 2, is considered to have a poor prognosis for spontaneous resolution. Black infants with severe bowing should be evaluated carefully for progression and for the presence of Blount's disease.

Knock-knees of mild to moderate degree up to the age of 7 years may be considered within normal limits. Asymmetry or a tibiofemoral angle of $> 15°$ of valgus or association with short stature are indications for orthopedic intervention, as spontaneous resolution is unlikely. A 10-year-old child with more than 3 inches between the medial malleoli is not likely to correct spontaneously.

Severe varus deformity that requires intervention may be managed by either a long leg brace with lateral pull strap, frame brace, or Blount brace. Severe valgus deformity on the other hand may require surgical intervention with procedures designed to alter the medial distal femoral and medial proximal tibial epiphyses.

SUMMARY

We have attempted to show that the majority of conditions encountered in gait disturbances in children are either extreme variations of normal physiologic developmental stages or secondary to positional, familial, or other environmental factors. Most of those conditions can be managed by the informed pediatrician with a minimum of invasive, investigational technology or treatment, as the conditions are most often self-limited or resolve spontaneously, producing little if any lasting functional deformity. However, the pediatrician must be able to recognize the extreme variants and range of normal phenomena in order to counsel and reassure parents, on the one hand, and to seek orthopedic consultation and joint management, on the other, if indicated. We seek here to dispel some of the myths, jargon, and fears so often associated with normal variations of gait which respond no better to unproven treatment regimens than to tincture of time.

REFERENCES

Clarren, Smith: Congenital deformities. Pediatr Clin North Am 24:665, 1977

Ferguson AB Jr: Pathology and treatment of Legg-Perthes disease. Pediatr Am 272, 1976

Hensiger RN: Congential dislocation of the hip. Ciba Clin Symp 31:5, 1979

McDade Bow legs and knock knees, Pediatr Clin North Am 24:825, 1977

Staheli LT: Torsional deformity. Pediatr Clin North Am 24:799, 1977

Staheli, T: Torsional deformities in children. J Cont Ed Pediatr 20:11, 1978

Staheli LT, Griffin L: Corrective shoes for children: a survey of current practice. Pediatrics 65:13, 1980

Cross-References to *Pediatrics,* 17th ed.

THIRTY-FIVE

Eye Problems

Frederick M. Wang

The accurate evaluation and proper management of ocular disorders is essential. It may be sightsaving or even lifesaving.

The pediatrician's role in the eye care of children includes (1) the early recognition of asymptomatic ocular pathology, (2) the accurate assessment of ocular symptoms and signs, (3) timely ophthalmologic referral, (4) emergency treatment, and (5) treatment of those conditions a pediatrician may elect to manage. This chapter provides guidelines for the pediatrician to fulfill this role. Many important conditions, such as cloudy cornea, cataract, leukokoria, or exophthalmos, obviously require ophthalmologic referral. Detailed discussion of conditions where direct ophthalmologic referral is indicated is beyond the scope of this chapter.

ROUTINE OCULAR CARE AND AMBLYOPIA

The paramount role of the pediatrician in eye care is the early identification of those conditions likely to go unrecognized by patients and relatives. Poor visual acuity in the very young or slowly diminishing visual acuity in older children may go unnoticed. As the eyes are paired structures, significant uniocular pathology may exist without recognition by child or parent. Routine ocular screening is, therefore, indicated.

Definition

Routine ocular screening is a regular plan of health maintenance designed to elicit underlying pathology and amblyopia. Routine screening of newborn and preschool children is of particular import, for at these ages the yield is greatest and the prognosis for remediation is best.

Amblyopia, "lazy eye," is a condition where unstimulated cells of the visual pathway are literally lost over time with resultant loss of visual acuity. This process can occur through age 9, at which age the visual pathways are fully developed. It is found in 2–3% of the population and represents the most common cause of uniocular blindness.

ETIOLOGIES

Any process that causes a poor visual image from one eye will lead to an amblyopia of that eye. Such processes include (1) strabismus where one eye is suppressed to avoid diplopia and visual confusion, (2) anisometropia, a disparity in refractive errors between the two eyes, and (3) anything that blocks light (ex anopsia) from reaching the retina (e.g., ptosis, opacities of the optical pathway such as a cloudy cornea or cataract).

Certain conditions are so frequently associated with ocular pathology that ophthalmologic referral is indicated even without ocular signs or symptoms present (Table 1).

TABLE 1. INDICATIONS FOR OPHTHALMOLOGIC REFERRAL IN THE ABSENCE OF OCULAR SYMP-TOMS OR SIGNS

Signs	History	Systemic Conditions
Torticollis	Prematurity (shortage of oxygen)	Diabetes
Bony orbital and cranial anomalies	Drugs	Juvenile rheumatoid
Low-set ears	Chronic steroids	arthritis
Pierre Robin syndrome	Diodohydroxyquin	Systemic immune disease
Dwarfism	Ethambutol	Akylosing spondylitis
Hydrocephalus	Long-term phenothiazines	Enzymatic defects
Periorbital vascular hamartomas	Family history	Chromosomal abnormalities
Sensorineural deafness	Strabismus	Sickle hemoglobinopathies
Hematuria	Amblyopia	Phakomatoses
	High refractive error	Dysautonomia
	Congenital ocular disorders	Ectodermal dysplasias
	Night blindness	Marfan's syndrome
	Retinal disease, early acquired	Infectious diseases, congenital or acquired
		TORCH
		Syphilis

Differential Diagnosis

History. For infants, a history of age-appropriate visual behavior should be elicited: following to the midline by 6 weeks, following past the midline by 2 months, reaching for objects by 4 months, and a responsive smile by 3–4 months. Acuity in infants has been shown by recent techniques to be in the range of 20/400 during the first month of life, increasing to 20/40 by 12 months and 20/20 by age 18–24 months.

For older children, difficulty seeing the blackboard, the need to be in close proximity to objects of visual regard, "tired" eyes, or headache with visual use signal the need for visual examination. Specific dysfunctions, for example, difficulty with night vision, obviously require ophthalmologic referral.

Physical Examination. A systematic approach to routine ocular examination will uncover most ocular pathology. This process entails general observation, measurement of visual acuity, assessment of ocular alignment, testing pupillary reflexes, and ophthalmos-copy. These examinations require a minimum of equipment: a small toy, illiterate E eye chart and demonstration case, a standard Snellen letter and number chart, an eye occluder, a penlight, and an ophthalmoscope.

Accurate assessment of visual acuity is the most important part of the examination. Visual system dysfunction anywhere from the cornea to the cerebral cortex often diminishes visual acuity. For infants, fixation behavior and following of silent objects is usually elicited by the sixth week. Rarely, this takes up to 6 months. Acuity should first be tested binocularly and then monocularly. Monocular testing is easily accomplished with the child seated on the mother's lap, the examiner placing his or her fingers on the child's head and occluding an eye with the thumb while observing ocular fixation and following. An excellent clue to monocular decreased vision is avoidance movement (crying, head movement, or attempts to remove the thumb) when the eye with better vision is occluded. Another clue is nystagmoid or random purposeless eye movement.

In addition to observing them for fixation and following behavior, preschool children (3–4 years old) can often be tested with picture, matching, or illiterate E charts. The occluder should be held by the examiner. Children are extremely clever at peeking around a self-held occluder or looking through the fingers of their occluding hand. Having the parent point to the letters may be helpful.

School-aged children are similarly tested with Snellen number or letter charts.

Responses to testing for visual acuity are also functions of attention, cooperation, intelligence, and motivation. Children frequently tire of the testing. To help avoid this effect, testing of each eye should begin with the 20/50 line. In retesting, test the poorer eye first.

In addition to testing visual acuity, the following examinations should be done:

- Observe the ocular structures: note ocular comfort, ocular symmetry, lid position, form, and symmetry, lash direction, tear film symmetry, whiteness of the conjunctiva and sclera, and corneal size and clarity.
- Test ocular alignment as described under Strabismus in this chapter.
- With the penlight, observe the pupillary sizes, equality, and reactions.
- With the ophthalmoscope, observe each fundal red reflex. Any opacity of the optical pathway will obstruct this red reflex. The optic nerves, retinal vessels, and maculae should be observed. This is difficult or impossible through the undilated pupil of an uncooperative youngster and is not as critical to screening as the aforementioned portions of the examination.

Management

Referral for ophthalmologic evaluation is indicated for the entities listed in Table 1. The frequency of asymptomatic ocular pathology in these conditions is high enough to warrant full ocular examination.

Children not demonstrating age-appropriate visual behavior or acuity (Table 2) should be referred to the ophthalmologist, as should children with significant ocular signs or symptoms.

The ophthalmologist will diagnose the condition and institute appropriate therapy. For many conditions early referral has great prognostic implication. For example, monocular congenital cataract if treated in the neonatal period has a far better visual prognosis than if removed after the first month or two of life. Many systemic conditions present with ocular symptoms or signs, and the ophthalmologist and pediatrician should coordinate diagnostic and treatment regimens.

Amblyopia is treated, after best correcting any underlying ocular condition, by forcing the patient to use the amblyopic eye by occluding the fellow eye. Early diagnosis is of prognostic significance. Amblyopia is more easily reversed in the young. Proper educational placement of children with low vision

TABLE 2. VISUAL ACUITY INDICATIONS FOR REFERRAL (CRITERIA FOR EITHER EYE)

Infants and Toddlers
 Poor fixation or following behavior
 Nystagmus or random purposeless eye movements
 Avoidance movements

Preschool
 All the above
 E, letter-matching, or picture charts
  Any age: a difference of more than one line between the two eyes
  3 year old: less than 20/40
  4 year old: less than 20/30
  5 year old: less than 20/30

School Age
 Snellen number or letter charts
  Any age: difference of more than one line between the two eyes
  6 year old: less than 20/30
  7 year old and older: less than 20/20

should be coordinated by pediatrician, ophthalmologist, and educators.

STRABISMUS

The early detection of strabismus by pediatricians is both challenging and rewarding. It has been estimated that 3–4% of children have strabismus. Unrecognized strabismus may result in (1) failure to diagnose serious ocular and neurologic pathology, (2) amblyopia, (3) permanent loss of binocular function, (4) abnormal head positions, resulting in secondary musculoskeletal changes, and (5) cosmetic problems with psychologic sequelae.

Definition

Strabismus (Gr. *strabismos* to squint) is the term for ocular misalignment. Strabismus exists if both eyes are not directed to the object of conscious regard. Such misalignment may (1) be horizontal, vertical, or torsional, (2) be congenital or acquired, (3) be constant or intermittent, (4) be limited to one eye, or the viewing eye may alternate, (5) change with viewing distance, (6) be present only in certain positions of gaze, or (7) change with gaze.

Ocular alignment is described in a nomenclature consisting of a prefix and suffix (Table 3, Figs. 1 and 2). Deviations remaining relatively constant in various gaze positions are *comitant*, while those which change with gaze are termed *incomitant*.

Etiologies of Strabismus

Ocular alignment is influenced by anatomic and physiologic factors. These include orbital anatomy and ocular position within the orbits, supranuclear control of cranial nerve tone to the extraocular muscles, and a CNS binocular fusional viewing feedback mechanism. Near viewing stimulates the obligatory synkinetic triad of (1) *accommodation*—focusing by increasing the power of the lens, (2) *convergence*, and (3) *pupillary constriction*. A balance of accommodation and accommodative-convergence maintains alignment at near.

Any dysfunction of these alignment mechanisms, if uncompensated, results in a strabismus. If the compensation is intermittent, so will be the strabismus. Compensation may require effort and be compromised by illness, fatigue, or stress.

The etiology of most strabismus, although unknown, is presumed to be dysfunction of motor or sensory central nervous system control of ocular alignment. Strabismus due to deficiency in specific alignment factors, such as cranial nerve palsy, myasthenia gravis, or orbital structural abnormality, occurs with much lower frequency.

Differential Diagnosis
History. Because of its possible intermittency, any history of ocular deviation should be carefully regarded. In general parents and relatives are reliable observers.

TABLE 3. STRABISMUS NOMENCLATURE

Prefix		Suffix		Examples	
Ortho:	eyes straight	*Phoria:*	tendency to turn, but	Esotropia:	eye involved turns in
Eso:	eye turns in		eyes are straight	Exophoria:	eye has tendency to
Exo:	eye turns out		when used together		turn out but eyes are
Hyper:	eye turns up		(latent deviation)		straight when used
Hypo:	eye turns down	*Tropia:*	eye is deviated (manifest deviation)		together

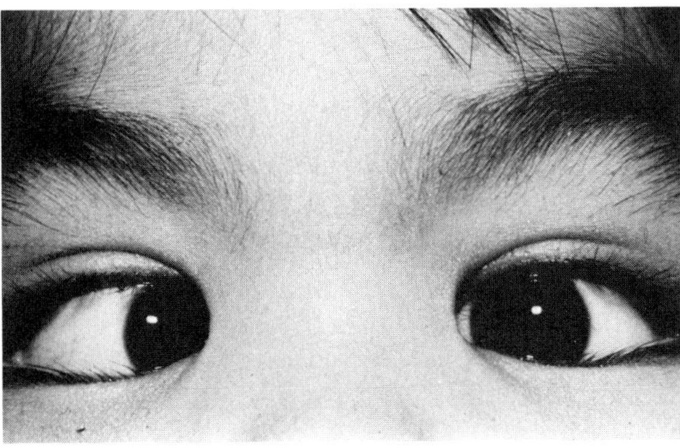

Figure 1. Esotropia. Left eye viewing, right eye deviated inward.

Questions helpful in evaluation include:

- Developmental history—children with problems in supranuclear tone or other cranial pathology have a higher likelihood of strabismus.
- Is there a family history of ocular deviation? Many of the conditions associated with strabismus have a familial predisposition, including orbital anatomy, ocular muscle tone, refractive errors, and binocular functioning.
- What is the nature of the deviation? The pseudoepicanthic fold produced by immature development of the nasal bridge in most infants covers a variable portion of the medial sclera. This may present an esotropic appearance (pseudoesotropia) as more sclera is visible laterally (Fig. 3). A clue to this condition is a history of apparent worsening in side gaze, at which time the medial sclera is further covered.
- Is the deviation constant or intermittent? If intermittent, when does it occur? Is the deviation present now? Avoid false reassurance as an intermittent esotropia may not be present at the time of examination even though an esotropic appearance is found due to a pseudoesotropia. Intermittent strabismus may be present only with stress, fatigue, or illness.
- When was the deviation first observed? Any

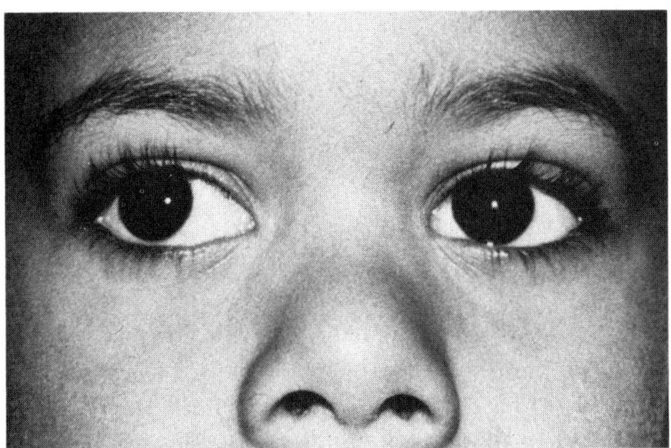

Figure 2. Exotropia. Left eye viewing, right eye deviated outward.

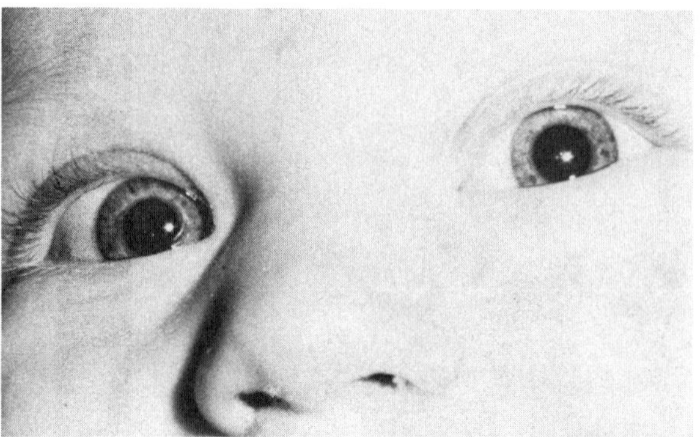

Figure 3. Pseudoesotropia. Ocular alignment is normal. The broad nasal bridge and epicanthic folds create the illusion of an right esotropia as no sclera is visible nasally in the right eye.

constant ocular deviation at any age, even in the neonate, is of significance. Until muscular visual development occurs, between 2 and 5 months, transitory convergent and divergent deviation may be noted. Bell's phenomenon of upward and outward rotation when the eyelids are forcibly elevated may be mistaken for a strabismus in the very young. Once past the age of binocular development any deviation, even transient, is of significance when the child is ocularly attentive. Certain patterns of ocular deviation have a propensity for development at certain ages. Accommodative esotropia frequently presents in mid to late infancy, whereas intermittent exotropia appears more often around age 3 years.

- Does the child complain of diplopia? Is it horizontal, vertical, torsional, or some combination of these? Is it greater in certain fields of gaze, at distance or near? As children through early school age have adaptive mechanisms to avoid diplopia in longstanding strabismus, diplopia should be considered evidence of a recently acquired deviation. Attention should therefore be focused on cranial nerve, myoneural junction, or local orbital problems.

Physical Examination. With the child comfortably seated—with infants this is best in mother's lap—observations of (1) ocular alignment, (2) head postures, (3) epicanthic folds, (4) lid symmetry, and (5) ocular rotations are made. Visually interesting objects are presented at both near and far distances. Intermittent exotropia may be found only at far distance and accommodative esotropia only at near. For near observation a small toy or picture requiring detailed viewing to stimulate accommodation is preferred over a simple light source or large object.

The corneal light reflex test, although yielding both false positives and false negatives, is a useful and rapid means of assessing ocular alignment in the young child. The image of a penlight reflected from the cornea should appear almost centered on each pupil. Decentration indicates a tropia: outward decentration indicates esotropia; inward decentration indicates exotropia (Figs. 1 and 2).

The initial portions of the examination should be rapidly performed, as young children fatigue easily.

Visual acuity should next be carefully assessed as outlined above. Decreased acuity may be the cause (loss of binocular feedback) or result (amblyopia) of a strabismus. The cover test yields a more accurate assessment of ocular alignment than simple observation or corneal reflex testing, as it directly tests visual direction. With the child fixating on an object, covering one eye should produce no ocular movement of the fellow eye. If movement of the fellow eye occurs to take up fixation, a heterotropia is present. Outward movement of the noncovered eye indicates an esotropia, inward movement an exotropia (Fig. 4). Test both eyes at far and near distances in this manner.

To elicit heterophorias, binocularity must be interrupted. This is accomplished by covering one eye while the other is fixating on a target. The cover is then quickly switched to the fixating eye while any movement of the previously covered eye is noted. Alternating the cover from one eye to the other, while insuring fixating with the uncovered eye before switching, is known as the alternate cover test. Fixation movements outward indicate an esodeviation; inward an exodeviation. If the prior cover test was normal, a heterophoria exists (Fig. 5).

The cover test and alternate cover test should be performed with the head straight and the eyes in primary position. Certain incomitant deviations may be missed if the examination is performed with the child using a compensatory head posture.

Management

A history suggestive of intermittent strabismus or the demonstration of strabismus is reason for ophthalmologic referral.

The ophthalmologist will measure visual acuity, quantitate the deviation with the use of prisms, check rotations, assess the degree of comitancy, test the binocular status, uncover refractive causes of decreased acuity or accommodative misalignment, and rule out other ocular pathology.

The treatment of strabismus is directed toward (1) attaining the best individual ocular function, (2) possible restoration of binocular vision, and (3) cosmesis.

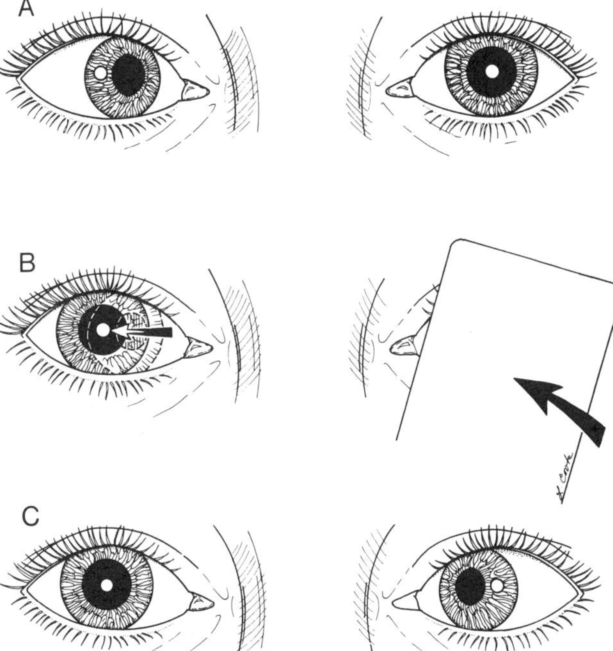

Figure 4. Heterotropia detection (example: esotropia). A. Esotropia with left eye viewing. Right eye turned in. B. Cover test: covering the viewing left eye results in an outward refixation movement of the right eye. C. Upon uncovering the left eye, the right eye maintains fixation; an alternating esotropia is present. (If upon uncovering the left eye an immediate return to left viewing (A) occurs, a right esotropia exists, and amblyopia of the right eye should be suspected.)

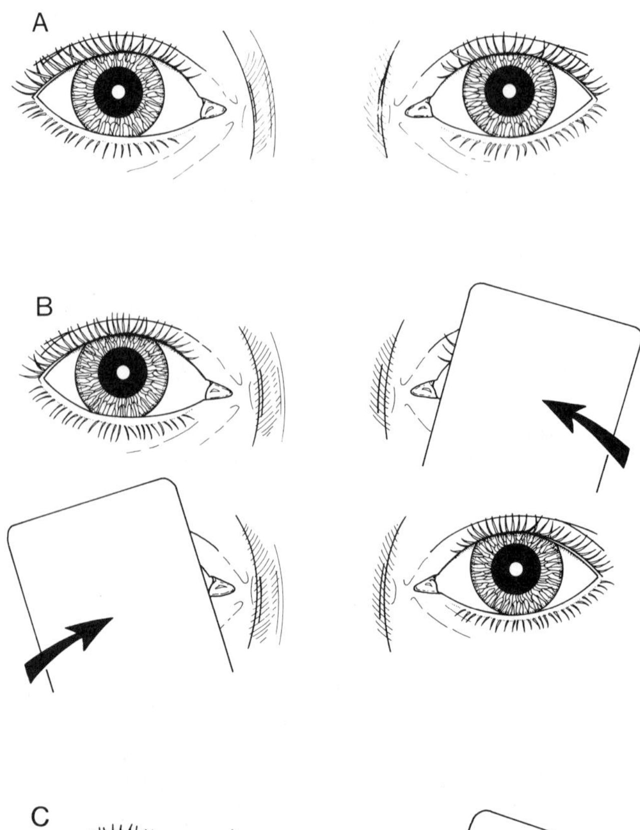

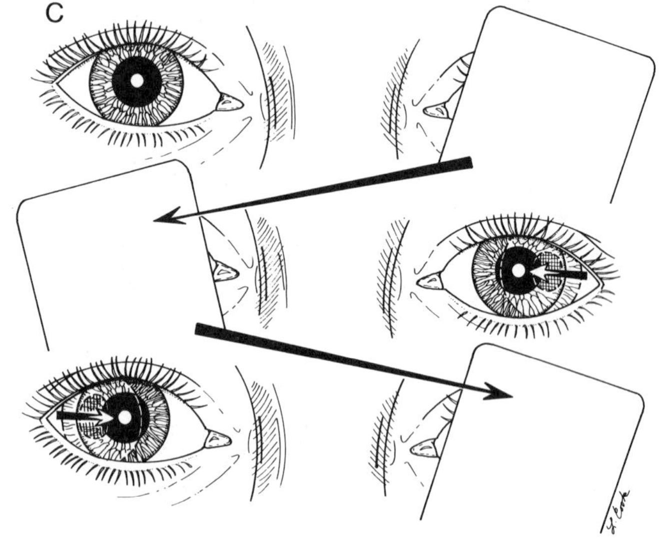

Figure 5. Heterophoria detection (example: exophoria) A. Ocular alignment appears normal. B. Cover test: covering either eye elicits no refixation movement of the fellow eye; therefore, no heterotropia is present. C. Alternate cover test: rapidly switching the cover from one eye to the other reveals inward refixation movement of the uncovered eye. The eye under cover had deviated outward; exodeviation exists. As no heterotropia is present (B) an exophoria exists.

Best individual ocular function is attained by correction of refractive errors, underlying pathology, and amblyopia. The child who freely alternates, thereby intermittently stimulating each eye, usually does not develop amblyopia. Amblyopia occurs in a strabismic setting if one eye is suppressed to avoid diplopia and visual confusion. Stimulation of an amblyopic eye by patching the fellow eye may reverse the process. The younger the patient, the more complete and rapid the response. By approximately 9 years of age, the visual pathways are fully developed, and the visual acuity is stable at whatever level has been achieved.

Restoration of binocularity is possible in the very young or in older children if they once possessed binocularity. Management is dependent upon the etiologic mechanism. Presumed abnormal supranuclear tonus, as present in congenital esotropia, requires surgical weakening (recession) or strengthening (resection) of the extraocular muscles. The obligatory accommodative-convergence of a farsighted child is relieved with plus (convex) lenses. Children with an overactive accommodative-convergence mechanism who manifest an esotropia at near are often helped by bifocals, which alleviate the need to accommodate. Anticholinesterase drops, such as phospholine iodide, lessen the accommodation but are more useful for diagnosis than long-term treatment. Eye exercises have a limited role in strabismic care. Exercises may strengthen convergence ability, helping keep the eyes straight in patients with convergence insufficiency.

Cosmetic considerations in patients with strabismus are important. Strabismic children may avoid direct eye contact as a response to the difficulty of others in establishing eye contact with them. This, coupled with peer teasing, frequently results in a poor self-image and other psychologic problems. Cosmetic surgery is indicated to avoid these sequelae.

Compensatory head postures may be corrected with extraocular muscle surgery. The position of fusion may be shifted to the head-straight posture by extraocular muscle realignment.

Incomitant deviations may be caused by nonparalytic ocular fibrosis or retraction syndromes or may herald a cranial nerve palsy, myoneurojunctional dysfunction, such as myasthenia gravis, or orbital problem. The presence of diplopia indicates an acquired etiology. The pediatrician and ophthalmologist should, in concert, evaluate and manage systemic conditions leading to strabismus.

PERIOCULAR AND OCULAR TRAUMA

Ocular trauma occurs all too frequently. The need for ocular protection for certain activities, such as racket sports or school workshops, should be emphasized by all who are providing pediatric care.

The pediatrician is often the first physician consulted after an ocular injury and must be able to assess the injury and determine if ophthalmologic consultation is necessary. Certain emergency measures may prove sightsaving.

Definition
Ocular trauma is injury inflicted upon the eye and periocular structures.

Classification and Etiologies of Periocular and Ocular Trauma
Ocular trauma may be usefully divided into major categories based upon the nature of the trauma (Table 4). Much overlap exists in the produced sequelae, depending on the severity of the trauma.

Diplopia, loss of full ocular rotations, or enophthalmos (do not be fooled by pseudoenophthalmos secondary to lid swelling) may indicate a fracture of the orbital wall with muscle entrapment. Skull x-rays with sinus views should be obtained. Tissue incarce-

TABLE 4. OCULAR TRAUMA

Blunt Trauma	**Lacerations**
Lid	Lid
Ecchymosis	Conjunctiva
Orbit	Cornea or sclera
Blowout fractures	Nonperforating
Globe	Perforating
Subconjunctival hemorrhage	**Foreign Bodies**
Hyphema	Extraocular
Iritis	Intraocular
Lens problems: cataract, dislocation	**Chemical Injuries and Burns**
Vitreous hemorrhage	Chemical
Retinal problems: edema, scarring, tears, detachment	Thermal
Optic nerve dysfunction	Ultraviolet
Abrasions	
Lid	
Cornea	

rated in and swelling about an orbital floor fracture may be seen as a teardrop sign in the superior maxillary sinus, or clouding of the sinus may be the only x-ray finding (Fig. 6). Other causes of traumatic diplopia should be investigated.

Hyphema, blood in the anterior chamber, is generally produced by a significant blow to the globe (Fig. 7). It may, especially in patients with sickle cell disease or trait, cause a dangerous rise in intraocular pressure. Visual acuity is usually decreased. An injury sufficient to produce a hyphema frequently damages other intraocular structures, such as the iris, filtration angle, lens, and retina. Rebleeding after apparent clearing or improvement may occur, usually 3–5 days after initial trauma. Damage to the filtration angle may produce glaucoma even years later. Retinal dialyses may also be a late sequela of such injuries.

Traumatic iritis, an inflammatory process in the anterior segment, should be suspected if a ciliary flush (see Periocular and Ocular Inflammation) is present. Pain and photophobia are present. Visual acuity is usually decreased.

Diminution of the red reflex after blunt trauma indicates some opacification of the optical media, such as hyphema, iritis, cataract, or vitreous hemorrhage.

Central retinal injury results in decreased acuity. Floaters, flashing lights, and a peripheral curtain in the visual field are symptoms associated with peripheral retinal trauma.

Trauma to the optic nerve will be signaled by visual and pupillary abnormalities.

Differential Diagnosis

History. Certain questions are helpful in evaluating and caring for ocular trauma.

- How did the injury occur? The how, when, where, and why of the trauma must be recorded, as it may become part of a legal proceeding.
- What was the nature of the traumatizing material, its composition, and the velocity of the impact? These factors obviously determine likely sequelae. In addition to ocular injury, large objects may damage intracranial, facial, and dental structures. Small, high-velocity missiles may produce ocular penetration without obvious traumatic external signs. Foreign bodies are more common with particulate or fragmenting materials.

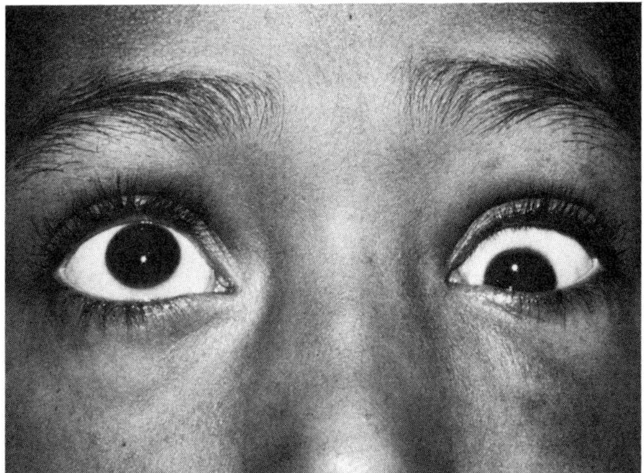

A

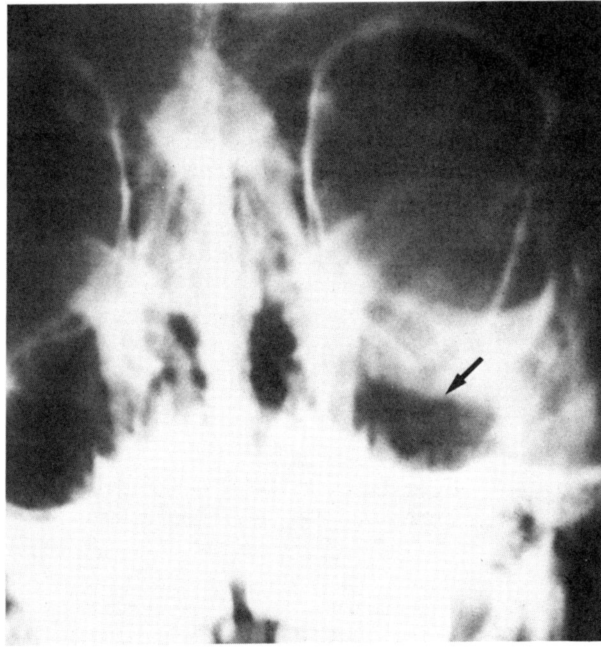

B

Figure 6. Blowout fracture. Left orbital floor. A. Tissue incarcerated in fracture prevents elevation of left eye. B. X-ray demonstrating the fracture with tissue incarceration (arrow).

The nature of the material producing a corneal abrasion determines the pathogens introduced.

- What hurts, and how much does it hurt? Corneal abrasions and intraocular injuries usually produce moderate to severe ocular pain. Abrasions usually produce a foreign body sensation, especially with lid movement. Concomitant facial and dental trauma should not be missed.
- With blunt trauma, a careful neurologic history must be obtained. With significant

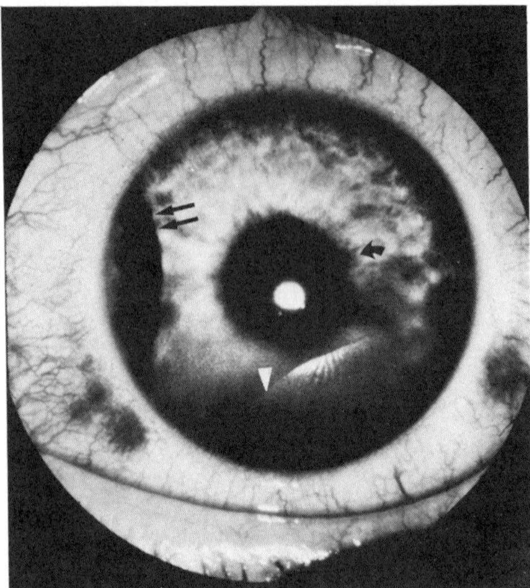

Figure 7. Hyphema. Note blood layered out inferiorly in the anterior chamber (white arrowhead), clot in the anterior chamber (double arrows), and irregular pupil due to a tear of the iris sphincter (curved arrow).

ocular trauma, serious neurologic sequelae may be overlooked.

- Is diplopia present? Diplopia may be produced by (1) orbital fracture, (2) hematoma of the orbit or extraocular muscles, (3) palsy of the third, fourth, or sixth cranial nerves at either an orbital or intracranial site, (4) damage to extraocular muscles, (5) intracranial skew deviation, or (6) decompensation of a preexisting ocular phoria, becoming a tropia. Rarely, monocular diplopia may be produced by subluxation of the lens or retinal edema or detachment.
- What is the past ophthalmic history? Avoid the pitfall of assuming that ocular dysfunction is secondary to the trauma. Poor visual acuity after an injury may be caused by the absence of spectacles which broke at the time of the injury. Poor acuity, strabismus, ptosis, or even proptosis may have antedated the trauma. Eyedrops beings used

before the trauma may produce dramatic pupillary changes.
- When did the child last eat? A patient with ocular trauma should not be fed until assessment has shown that no emergency surgery is required.

Physical Examination. Any periocular or ocular trauma should be assessed with a complete eye examination, as outlined in the first section of this chapter. Even seemingly minor lid lacerations may be associated with serious underlying ocular injury. The examination should include neurologic, facial, and dental structures when indicated.

An accurate measurement of visual acuity is of paramount importance, as it assesses the integrity of many components of the visual system. An attempt should be made to test acuity even if the lid is grossly swollen. First, try without forcibly opening the lid, as only a slip opening is necessary for acuity assessment. For painful conditions, such as corneal abrasions, which prevent lid opening a drop of a topical ocular anesthetic, e.g., proparacaine HCl 0.5%, may be safely employed to facilitate the examination. Any force required to open the lid should not transmit pressure to a possibly perforated globe. Commercially available lid speculum or lid retractors fashioned from paperclips should be employed. Acuity assessment of the fellow eye should be recorded.

Certain features of the complete examination require close scrutiny when evaluating ocular trauma.

Lids. The positions of the inner and outer lid fissures should be assessed, since the ligaments that hold them in place can be avulsed or disrupted. Integrity of the lid margins is vital to the critical function of tear distribution and is of particular cosmetic concern. The proximal lacrimal drainage system lies superficially and is easily traumatized. Therefore, any lid trauma medial to the lacrimal puncta requires careful ophthalmologic evaluation.

The Globe. The corneas, sclerae, anterior chambers, and pupils must be carefully examined. Perforation may be obvious if the globe is collapsed. More frequently, however, a perforation presents with a small bit of uveal tissue plugging the site. This usually appears as a small brown mound and should not be mistaken for a foreign body (Fig. 8).

The roundness, centricity, and reactivity of the pupils should be checked. Iris plugging a corneal perforation may cause pupillary distortion (Fig. 8). Direct trauma to the iris and anterior segment may produce either mydriasis or miosis. Other causes of anisocoria after trauma include intraorbital trauma to the ciliary nerves or ganglia, Horner's syndrome, and intracranial third-nerve palsy.

If the globe is intact, the conjunctiva is examined for the presence of foreign bodies.

The cornea is carefully examined for disruptions of the epithelium (abrasions). If a corneal abrasion is suspected and not seen with a penlight, a wetted fluorescein strip is touched to the inferior conjunctiva after instillation of a drop of anesthetic. After a few minutes to allow lacrimal washout, the cornea is examined, preferably with a blue light. The area of an abrasion will retain the fluorescein. Instillation of too much fluorescein or failure to wait for lacrimal washout will cause pooling of the flourescein on an intact corneal epithelium and may be mistaken for an abrasion.

The anterior chamber should be checked for the presence of blood (hyphema) (Fig. 7). In an upright patient, blood frequently layers out inferiorly. In a supine patient, it may produce only a pinkish coloration in front of the iris.

The quality and equality of the red reflex should be noted. It can be diminished by corneal, anterior chamber, lenticular, and vitreous abnormalities. A funduscopic examination is then performed.

Ocular Alignment and Rotations. A careful check of ocular alignment and rotations will help differentiate the etiology of traumatic diplopia. In some patients diplopia can only be elicited by checking ocular rotations, for it may not be present in primary position.

Laboratory Aids. X-rays of the orbital region are useful in fracture and foreign body diagnosis. The Caldwell and Waters views are preferred for orbital wall detail. An orbital wall fracture or tissue incarcerated in the fracture may be seen (Fig. 6B). Clouding of the maxillary sinus may be the only roentgenographic abnormality seen with orbital floor fracture. Hypocycloidal polytomography may further detail the fracture. The radiodensity of a foreign body determines the usefulness of x-ray for detection and localization. Computerized tomography is useful for accurate foreign body localization.

Ultrasound techniques are useful in ocular assessment when a cloudy media prevents visualization of the posterior pole, such as with a large hyphema or cataract. Lens dis-

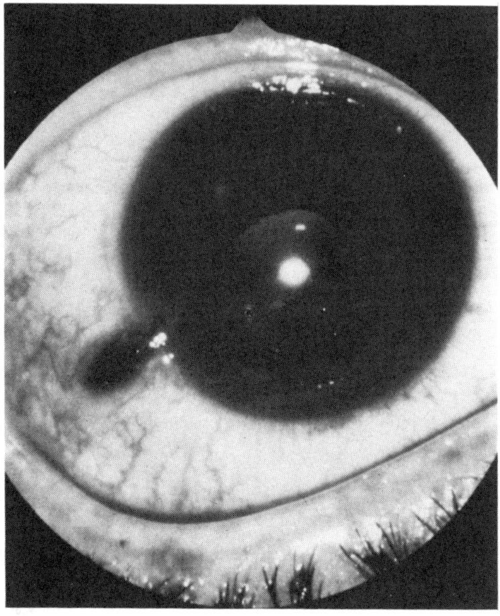

Figure 8. Ruptured globe. Iris prolapse through the corneoscleral wound distorts the pupil.

location, retinal detachment, and intraocular foreign body can be detected by ultrasound.

Management

A management plan is formulated following the determination of the nature and severity of injury. The pediatrician may elect to treat ecchymoses, superficial foreign bodies, abrasions, and lacerations not involving vital structures.

All patients with decreased acuity require ophthalmologic referral. Even with superficial corneal abrasion, referral may be indicated if there is any doubt about associated injuries.

Immediate measures for certain conditions may be necessary. The following guidelines for the assessment and treatment of ocular trauma are recommended.

Blunt Trauma. Lid swelling and ecchymosis may be managed with cold compresses for the first 24 hours and then warm compresses as necessary. Inform the parents that the ecchymosis may spread to adjacent areas.

Subconjunctival hemorrhage does not require therapy. Reassurance should be given that it will clear over a period of several weeks.

Abrasions. Treatment of corneal abrasions is directed toward relieving the ocular discomfort and prevention of infection. An antibiotic drop, such as 10% sulfacetamide, is instilled and a pressure patch is applied (Fig. 9). A pressure patch is created by placing two eye pads over the closed lid, placing one side of a 6-inch piece of paper tape on the central forehead, and applying the other end to a raised cheek. The cheek returning to its normal position tightens the tape. Three or four additional pieces of tape are applied between the same two points in a similar fashion, curv-

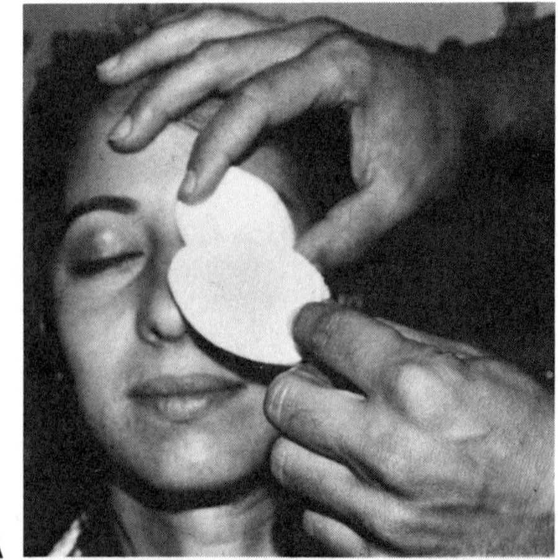

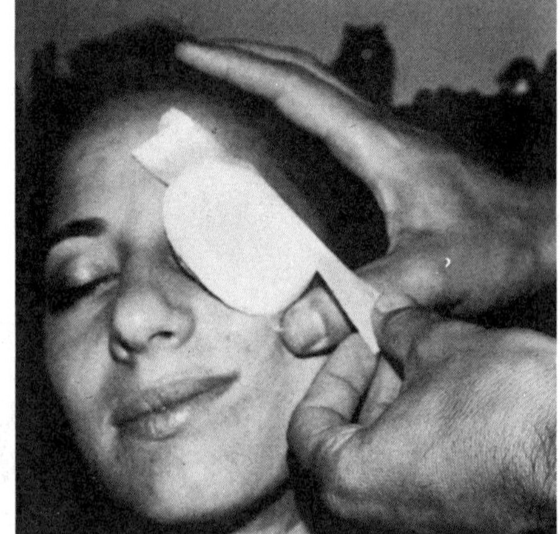

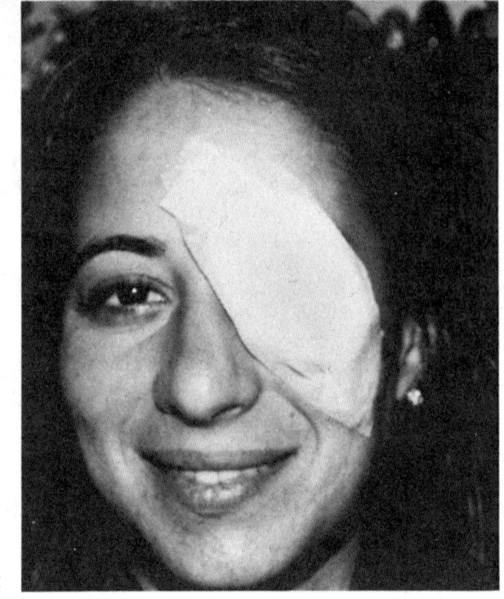

Figure 9. Pressure patch. A, B, C. Steps in application.

ing to cover the pads. This tight dressing prevents continued rubbing of the cornea by eliminating blinking of the lid.

The dressing should be removed the following day, and the abrasion should be reassessed. Symptomatic improvement, improved or stable visual acuity, and continued corneal clarity indicate satisfactory progress. If the abrasion persists, treatment with an antibiotic drop and pressure patch is again employed. This process should be continued daily until resolution. Unless there is progressive daily improvement, ophthalmogic referral is indicated.

A local anesthetic should *never* be given to the patient, as its chronic use leads to serious corneal injury.

Lacerations. If vital structures, such as the lid margin, lacrimal system, or globe, are involved, ophthalmologic referral is necessary.

Certain measures are indicated while awaiting consultation. Tetanus toxoid should be given as indicated. Lid lacerations, with an intact globe, should be irrigated with normal saline for cleansing and to remove foreign material. Moist saline soaks should be used to prevent tissue dehydration.

If penetration of the globe is suspected, an eye shield (not a patch) should be placed. The shield must rest on bony structures, not the eye. Prophylactic, systemic, high-dose, intravenous, broad-spectrum antibiotics, such as a cephalosporin or ampicillin and oxacillin, should be instituted. Tetanus toxoid is given as indicated. The patient should remain NPO pending ophthalmologic evaluation.

Foreign Bodies. Superficial foreign bodies are common. They usually present acutely with a painful sensation. The presence of a foreign body beneath the lid should be suspected when multiple or vertical corneal abrasions are noted. Corneal foreign bodies present much as corneal abrasions. A retained conjunctival foreign body may present with chronic ocular irritation.

Conjunctival and superficial corneal foreign bodies may be removed with irrigation or a moistened applicator. The use of a lid speculum and a drop of local anesthetic will facilitate the process. Metallic corneal foreign bodies often produce a rust ring about them and should be referred to an ophthalmologist. If the foreign body is deep or not easily removed, referral is indicated. In the interim, an antibiotic drop should be instilled.

Intraocular foreign bodies should be managed as described for perforating lacerations of the globe.

Chemical Injuries and Burns. Chemical burns are true ocular emergencies. Acid often coagulates protein, which limits its penetration. Alkali burns penetrate deeply, producing disastrous results. For any chemical injury, copious irrigation with water or saline should be instituted immediately. Local anesthetic drops and a lid speculum are useful in overcoming blepharospasm. Extension tubing from a hanging IV bottle makes an excellent nozzle. Irrigate with 1–2 liters of fluid over 20 minutes. Do not attempt to neutralize acids with alkalis or vice versa, as the heat produced by the chemical reaction is destructive. Following irrigation, a search for foreign material is made. Ophthalmologic referral is indicated.

Protected by the lids and moist ocular surface, the globes are relatively resistant to thermal burns. When the lashes are intact, the globes are rarely involved. The conjunctiva should be checked for foreign bodies and irrigated if necessary. The loose periocular tissues are frequently affected by thermal burns and burn edema. Subsequent retraction of the lids with exposure of the globe may occur and require frequent lubricating ointments. Temporary suturing of the lids (tarsorraphy) by an ophthalmologist may be indicated for corneal exposure.

Ultraviolet radiation, such as produced by a sunlamp, may cause intense ocular pain. Symptoms typically present 6–12 hours after exposure when superficial corneal erosion occurs. A cycloplegic drop, such as 1% cyclopentolate, an antibiotic drop, and a pressure patch (Fig. 9) usually lead to resolution in 12–36 hours.

PERIOCULAR AND OCULAR INFLAMMATION

Careful attention to the history, clinical setting, symptoms, signs, and therapeutic response of periocular and ocular inflammation will guide the pediatrician in the proper care of these conditions. Guidelines for the pediatrician to perform this analysis are presented in this section. The pediatrician may elect to care for many common inflammations; guidelines for this treatment are included in this section.

The improper early management of periocular and ocular inflammations may lead to serious sequelae. The ability of most pediatri-cians to examine the eye and surrounding structures fully is limited, and ophthalmologic referral is frequently indicated. A detailed discussion of the diagnosis and treatment of those conditions requiring referral is beyond the scope of this chapter.

Definition
An inflammatory response of ocular or periocular tissues may be caused by a host of infectious, immune, metabolic, and idiopathic conditions.

Classification and Etiologies of Periocular and Ocular Inflammation
Nontraumatic inflammation of the ocular and periocular structures is best categorized by site. The site of inflammation is of paramount diagnostic and management significance.

TABLE 5. PERIOCULAR AND OCULAR INFLAMMATIONS (NONTRAUMATIC) OF CHILDHOOD, INCLUDING COMMON ETIOLOGIC CONSIDERATIONS

Lids—Localized Inflammation
Blepharitis
  Seborrheic
  Eczematoid
  Infectious
    Bacterial: *Staphylococcus aureus*
    Viral: herpes simplex and herpes zoster, molluscum contagiosum
    Parasitic: mites and lice

Diffuse Periorbital and Orbital Inflammation
Periorbital (preseptal)
  Edema
    Allergic
      Insect bite
      Angioneurotic
      Local
    Parasitic: trichinella
    With systemic edematous conditions
    With contiguous sinusitis
  Cellulitis
    Bacterial: *S. aureus* (esp. posttraumatic), *Streptococcus pyogenes*, *Haemophilus influenzae*, *Peptococcus*, *Bacteroides*
    Viral: herpes simplex and herpes zoster, molluscum contagiosum

---

(*continued*)

Orbital
  Cellulitis
    Bacterial: *S. aureus, S. pyogenes, Streptococcus pneumoniae, H. influenzae*
    Mycotic: mucormycosis (acidotic or debilitated patient), *Candida albicans* (immunosuppressed)
  Pseudomotor
  Orbital myositis
  Infantile cortical hyperostosis
  Metabolic and endocrine
    Dysthyroid
    Acute glomerulonephritis
    Amyloid
  Tumor
    Nonneoplastic
      Hamartomas: vascular, lymphatic
      Choristomas: dermoids
      From contiguous structures: mucocele, encephalocele
      Orbital hemorrhage: hemophilia
      Parasitic cysts: *Echinococcus*
    Neoplastic
      Primary ocular
      Primary orbital
      Infiltrative: leukemia, lymphoma, histiocytosis
      Metastatic
      From contiguous structures: paranasal sinuses, bone, intracranial

Lacrimal Gland
Dacryoadenitis
  Viral: mumps, mononucleosis
  Bacterial: *S. aureus, S. pyogenes*
  Mycotic
  Sarcoidosis
  Neoplastic

Lacrimal Drainage System
Canaliculitis
  Viral: primary herpes simplex
  Bacterial: *S. aureus, S. pneumoniae,* arachnia propica
  Mycotic: *Actinomyces, Aspergillus, Candida*
  Toxic-pharmacologic: phospholine iodide
Dacryocystitis
  Bacterial: *S. pneumoniae, S. aureus, H. influenzae*
  Mycotic: *Aspergillus, C. albicans*

Conjunctiva
Conjunctivitis: See Tables 8, 9, and 10

Cornea
Superficial keratitis
  Infectious
    Viral: adenovirus, varicella, molluscum contagiosum, herpes simplex
    Chlamydial: trachoma, inclusion conjunctivitis
    Bacterial: with staphylococcal blepharitis, with many bacterial conjunctivitides
  Mechanical
    Lash
    Lid lesion
    Exposure

(*continued*)

Toxic-pharmacologic: idoxuridine, Ara-A
Neurotropic: (hypesthesia cranial nerve V)
Dry eye states
  Aqueous deficiency: decreased lacrimation
  Mucin deficiency: loss of conjunctival goblet cells secondary to generalized mucous membrane
    disorders (See Table 9)
Corneal ulcers
  Bacterial: *S. aureus, S. pneumoniae, Pseudomonas aeruginosa, Streptococcus epidermidis,* viridans
    streptococci, *Moraxella* sp., other Gram-negative rods
  Fungal: *Fusarium, Cephalosporium, Candida*
  Immune: herpes simplex, systemic immunologic dysfunction

Episclera and Sclera

Episcleritis
  Idiopathic
  Systemic immune diseases
  Viral: herpes zoster
  Gout
  Allergy
Scleritis
  Idiopathic
  Systemic immune disease: Behcet's syndrome, Wegener's granulomatosis, Takayasu's arterio-
    pathy, systemic lupus erythematosus, dermatomyositis
  Inflammatory bowel disease: regional enteritis, ulcerative colitis
  Metabolic: gout, porphyria, alkaptonuria, hypercalcemia, cystinosis
  Infections
    Viral: herpes zoster
    Bacterial: varied
  Allergic
  Erythema nodosum

Anterior Uveal Tract

Iritis
  Idiopathic
  Systemic immune disease: juvenile rheumatoid arthritis, ankylosing spondylitis, Behcet's syndrome
  Fuchs' heterochromic cyclitis
  Sarcoid
  Keratouveitis: adenovirus, herpes simplex, syphilis, tuberculosis, herpes zoster
  Viral: infectious mononucleosis, influenza
  With posterior uveitis

Posterior Inflammations

Vitritis, retinitis, choroiditis
  Viral: congenital and acquired cytomegalic inclusion disease, congenital herpes, congenital rubella
  Bacterial: tuberculosis, various in endophthalmitis
  Mycotic: *C. albicans,* histoplasmosis, coccidioidomycosis
  Parasitic: toxoplasmosis (esp. congenital), *Toxocara canis*
  Tumor: retinoblastoma, leukemia, lymphoma, reticulum cell sarcoma
  Metabolic: amyloid
  Idiopathic
Optic neuritis
  Demyelinative diseases: viral and postviral, multiple sclerosis, other primary metabolic types
  Contiguous inflammations: meninges, orbit, paranasal sinuses
  Granulomatous inflammations: sarcoidosis, tuberculosis, mycotic, syphilis
  Intraocular inflammations
  Metabolic: drugs, nutritional deficiencies, toxins

TABLE 6. DIAGNOSTIC CONSIDERATIONS IN NONTRAUMATIC PERIOCULAR AND OCULAR INFLAMMATION

Sign	Examine Further For	Diagnostic Considerations

Decreased visual acuity	Clarity of media
	  Corneal clarity
	  Red reflex and quality fundus image
	Pupillary reactions
	Optic nerve appearance
		Keratitis
		Intraocular inflammation
		  Iritis
		  Vitritis
		  Retinopathy
		Optic neuritis

Localized lid swelling	Site Mass Inflammatory signs Skin lesions Seborrhea, scalp Parasites, local	Blepharitis Hordeolum Chalazion

Diffuse lid swelling	Inflammatory signs
	Adenopathy
	Sinusitis
	Skin lesions
	  Antecedent trauma
	  Bites
	  Infection
	  Generalized rashes
	Dental infection
	Generalized edema
	Evidence of orbital inflammation
	  Proptosis
	  Restricted rotations
	  Marked chemosis
	  Pupillary abnormalities
		Periorbital (preseptal)
		  inflammation
		Orbital inflammation

Red eye
(conjunctival hyperemia)
	Evidence of intraocular inflammation
	  Decreased acuity
	  Photophobia, blepharospasm, tearing
	  Ocular pain
	  Ciliary flush
	  Pupillary abnormalities
	  Poor red reflex
	Discharge characteristics
	Lacrimal system infection
	Lid and lash abnormalities
	Diffuse skin and mucus
	Systemic disease
		Conjunctivitis
		Keratitis
		Episcleritis and scleritis
		Iritis
		Glaucoma, acute

Pupillary abnormality		Intraocular inflammation Optic nerve dysfunction Orbital inflammation Pharmacologic
Poor red reflex		Keratitis Intraocular inflammation Cataract

The major categories of nontraumatic periocular and ocular inflammations of childhood are listed in Tables 5 and 6.

Lids—Localized Inflammation.

Blepharitis. Inflammation of the lid margins is most commonly due to seborrheic, eczematoid, or infectious processes.

Seborrheic blepharitis is characterized by overactivity of sebaceous glands, producing marginal inflammation with greasy, scaly deposits. The deposits represent both sebum and epithelial debris. Examination of the scalp and retroauricular region often reveals a generalized seborrheic diathesis.

Infectious blepharitis is most commonly due to staphylococci. It may be primary or secondary to seborrheic or eczematoid involvement. Marginal inflammation and accumulations of material at the base of the cilia, collarettes, are characteristic. Concomitant conjunctivitis, occasionally phlyctenular, is frequent.

Molluscum contagiosum is an inflammatory mass presumably viral in origin. It usually presents as multiple, small, whitish, umbilicated firm papules. If the lid margin is involved, a significant chronic keratoconjunctivitis may occur.

Herpes simplex infection may affect the eyelids with vesicles, swelling, and erythema. Preauricular adenopathy is frequently found.

Crab lice and mites occasionally produce marginal irritation.

Hordeolum. This is an acute inflammation of the glands of the lid. Involvement of the tarsal meibomian glands, an internal hordeolum, usually represents a staphylococcal abscess. Infection of the superficial sebaceous and sweat glands at the lid margin produces an external hordeolum (stye), also commonly staphylococcal in origin.

Chalazion. This is a granulomatous, usually nontender inflammation of a meibomian gland (Fig. 10).

Diffuse Periorbital (Preseptal) and Orbital Inflammation. The differentiation of periorbital (preseptal) from orbital (postseptal) inflammation is critical for proper diagnosis and management.

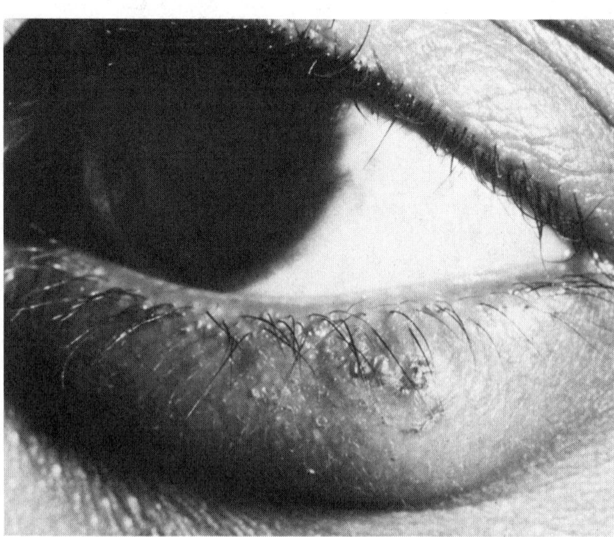

Figure 10. Chalazion.

The orbital septum is a fibrous membrane arising from the periocular periosteum and attaching to various lid structures superficial to the conjunctiva. It separates the skin and subcutaneous tissues from the intraorbital structures. The septum acts as a barrier to inflammatory processes, preventing them from entering the orbit.

Signs of orbital inflammation include marked conjunctival swelling (chemosis), proptosis, and limitation of ocular rotations (Fig. 11). The process may affect the globe, producing intraocular inflammation. It may also affect intraorbital vessels and nerves, producing optic neuritis, corneal hyperthesia, and pupillary abnormalities. Pain on ocular movement and diplopia are often noted. These signs and symptoms are not found with preseptal inflammations. A CT scan may be helpful if the localization of the inflammation is in doubt.

Periorbital (Preseptal) Inflammation. Preseptal lid swelling results from a number of inflammatory processes (Table 5). It may be associated with systemic (e.g., nephrotic syndrome) or angioneurotic edemas. Inflammation may also be caused by local toxins (e.g.,

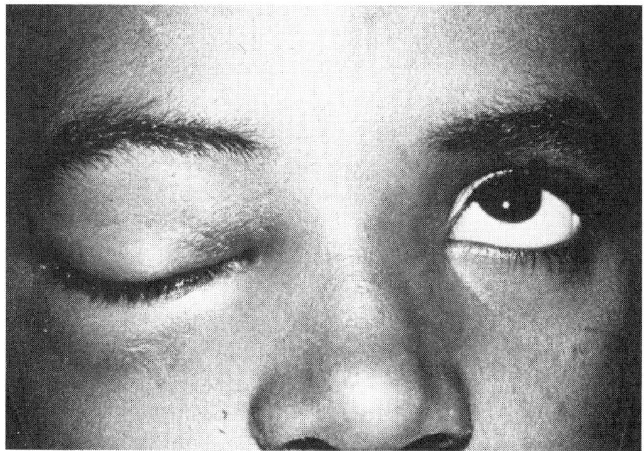

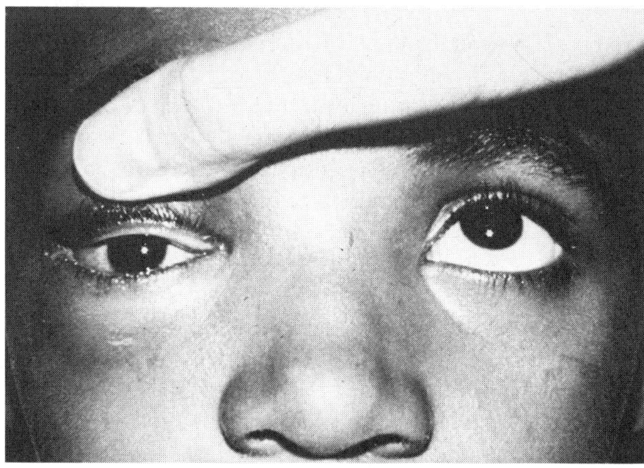

Figure 11. Orbital cellulitis. A. Right lid erythematous and swollen shut. B. Failure of elevation of right eye due to orbital inflammation.

contact dermatitis or insect bite), contiguous inflammatory processes (e.g., sinusitis), parasitic infestations (e.g., trichinosis), or an infectious cellulitis.

Preseptal cellulitis may be secondary to conjunctivitis, local skin infection (e.g., impetigo, herpes) or gland infection (e.g., hordeolum), antecedent trauma, or hematogenous spread. The lid is warm, red, and tender. Mild to moderate conjunctival swelling with a mucoid to purulent discharge may be present. The temperature is usually normal or slightly elevated. The white blood count is usually mildly elevated. Signs of orbital involvement, such as marked chemosis, pain on rotations, limited rotations, and proptosis, are absent.

Preseptal cellulitis secondary to antecedent trauma or contiguous skin infection is most commonly due to *Staphylococcus aureus* and occasionally to anaerobes.

Without antecedent trauma, *S. aureus* group A, *Streptococcus pyogenes*, and *Haemophilus influenzae* are common. *H. influenzae* is more common between 6 months and 4 years and may produce a characteristic, sharply demarcated, purple coloration. Erysipelas may be found with group A streptococcus.

Microbiologic work-up should include gram stains and cultures of any drainage material. Blood cultures are indicated. In severe cases, needling of the preseptal space may be indicated to obtain a culture. Instillation and aspiration of unpreserved saline is employed if pus is not obtained. Utmost care must be exercised to avoid septal penetration when needling.

Orbital Inflammation. Knowledge of the etiology of an orbital inflammatory process is imperative for proper management. The history and physical examination will limit the differential diagnosis (Table 5).

Orbital cellulitis presents as an acute inflammatory process, usually associated with a high fever in a child who appears ill. Signs of orbital involvement include marked conjunctival swelling, proptosis, and limitation of ocular rotations (Fig. 11). Marked swelling, redness, heat, and tenderness are often present. Contiguous paranasal sinusitis or antecedent trauma penetrating the orbital septum are the most common etiologies. Less frequently, posterior extension of a preseptal cellulitis, hematogenous spread, dental abscess, or a contiguous osteomyelitis is responsible.

Laboratory studies should include a CBC and blood cultures. Microbiologic stains and cultures of any drainage should be obtained. X-rays of the paranasal sinuses and orbits and CT scans are usually indicated.

S. aureus is the most common pathogen in posttraumatic orbital cellulitis. *S. aureus, S. pyogenes, Streptococcus pneumoniae,* and *H. influenzae* (especially in young children) are most common with contiguous sinusitis. Anaerobes, Gram-negative aerobes, and fungi (especially in immunosuppressed, acidotic, and debilitated children) are occasionally causative.

Complications of orbital cellulitis include cavernous sinus thrombosis, optic neuritis, central retinal artery occlusion, and subperiosteal, subdural, and brain abscesses. With current antimicrobial therapy these complications have become less common.

Orbital pseudotumor is an inflammatory orbital process which is often misdiagnosed as a cellulitis. It may be unilateral or bilateral. Patients typically have the onset of periocular pain, swelling (especially early morning), chemosis, conjunctival injection, and restricted ocular rotations. Photophobia, diplopia, pain on motion, iritis, and proptosis may be present. The inflammatory reaction and systemic findings are usually less than with an orbital cellulitis. Sinus x-rays are usually clear, an important distinguishing feature. The course is more chronic than with orbital cellulitis and may be recurrent.

The Red Eye, Nontraumatic Ocular Inflammation: Conjunctivitis, Keratitis, Episcleritis and Scleritis, and Iritis. The nontraumatized red eye is very commonly encountered in pediatric practice. The vast majority of these patients have a conjunctivitis. Conjunctivitis is so common that all too often other serious inflammatory states are overlooked. Attention to the patient's symptoms and signs will prevent this pitfall. Conjunctival inflammation occurs with keratitis (corneal inflammation), episcleritis and scleritis, and iritis (inflammation of the anterior uveal tract). Deeper inflammation, therefore, must be ruled out even though conjunctivitis is present. Based on the history and examination, a differentiation can usually be made (Table 7). If any doubt exists, a slitlamp examination is indicated.

Conjunctivitis. The conjunctival mucous membranes react to a diversity of stimuli with an inflammatory response (Tables 8 and 9, Fig. 12). Certain features of the inflammatory response are helpful with the differential diagnosis (Table 8, Fig. 13, Fig. 14).

TABLE 7. DIFFERENTIAL DIAGNOSIS OF THE RED EYE

	Conjunctivitis	Keratitis	Episcleritis and Scleritis	Iritis
Visual acuity	Normal	Normal to decreased	Normal	Minimal to markedly decreased
Pain	None to mild sandy sensation	None to moderately severe	None to mildly severe	Mild to markedly severe
Photophobia	None to mild	None to moderate	None to mild	Mild to severe
Vascular congestion	Superficial conjunctival vessels Discrete vessels Red Diffuse distribution Intense in fornices, fade to cornea Move with conjunctiva	Superficial conjunctival and ciliary flush	Vessels of episclera and sclera Less discrete vessels Pink Localized Bulbar Does not move with conjunctiva	Ciliary flush Not discrete Pink Circumcorneal Less to fornices Does not move with conjunctiva
Cornea	Clear	Involved, may stain with fluorescein	Clear	Usually clear, may have deposits on posterior surface
Pupil	Normal	Normal	Normal	May be abnormal, often smaller with diminished response
Discharge	Mucoid or purulent	Variable	None to mild and clear	Increased, clear

TABLE 8. DISTINGUISHING FEATURES OF CONJUNCTIVAL INFLAMMATION

Feature	Description	Common Etiologies
Papillae (Fig. 13)	Small mounds consisting of a central vessel surrounded by inflammatory cells	Subacute and chronic conjunctivitis, giant papillae, vernal, soft contact lenses
Follicles (Fig. 14)	Small mounds consisting of an avascular aggregation of lymphocytes	Acute: viral, chlamydial Chronic: chlamydial, molluscum contagiosum
Phlyctenules	White nodular immunologic conjunctival response usually near limbus (may be on cornea) with adjacent vascular congestion, evolves into microabscess, heals 10–14 days	*S. aureus*—often associated with chronic lid involvement, tuberculosis, malnutrition
Pseudomembrane	Polymorphonuclear leukocytes in a fibrin meshwork, does not bleed when removed	Viral: especially EKC, (usually adenovirus 8) gonococcus *S. pyogenes,* erythema multiforme
True membrane	Arises from subconjunctival exudation, bleeds when removed	Diphtheria, erythema multiforme

Granulomas	Epithelioid nodules	Parinaud's syndrome
		  Cat-scratch
		  Tularemia
		  Sporotrichosis
		  Tuberculosis
		  Primary syphilis
		  Coccidioidomycosis
		  Other infectious agents less commonly
		Sarcoidoisis

Subconjunctival hemorrhages		EKC (epidemic keratoconjunctiviris) adenovirus *S. pneumoniae* *S. pyogenes* *Haemophilus* sp.
Preauricular adenopathy		Frequently: viral, chlamydial Occasionally: severe bacterial

Various etiologies result in clinically indistinguishable inflammatory reactions. Conjunctival cytology, microbiologic studies, and therapeutic trials are often necessary for differentiation. Cultures are of value if significant bacterial infection is suspected. Gram stain correlation is important, as an isolated culture may yield a pathogen which is either a part of the normal conjunctival flora or a superficial secondary invader.

Neonatal conjunctivitis (ophthalmia neonatorum) may represent a visual threat. Table 10 outlines the diagnosis and management. Ophthalmologic referral is indicated.

TABLE 9. DIFFERENTIAL DIAGNOSIS OF CONJUNCTIVITIS IN CHILDHOOD

Etiology	Distinguishing Features
Infectious	
Viral	Mucoid discharge
	Preauricular nodes
	Acute follicular reaction
Adenovirus types	
Pharyngoconjunctival fever (PCF)	Epidemiology: human contacts, swimming pools, summer, fall; fever, sore throat
	No pseudomembrane
	Keratitis: mild and transient
Epidemic keratoconjunctivitis (EKC)	Epidemiology: contacts, doctor's office non-seasonal; no systemic symptoms
	Pseudomembrane
	Occasional subconjunctival hemorrhage
	Keratitis: often moderate, subepithelial infiltrates
Herpes simplex Type 1 (occ. type 2)	Epidemiology: skin lesions, contacts
	Keratitis: dendritic, ulcerative
Molluscum contagiosum	Associated keratitis with marginal lid lesions
With viral exanthems	Usually no follicles
Measles	Occasionally conjunctival vesicles
Varicella	Keratitis may occur
Chlamydial	
Neonatal	No follicles (Table 10)
Trachoma	Epidemiology: crowding, poor sanitation
	Chronic follicles
	Scarring
Inclusion conjunctivitis	Epidemiology: human contacts (may be venereal)
	Preauricular nodes
	Follicles: mucopurulent discharge
	Keratitis may occur, corneal infiltrates
Bacterial	Mucopurulent to purulent discharge
	Papillae when resolving
	Usually no preauricular adenopathy
S. pneumoniae	Epidemiology: schools, fall, winter
	Course: spontaneously subsides 7–10 days
	Occasionally subconjunctival hemorrhages
	Rapid response to therapy
H. influenzae and *Haemophilus aegyptius*	Epidemiology: family, schools
	More inflammation than *S. pneumoniae*
	Occasionally subconjunctival hemorrhages
	Course: self-limiting, 3 weeks
	Moderate response to therapy
S. aureus	Epidemiology: poor hygiene
	Chronic lid infection
	Occasionally phlyctenular
	Course: chronic, does not subside spontaneously

(*continued*)

TABLE 9 (*Continued*)

Etiology	Distinguishing Features
Group A *S. pyogenes*	Very acute
	Severe
	Purulent
	Pseudomembrane
	Occasionally subconjunctival hemorrhages
Gonococcus	Epidemiology: contact (venereal)
	Hyperacute
	Hyperpurulent
Toxic-metabolic	Usually chronic follicular
Pharmacologic (eyedrops)	May be sensitivity to preservative
Environmental irritants	Epidemiology: fumes, pollutants
Thyroid disease	Chronic
	Observe for systemic symptoms (may be absent)
Vernal (atopic)	Epidemiology: atopic diathesis
	Family history of atopy
	Seasonal
	Watery or mucoid discharge
	Papillae (may be giant)
Generalized mucous membrane disorders	Diagnosis by system and generalized dermatologic findings
Erythema multiforme	
Mucocutaneous lymph node syndrome	
Reiter's syndrome	
Anaphylactoid purpura	
Dermatitis herpetiformis	
Toxic epidermal necrolysis	
Icthyosis	
Acrodermatitis enteropathica	
Epidermolysis bullosa	
Benign chronic familial pemphigus	

Sequelae are unusual following conjunctivitis due to typical bacteria, viruses, allergies, and irritants. Severe conjunctivitis, especially those associated with generalized mucous membrane conditions, may result in scarring with symblepharon formation, loss of conjunctival goblet cells and obstruction of lacrimal secretion resulting in dry eye states, and affectations of contiguous lid and ocular structures.

Other Ocular Inflammations. Etiologies for inflammation of the cornea (keratitis) (Fig. 15), episclera and sclera, and anterior uveal tract (iritis) (Fig. 16) are listed in Table 5. These conditions may be differentiated from conjunctivitis by the signs and symptoms listed in Table 6. Causes of posterior ocular inflammations are listed in Table 5. These may present with a red eye, pain, and decreased visual acuity (Fig. 17).

Differential Diagnosis

History. Certain questions are particularly useful for the pediatrician's assessment of periocular and ocular inflammation. Those below will help guide the pediatrician to either proper treatment or timely referral.

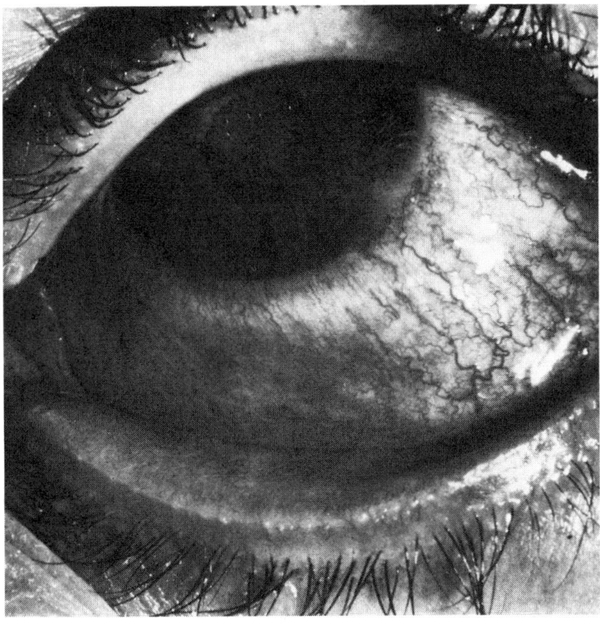

Figure 12. Conjunctivitis. The inflammation is diffuse, becoming more intense toward the lids. Note the dilated discrete superficial vessels.

• What is the course (time of onset, site of onset, progress of symptoms) of the inflammation? Is it recurrent? The pediatrician may elect to manage certain inflammations. Chronic or recurrent inflammation may be secondary to anatomic abnormalities, masses, unusual infectious agents, systemic conditions, or serious underlying ocular pathology and require ophthalmologic referral.

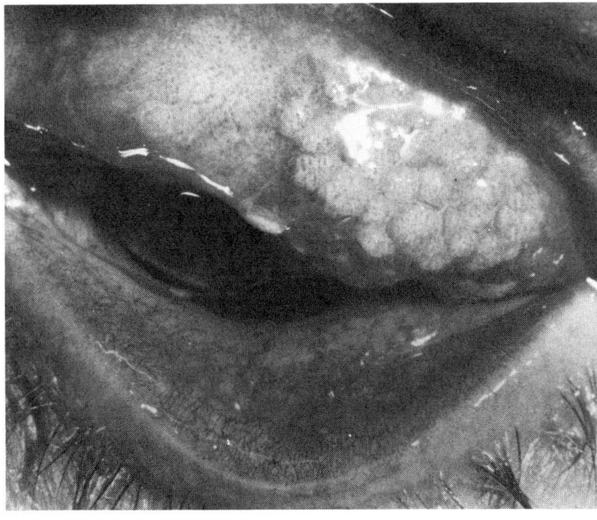

Figure 13. Papillae of conjunctiva.

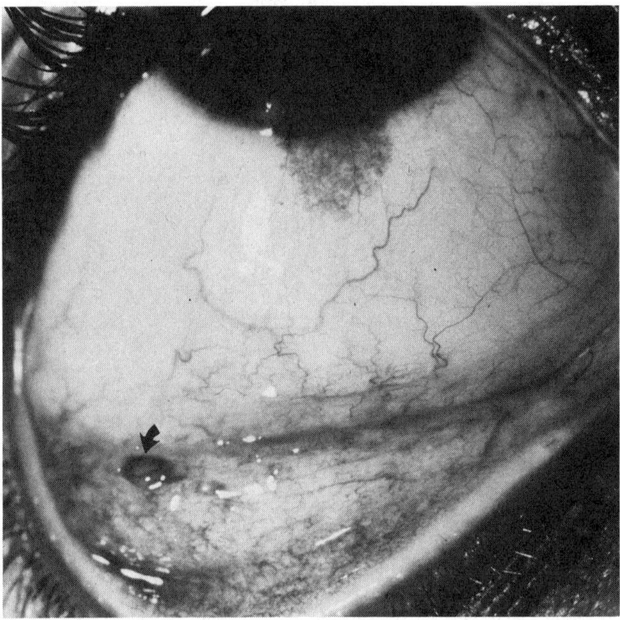

Figure 14. Follicles of conjunctiva (arrow).

- Is visual acuity decreased? What is the severity of any discomfort? Is photophobia present? Decreased acuity, significant ocular discomfort, ocular pain, or photophobia herald inflammatory processes of the cornea or intraocular structures and require ophthalmologic referral.
- Is a discharge present? What is its course and nature? Conjunctivitides often present with a mucoid or purulent discharge de-

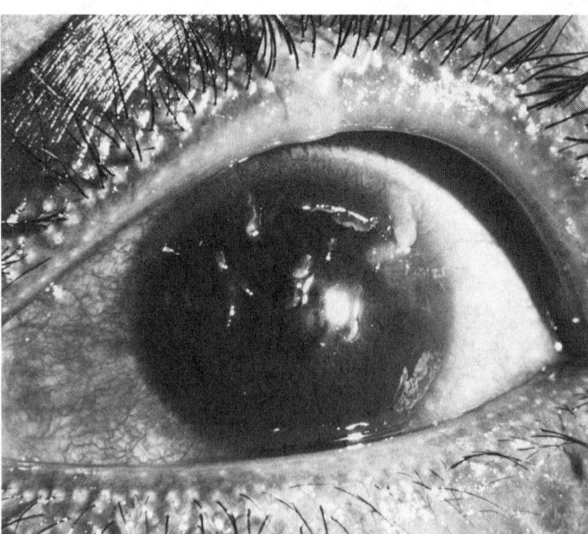

Figure 15. Keratitis. Note irregularity of superior corneal epithelium. This is a filamentary keratitis due to changes in tear components.

TABLE 10. NEONATAL CONJUNCTIVITIS

Etiology	Onset	Discharge	Microbiologic Work-up	Treatment
	Except for silver nitrate, not a reliable guide	Not a reliable guide	Gram stain Giemsa stain Culture (include for gonococcus) Chlamydial culture when indicated	
Silver nitrate	First 24 hr	Mucoid-mucopurulent	Negative	None necessary Irrigation
Gonococcal	24–72 hr	Copious pus	Bacteria on stains and culture Determine penicillin sensitivity Test for syphilis	Isolate patient at least 24 hr Aqueous crystalline penicillin G 50,000 U/kg/day IV given in 2 divided doses for 7 days Frequent saline irrigation until discharge clears
Bacterial	After 72 hr	Mucopurulent-purulent	Bacteria on stains and culture	10–30% sulfacetamide 4 times daily, continue for 3 days after clinical resolution
Chlamydial	2–14 days (peak 5–12 days)	Mucopurulent	Inclusions on Giemsa stain Culture mother	30% sulfacetamide 4 times daily for 3–6 weeks Alternatives: 1% tetracycline ointment Erythromycin ointment or oral Watch for pneumonitis Consider systemic sulfonamide or erythromycin for 3 weeks

pending upon the inciting pathogen. Deeper ocular inflammations and lacrimal obstruction may yield only a clear discharge.

- Is the condition bilateral? Certain infectious, irritant, and systemic conditions are more likely bilateral.
- Are there associated dermatologic, craniofacial, or systemic symptoms? Does the patient have a systemic disease? Periocular and ocular inflammation may be part of a wider process, contiguous or disseminated. Orbital inflammation may produce a septic picture.
- Has there been exposure to others with inflammatory processes or certain physical environments? Is any therapy being employed? Inflammations are often con-

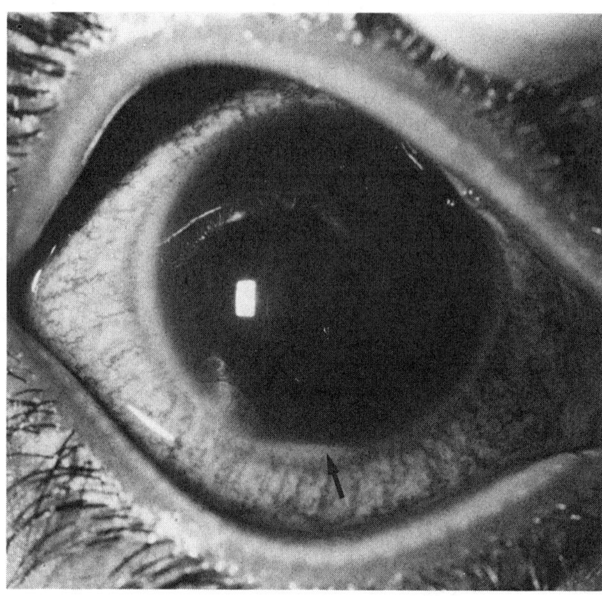

Figure 16. Iritis. Note the circumcorneal (ciliary flush) with less inflammation toward the lids. The anterior chamber reaction is here so severe that a discrete layer of inflammatory cells, a hypopyon, is seen inferiorly (arrow).

tracted by exposure to ocular pathogens harbored by other persons or the environment, such as stagnant pools or areas with parasites. Eyedrops and their preservatives may produce local sensitivity.

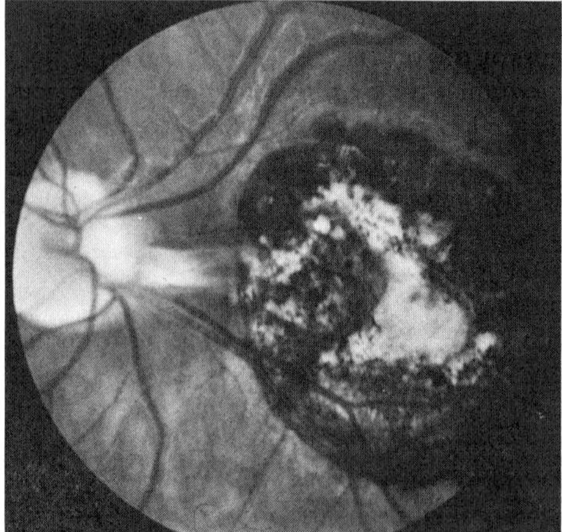

Figure 17. Chorioretinal scar in the posterior pole due to toxoplasmosis.

- Is diplopia present? This indicates orbital or intracranial inflammation.
- What is the past ocular history? Knowledge of the ocular status prior to the inflammatory process is necessary to determine what findings are new.

Physical Examination. The pediatrician's complete ocular examination as described in the first section of this chapter is indicated. Certain features and extensions of the examination will help determine the sites and nature of the inflammatory involvement. These are listed in Tables 6, 7, 8, 9, and 10.

Laboratory Aids. Periocular and ocular tissues react only in a limited number of ways to the diversity of inflammatory stimuli. Proper use of ancillary tests will help delineate the nature, etiology, and extent of the inflammatory process.

Exfoliative cytology is useful in differentiating types of conjunctival and corneal inflammations. Gram (microorganisms) and Giemsa (cytology, inclusions) stains should be employed. Polymorphonuclear leukocytes indicate acute inflammation, lymphocytes subacute or chronic inflammation, eosinophils an allergic reaction, and plasma cells an immune response. Bacteria, fungi, and various types of viral inclusion bodies may be observed.

Cultures of drained, exfoliated, aspirated, or biopsied material may yield the specific inflammatory pathogen. Proper medium to support growth of possible pathogens is necessary. Special media are needed for certain bacteria (e.g., *H. influenzae, Neisseria gonorrheae*), viruses, chlamydia, and fungi. Cytologic correlation of a positive culture will prevent mistaking a component of the normal flora or a secondary invader as an inciting pathogen.

Serologic studies are important adjuncts for the diagnosis of viral, chlamydial, parasitic, and immune inflammations.

X-rays, CT scans, and ultrasound recordings of the periocular region may delineate the extent of an inflammatory process. These tests may be useful in differentiating between a periorbital and an orbital cellulitis. These tests are indicated when contiguous inflammatory processes, such as paranasal sinusitis or osteomyelitis, are suspected.

Systemic effects of periocular and ocular inflammation may be monitored with CBC, ESR, and other acute phase reactants. Blood cultures should be performed if systemic involvement is suspected.

Management
Lids—Localized Inflammation.
Blepharitis. Treatment of seborrheic blepharitis is directed toward improved cleanliness, regularly removing the marginal scales mechanically with a moist applicator, and the regular use of mild keratolytic anti-dandruff shampoos.

Eczematoid or psoriatic conditions that affect the lid margins are treated with mild steroid preparations three or four times daily. Chronic application should be avoided.

Infectious blepharitis is most commonly caused by staphylococci. It may be primary or secondary to seborrheic or eczematoid involvement. Improved hygiene, applicator debridement, and a sulfonamide ointment are indicated. Erythromycin ointment should be substituted if sulfonamides fail. A combination of a sulfonamide and a steroid may be used for the first few days to decrease any eczematoid component.

Molluscum contagiosum of the lid is usually a benign, self-limiting condition that heals without scarring. If the lid margin is involved a significant chronic keratoconjunctivitis may occur. Simple curettage is then indicated. Herpes simplex lid infections require ophthalmologic referral. Prophylaxis with an antiviral agent to prevent corneal involvement may be indicated.

For crab lice and mites an application of 0.5% physostigmine ointment is curative. Other sites of infestation must be treated appropriately.

Hordeolum. Treatment of hordeolum consists of warm compresses 4–6 times daily for 15 minutes, followed by a sulfonamide drop. Incision and drainage by an ophthalmologist may be necessary.

Chalazion. Treatment with frequent warm compresses, for weeks if necessary, is recommended. Incision and drainage may be necessary.

Diffuse Periorbital (Preseptal) and Orbital Inflammation. Treatment of preseptal cellulitis includes drainage of the preseptal space if abscess is present and appropriate antibiotic therapy. Antibiotic therapy is initially based on clinical setting (posttraumatic or hematogenous), signs (e.g., color), the patient's age, and Gram stain. Initial treatment with ampicillin and oxacillin is employed where no pathogen is identified. If *H. influenzae* is strongly suspected, chloramphenicol is added. The intravenous route should be employed for moderate to severe infection. With sufficient clinical improvement, the oral route may be substituted after 48–72 hours. Treatment should continue for a minimum of 10 days.

Therapy of orbital cellulitis is directed toward treating any underlying conditions and instituting appropriate antibiotic therapy. Sinus drainage and nasal decongestants, removal of retained orbital foreign materials, and drainage of dental abscesses may be indicated. Ophthalmologic and often otolaryngologic referral is indicated.

High-dose intravenous antibiotic therapy should be instituted. After 5–7 days the oral route may be substituted if sufficient improvement has occurred. Antibiotics should be continued for a minimum of 10 days. Selection of antibiotics is based on the microbiologic studies, clinical setting, underlying etiology, and the patient's age. Where no clear-cut indication of the offending organism is found, ampicillin or chloramphenicol and oxacillin should be used. Ocular lubricants are instilled if corneal exposure secondary to proptosis and lid involvement exists.

Orbital pseudotumor is responsive to systemic steroid therapy.

The Red Eye.
Conjunctivitis. Treatment of conjunctivitis with an ocular antibiotic, such as 10% sulfacetamide four times daily, will result in rapid eradication of most simple bacterial infections. It will provide lubrication and prevent secondary infection in viral and simple irritant conjunctivitides. Treatment should be continued for 7 days or 3 days after clinical resolution. If progressive improvement leading to resolution does not occur, ophthalmologic referral is indicated.

Conjunctivitis which is chronic, recurrent, hyperacute, or associated with lid, lacrimal, or systemic conditions requires ophthalmologic evaluation. Steroid therapy is indicated for some of these conditions but

should only be instituted after ophthalmologic consultation. Therapy for neonatal conjunctivitis (ophthalmia neonatorum) is outlined in Table 10.

Other Ocular Inflammation. For superficial keratitis, episcleritis and scleritis, and intraocular inflammations, ophthalmologic referral is indicated.

EXCESSIVE TEARING IN INFANCY

Excessive tearing in infancy is common. It is produced by increased lacrimation or obstruction to lacrimal drainage. Because obstructive causes occur more frequently, serious pathology underlying increased lacrimation is often overlooked.

Definition
Excessive tearing may manifest as a moist-appearing eye with a large tear film, moist lashes, and tears rolling down the cheek (epiphora).

Classification and Etiologies
Increased Lacrimation. Increased lacrimation results from increased intraocular pressure (glaucoma), chronic irritation, or chronic inflammatory states. Concomitant photophobia is frequently found with these conditions.

Lacrimal Obstruction. Lacrimal drainage may be obstructed at any point from puncta to inferior turbinate. It is unassociated with photophobia, corneal enlargement, or haze. Most often it is due to a membrane obstructing the distal nasolacrimal duct.

Differential Diagnosis
History. Certain questions are helpful in making decisions about diagnosis and management:

- Is photophobia present? Photophobia signals ocular causes of increased lacrimation. Glaucoma must be ruled out.
- When was the tearing first noted? Has it been persistent? Has there been a purulent discharge? As discussed below, these answers help with decisions about management.
- Is there a similar family history? Congenital glaucoma may be recessively inherited.

Physical Examination. Photophobia, abnormal corneal size or clarity, decreased visual acuity, presence of a ciliary flush, abnormal pupillary sizes and reactions, and altered quality and symmetry of the red reflex all suggest glaucoma.

The lid and lash anatomy should be examined for causes of mechanical irritation and the conjunctiva for evidence of a chronic inflammatory condition.

The position and patency of the puncta should be noted. Pressure on the lacrimal sac just behind the inferomedial orbital rim will often produce an efflux of retained sac contents from the puncta in nasolacrimal duct obstruction. The nose should be examined for inflammatory, structural, and mass abnormalities which may obstruct drainage. The hydration of the nasal mucous membranes should be noted. Tearing without rhinorrhea is suggestive of lacrimal obstruction.

Management

Increased Lacrimation. Excessive lacrimation requires ophthalmologic evaluation for a detailed examination for causes of irritation or inflammation and assessment of intraocular pressure.

Lacrimal Obstruction. Massage of the nasolacrimal sac a few times daily prevents fluid stagnation and may help relieve the obstruction. Infection of the nonflowing tears occurs commonly. Acute episodes should be treated with an antibiotic drop, such as 10% sulfacetamide four times daily.

Probing the system usually produces permanent resolution. Since 80% of nasolacrimal duct obstructions resolve spontaneously by 8 months, the question of when to probe is dependent upon a number of factors. Intermittent obstructions more frequently resolve spontaneously than persistent ones. Chronic inflammation increases the risk of unsuccessful probing. If repeated probing is unsuccessful, much more extensive surgery is necessary to establish patency. Weighing these facts, some ophthalmologists advise early probing, while others prefer to wait until the patient is 1 year old. Arguments may be made for either regimen.

REFERENCES

Routine Ocular Care and Amblyopia

Friendly DS: Preschool visual acuity screening tests. Trans. Am Ophthalmol Soc 76:383, 1978

Friendly DS: Eye disorders in neonates. In Avery GB (ed): Neonatology: Pathophysiology and Management of the Newborn. Philadelphia, Lippincott, 1975, pp. 973–989

Pollard ZF: Are we missing ambylopia? The answer: preschool screening. Pediatrics 60:603, 1977

Vision Screening of Preschool Children. American Academy of Pediatrics, Committee on Children with Handicaps. Pediatrics 50:966, 1972

Strabismus

Adler R, Goldstein SH: Strabismus screening in pediatrics. J Pediatr 84:730, 1974

Noorden GK von: Binocular Vision and Ocular Motility. St. Louis, Mosby, 1980

Noorden GK von, Maumenee AE: Atlas of Strabismus, 2nd ed. St. Louis, Mosby, 1973

Parks MM: Ocular motility and strabismus. In Duane TD: Clinical Ophthalmology. Hagerstown, Harper & Row, 1979 (revision), Vol I, Chap 1–20

Periocular and Ocular Trauma

Paton D, Goldberg MF: Management of Ocular Injuries. Philadelphia, Saunders, 1976

Pilger IS: Medical treatment of traumatic hyphema. Surv Ophthalmol 20:28, 1975

Periocular and Ocular Inflammation

American Academy of Pediatrics, Committees on Drugs, Fetus and Newborn, and Infectious Disease. Prophylaxia and Treatment of Neonatal Gonococcal Infections. Pediatrics 65:1047, 1980

Binder PS: Herpes simplex keratitis. Surv Ophthalmol 21:313, 1977

Brook I: Anaerobic and aerobic bacterial flora of acute conjunctivitis in children. Arch Ophthalmol 98:833, 1980

Chavis RM, Graner A, Wright JE: Inflammatory orbital pseudotumor. Arch Ophthalmol 96:1817, 1978

Duane TD (ed): Clinical Ophthalmology. External Diseases of the Uvea. Hagerstown, Harper & Row, 1980 (revision), vol 4

Fulginiti VA: Common wisdom and new findings in sinusitis. Pediatrics 66:638, 1980

Gellady AM, Shulmon ST, Ayoub EM: Periorbital and orbital cellulitis in children. Pediatrics 61:272, 1978

Gigliotti F, Williams WT, Hayden FG, et al.: Etiology of acute conjunctivitis in children. J Pediatr 98:531, 1981

Goldberg F, Berne AS, Oski FA: Differentiation of orbital cellulitis from preseptal cellulitis by computed tomography. Pediatrics 62:1000, 1978

Healy GB: Acute sinusitis in childhood. N Engl J Med 304:779, 1981

Mottow LS, Jakobiec FA: Idiopathic inflammatory orbital pseudotumor in childhood. Arch Ophthalmol 96:1410, 1978

Nichols RL: Infections with *Chlamydia trachomatis*. Pediatrics 64:270, 1979

Wald ER, Milmoe GJ, Bowen A, et al.: Acute maxillary sinusitis in children. N Engl J Med 304:749, 1981

Excessive Tearing in Infancy

Petersen RA, Robb RM: The natural course of congenital obstruction of the nasolacrimal duct. J Pediatr Ophthalmol Strabismus 15:246, 1978

Cross-Reference to *Pediatrics,* 17th ed.

THIRTY-SIX

Menstrual Disorders in the Adolescent Girl

Susan M. Coupey

Since the current average age at menarche in the United States is approximately 12.5 years, the pediatrician is called upon to diagnose and treat disorders of menstruation. Abnormalities of the menstrual cycle are frequent at both ends of the reproductive years, and young adolescent girls often present to the clinician with painful menstruation (dysmenorrhea), excessive uterine bleeding (menorrhagia), or irregular, infrequent menses (oligomenorrhea and secondary amenorrhea). In addition, there has been an increase in the number of adolescents who are sexually active, a behavioral expression of earlier physiologic maturation. Pediatricians must consider the consequences of sexual behavior, pregnancy, and sexually transmitted disease in the differential diagnosis of menstrual abnormalities in adolescent girls.

DYSMENORRHEA

The symptom of dysmenorrhea or painful menstrual periods is very common among adolescent girls and is a leading cause of school absenteeism in this population. In the National Health Examination Survey 60% of 12–17-year-old girls reported dysmenor-

rhea, and 14% missed school frequently due to this symptom.

When an adolescent girl complains of menstrual cramps, the physician must differentiate between the very common primary dysmenorrhea, thought to be initiated by prostaglandin-induced uterine contractions, and other less frequent but often more serious causes of painful menstruation. A careful history and physical examination including a genital examination are mandatory before any treatment is prescribed. Occasionally, ultrasonography, examination under anesthesia, or laparoscopy may be necessary for diagnosis.

Definition

Dysmenorrhea is defined as crampy lower abdominal or back pain that occasionally radiates down the thighs and is associated with menstrual flow. Nausea, vomiting, diarrhea, headache, and depression sometimes accompany the pain.

The severity of the pain is described as mild, moderate, or severe. Mild dysmenorrhea occurs on the first day of bleeding, lasts only a few hours, and does not interfere appreciably with the daily routine of the adolescent. Moderate dysmenorrhea often lasts for

2 or 3 days and may interfere with the daily routine on the first day of pain. For example, the patient may report that she needs to lie down in the nurse's office at school. She may even have to leave school early or miss a day of school, although usually not every month. Associated symptoms of nausea, diarrhea, and headache can be present but are mild. Severe dysmenorrhea can last anywhere from 2 to 7 days, interferes with daily routine to a significant extent, and frequently occurs with symptoms of gastrointestinal upset.

Etiology

Dysmenorrhea is classified as primary or secondary depending upon the presence or absence of organic pelvic pathology. Primary dysmenorrhea usually does not develop in adolescents until 4–18 months after the menarche, when regular ovulatory menses begin, and it occurs only with ovulatory cycles. The diagnosis of primary dysmenorrhea is based upon a typical history of menstrual pain in the absence of pelvic pathology or other known causes of dysmenorrhea. The etiology is thought to be due to either excessive secretion of prostaglandins by the secretory endometrium or a hypersensitivity of myometrial receptors to normal levels of prostaglandins, causing painful myometrial contractions. Elevated levels of prostaglandins have been demonstrated in the menstrual blood of women with primary dysmenorrhea. In addition, plasma removed from women at a time when they were experiencing dysmenorrhea reproduced the crampy pain and associated symptoms when reinfused into the same women at a time when they were asymptomatic and not menstruating. This study suggests the presence of a circulating factor capable of inducing symptoms of dysmenorrhea.

Moderate to severe dysmenorrhea, especially if it has occurred since the very first menstrual period, is more likely to be secondary to organic pathology or significant psychologic disturbance (Table 1). In an adolescent with an isolated, atypical, painful menstrual period, acute causes of secondary dysmenorrhea must be excluded. The most common causes are threatened abortion and gonococcal or nongonococcal endometritis and/or salpingitis.

Endometriosis, while not common in teenagers, is now being diagnosed more frequently in this age group and should be suspected in older adolescents with a history of increasingly severe menstrual cramps over several cycles. Adnexal masses or nodularity of the uterosacral ligaments or rectovaginal septum are usually absent on physical examination. There is generally significant tenderness of pelvic structures around the time of the menses, which often disappears during the rest of the cycle. Genital tract malforma-

TABLE 1. ETIOLOGY OF SECONDARY DYSMENORRHEA IN ADOLESCENTS

Complications of pregnancy	Endometriosis
Threatened abortion	Psychologic stress
Ectopic gestation	School phobia
Genital tract infections	Rape-trauma syndrome
Acute endometritis and/or salpingitis due to sexually transmitted disease	Systemic disease
Chronic salpingitis	Acute intermittent porphyria
Septic abortion	Iatrogenic
Genital tract malformations	Intrauterine device
Vaginal septum	
Rudimentary uterine horn	
Cervical stenosis	

tions are uncommon causes of painful menses, but when present they frequently require surgical correction.

Psychologic stress as the primary etiology for dysmenorrhea is relatively rare in teenagers. Some adolescents with mild primary dysmenorrhea, however, will have a strong psychologic overlay with decreased pain tolerance and much anxiety centered around the menses. Many of these patients will respond favorably to examination, explanation, and reassurance, with or without analgesic or prostaglandin synthetase inhibitor therapy. Occasionally, the pain and anxiety are signs of deeper stresses, such as school phobia or the rape-trauma syndrome. Menstrual cramps can be the presenting symptom of school phobia, usually occurring in junior high school girls aged 12, 13, or 14 years. The diagnosis is suggested when there is a discrepancy between the severity of the reported symptoms and the loss of school days and is supported by finding a family structure or recent event which makes it difficult for the adolescent to leave home. Teenagers with the rape-trauma syndrome can present with a functional complaint several months after the traumatic event. Often the complaint is centered in the genital area and can manifest as dysmenorrhea. If the physician thinks that a rape may have occurred, it is helpful to include a question in the routine sexual history such as: "Has anyone ever done anything to you sexually that you didn't want him to do?" Usually, the symptom can be alleviated when the adolescent is given the opportunity to share her secret and work through her feelings of guilt and fears of physical damage. This therapy may be accomplished by the primary physician or by referral to a psychiatrist, psychologist, or social worker.

Differential Diagnosis

History. Sexual behavior must always be part of the history elicited because of the frequency of significant medical complications associated with sexual intercourse among teenagers. The physician should ascertain whether the adolescent is sexually inexperienced, a sexual beginner but still a virgin, or has experienced sexual intercourse. Certain diagnostic considerations, such as complications of pregnancy or sexually transmitted disease, are less likely in the adolescent who denies intercourse behavior. It should be obvious that this very necessary yet very sensitive part of the history should be taken from the adolescent alone without either parent present and with the assurance of confidentiality within the physician-patient relationship.

Useful questions include:

- Have you had painful menstrual periods before? An isolated abnormal period suggests acute secondary causes for the dysmenorrhea, e.g., infection or a complication of pregnancy.
- When does the pain start—before, with, or after the blood flow? In common primary dysmenorrhea the pain starts on the first day of blood flow. An atypical pattern of pain suggests secondary dysmenorrhea.
- Describe the pain for me. Where is it located? Does it come and go or is it always there? Atypical location, duration, or intensity of pain suggests secondary dysmenorrhea, e.g., from endometriosis or a genital tract malformation.
- How long does the pain last? Pain lasting more than 3 days is uncommon in primary dysmenorrhea and more common in endometriosis.
- Are there any associated symptoms, such as nausea, vomiting, or diarrhea? If these are present, the dysmenorrhea falls into the moderate or severe category.
- What do you do when you get the pain? Are you able to continue with your activities? Do you go to bed? Have you had to miss school (work) because of pain? Pain that significantly interferes with daily routine is more likely to be due to organic or psychologic pathology.
- Does anything make the pain worse or better? Have you tried taking any medicine for

it? Primary dysmenorrhea typically improves with exercise and analgesics. Pelvic infections and endometriosis are usually accompanied by dyspareunia.

- How old were you when you started having your menstrual periods? Did the pain begin with your first period? Primary dysmenorrhea usually does not start at the menarche because initial menstrual periods are usually anovulatory. Genital tract malformations with obstruction to blood flow often produce pain with the first menses.
- Are your periods usually regular? Regular periods imply the establishment of ovulatory cycles. Endometriosis can be associated with menstrual irregularities.
- When was your last period? Complications of pregnancy usually occur after at least one missed period.
- Does anyone else in your family have menstrual cramps? Primary dysmenorrhea tends to run in families.
- Do you have cramps or abdominal pain at times of the month when you are not having your menstrual period? Pain from endometriosis, pelvic infection, or of psychologic origin is sometimes present at other times of the month.

Physical Examination. In general, every adolescent who has sufficient dysmenorrhea to seek a physician's help requires a pelvic examination. Occasionally, in very young adolescents in whom the symptom of mild dysmenorrhea is elicited as an incidental finding, genital examination and inspection of the vaginal introitus without vaginal or rectal examination is sufficient, especially since nothing stronger than aspirin or acetaminophen need be prescribed. All adolescents complaining of moderate or severe dysmenorrhea require an examination of internal pelvic structures as well as a complete physical examination. Any virginal adolescent whose vagina admits one finger (and most do) can, if properly prepared and relaxed, undergo a speculum and bimanual examination. If vaginal examination is not possible, a rectoabdominal ex-

amination can contribute much information about uterine or adnexal tenderness or masses. An examination under anesthesia may be indicated if pelvic pathology is strongly suspected and an adequate pelvic examination in the office cannot be performed.

Signs to note during physical examination:

1. Look for lower abdominal tenderness or a mass that may signify pelvic pathology, such as infection, or pregnancy.
2. Assure that the structures of the vulva, vagina, and cervix look normal and that there is no complete or partial vaginal septum, duplication of the cervix, or other congenital structural anomaly.
3. Observe the quality (color, consistency, amount, odor) of the vaginal discharge. If abnormal, it may signify infection.
4. Observe the appearance of the cervix. Bluish color is associated with early pregnancy. Petechiae, swelling, and discharge are associated with infection. An open cervical os with an enlarged uterus suggests threatened abortion. Purulent cervical discharge and a tender uterus suggest endometritis.
5. On bimanual examination, check for tenderness of the cervix, uterus, or of the tubes and ovaries. Tenderness is associated with cervicitis, endometritis, salpingitis, endometriosis, and ectopic pregnancy.
6. Check for masses in the adnexal regions and for size of the uterus. An enlarged uterus is associated with pregnancy. Adnexal masses can be due to infection (tubovarian abscess), pregnancy (ectopic), cysts (chocolate cyst of endometriosis), and congenital malformations (rudimentary uterine horn, vaginal duplication with occlusion).

Laboratory Investigation.

1. Serum-beta-subunit human chorionic gonadotropin (HCG) or urine pregnancy test if pregnancy is suspected.

2. Endocervical, rectal, and pharyngeal cultures for *Neisseria gonorrhoeae* and endocervical cultures for *Chlamydia trachomatis,* if infection is suspected.
3. Pelvic ultrasonography to help rule out congenital malformations, ectopic pregnancy, cysts, abscesses, or intrauterine devices.
4. Laparoscopy with biopsy if endometriosis is a strong consideration.

Management

Practicing pediatricians who are comfortable with their ability to conduct an adequate pelvic examination can manage most cases of mild to moderate primary dysmenorrhea. If the pain is not severe and has occurred with several menstrual cycles and if the pelvic examination is normal, primary dysmenorrhea is very likely. Treatment with simple analgesics or prostaglandin synthetase inhibitors, such as acetylsalicylic acid, indomethacin, naproxen, ibuprofen, or mefenamic acid, is usually effective (Table 2). All of these drugs are effective in controlling the painful uterine contractions. Acetylsalicylic acid has the

disadvantage of having to be taken 2 days before menses begin and, therefore, demands regular cycles and obsessive record keeping, neither of which is an especially common trait of most adolescents. Mefenamic acid (Ponstel) has the theoretical advantage of inhibiting prostaglandin activity as well as blocking prostaglandin synthesis and, therefore, would be expected to be effective more rapidly. In clinical practice, there does not seem to be much difference among these drugs either in their effectiveness or in the frequency of side effects. The major side effects of all these medications are nausea and other gastrointestinal complaints. These drugs should never be taken for more than 3 days each cycle in order to avoid the more serious effects that have been reported with long-term use.

For the sexually active girl or one in whom the above listed medications are ineffective, ovulation suppression with a low-dose combination oral contraceptive is often successful. Any one of the oral contraceptives containing 35 μg of ethinyl estradiol or 50 μg of mestranol combined with a synthetic progestagen is appropriate. A 28-day dosage schedule is easier for adolescents to remember than the 21-day schedule.

If the pain is atypical in its distribution, intensity, duration, or onset or if there are abnormal pelvic examination findings, secondary dysmenorrhea should be considered. Most of these secondary conditions should be managed by a consultant gynecologist. However, sexually transmitted infections can be managed by the primary care physician. If sexually transmitted endometritis is suspected and there is no adnexal tenderness to suggest salpingitis, antibiotic treatment is indicated. This consists of 4.8 million units of procaine penicillin IM and 1 g of probenecid orally, followed by 500 mg of ampicillin po qid for 10 days or tetracycline hydrochloride 500 mg qid for 10 days. If salpingitis is suspected because of fever, elevated white blood cell count, elevated erythrocyte sedimentation rate, or bilateral adnexal tenderness, it is

TABLE 2. TREATMENT OF PRIMARY DYSMENORRHEA

Drug	Dosage	Day of Cycle*
Acetylsalicyclic acid (aspirin)	650 mg po q6h	−2 to +3
Indomethacin (Indocin)	50 mg po tid	1 to +3
Naproxen sodium (Anaprox)	550 mg initially, then 275 mg q6h	1 to +3
Ibuprofen (Motrin)	400 mg po q6h	1 to +3
Mefenamic acid (Ponstel)	500 mg initially, then 250 mg po q6h	1 to +3

*Day 1 is first day of menstrual flow.

best to admit the teenager to the hospital for intravenous antibiotic therapy.

Gynecologic consultation must be sought for suspected threatened abortion or ectopic pregnancy and for diagnosis and management of suspected endometriosis or congenital genital tract anomalies. If psychologic stress is considered to be a significant factor in the etiology of the pain, a consultation with a psychiatrist or clinical psychologist for diagnostic confirmation and therapeutic recommendation is very helpful.

EXCESSIVE MENSTRUAL BLEEDING

Most adolescent girls have one or two menstrual periods with heavy bleeding during the first year after the menarche. Commonly, these unusually heavy periods stop without any therapy and are not associated with a fall in hematocrit. Occasionally, a young girl will have a massive uterine hemorrhage or frequent episodes of excessive menstrual blood loss and will require thorough evaluation, pharmacologic therapy, and, possibly, blood transfusion. Adolescents almost never require dilatation and curettage for either diagnosis or treatment of excessive uterine bleeding except when it is associated with incomplete abortion or in the rare instance when hormonal therapy fails.

Definition

Excessive menstrual bleeding or menorrhagia can be categorized in terms of (1) the amount of blood lost per day, (2) the number of days of vaginal bleeding, and (3) the frequency of episodes of bleeding. It is difficult to quantify the amount of blood lost per day. However, a girl who bleeds enough to soak through more than six full-sized pads per day or passes clots can be said to be bleeding heavily. If this amount of bleeding continues for more than 3 days or tapers off and then resumes within a few days, it is clearly excessive. Any vaginal bleeding that leads to an acute

fall in hematocrit or signs of hemodynamic compromise (tachycardia, postural hypotension) requires immediate investigation and therapy.

Etiology

The most common reason for prolonged heavy bleeding in teenagers is anovulation. This form of menorrhagia is called "dysfunctional uterine bleeding." More than half of the cycles in the first 2 years after the menarche are anovulatory. A follicle is stimulated to mature under the influence of follicle-stimulating hormone (FSH), but in the absence of the midcycle surge of luteinizing hormone (LH), it fails to rupture and release its ovum. Eventually, estrogen production decreases, and withdrawal bleeding occurs. In most cases, this process is of no medical significance and can be considered part of the normal maturation process of the hypothalamic/pituitary/ovarian axis. However, these anovulatory cycles are often short, and vaginal bleeding can occur at 2–3-week intervals, leading to significant blood loss in a few months. In some cases, the unruptured follicle persists for a longer time, 6–8 weeks, producing large amounts of estrogen which, in turn, stimulates the formation of a hyperplastic, proliferative endometrium. When estrogen production eventually diminishes, the resulting withdrawal bleeding can be excessive.

While dysfunctional uterine bleeding is the most common cause of excessive menstrual bleeding in the adolescent girl, a variety of other pathologic entities should be considered (Table 3).

Differential Diagnosis

History. The history should be directed at determining the amount and frequency of the vaginal bleeding, the presence or absence of associated symptoms, the sexual behavior of the adolescent, whether pregnancy is a possibility, and any medications that may have been taken. This history should be ob-

TABLE 3. ETIOLOGY OF EXCESSIVE MENSTRUAL BLEEDING IN ADOLESCENTS

Dysfunctional uterine bleeding	Endocrine disorders
Complications of pregnancy	Hypothyroidism
Abortion	Adrenal disorders
Ectopic pregnancy	Polycystic ovary syndrome
Blood dyscrasias	Diabetes mellitus
Clotting disorders, e.g., von Willebrand's disease	Infection
Thrombocytopenia	Sexually transmitted
Leukemia	Postabortion
Cysts and neoplasms	Trauma
Cervical or endometrial polyps	Foreign body
Vaginal adenosis or clear cell adenocarcinoma	Coital trauma
Uterine leiomyomas (fibroids)	Drugs
Trophoblastic disease	Misuse of oral contraceptives
Ovarian cysts or tumors	Anticoagulant drugs

tained in private without the parents present. Pertinent questions include:

- When was your last menstrual period? Was it normal for you? Significant dysfunctional uterine bleeding often follows a 6–12-week period of amenorrhea, as do complications of pregnancy and endocrine disorders associated with anovulation, such as polycystic ovary syndrome and certain adrenal disorders. A clotting disorder, such as von Willebrand's disease, will more likely present as excessive bleeding from the first menstrual period.
- About how many pads per day are you using? Are they soaked through when you change them? Have you passed any blood clots? More than six soaked pads per day or passage of clots signifies heavy bleeding.
- How old were you when you started menstruating? Anovulatory dysfunctional uterine bleeding is common within 3 years of the menarche.
- Are your periods usually regular? Anovulatory cycles can be short, occurring at less than 3-week intervals and leading to a significant blood loss over a 2–3-month interval. They can also be associated with a longer period of amenorrhea followed by very

heavy bleeding. Ovarian cysts or tumors, uterine leiomyomas, pregnancy, and endocrine disorders can all be associated with irregular menses.
- Have you had any abdominal pain? Does it occur only with the bleeding or at other times as well? Anovulatory bleeding is painless. Abdominal pain associated with excessive bleeding suggests other diagnoses, such as infection, complications of pregnancy, or ovarian neoplasms and cysts, which can produce lower abdominal pressure symptoms and chronic pain.
- Have you fainted or felt lightheaded or dizzy recently? Syncope or near-syncope can be associated with massive acute blood loss. Syncope can be the presenting symptom of early pregnancy in the adolescent.
- Have you felt nauseated? Are your breasts swollen or tender? These are early signs of pregnancy.
- Is it possible that you may be pregnant? This question should be asked if there is any suspicion on the part of the physician. If the teenager answers no, ask why not. The answer to this second question may surprise you!
- Have you had any other episodes of excessive bleeding? The patient may have had

hemorrhaging after a tonsillectomy or other procedure or in association with trauma. This would suggest a clotting disorder.

- Are you taking any medications? Intermittent or irregular use of oral contraceptives can produce frequent episodes of withdrawal bleeding. Excessive anticoagulant therapy can lead to uterine hemorrhage.
- Did your mother take any hormones during her pregnancy with you? Maternal diethylstilbestrol ingestion is associated with vaginal adenosis and clear cell adenocarcinoma of the vagina and cervix in their daughters.

Physical Examination. As with other menstrual disorders, a complete physical examination including a pelvic examination is necessary in the teenager with clinically significant excessive menstrual bleeding. The comments on pelvic examinations in virginal adolescents in the previous section on dysmenorrhea apply equally well in this case.

Signs to note during physical examination:

1. Vital signs: a resting tachycardia or postural hypotension is associated with massive, acute blood loss. Fever should suggest infection.
2. Pallor is a sign of anemia.
3. Hirsutism and obesity may be associated with adrenal disorders or polycystic ovary syndrome.
4. Petechiae or purpura are signs of blood dyscrasia.
5. Breast engorgement may be associated with pregnancy or an estrogen-producing ovarian neoplasm or cyst.
6. An abdominal mass may be present with pregnancy or a large ovarian tumor or cyst.
7. Lower abdominal tenderness is found with pelvic infection.
8. Careful pelvic examination to detect vaginal or cervical tumors, polyps or signs of trauma, uterine enlargement (pregnancy,

fibroids), or adnexal masses should be performed. This examination also allows for objective quantification of the amount of bleeding by the physician.

Laboratory Investigation.

1. Hemoglobin or hematocrit determination.
2. PT, PTT, platelets, and bleeding time may be indicated if a clotting disorder is suspected.
3. Serum beta-subunit HCG or urine pregnancy test may be indicated.
4. If an endocrine disorder is suspected, such studies as thyroid function tests, serum gonadotropins, and other hormonal tests may be required.
5. A blood test for syphilis (VDRL) and cultures of the endocervix for _N. gonorrhoeae_ and _C. trachomatis_ should be done on all sexually active girls.

Management

Most cases of excessive menstrual bleeding in the adolescent can be managed by the primary care physician if the pelvic examination reveals no abnormality and a diagnosis of dysfunctional uterine bleeding is made. Ongoing uterine hemorrhage with hemodynamic compromise or a significant fall in hematocrit demands immediate hospitalization and hormonal therapy. Intravenous Premarin 25 mg every 4 hours until bleeding stops or for a total of not more than four doses is usually effective. Dilatation and curettage may be necessary if Premarin is ineffective; such patients are usually found to have endometrial pathology. Intravenous Premarin therapy should be followed by a high-dose progestogen-estrogen combination oral contraceptive pill (e.g., Enovid 5 mg, Norinyl 2 mg) qid for 7 days. The patient should then be placed on a low-dose combination oral contraceptive pill for 3 months. If the bleeding has been prolonged but not massive and there is no hemodynamic compromise and only mild to moderate anemia, the girl can be treated as an outpatient with a 7-day course of high-dose combination progestogen-estrogen therapy as outlined above, followed by a 3-month course of low-dose combination oral contraceptive therapy. The sexually active teenager should continue on oral contraceptives. All teenagers with significant dysfunctional uterine bleeding should be followed closely, since this is frequently a continuing problem. Iron therapy should be given to correct anemia and replenish iron stores.

Acute secondary causes of excessive menstrual bleeding, such as complications of pregnancy and infection, are usually accompanied by lower abdominal pain and are obvious on pelvic examination. Diagnosis is confirmed by the appropriate laboratory tests as noted above. Pubertal girls who present with massive uterine bleeding at the menarche or within the first 2 years of menses should be investigated thoroughly for blood dyscrasias. Coagulation disorders are frequently present in those girls who require hospitalization and transfusion. These are, most commonly, von Willebrand's disease or idiopathic thrombocytopenic purpura. If one of these disorders is diagnosed, hematologic consultation would be appropriate to determine management.

Polycystic ovary syndrome is associated with ovulatory dysfunction and infrequent menses (oligomenorrhea). However, excessive uterine bleeding can also occur due to unopposed estrogen stimulation, causing a hyperplastic endometrium. This syndrome should be suspected in teenagers who are overweight and who continue to have irregular periods beyond 2 years after their menarche. These girls may also be mildly hirsute. Enlarged cystic ovaries can often be palpated on bimanual pelvic examination and demonstrated by pelvic ultrasonography. Serum luteinizing hormone levels are chronically elevated, while follicle-stimulating hormone levels are normal. Serum testosterone and

androstendione levels are usually in the high normal range or minimally elevated. Twenty-four-hour urinary 17-ketosteroids are most frequently normal. Low-dose combination oral contraceptive therapy is indicated to suppress androgen production by the ovary and to allow for regular shedding of the endometrium.

Other causes of excessive menstrual bleeding in adolescents include trauma, foreign body, and drugs. These can be excluded by history and pelvic examination. Hypothyroidism may be accompanied by few physical signs and serum T_4 and TSH concentrations should be measured if there is no obvious cause of the bleeding.

OLIGOMENORRHEA AND SECONDARY AMENORRHEA

Irregular menstrual periods are common in adolescent girls within the first 2 years of the menarche. It takes an average of 15 months to complete the first 10 menstrual cycles. As the gynecologic age (chronologic age minus age at menarche) increases, however, the menses most often become more regular. If they do not, pathology should be suspected.

The most common cause of missed menstrual periods in the adolescent is pregnancy. Even those who routinely care for adolescents have failed, on occasion. to recall this fact and have, therefore, experienced unnecessary delay in diagnosing pregnancy. For example, one of our patients, a 15-year-old girl, who vehemently denied sexual activity, was evaluated for 2 months of amenorrhea with hormonal studies because of her past history of precocious puberty. She had a markedly elevated dehydroepiandrosterone sulfate level and was sent for abdominal ultrasonography in search of an adrenal tumor. An intrauterine gestation was revealed. Pelvic examination and urine pregnancy testing, two less complicated and less costly procedures, may have saved the needless delay in diagnosis. Many younger adolescents, employing the magical thinking of childhood, firmly believe that they cannot become pregnant and will deny the possibility if questioned. A urine pregnancy test is simple to obtain, inexpensive, and should be part of the initial work-up of every adolescent with oligomenorrhea or secondary amenorrhea.

Definition

Oligomenorrhea means infrequent menstrual periods. A postmenarchal adolescent who has missed 2 or more periods can be said to be oligomenorrheic. Teenagers with oligomenorrhea have irregular patterns of bleeding as well as infrequent menses and may, for example, miss 2 periods, have a normal period, miss 4 periods, then have 2 normal periods in a row.

Secondary amenorrhea is defined as 6 consecutive months of absent menses after at least 1 normal menstrual period. Conditions that lead to secondary amenorrhea often begin with an episode of oligomenorrhea. Thus, the differential diagnoses for these two symptoms will be discussed together.

Etiology

Physiologic oligomenorrhea is the norm for girls with a gynecologic age of 2 years or less. This is due to developmental immaturity of the hypothalamic/pituitary/ovarian axis with failure of regular ovulation. This diagnosis should not be made if the girl is 3 years or more beyond the menarche. For an average maturing girl with menarche at 12.5 years, the period of physiologic oligomenorrhea should be over by age 15.5 years. For early maturers this period can be complete by age 13 years. In physiologically mature adolescent girls the most common cause of oligomenorrhea or secondary amenorrhea (besides pregnancy) is the hypothalamic suppression that occurs with weight loss, psychologic stress, or vigorous athletic training. It is important to make these diagnoses accurately. Hormonal therapy generally should not be given. In the case of anorexia nervosa,

an increasingly prevalent illness among teenagers, early diagnosis and treatment greatly improve the prognosis. The diagnosis of these conditions is made by history and physical examination and confirmed by a few selected laboratory tests. Other less common etiologies for oligomenorrhea or secondary amenorrhea are listed in Table 4 in approximate descending order of frequency of occurrence in adolescents.

Differential Diagnosis

History. Many of the questions listed in the sections on dysmenorrhea and excessive menstrual bleeding are applicable to these patients. As with other menstrual disorders, questions designed to establish the age at menarche, date of last menstrual period, previous pattern of menstrual periods, presence of other significant illness, medical and nonmedical drug history, and sexual behavior of the adolescent are mandatory. Other useful questions to ask the teenager when investigating oligomenorrhea or secondary amenorrhea include:

- Have you gained or lost a lot of weight recently? Rapid weight loss, even if the patient is not too thin, can be associated with absent menses. If the patient looks very thin, further questions regarding her dietary habits and self-image can help in the diagnosis of anorexia nervosa. Some obese adolescents become oligomenorrheic for reasons that are unclear and will regain their menses with weight loss. Polycystic ovary syndrome is associated with obesity.
- Do you participate in competitive sports or train vigorously for some physical activity? Some highly trained female athletes become amenorrheic possibly due to a redistribution of the ratio of lean body mass to fat.
- Have you recently gone to live away from home? Has anything happened lately in your life that upset you? Emotional stress is a well-known cause of amenorrhea in sus-

TABLE 4. ETIOLOGY OF OLIGOMENORRHEA AND SECONDARY AMENORRHEA IN ADOLESCENTS

Developmental immaturity of the hypothalamic/pituitary/ovarian axis
Pregnancy
Eating disorders
  Anorexia nervosa
  Rapid weight loss
  Obesity
Psychologic stress
  Separation anxiety (camp, college, boarding school)
  Major family or life stress
Rigorous athletic training
  Distance runners
  Gymnasts
  Dancers
Polycystic ovary syndrome
Other endocrinopathy
  Thyroid disorder
  Adrenal disorder
  Amenorrhea-galactorrhea syndrome (hyperprolactinemia)
  Androgen-producing neoplasm
	Systemic disease
	  Tuberculosis
	  Systemic lupus erythematosus
	  Chronic active hepatitis
	  Inflammatory bowel disease
	Hypothalamic/pituitary failure
	  Idiopathic
	  Space-occupying lesions (craniopharyngioma, meningioma)
	  Inflammatory lesions (tuberculosis, sarcoid, histiocytosis X)
	Premature ovarian failure
	  Idiopathic
	  Gonadal dysgenesis
	Drugs
	  Post birth control pill amenorrhea
	  Opiate addiction

ceptible adolescents via hypothalamic suppression. Amenorrhea in college freshmen is very common.

- Have you had any headaches or problems with your eyes recently? Pituitary neoplasms and other space-occupying lesions can cause headache and visual field deficits as well as various endocrine deficiency syndromes.
- Have you noticed any fluid coming from your breasts? Galactorrhea is sometimes found with CNS lesions. It is also a feature of the galactorrhea-amenorrhea syndrome associated with prolactin-producing pituitary adenomas. Some girls will have a nipple discharge in early pregnancy.

Physical Examination. The general rule that pelvic examination is necessary in the investigation of all menstrual disorders in teenagers applies also in these patients. An exception can be made for the virginal, early pubertal girl (Tanner stage 2,3, or 4) who has no indication of any other illness, who is within 2 years of her menarche, and who has a negative urine pregnancy test. The diagnosis in this case would be developmental immaturity of the hypothalamic/pituitary/ovarian axis. An adolescent who is virginal and clearly meets the psychologic and physiologic criteria for a diagnosis of anorexia nervosa probably does not require pelvic examination either.

Signs to note during physical examination:

1. Height and weight: short stature can be associated with gonadal dysgenesis, which usually presents as primary amenorrhea but can occasionally present as secondary amenorrhea. Obesity is often a feature of the polycystic ovary syndrome and, even in the absence of cystic ovaries, can be associated with oligomenorrhea. Excessive

weight loss is often accompanied by amenorrhea and may be a sign of anorexia nervosa.

2. Vital signs: anorexia nervosa, hypothyroidism, and athletic training can be accompanied by a slow heart rate. Hypertension is noted in some adrenal disorders, e.g., Cushing's syndrome.

3. Tanner stage: the menarche usually occurs at breast and pubic hair stage 4 but occasionally can occur as early as Tanner stage 2, in which case irregular infrequent menses can continue longer than 2 years after menarche and still be attributed to developmental immaturity of the hypothalamic/pituitary/ovarian axis. If a girl is clearly Tanner stage 5 and has been so for at least a year, her oligomenorrhea or amenorrhea is much less likely to be due to developmental immaturity.

4. Breast examination: engorged, tender breasts often accompany pregnancy. The nipple should be milked gently for fluid, since galactorrhea may not be observed or reported by the patient.

5. Skin: acne and hirsutism of cheeks, chin, midline chest, or midline abdomen may be signs of polycystic ovary syndrome, adrenal disorder, or androgen-producing neoplasm. Abdominal striae would suggest Cushing's disease or pregnancy.

6. Pelvic examination may reveal the bluish cervix and enlarged uterus of pregnancy, bilateral ovarian enlargement suggestive of polycystic ovary syndrome, or atrophic vaginal mucosa and scant discharge suggesting ovarian or hypothalamic/pituitary failure.

Laboratory Tests

1. Serum beta-subunit HCG or urine pregnancy test.

2. Complete blood count and erythrocyte sedimentation rate if occult systemic disease is suspected (ESR is elevated in pregnancy).

3. Thyroid function studies may be indicated if endocrinopathy is suspected.

4. Serum gonadotropins, FSH and LH, are elevated in ovarian failure (e.g., gonadal dysgenesis) and decreased in hypothalamic suppression syndromes (e.g., anorexia nervosa, stress-related amenorrhea). LH is elevated and FSH is normal in polycystic ovary syndrome.

5. Serum prolactin is elevated when there is a prolactin-producing pituitary adenoma (micro or macro) and in various disorders of the hypothalamus when the secretion of prolactin-inhibiting factor is decreased.

6. Assessment of androgen hormone production may be indicated if there are signs of virilization. This can be evaluated by measuring serum androgens (testosterone, Δ4-androstenedione, dehydroepiandrosterone) and/or 24-hour urinary excretion of androgenic metabolites as 17-ketosteroids.

7. Lateral skull x-ray, high resolution CT scan of the sella turcica, and pelvic ultrasonography all may be useful studies in selected cases.

Management

Developmental immaturity of the hypothalamic/pituitary/ovarian axis is a diagnosis of exclusion. In most cases, this diagnosis should not be made in an adolescent who is 3 years or more beyond her menarche, regardless of her chronologic age. No treatment should be given for this type of irregular menses. Pregnancy is always a consideration in every adolescent presenting with a history of one or more missed menstrual periods and should be excluded by urine pregnancy test and abdominal and pelvic examination. Management of adolescent pregnancy is beyond the scope of this chapter, and the reader is referred to the Kreutner and Hollingsworth text for an excellent discussion of this topic.

Girls with anorexia nervosa frequently present with the initial complaint of secondary amenorrhea, occasionally even before marked weight loss has occurred. These patients usually come from middle and upper socioeconomic class families, are compulsive, high-achieving, "good daughters," and have an altered body image, believing they are fat when they are actually very thin. They are obsessed with food and have bizarre eating patterns, often with binging and self-induced vomiting. These teenagers and their families require intensive long-term psychotherapy. When severely malnourished, they require hospitalization for nutritional support. This diagnosis can be made by history and physical examination, and these patients should not be given hormonal medication to induce menses.

Those girls in whom amenorrhea is thought to be due to psychologic stress or athletic training may be safely observed for 6 months. If amenorrhea persists throughout the 6 months, further evaluation is indicated. Such evaluation would include demonstration of hypothalamic suppression by measurement of serum gonadotropins (FSH and LH) and exclusion of hypothyroidism, hyperprolactinemia, and excessive androgen production. In addition, a lateral skull x-ray to confirm that the sella turcica is normal is of value. If no other pathology is found, these girls should not be treated with hormones to bring on the menses. The menstrual periods will resume when the stress is alleviated or there is a break in the athletic training. If there is evidence of psychopathology, psychotherapy may be of value.

Obese adolescents who have been oligomenorrheic for 1 year or amenorrheic for 6 months or are hirsuit should undergo a similar hormonal investigation. In addition, they should have pelvic ultrasonography to exclude enlarged ovaries with multiple small cysts unless the examiner is satisfied that pelvic examination has been adequate for this purpose. It is often difficult to feel enlarged ovaries in an obese teenager, especially if she is virginal. If the polycystic ovary syndrome is suspected or any of the hormonal studies are

abnormal, the patient should be referred to either an endocrinologist or a gynecologist for further investigation and therapy.

Some adolescents with gonadal dysgenesis can undergo normal pubertal development with menarche, then present with secondary amenorrhea due to ovarian failure. These girls often have the karyotype of XX/XO mosaic. They usually have short stature and may have some other stigmata of Turner's syndrome (webbed neck, widely spaced nipples, low hairline, short fourth metacarpals, increased carrying angle of arms). Pelvic examination may reveal poor estrogenization of the vagina and a small uterus. Vaginal smear will show no estrogen effect, and serum FSH and LH will be elevated. A karyotype is necessary for diagnosis, and estrogen and progestogen cyclic therapy is indicated. This treatment is probably best supervised by an endocrinologist or a gynecologist.

Patients with secondary amenorrhea who have signs or symptoms of central nervous system disease (severe headaches, visual field deficits), evidence of other hormonal deficit (hypothyroidism, diabetes insipidus, adrenal insufficiency), or hyperprolactinemia require thorough investigation. Space-occupying lesions must be excluded. Releasing factor and other provocative tests to further explore pituitary function may be indicated. These investigations are best carried out by a neurologist and an endocrinologist, and management depends on the diagnosis.

BIBLIOGRAPHY

Altchek A: Dysfunctional uterine bleeding in adolescence. Clin Obstet Gynecol 20:633, 1977

Apter D, Viinikka L, Vihko R: Hormonal pattern of adolescent menstrual cycles. J Clin Endocrinol Metab 47:944, 1978

Chan WY, Yusoff DM, Fuchs F: Prostaglandins in primary dysmenorrhea. Amer J Med 70:535, 1981

Claessens EA, Cowell CA: Acute adolescent menorrhagia. Am J Obstet Gynecol 139: 277, 1981

Emans SJ, Grace E, Goldstein DP: Oligomenorrhea in adolescent girls. J Pediatr 97:815, 1980

Kreutner AKK, Hollingsworth DR (eds): Adolescent Obstetrics and Gynecology. Chicago, Year Book, 1978

Cross-Reference to *Pediatrics,* 17th ed.

THIRTY-SEVEN

Sexually Transmitted Diseases

Walter D. Rosenfeld and Nathan Litman

Between 1971 and 1979 the prevalence of sexual activity among adolescent girls increased dramatically, with over a third having had a sexual experience by age 16. A survey made in 1979 revealed that 70% of boys between the ages of 17 and 21 years had had sexual intercourse. It has become apparent that a pattern of earlier and more frequent sexual activity has emerged among adolescents. Barrier contraceptives, such as the condom, which afford some degree of protection against transmission of pathogens, are not popular among teenagers. The increase in sexual activity with the limited use of barrier methods has resulted in a sharp rise in the incidence of sexually transmitted diseases in adolescents. It is common for adolescents to have inaccurate information about sexually transmitted diseases. They should be informed about the nature of their infection and the fact that it can occur again if they are reexposed.

Sexually transmitted diseases (STD) are a group of unrelated infections caused by diverse microorganisms that are transmitted by intimate, usually genital, contact. These are now the most common of all the reportable infectious diseases in the United States. In 1980, there were over 1 million cases of gonorrhea reported to the Centers for Disease Control (CDC). Though the number of reported cases of gonococcal infection in the United States tripled between 1950 and 1975, this dramatic rise is to some degree overshadowed by the fivefold increase in incidence noted in 15–19-year-old girls in the decade between 1965 and 1975. Nongonococcal urethritis is not a reportable disease, but it appears to be at least as common as gonorrhea. There are over 850,000 patients per year with pelvic inflammatory disease, a problem for which sexually active adolescent females are at significantly greater risk than their adult counterparts. The CDC estimates that between 200,000 and 500,000 persons annually suffer an initial episode of genital herpes and that recurrent episodes exceed several million per year. There has been a resurgence in the incidence of syphilis, which had declined following World War II and reached its nadir in the 1950s. Genital lice, scabies, trichomoniasis, and nonspecific vaginitis are all common sexually transmitted infections.

Adolescents with an STD may present to the clinician in a variety of ways. The chief complaint may clearly suggest the presence

Supported in part by a grant from the Robert Wood Johnson Foundation, Princeton, New Jersey.

of an STD, as in those instances in which there is a sore on the external genitalia or a urethral or vaginal discharge. Nevertheless, gonococcal and syphilitic infections are often asymptomatic, and patients with pelvic inflammatory disease may have only nonspecific lower abdominal pain. Pediatricians must be prepared to investigate the possibility of an STD in the evaluation of teenagers with vague complaints. The physician should routinely inquire about sexual activity and contraceptive use, even in those adolescents who are being seen for clearly unrelated conditions (Table 1). Such inquiries are frequently the means by which STD and other problems related to sexuality are identified.

An important aspect in the management of any of these infections is to be certain that another STD is not present and that the patient's sexual contacts are examined and treated. Patients and contacts should have a serologic test for syphilis and a urethral or cervical culture for *Neisseria gonorrhoeae*. Even if evidence of current infection is absent, sexual exposure to a person with any of the following diseases warrants treatment: gonorrhea, chlamydial infection, syphilis, trichomoniasis, scabies, pubic lice, lymphogranuloma venereum, chancroid, and granuloma inguinale.

To facilitate candid communication regarding sexual activity, the adolescent should be interviewed in the absence of parents, with confidentiality assured. If parents are present initially, it may be helpful to elicit some data from them and then request that they remain in the waiting area for the remainder of the history and physical examination. This avoids the awkward situation of having to ask the parents to leave the room only when the sexual history is sought.

In adolescents an STD is primarily an infection resulting from voluntary sexual activity. In contrast, when STD is identified in a prepubertal child, it should be evaluated as evidence of probable molestation. The clinical manifestations and management of the neonate who has acquired an STD by transmission from its mother, either during pregnancy or delivery, is beyond the scope of this chapter.

TABLE 1. SCREENING PROCEDURES FOR SEXUALLY ACTIVE ADOLESCENTS*

1. Historical information regarding menstruation, pregnancy, use of contraceptives, sexual practices, sexual preference, number of partners, and the existence of sexually transmitted disease in sexual contacts
2. Examination of genitalia for evidence of external lesions, urethral or vaginal discharge, and inguinal adenopathy
3. Pelvic examination, including Pap smear
4. Urethral or cervical culture for gonorrhea, other sites as appropriate
5. Urinalysis
6. Serologic test for syphilis

*Frequency of screening depends on number of sexual partners, relative incidence of sexually transmitted diseases in the community, and presence of any sexually transmitted disease in the adolescent.

URETHRAL DISCHARGE (URETHRITIS)

Definition of the Problem

Urethritis is an inflammatory process of the urethra that occurs most frequently in males. Though dysuria and frequency are common, most affected patients complain of a urethral discharge. A minority of patients have no symptoms and either are identified as contacts of females with cervicitis or are found incidentally to have pyuria. With only rare exceptions, urethritis should be thought of and approached clinically as a sexually transmitted disease.

Etiology

Although numerous microorganisms have been suggested as possible etiologic agents, only a few are known to cause urethritis (Table 2). *N. gonorrhoeae* and *Chlamydia tra-*

TABLE 2. ETIOLOGY OF URETHRITIS

Infectious	Noninfectious
Common	All uncommon
N. gonorrhoeae	Trauma
C. trachomatis	Self-induced
U. urealyticum	(e.g., penile
Uncommon	stripping)
T. vaginalis	Iatrogenic (e.g.,
Herpes simplex	Foley catheter)
virus	Foreign body
Treponema	Crystalluria
pallidum	Reiter's syndrome*
Candida albicans	
Reiter's syndrome*	

*Whether or not infection plays a role in the pathogenesis of this entity is unclear at present.

chomatis are the most important causes of this infection. Nongonococcal urethritis (NGU) includes all cases of urethritis in which the gonococcus cannot be implicated and probably occurs at least as commonly as gonorrhea. The incidence of these two entities varies, depending upon the population studied. Although the term NGU implies a diagnosis of exclusion, there are specific organisms that are known to be causative. *C. trachomatis* is the organism most often identified in males with NGU, accounting for 40–50% of cases. *Ureaplasma urealyticum,* formerly known as T strain mycoplasma, is another, less frequent cause of urethritis. *Trichomonas vaginalis, Candida albicans,* herpes simplex virus, and meatal syphilitic chancres all are associated with a limited number of cases, probably less than 5%.

Noninfectious causes of urethritis are uncommon. They should be suspected when there is a suggestive history or physical finding or in patients who seem to be unresponsive to antibiotic treatment. Reiter's syndrome, comprised of the triad of NGU, arthritis, and eye involvement (either conjunctivitis or uveitis), is of unknown etiology. Iatrogenic or self-induced trauma and the presence of a foreign body within the urethra are occasional causes of urethritis. Urethral strictures may be idiopathic or may result from either trauma or prior infection. Contact with chemicals, especially vaginal spermicidal suppositories, creams, or jellies, may cause a mild transient urethritis. Rarely, patients have a heavy precipitation of crystals in the urine, causing local irritation. Finally, an adolescent occasionally presents with symptoms of urethritis in the absence of any identifiable pathology. This is often related to a specific preceding traumatic event (e.g., a homosexual contact, contact with a prostitute), or to heightened anxiety concerning sexuality.

Differential Diagnosis

History. Patients should be asked about the presence of a urethral discharge. Any quantity of exudate is diagnostic of urethritis. However, the lack of a discharge in a male complaining of lower urinary tract symptoms, such as frequency and dysuria, by no means makes urethritis an unlikely possibility. The essential aspect of clinical management is to distinguish gonococcal urethritis from NGU. A description of both the quantity and the quality of the discharge should be sought. Gonococcal urethritis tends to produce a discharge that is purulent, thick, and copious, whereas the discharge in NGU is more often mucoid and thin and may be scant. It is often helpful to know when the symptoms began in relation to the sexual contact and the time of presentation. Gonorrhea has a shorter incubation period (2–7 days) than NGU (10–20 days). In addition, patients with gonorrhea tend to have more severe symptoms and, therefore, come to medical attention sooner (2–4 days) than those with NGU (5–7 days).

Information should be sought in regard to a prior history of a sexually transmitted disease, what medication was used and for how long, whether there were one or more sexual contacts, and whether contacts were treated with an effective antibiotic regimen. The patient should be asked if his partner has had a recently diagnosed vaginal or "pelvic" infection and, if not, if she has any suggestive symptoms.

If the history is atypical (e.g., denial of any sexual activity), other data may help support the establishment of one of the more uncommon diagnoses.

- Has there been local trauma, such as the insertion of a foreign body (iatrogenic or self-induced), causing urethral inflammation?
- Has the patient had signs or symptoms of arthritis, which might suggest Reiter's syndrome? (This could also be compatible with disseminated gonococcal infection, which commonly presents with arthritis).

The above information may serve as a clue to diagnosis.

It should be kept in mind that there are many exceptions to the classic clinical presentation associated with the various types of urethritis, and a definitive diagnosis can be made only with the aid of information from the laboratory.

Physical Examination. The physical examination is helpful both in further clarifying the nature of the discharge and in discovering associated or coincidental pathologic findings. The urethral meatus should be examined for dried crusts, erythema, and the presence of a discharge. Other lesions seen on the glans, penile shaft, or surrounding skin, such as herpetic vesicles or a chancre, may also be present in the urethra and therefore provide a clue to etiology. If there is no spontaneous discharge, the urethra should be stripped by gently squeezing the base of the penis between the thumb and forefinger while moving the examining hand toward the meatus. Attempts to obtain a discharge should include several repetitions of this procedure and, finally, prostatic massage. If these techniques still fail to produce a discharge, a calcium alginate swab should be inserted 2 cm into the urethra to obtain a specimen for culture and gram stain.

There may be coexisting epididymitis, especially if the urethritis has gone untreated for some time. Presence of inguinal adenopathy may be seen with any genital infection, but if it is marked, it should arouse suspicion of the possible coexistence of another STD with urethritis.

Laboratory Procedures. Laboratory procedures, particularly the gram stain, are crucial to making a specific diagnosis and choosing treatment (Fig. 1). As mentioned previously, patients with an obvious urethral discharge should be assumed to have urethritis. A gram stain of the discharge enables the clinician to distinguish between gonorrhea and NGU. Typical gram-negative diplococci seen within the cytoplasm of polymorphonuclear cells are considered diagnostic of gonococcal urethritis (Fig. 2). If these organisms are not observed microscopically, the patient can be assumed to have NGU. A third situation occurs when organisms are seen but are either atypical in appearance or not intracellular. This is an equivocal finding, and, though consistent with either entity, it is usually indicative of NGU.

A specimen should be streaked directly onto Thayer-Martin or other appropriate culture medium that selectively favors the growth of *N. gonorrhoeae*. The culture must be incubated in a carbon dioxide environment at 37C. Even though the results of the gram stain usually are accurate, the culture may be helpful in planning treatment for the partner, identifying strains of penicillin-resistant gonorrhea, and clarifying the diagnosis when the smear is equivocal.

The identification of *Chlamydia*, which must be grown in a special tissue culture, is a procedure that is relatively expensive, slow, and not generally available in most clinical settings. In addition, since this pathogen can be identified in only 40–50% of patients with NGU and most nonchlamydial NGU responds to the drugs used against *Chlamydia*, it is probably unnecessary to culture in most cases. However, in those individuals with

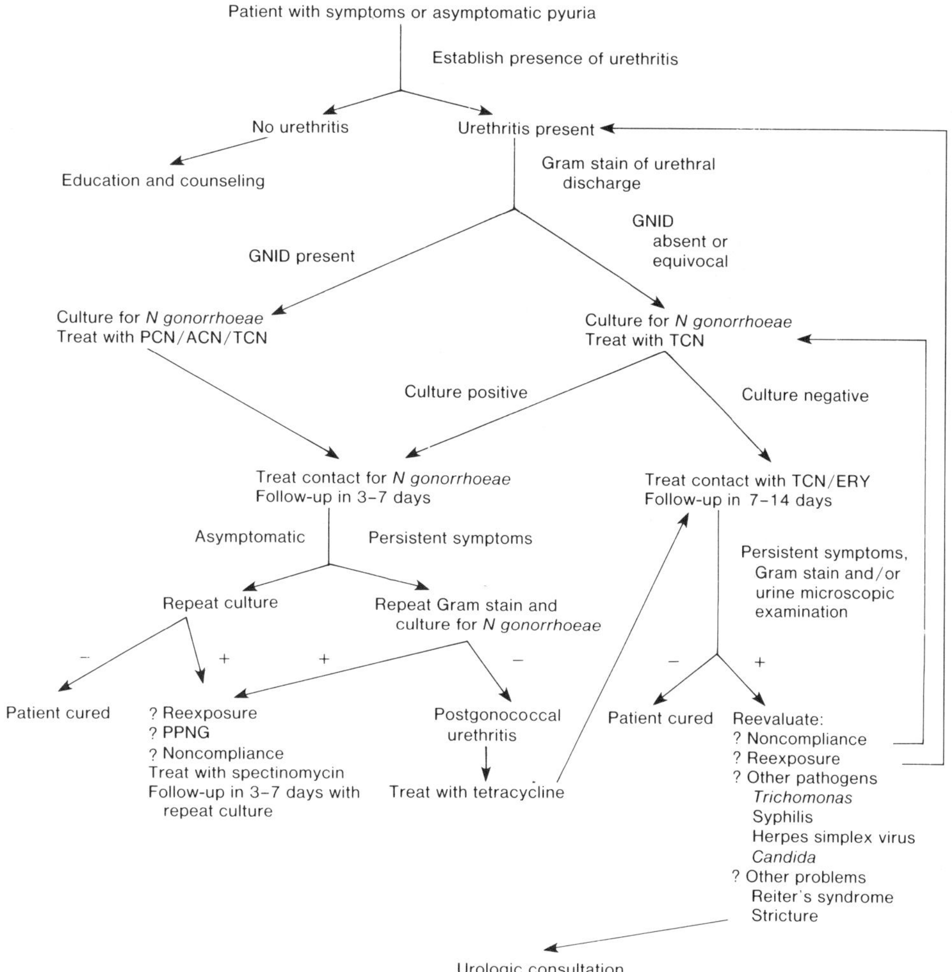

Figure 1. Evaluation and management of the patient with urethritis. *(From Rosenfeld WD, Litman N: Urogenital tract infections in male adolescents. PIR 4(8):259, 1983.)*

multiple recurrences or persistent infection, cultures for *Chlamydia* may be helpful.

With some of the less common etiologies, such as herpes simplex or syphilis, positive laboratory tests (e.g., viral culture, darkfield examination, VDRL) may identify the cause of urethritis. *T. vaginalis* is so uncommon as a cause of symptomatic urethritis in males that it is generally not considered unless the patient's sexual contact has had a recent diag-nosis of trichomonal vaginitis. Under this circumstance or when a patient has failed to respond to a standard treatment regimen for urethritis, a normal saline wet preparation of the urethral exudate should be examined microscopically for the presence of motile trichomonads. Budding yeast forms may also be seen in the rare patient with candidal urethritis. Again, confirmation of this diagnosis is usually sought in patients with a fun-

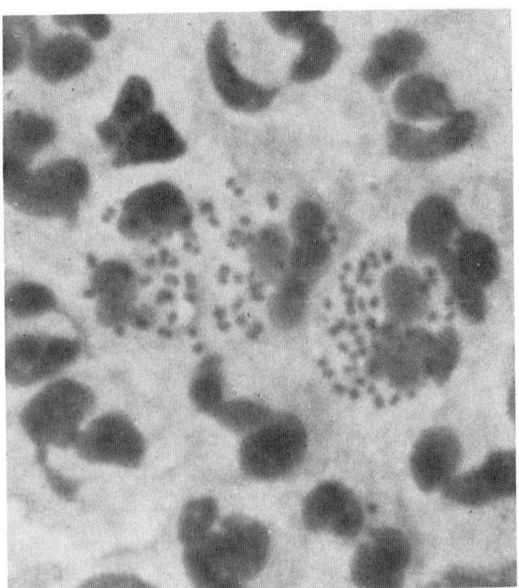

Figure 2. Gram stain diagnostic of gonococcal urethritis.

gal skin rash, when there is no response to the usual therapy, or when suspicion is aroused because of the presence of candidal vaginitis in the sexual partner.

In some cases, where the symptoms are mild or intermittent and little or no discharge is present, even the very diagnosis of urethritis may be called into question. Here, specimens obtained after penile stripping or prostatic massage are gram stained, and the number of polymorphonuclear leukocytes is quantified. Five or more cells per oil-immersion field correlates well with the presence of urethritis. Another technique is to compare the first 10 ml of an overnight urine with a midstream specimen. Equal aliquots are centrifuged separately, and the sediments are examined. The presence of 15 or more cells per high power microscopic field in the initial specimen, with fewer in the midstream fraction, indicates urethritis.

Though some hematuria can be seen with urethritis, a large amount is more likely to be due to trauma, a foreign body, or cystitis. It should be kept in mind that concurrent, multiple, sexually transmitted infec-

tions do occur. The combination of gonococcal urethritis and NGU is not uncommon in males. Patients with a discharge and an obvious external lesion (e.g., syphilitic chancre on the glans) should have a complete evaluation, including a gram stain of the exudate, as it is quite likely that they have two infections.

Management

As with other infectious diseases, the choice of antibiotic in patients with urethritis ideally is made after specific susceptibilities of an isolated pathogen have been determined. However, positive identification by culture and sensitivity testing is not possible at the time patients initially come for care. Even under optimal circumstances, when a reliable and efficient laboratory facility is available, results are usually available no sooner than 48–72 hours after a specimen has been obtained. As the majority of patients with urethritis are at least mildly uncomfortable and anxious, it is desirable to begin therapy at the time of their initial visit before culture results are known. In addition, prompt treatment decreases the opportunity for further dissemination of the disease and increases the probability of cure by diminishing the impact of a patient's failing to keep a return appointment. Fortunately, appropriate and effective antibiotic therapy can usually be prescribed on the basis of the gram stain.

For gonococcal urethritis, the drug of choice is aqueous procaine penicillin G. A dose of 4.8 million units is given intramuscularly, 2.4 million units injected at each of two sites, with simultaneous oral administration of 1 g of probenecid (Table 3). This dosage regimen is highly effective and completely avoids potential problems of compliance. Alternative regimens are used when an intramuscular injection is undesirable or refused, penicillin allergy is present, or when it is considered necessary to provide adequate coverage for coexistent NGU. Tetracycline HCl 500 mg orally 4 times daily for 5 days is the treatment of choice in the penicillin-allergic patient. Spectinomycin or cefoxitin

TABLE 3. TREATMENT OF GONOCOCCAL URETHRITIS

Drug	Dose	Duration of Treatment
Procaine penicillin G*	4.8 million units IM	Once
plus probenecid	1 g orally	
Ampicillin*[†]	3.5 g orally	Once
or		
amoxicillin*[†] plus	3.0 g orally	Once
probenecid	1 g orally	
Tetracycline HCl*[‡]	500 mg orally qid	5 days
Spectinomycin[†§]	2 g IM	Once
Cefoxitin[†§] plus	2 g IM	Once
probenecid	1 g orally	

*Aborts incubating syphilis.
[†]Will not eradicate pharyngeal gonorrhea.
[‡]Effective for NGU if used for 7–10 days.
[§]Effective against PPNG.

with probenecid is indicated when a patient is thought to be infected by penicillinase-producing *N. gonorrhoeae* (e.g., when diagnosed in the sexual partner or in geographic areas where its prevalence is high, such as parts of Southern California). The presence of penicillinase-producing *N. gonorrhoeae* should be suspected when a consort of the patient is known to have such an infection or in treated patients with persistent *gonococcal* urethritis where problems with medication compliance and reinfection can be excluded. It is crucial in these cases to document the presence of the penicillin-resistant gonococci with culture and sensitivity testing.

NGU is best treated with one of the tetracyclines (Table 4). Both *C. trachomatis* and *U. urealyticum* are sensitive to these antibiotics. Even when neither of these organisms can be implicated as the etiologic agent, tetracycline is usually effective. Tetracycline HCl 500 mg orally 4 times daily for 7–10 days is effective and is relatively inexpensive. It has the disadvantages of frequent administration and diminished absorption if taken with dairy products or other food. The long-acting tetracyclines, minocycline, and doxycycline, while somewhat more costly, need be administered only twice daily without dietary restrictions. Another significant advantage of all the tetracyclines is that in the doses used to treat NGU, they will also provide ade-

TABLE 4. TREATMENT OF NONGONOCOCCAL URETHRITIS

Drug	Dose	Duration of Treatment
Tetracycline*[†‡]	500 mg orally qid	7–10 days
Doxycycline*[†‡]	100 mg orally bid	7–10 days
Erythromycin[‡§]	500 mg orally qid	7–10 days

*Contraindicated in children less than 8 years old and pregnant women.
[†]Effective for gonococcal urethritis.
[‡]Aborts incubating syphilis.
[§]High incidence of gastrointestinal side effects at this dose may necessitate use of 250 mg qid for 14 days with careful follow-up.

quate coverage for gonorrhea. For this reason, they should be used when distinction between these two diagnoses is uncertain, as in cases where the gram stain is equivocal.

Postgonococcal urethritis is an entity that occurs in some patients who have been treated with a penicillin for gonococcal urethritis. Affected patients report a persistent or new discharge after a diminution or resolution of their original symptoms. The explanation of this sequence of events is that there has been simultaneous infection with *N. gonorrhoeae* and one of the agents of NGU (usually *C. trachomatis*). The incubation period for *Chlamydia* is longer than that for gonorrhea. The initial discharge, secondary to gonococcal infection, responds to the penicillin, while the microorganisms responsible for postgonococcal urethritis are insensitive to this antibiotic. For this reason, some prefer to use oral tetracycline for 7–10 days in all patients with urethritis, even when the initial gram stain indicates gonococcal infection.

Clinicians should be aware of some problems associated with all of these antibiotics. A major disadvantage of the tetracyclines and erythromycin is that they require patient compliance. Penicillin is given intramuscularly, and treatment with ampicillin or amoxicillin can be completed while the patient is still in the office or clinic, since they are given as a single dose. The tetracyclines, because they interfere with tooth development, are contraindicated in children less than 8 years old and in pregnant women. In addition, both the tetracyclines and erythromycin cause unpleasant gastrointestinal side effects in many patients.

Undiagnosed coexisting infections may be adequately treated or masked by some of the regimens used for urethritis. Patients who have contracted syphilis but who are seen before a chancre appears will be cured by some but not all of the above treatments for urethritis. Pharyngeal gonorrhea, which is usually overlooked, is often not eliminated with ampicillin, amoxicillin, spectinomycin, or cefoxitin.

Patients should be advised to abstain from sexual activity until resolution of the infection is documented. Those with gonorrhea can be reevaluated 3–7 days after completion of treatment, while patients with NGU should be seen 1–2 weeks after finishing their course of antibiotic. The test of cure visit should include a clinical assessment as well as a culture for the gonococcus (in those with gonorrhea) and a microscopic examination of the urine or smear obtained from the urethra. The evaluation of treatment failures must be systematic and complete, including questioning of the accuracy of the original diagnosis. Other common problems include poor compliance with medication, reexposure to an untreated contact, and postgonococcal urethritis. Situations less frequently encountered are infection with *Trichomonas, Candida,* herpes, syphilis, or penicillinase-producing *N. gonorrhoeae.* Recommendations for management of these infections are addressed in the sections on vaginal discharge and genital lesions.

Those patients whose persistent urethritis cannot be explained on the basis of any of the above should receive a trial of an alternative treatment regimen. Some of these patients have a prostatic focus of infection from which the organisms are not completely eliminated and may require a prolonged period of antibiotic treatment. It is essential to reexamine these patients to confirm that their infection has cleared. Urologic consultation is usually unnecessary except for those with unexplained, persistent, or recurrent infection.

SCROTAL SWELLING AND PAIN (EPIDIDYMITIS)

Definition of the Problem

In infancy and early childhood, the most frequent diagnosis in patients presenting with scrotal swelling and pain is an incarcerated inguinal hernia. In the older child and adolescent, however, that diagnosis is uncommon. Trauma, testicular torsion, and epididymitis (usually due to a sexually transmitted pathogen) are the common entities in teenage patients.

Etiology

Epididymitis is most commonly a result of the retrograde migration of microorganisms causing urethritis from the urethra via the vas deferens to the epididymis (Table 5). The pathogens most often implicated under these circumstances are *N. gonorrhoeae* and *C. trachomatis*. Less common pathogenetic processes causing epididymitis include the spread of microorganisms to the epididymis from a bacteremia or viremia and the reflux of infected urine into the epididymis in patients with either anatomic or functional urethral obstruction.

Differential Diagnosis

History. The diagnosis of epididymitis due to sexually transmitted pathogens can be made on the basis of a characteristic history and physical examination. The differential diagnosis includes trauma, testicular torsion, and epididymitis secondary to other etiologies. Hydroceles, varicoceles, and spermatoceles are usually painless and easily identified. Testicular tumors, though rare, should

TABLE 5. ETIOLOGY OF SCROTAL SWELLING AND PAIN

Epididymitis
  Sexually transmitted
    N. gonorrhoeae
    C. trachomatis
    Others?
  Secondary to anatomic or functional urethral obstruction
  Secondary to viremia or bacteremia
Testicular torsion
Testicular trauma
Hydrocele
Varicocele
Spermatocele
Testicular tumor

also be considered as a cause of painless scrotal swelling.

Traumatic epididymo-orchitis is usually diagnosed on the basis of a history of injury. Torsion should be suspected in younger patients (usually 7–14 years) with an acute onset of pain and absence of other genitourinary tract symptoms. The history may reveal a known genitourinary tract abnormality, suggesting epididymitis not associated with a sexually transmitted disease. The patient with acute epididymitis due to a sexually transmitted pathogen has an insidious onset of a dull aching in the scrotum. The teenager usually will have noticed dysuria or urethral discharge.

Physical Examination. The physical examination may provide evidence of a systemic illness (e.g., mumps) as an etiology. Most patients with epididymitis due to a sexually transmitted disease are afebrile and not acutely ill. The scrotum on the affected side appears erythematous and swollen. The epididymis is in the normal posterolateral position in relation to the testis but is enlarged and tender. The testis can usually be distinguished from the epididymis and recognized as not being inflamed. The ipsilateral vas deferens is sometimes tender to palpation. Elevation and support of the scrotum may relieve the discomfort.

Torsion of the testis should be suspected if there is inguinal pain, tender enlargement of the involved gonad, and scrotal edema. The testis is rotated, and the spermatic cord is shortened, causing the gonad to be retracted. There is no relief of pain with elevation and support of the scrotum.

Laboratory Procedures. Among epididymitis, testicular torsion, and trauma, pyuria is present only in patients with epididymitis secondary to a sexually transmitted disease or urethral obstruction. A urethral discharge is present only in those patients with a sexually transmitted disease-associated epididymitis. A urethral discharge should be sought, and, if present, gram stain and cultures of the discharge (or urethra) should be obtained to identify the organism and differentiate epididymitis secondary to gonococcal and nongonococcal urethritis.

Despite the differences cited, the presenting symptoms and signs often do not permit distinction between torsion of the testis and epididymitis. If this is the case, there is an urgent need for urologic consultation to establish the correct diagnosis, since prompt surgical intervention is required for treatment of torsion.

Management

Patients with gonococcal epididymitis should be treated with any of the standard initial regimens for uncomplicated gonorrhea, followed by ampicillin, amoxicillin, or tetracycline in a dose of 500 mg 4 times a day for 10–14 days. For epididymitis associated with NGU, tetracycline or erythromycin 500 mg 4 times a day for 10–14 days is indicated. In epididymitis not associated with a sexually transmitted pathogen, treatment with ampicillin or tetracycline can be started while awaiting culture results. Cultures of an epididymal aspirate can be useful in guiding therapy when the pathogen cannot be identified by other techniques and in patients who have failed to respond to treatment. Consultation with a urologist should be sought for patients with unresponsive or recurrent epididymitis.

VAGINAL DISCHARGE (VAGINITIS)

Definition of the Problem

Vaginitis is encountered in all age groups, from infancy through adult life. Most commonly, it is marked by an abnormal discharge, although itching, burning, pain, or dysuria may also be presenting complaints. The vaginal environment undergoes a series of alterations during the progression from childhood through adolescence and into adulthood. In the prepubertal child the vagina lacks glycogen and lactobacilli, has a neutral pH, and is atrophic, with a thin layer of epithelial cells. At puberty the presence of estrogen results in marked changes in the local environment. Vulvar sebaceous gland activity increases, the layers of vaginal epithelial cells become thickened, and the cellular glycogen content rises. Although a variety of anaerobic and aerobic bacteria are present, lactobacilli become the dominant flora. The lactobacilli utilize glycogen to produce lactic acid, which lowers the vaginal pH to 3.5–4.5. As these changes are generally protective, some vaginal infections in postpubertal girls (e.g., candidiasis, nonspecific vaginitis) occur more frequently when external factors are introduced (e.g., systemic antibiotics) which upset the natural equilibrium. In addition, the potential for the introduction of pathogens (e.g., *T. vaginalis*) occurs in girls who are sexually active.

Normal vaginal secretions may at times be confused with the discharge resulting from a vaginal infection. Physiologic leukorrhea is a mixture of desquamated epithelial cells and endocervical mucus. The volume of these secretions increases in the presence of estrogen or when there is a cervical eversion. However the discharge is neither irritating nor foul-smelling. Most often, no treatment is necessary beyond reassurance, although an occasional teenager with a copious discharge will require a pad or tampon to keep her clothes dry.

Etiology (Table 6)

Candidiasis (Moniliasis). This yeast infection is caused by *C. albicans*. The discharge is white and thick, with a creamy or cheesy consistency, and extremely pruritic. It is often associated with a fair degree of inflammation and edema of the vaginal wall and labia. A typical erythematous, confluent maculopapular rash with satellite lesions is at times seen

TABLE 6. CLINICAL FEATURES OF VAGINITIS

	Quantity	Consistency	Odor	Vulvovaginal Inflammation	Dyspareunia
Physiologic leukorrhea	0 to ++	Mucoid	0	0	0
Candidiasis	0 to +++	Cheesy or creamy white	0	0 to +++	+/−
Trichomoniasis	0 to ++	Yellow, frothy	+++	0 to +++	++
Nonspecific vaginitis	+ to ++	Frothy	++ (Fishy)	+/−	0
Foreign body	++	Bloody or purulent	++++	+/−	+/−

on the skin of the surrounding perineal area. Although *Candida* is present in up to 25% of asymptomatic women, candidal vaginitis may result from sexual transmission or when overgrowth of organisms is fostered by the use of systemic, broad-spectrum antibiotics or oral contraceptives, obesity, or diabetes mellitus.

Trichomoniasis. *T. vaginalis* is a flagellated protozoan that is always considered a pathogen but is occasionally present in individuals who are asymptomatic. It commonly results in a copious, yellow, frothy, malodorous discharge and may cause vulvar irritation. Some patients complain of dysuria and dyspareunia. It is most often sexually transmitted but may also be acquired through close physical contact without sexual intercourse.

Nonspecific Vaginitis. *Gardnerella vaginalis* is thought to be the agent responsible for this condition. Though the mechanism is not known, recent studies support the hypothesis that this organism acts synergistically with the anaerobic flora present in the vagina to cause vaginitis. The discharge, which is often slight in quantity, is gray and frothy and usually does not cause irritation, itching, or dyspareunia. It has a characteristic fishy odor caused by the liberation of amines by the anaerobes. Although nonspecific vaginitis is as-sociated with sexual intercourse, the role of the male contact is unclear.

Foreign Body, Chemical Irritants. While vaginal foreign bodies are more commonly encountered in prepubertal girls, they are occasionally found in adolescents. Lost tampons and objects used for masturbation are among the most frequent offending items. A foreign body should be considered whenever there is a persistent foul-smelling or bloody discharge. Chemicals, such as feminine hygiene products, contraceptive jellies and creams, powders, perfumes, and soaps, may cause a local vulvitis or vaginitis. These may result in a great deal of discomfort, and, though the inflammation is usually self-limited, repeated contact may result in a persistent problem.

Gonorrhea and Other Infections. *N. gonorrhoeae* causes a true vaginitis with a profuse purulent discharge only in prepubertal girls. However, in adolescents it may produce a vaginal discharge secondary to cervicitis. It is essential, therefore, to perform a speculum examination and to obtain cervical cultures for gonorrhea in all sexually active girls complaining of an abnormal discharge. Other entities, such as herpes genitalis and condyloma acuminata, may be seen in association with a discharge or discomfort. As these infections are more commonly identified as lesions in the vulvar area, they are discussed in the section on Genital Lesions.

Differential Diagnosis

History. Information is needed regarding the characteristics of the discharge as well as other symptoms of vaginal irritation. The quantity (scanty to copious with persistent staining of undergarments), consistency (thick, thin, mucoid, cheesy), and color (yellow, white, bloody) need to be ascertained. Some patients deny having any discharge but will complain of a foul odor or burning and itching inside or outside the vagina. For others, the most significant manifestation of vaginitis is superficial pain with intercourse (as compared with the deep dyspareunia seen in salpingitis). Presence of urinary symptoms, such as dysuria and frequency, should not mislead the examiner into prematurely diagnosing a urinary tract infection, especially when other symptoms of vaginitis are present. In fact, several studies have demonstrated that adolescent or adult females with dysuria are more likely to have a vaginal or cervical infection than a urinary infection.

A particularly heavy physiologic discharge may occur prior to and immediately following the menarche. Menstrual irregularities, such as menorrhagia or severe dysmenorrhea in association with a purulent discharge, may be an indication of gonococcal or nongonococcal cervicitis or salpingitis. The patient should be asked about chronic illness (e.g., diabetes mellitus) and recent use of systemic antibiotics. Sexual activity and the use of contraception should be ascertained. Contraceptive cream, jelly, or foam used with or without a diaphragm may be a source of chemical or allergic irritation. Oral contraceptive use facilitates overgrowth of *Candida.*

Physical Examination. It is not possible to identify accurately the type of vaginitis or even to be certain that infection exists on the basis of historical information alone. Some patients will be extremely concerned about a small amount of physiologic leukorrhea, while others will have a copious abnormal discharge incidentally found during a routine pelvic examination.

The pelvic examination should include a careful inspection of the perineal skin and labia for a rash. A rash is seen most often in the presence of vaginal candidiasis but can occur any time the perineum is exposed to heat, moisture, or scratching. A vaginal speculum is used to permit visualization of the vaginal walls and cervix and to detect a discharge or a foreign body. Water alone should be used to ease the insertion of the speculum, as the lubricating gels contain bacteriostatic agents that may render cultures negative or distort the appearance of cells to be examined microscopically. Even in virginal girls, if the introitus permits insertion of one finger, a small speculum can be used, affording a more complete inspection. When this is not possible, a saline-moistened cotton swab can be used to obtain specimens from the vagina, and a digital rectal examination may disclose the presence of a foreign body.

With both trichomoniasis and candidiasis, the vaginal wall is often erythematous, though adherent white plaques are characteristic of the latter. The discharge, which will often pool in the posterior vaginal fornix, should be described in terms of quantity, consistency, color, presence of bubbles, and odor. The appearance of the cervix should be noted, particularly in regard to the presence of erosion or eversion and whether there is a mucous (physiologic) or purulent (gonococcal, chlamydial, trichomonal) discharge from the os.

Laboratory Procedures. The initial laboratory assessment is performed concurrently with the vaginal examination. Almost without exception, sexually active teenagers with vaginitis should have an endocervical culture in a search for concurrent cervicitis due to *N. gonorrhoeae.* To detect gonorrhea, a calcium alginate or cotton swab is inserted into the endocervix and plated on Thayer-Martin medium. Culture techniques to determine the various causes of vaginitis are not helpful except in the case of candidiasis, where the use of Nickerson medium is simple and fairly reliable. It should be noted that as many as 25–30% of normal women will have positive vaginal cultures for yeast, so that the use of this culture is not warranted in patients without signs or symptoms of vaginitis.

The most important aspect of the laboratory evaluation for vaginitis is the microscopic examination of a wet preparation. This is obtained from the vaginal pool and is placed either on a glass slide or in a small tube with about 0.5 ml bacteriostatic saline. The latter technique avoids the possibility that the specimen will dry out before the examiner is able to look at it under the microscope. In addition, applying the swab to litmus paper will ascertain the vaginal pH. A Papanicolaou (Pap) smear should be considered in sexually active teenagers and may reveal trichomonads, yeast, or the viral inclusion bodies associated with herpes genitalis not detected by either the culture or the wet preparation. It should be noted that the identification of an etiology for the vaginitis does not negate the possibility of a second causative agent or the presence of gonococcal cervicitis. Sexually transmitted diseases are often found in combination. The laboratory findings associated with each etiology are shown in Table 7.

Physiologic Leukorrhea. In physiologic leukorrhea there is no odor to the secretions, which on microscopic examination have few leukocytes, a small number of bacteria, and normal vaginal epithelial cells with sharp borders.

Candidiasis. Budding yeast and pseudohyphae at times can be seen. If 10% potassium hydroxide (KOH) is added to the specimen, the vaginal cells are lysed, making it easier to identify the yeast.

Trichomoniasis. When suspended in saline, trichomonads appear as motile, flagellated organisms. When active inflammation is present, many leukocytes and vaginal epithelial cells are also seen. If examined promptly, the wet preparation is positive in 75–90% of cases.

Nonspecific Vaginitis. This is the most difficult diagnosis to make. The wet preparation in this condition shows relatively few leukocytes and many small bacteria, which attach to the vaginal epithelial cells. The cytoplasm of these cells appears stippled with indistinct borders due to the presence of bacteria. These are called "clue cells." In addition to an elevated pH, the discharge has a characteristic fishy odor that is enhanced by the addition of KOH.

TABLE 7. VAGINITIS: MICROSCOPIC APPEARANCE OF THE DISCHARGE

	pH	Epithelial Cells	Leukocytes	Other
Physiologic leukorrhea	<4.5	Few present, sharp borders	Few	—
Candidiasis	<4.5	Many	Moderate	Budding yeast, pseudohyphae
Trichomoniasis	5–7	Many	Many	Motile trichomonads
Nonspecific vaginitis	5–6	Clue cells	Few	Many bacteria

TABLE 8. TREATMENT OF VAGINITIS

	Antibiotic	Dose
Candidiasis	Miconazole or clotrimazole	1 tablet or applicatorful intravaginally daily for 7–14 days
	Alternative: nystatin	One tablet intravaginally twice daily for 7–14 days
Trichomoniasis	Metronidazole*	2 g orally in one dose
	Alternative: metronidazole*	250 mg orally 3 times daily for 7 days
Nonspecific vaginitis	Metronidazole*	500 mg orally twice daily for 7 days
	Alternative: ampicillin	500 mg orally 4 times daily for 7 days

*Should not be used during pregnancy.

Management

Once the etiology of vaginitis has been determined, specific treatment can be initiated (Table 8).

Candidiasis. Either miconazole or clotrimazole is effective when administered intravaginally once daily for 7–14 days. Both drugs are available as either a cream or a suppository. These drugs are more effective than nystatin, which has the additional disadvantage of requiring twice daily application. Most patients can be treated adequately in 1 week, but some with multiple recurrences or underlying problems, such as diabetes mellitus, may require 2 weeks or more of therapy. Lesions on the vulva or perineal skin should respond to the simultaneous topical application of any of these medications. Sexual contacts need not be treated unless they have candidal skin infection, in which case topical medication is indicated.

Trichomoniasis. Metronidazole is the only medication available in the United States that is effective for the treatment of trichomoniasis. It is administered as a single dose of 2 g orally. In the past, an alternative regimen of 250 mg 3 times daily for 7 days

was utilized. The advantages of the single-dose treatment are an increased likelihood of compliance, lower cost to the patient, and, possibly, a reduced chance of overgrowth with *Candida*. Common adverse side effects include nausea, vomiting, and epigastric pain. Patients should be advised against the use of alcohol during therapy, since metronidazole has a disulfiram-like action and may result in flushing as well as marked gastrointestinal tract reactions. Because metronidazole has been implicated as a carcinogen in rodents, it is contraindicated during the first trimester of pregnancy and probably should be avoided throughout pregnancy. With rare exceptions, trichomoniasis should be considered a sexually transmitted disease, and, therefore, all male sexual contacts (who are usually asymptomatic) should be treated simultaneously with the same regimen of metronidazole.

Nonspecific Vaginitis. A variety of drugs has been used to treat nonspecific vaginitis. Local sulfonamide creams, for some time the most widely used therapy, have been shown to be ineffective. Ampicillin, which is administered in a dose of 500 mg orally 4 times daily for 7 days, also has a high failure rate. Metronidazole, which is now the drug of choice, is thought to be effective at least in part due to its activity against anaerobes. The current recommendation is a 7-day course of metronidazole at either 500 mg twice daily or 250 mg 3 times a day. Although controversy exists as to the appropriate management of sexual contacts, current recommendations would suggest treatment only for partners of patients with recurrent or persistant nonspecific vaginitis. For these male contacts, ampicillin (500 mg 4-times a day for 1 week) would appear to be the drug of choice, although a 7-day course of metronidazole is also acceptable.

PELVIC PAIN

Definition of the Problem

Although abdominal pain in children of either sex has multiple etiologies, the evaluation of this symptom is even more complex in the adolescent female. A number of gynecologic conditions, including salpingitis, must be considered in the teenage girl complaining of lower abdominal or pelvic pain. Pelvic inflammatory disease (PID) is a broad term used to denote infection of the fallopian tubes (salpingitis), with possible involvement of the ovaries or surrounding peritoneal cavity. Acute salpingitis is among the more important etiologies of pelvic pain in adolescent females in terms of incidence, morbidity, and potential sequelae, such as infertility and chronic pain.

Etiology

There are numerous etiologies for pelvic pain in female adolescents, including problems in several organ systems (Table 9). In addition to acute salpingitis, the conditions that are most important in terms of incidence and morbidity include acute appendicitis, ectopic pregnancy, spontaneous abortion, rupture or torsion of an ovarian cyst, and ovarian neoplasm.

N. gonorrhoeae has long been recognized as a frequent cause of acute salpingitis. While the isolation of a microorganism from the endocervix does not necessarily implicate it as the cause of concurrent upper genital tract disease, studies in adults have demonstrated the presence of the gonococcus in the cervix

---

TABLE 9. ETIOLOGY OF PELVIC PAIN IN ADOLESCENT FEMALES*

Gynecologic	*Urinary tract*
Intrauterine pregnancy	Acute pyelonephritis or cystitis
Ectopic pregnancy	Nephrolithiasis
Threatened abortion	*Gastrointestinal tract*
Septic abortion	Acute appendicitis
Endometritis	Gastroenteritis
Acute salpingitis	Inflammatory bowel disease
Tubo-ovarian abscess	Intestinal obstruction
Ovarian cyst	Mesenteric lymphadenitis
Ruptured	Peritonitis
With torsion	*Other*
Ovarian neoplasm	Functional
Mittleschmerz	
Dysmenorrhea	
Endometriosis	
Pelvic thrombophlebitis	

*Pelvic pain signifies *lower* abdominal pain.

of 33–81% of patients with acute salpingitis. A number of other studies utilizing culdocentesis or laparoscopy have confirmed the frequent association of this pathogen with salpingitis.

C. trachomatis, a microorganism that exists as an intracellular parasite, has received a great deal of attention over recent years as a cause of sexually transmitted genital tract disease in both males and females. It is often responsible for many of the same conditions attributed to *N. gonorrhoeae*. At present, its incidence in acute salpingitis is not known, although it does seem to be involved frequently and perhaps to an even greater extent in adolescents than in adult women.

A multitude of other organisms has been associated with salpingitis, including Enterobacteriaceae, *U. urealyticum*, and anaerobic bacteria. In addition, it is clear that at times infection is polymicrobial. It has been postulated that some microorganisms are capable of causing infection only after the fallopian tubes have been damaged by prior infection with more virulent bacteria, such as *N. gonorrhoeae*.

Host factors play an important role in the development of salpingitis. *Age* seems to be a determinant for risk. A sexually active, 15-year-old female has been estimated to have a 10-fold greater chance of developing acute salpingitis than has a 24-year-old woman. As the *number of sexual partners* increases, so does the potential for exposure to pathogens associated with infection, and recent studies have shown a trend toward sexually active teenagers having a greater number of partners. Girls who have had *previous episodes of gonococcal salpingitis* are also at increased risk. This may simply represent a statistical association with other risk factors or may relate to an alteration of the involved tissues due to damage done during the initial episode. Use of an *intrauterine device* is an additional factor associated with an increased probability for upper genital tract disease.

Differential Diagnosis

History. Establishing the diagnosis of acute salpingitis is often quite difficult. The clinical presentation can be variable, often without all of the classic findings. The microorganisms responsible are frequently difficult to isolate. Salpingitis may be confused with other processes that can cause similar signs and symptoms. A careful and complete evaluation is required to distinguish acute salpingitis from other clinical entities.

The history often enables the clinician to determine whether disease involves primarily the genital tract or includes another organ system. For example, the diagnosis of inflammatory bowel disease may be suggested when there is a history of chronic constitutional symptoms with abdominal pain, especially when diarrhea or bloody stools are reported. Presence of lower urinary tract symptoms, such as frequency, urgency, dysuria, and hematuria, should alert the physician to the possibility of a urinary tract infection, although these complaints can also be encountered in patients with acute salpingitis. In teenagers whose symptoms cannot be attributed to an organic etiology and who have a history of psychosocial dysfunction, a diagnosis of functional abdominal pain should be considered.

The classic presentation of *acute salpingitis* includes bilateral lower abdominal pain, an abnormal vaginal discharge, and moderate fever, all having their onset within 1 week of the menses in a girl who is sexually active (Table 10). Menses are frequently abnormal, with increased blood loss and severity of cramps. History of a new sexual partner, multiple consorts, dyspareunia, use of an intrauterine device, and prior episodes of salpingitis should be sought, as they are frequently found in patients with salpingitis.

Acute appendicitis may at times be difficult to distinguish from salpingitis. In the former, the sequence is fairly consistent. Pain is usually the initial symptom. It most often begins

TABLE 10. CLINICAL FEATURES OF ENTITIES CAUSING PELVIC PAIN

	Menstrual Irregularity	Fever	Cervical Discharge	Usual Initial Manifestation
Acute salpingitis	Yes, with or without menorrhagia	Mild to moderate	Yes	Unilateral or bilateral lower quadrant pain
Acute appendicitis	No	Mild	No	Epigastric pain
Ectopic pregnancy	H/O missed or atypical menses. Menorrhagia with fall in HCT	No	No	Pain and vaginal bleeding
Spontaneous or threatened abortion	H/O missed menses, menorrhagia	No	No	Vaginal bleeding
Ovarian cyst	Sometimes	No	No	Pain or menstrual irregularity
Ovarian neoplasm	Sometimes	No	No	Pelvic mass

in the periumbilical area with subsequent migration to the right lower quadrant. This is followed by nausea, vomiting, anorexia, and a low-grade fever. The above description varies depending on how long the process has been taking place, the location of the appendix, and whether or not it has ruptured.

The possibility of a *complication of pregnancy* should be high on the list of considerations in the patient with pelvic pain who has been having intercourse, without contraception, particularly when menses in the past month or two have been absent or light. A ruptured ectopic pregnancy and a spontaneous or threatened abortion are characterized by nausea, vomiting, and vaginal bleeding. There may be a history of syncope in patients with either of these problems, though in the former, frank shock due to hypovolemia can occur. Patients should be asked about a history of prior episodes of salpingitis and use of an intrauterine device, as these are both risk factors for development of an ectopic pregnancy.

Ovarian cysts are common and may give rise to pain if they rupture, become very large, or undergo torsion. Menstrual irregularities, including delayed menses as well as menorrhagia, are frequent concomitants of these cysts. Both benign and malignant *neoplasms* of the ovary occur uncommonly in adolescents but have great importance in terms of associated morbidity. While some patients have nausea, vomiting, urinary frequency, or pelvic pain, many present for care only after the tumor has grown to a very large size, causing a noticeable increase in their abdominal girth.

Physical Examination. The physical examination is influenced to some extent by the historical information obtained, though at times findings discovered during the examination (such as tenderness on the left side in a patient complaining of right lower quadrant pain) will remind the examiner that the history may be incomplete. Some adolescents with acute salpingitis have a toxic appearance, difficulty with ambulation, and a marked elevation of temperature, while others may not seem terribly ill. Direct, and sometimes rebound, tenderness in one or both lower quadrants is consistently present. Any teenager with possible PID must have a pelvic examination. In fact, this procedure can be safely postponed only with patients who have not been sexually active and in whom an acute abdominal condition clearly does not exist. A speculum (lubricated with water only) should be used to visualize the cervical os, where an erosion or a purulent discharge may be seen with salpingitis. A gram stain and culture for gonorrhea are obtained from the endocervix. The bimanual examination reveals tenderness with movement of the cervix and with palpation of the uterus or adnexa. An adnexal mass may also be appreciated.

Patients with acute appendicitis typically have a low-grade fever, right lower quadrant tenderness, and localized peritoneal irritation, with positive obturator and psoas signs, and rebound tenderness. Bowel sounds are usually diminished or absent, and the rectal examination elicits increased pain on the right. Adolescents with an ectopic pregnancy that has not ruptured are afebrile, with unilateral lower quadrant tenderness, and have a tender adnexal mass palpable on pelvic examination. Those patients in whom rupture has occurred may present with hypotension and profuse vaginal bleeding. A teenager with a spontaneous abortion usually displays all the signs of early pregnancy, including a softened and bluish cervix and uterine enlargement, in addition to having bleeding. An ovarian cyst or neoplasm is manifested as an adnexal mass and is associated with tenderness, peritoneal signs, or bleeding if rupture, torsion, or infarction has occurred.

Laboratory Procedures. Laboratory tests are used to supplement the history and physical examination. However, it is the exception rather than the rule when they are diagnostic. Essential tests to be done include a complete blood count, erythrocyte sedimentation rate, and a urinalysis of a clean-voided specimen. If vaginal bleeding has been present, a hematocrit obtained early in the course is useful to serve as a baseline. It may also give some estimate as to the severity of blood loss. Commonly, acute appendicitis must be distinguished from acute salpingitis. In the early stages of acute appendicitis there is usually only mild elevation of the white blood cell count with a normal or slightly raised sedimentation rate. A patient with acute salpingitis, in contrast, is more likely to present with a significant elevation of both. It must be stressed that the findings often are at variance with the classic picture and may be altered by the extent of involvement at the time of presentation, previous treatment with antibiotics, and perhaps by the specific microorganism involved.

The presence of white blood cells in the urinalysis may be due to contamination from a vaginal discharge, a true urinary tract infection, or inflammation of a ureter or the bladder by a nearby infected structure. A midstream clean-voided urine specimen for culture and sensitivity should be obtained when there is significant pyuria.

Patients who are sexually active should have a gram stain of material obtained from the endocervix and cultures for gonorrhea taken from the rectum and pharynx as well as the endocervix. If pregnancy is a possibility, a test for this should be performed prior to any x-ray studies. In nonpregnant patients a plain film of the abdomen may be useful and may reveal a mass or a fecalith. If ultrasonography is available, it can be extremely helpful in detecting pregnancy (both ectopic and intrauterine), a pelvic mass, or fluid in the cul-de-sac, indicative of either infection or bleeding.

Management

If acute appendicitis seems likely, prompt surgical consultation is indicated. In some patients, even after a thorough investigation, this diagnosis cannot be excluded, and a laparotomy will be necessary. In other situations, it may be difficult to distinguish between acute salpingitis and a ruptured ectopic pregnancy. If the latter is suspected, gynecologic consultation should be sought. Culdocentesis, performed by a gynecologist, may be helpful. The presence of blood is suggestive of a ruptured fallopian tube, implying the presence of an ectopic gestation. Pus is diagnostic of infection. If a small, uncomplicated ovarian cyst is suspected from the clinical or ultrasonographic findings, it is appropriate to observe a patient with mild symptoms and repeat the ultrasonogram in 2–3 months. Severe symptoms associated with a cyst may be indicative of torsion, rupture, or hemorrhage. In these instances, as well as in the case of a suspected neoplasm, consultation with an experienced surgeon or gynecologist is indicated. Laparoscopy or laparotomy may be necessary for both diagnosis and treatment.

Once the diagnosis of acute salpingitis has been made, antibiotic treatment should be initiated promptly. The need for hospitalization and parenteral therapy is clear in patients with high fever, severe pain, vomiting, and a toxic appearance. However, it is becoming more widely accepted that all adolescents with acute salpingitis, regardless of the severity of their symptoms, should be treated as inpatients in the hope of reducing the associated morbidity. The rationale for this approach is based on the high incidence of sequelae, the risk of infertility following infection, and the experience that teenagers have more problems with compliance with ambulatory regimens than do other age groups.

The severity and duration of signs and symptoms are primary determinants of the choice of an antibiotic regimen. Bacteriologic information gathered from the endocervical gram stain and culture is an aid in further refining therapy. The disadvantages of outpatient therapy have already been noted. However, such management might be considered in the minimally ill adolescent with symptoms present no longer than 2–3 days.

In teenagers with mild symptoms and an endocervical smear demonstrating intracellular gram-negative diplococci characteristic of *N. gonorrhoeae*, recommended outpatient treatment would include the administration of aqueous procaine penicillin G (APPG) 4.8 million units intramuscularly with 1 g probenecid orally and then oral ampicillin 500 mg 4 times daily for a total of 10 days. (Ampicillin 3.5 g or amoxicillin 3.0 g orally with probenecid may be used in place of the procaine penicillin and should also be followed by 10 days of oral ampicillin.) In those teenagers in whom *N. gonorrhoeae* cannot be demonstrated, tetracycline 500 mg orally qid should be administered for 10–14 days. For patients with mild symptoms who are hospitalized, aqueous penicillin G 20 million units/day intravenously is administered for 10 days. Those patients on intravenous penicillin alone, who have uncomplicated infection, an excellent clinical response, and cannot or will not remain in the hospital for their full course, can be changed to oral ampicillin 2 g/day for the duration of their therapy. Oral phenoxymethyl penicillin V has a different spectrum of activity from penicillin G and is inadequate for this situation.

Patients who are moderately ill upon presentation should be hospitalized and treated with either ampicillin 200 mg/kg/day intravenously and an aminoglycoside, such as gentamicin 5 mg/kg/day or, alternatively, a three-drug regimen consisting of clindamycin 30–40 mg/kg/day, ampicillin, and gentamicin. Clearly, those adolescents with more severe symptomatology or a suspected tuboovarian abscess require hospitalization and broad-spectrum antibiotic coverage, such as the above three-drug regimen. Such treatment provides ample activity against anaerobic organisms.

Metronidazole 30 mg/kg/day is being used increasingly as a substitute for clindamycin, as it provides excellent coverage for anaerobes as well as effective penetration into tissues. Cefoxitin 100 mg/kg/day, a broad-spectrum antibiotic with activity against gram-negative organisms, anaerobes, and *N. gonorrhoeae* (including penicillinase-producing *N. gonorrhoeae*), may be appropriate as single-drug therapy in some situations, especially in patients with penicillin allergy. The addition of an oral tetracycline to any of the above inpatient or outpatient regimens should be considered, since recent studies have demonstrated a high prevalence rate of *C. trachomatis* in patients with salpingitis, and routine culture techniques may fail to detect this organism. Erythromycin 1–2 g/day can be utilized as an alternative to tetracycline.

There should be a rapid response to therapy, within 24 to 48 hours, as assessed by monitoring the patient's temperature, pain, abdominal tenderness, findings on pelvic examination, white blood cell count, and ESR. These examinations should be used at the end of the treatment period also, to determine whether the therapy has been adequate.

At any point in the course, if there is a question about the correct diagnosis, surgical consultation should be sought. When a mass is palpated in the adnexa in a patient with salpingitis, a tubo-ovarian abscess should be suspected and confirmed by ultrasonography. However, this is a rare exception to the surgeons' rule that all abscesses need to be incised and drained. Most tubo-ovarian abscesses respond to medical therapy if appropriate antibiotics are used for a long enough period of time. The possibility that the infection may disseminate via the blood or spread to nearby structures, such as the liver, causing a perihepatitis (Fitz-Hugh-Curtis syndrome), should be remembered. This complication usually occurs prior to the initiation of therapy and should be considered in patients who present with right upper quadrant pain. Affected patients may require laparoscopy, both for confirmation of the diagnosis and to lyse adhesions that form between the capsule of the liver and the peritoneum or other structures.

Crucial to the management of all tubal infections is an appreciation of the limitations of currently utilized methods of ascertaining the causative organism. Normal vaginal flora may contain saprophytic species of *Neisseria* that can be mistaken for the gonococcus on gram stain. Organisms cultured from the endocervix may not correlate with those found on culdocentesis, which in turn may differ from laparoscopic samples from the serosal surface of the salpinx. All such information may be at variance with results obtained directly from the site of infection within the tubes. In addition, the frequency with which polymicrobial infections are encountered, particularly in adolescents with recurrent disease, is a further impediment to the dogmatic application of any single-drug regimen. Hence, regardless of the initial antibiotic regimen, patients must be reevaluated frequently, and therapy must be adjusted promptly if there is evidence of a lack of adequate clinical improvement.

One must be cautious about statements concerning future potential for fertility following salpingitis. Subsequent fertility or infertility is almost never a certainty, though well-intentioned professionals may leave the teenager with the gloomy prospect that they no longer have any reproductive potential. Many of these adolescents begin to test this possibility and return with a pregnancy. These fears need to be addressed when giving contraceptive advice to patients with salpingitis.

GENITAL LESIONS

Definition of the Problem

The skin at the genital area is subject to a variety of nonvenereal infections and noninfectious conditions that may involve only the genital region or occur as part of a more generalized eruption. Nonvenereal anogenital lesions may coexist with sexually transmitted diseases. Pyogenic infections, balanitis, seborrheic dermatitis, allergic reactions, psoriasis, and lichen planus are the most frequent of the nonvenereal processes. However, among adolescents, sexually transmitted diseases are the most common causes of genital lesions.

The differential diagnosis of genital lesions may be subdivided into several groups of clinically recognizable dermatologic findings (Table 11). Several of these disease entities appear under more than one category. For instance, genital herpes, in which progression from a vesicle to an ulcer to a crusted lesion occurs over a several day period, is listed under each of these descriptions. In syphilis, the primary chancre is an ulcer, whereas the condyloma lata of the secondary stage are papules. Most of these infections are more easily recognized in the male, because in the female, the site of infection may be the vagina or cervix without an obvious external lesion. In addition, due to the local moist environment, the external lesions in females are frequently macerated or secondarily infected, leading to further diagnostic confusion. Male homosexuals, as well as females who engage in rectal intercourse, may present with anal lesions. Less commonly, other body areas, such as the fingers, mouth, or breasts, may be the primary site of involvement of the sexually transmitted pathogen

Etiology

Genital Herpes. Although not a reportable infectious disease, herpes simplex virus (HSV) is the most common cause of genital lesions, with estimates of the incidence of new cases in the United States ranging up to 500,000 annually. In addition, as genital herpes is a recurrent condition, the prevalence of this infection is higher than that of gonorrhea. Man is the only natural host for and reservoir of HSV. Like the other herpes viruses, after a primary infection, HSV may become latent and subsequently reactivate despite the presence of circulating antibodies. Herpes simplex type 2 is responsible for approximately 90% of the genital infections, with type 1 (commonly associated with oral infections) accounting for the remaining 10%.

TABLE 11. GENITAL LESIONS

Ulcers, erosions, and chancres	*Vesicles*
Genital herpes simplex	Genital herpes simplex
Syphilis (primary stage, chancre; secondary stage, mucous patch)	Stevens–Johnson Syndrome
	Lymphogranuloma venereum
Lymphogranuloma venereum	*Miscellaneous*
Chancroid	Crusts
Trauma	Genital herpes simplex
Behcet's disease	Scabies
Granuloma inguinale	Nits
Malignancy	Pubic lice
Stevens–Johnson syndrome	Edema
Papules and warts	Trauma
Condyloma acuminata (venereal warts)	Linear tracks
Condyloma lata (secondary syphilis)	Scabies
Molluscum contagiosum	Papulosquamous lesions
Scabies	Secondary syphilis
Pearly penile papules	Psoriasis
Candidiasis	Reiter's syndrome
Lymphogranuloma venereum	Seborrheic dermatitis
Kaposi's sarcoma	Candidiasis

Primary genital herpes develops 2–12 days after sexual exposure to the virus. The primary or initial infection produces a more severe clinical illness than a recurrent episode. Local pruritus and pain may precede the genital lesions. Erythematous maculopapules progress to small vesicles (1–5 mm in diameter) which are typically grouped on an erythematous base. The vesicles break down to multiple superficial ulcerations that are exquisitely painful and may coalesce to ulcers 2 cm in diameter. Particularly in women, the eruption may spread in a wavelike fashion to involve the entire perineum, with new lesions appearing as older ones are healing. At this stage of the illness, patients may exhibit difficulty in ambulating due to the pain or may walk bowlegged so as to avoid the minor friction that exacerbates their discomfort. Severe dysuria may result in urinary retention, and sexual contact produces dyspareunia. Tender inguinal adenopathy is present in nearly all of the patients. The lesions heal with dry crusting and subsequent underlying reepithelialization. Ulcers in moist areas become macerated and tend to heal slowly. The primary infection resolves in 2–6 weeks.

The most common sites of involvement in men are the glans, foreskin, and shaft of the penis. In women, infection usually occurs on the vulva, perineum, vagina, and cervix, and may be accompanied by a vaginal discharge. In both sexes, anorectal herpes may occur with symptoms of rectal pain, pruritus, or tenesmus. Secondary bacterial infection of genital or perianal lesions is not uncommon. Local manifestations are accompanied by constitutional complaints of fever, anorexia, myalgia, malaise, and headache. Infrequently, aseptic meningitis due to herpes simplex develops.

Recurrent genital herpes develops in approximately 60% of those who have had a primary infection. The pathogenesis of the recurrence is reactivation of latent endogenous herpes virus in the sacral sensory ganglia. Half of patients with recurrent disease have an episode as often as once per month and another third have a recurrence every 2–4 months. As the interval from the primary infection increases, the frequency of recurrence diminishes. A characteristic prodrome described as a localized paresthesia, itching, burning, or hypersensitivity at the site of the subsequent lesion is experienced by nearly half of patients with recurrent disease. Less commonly, the prodrome consists of an ipsilateral neuralgia. Many patients can identify a triggering or precipitating factor for their recurrent lesions, including fever, trauma, emotional stress, menstruation, and sexual intercourse.

Recurrent genital herpes is milder than the primary infection, with fewer lesions, less pain, and an overall shorter duration (approximately 7–10 days from onset to healing). The tiny grouped vesicles on an erythematous base tend to reappear at the same location with each episode. Systemic manifestations usually are absent, and less than half of the patients have inguinal adenopathy.

The patient with active genital lesions is highly contagious. However, even during asymptomatic intervals, the patient may shed virus in genital secretions and infect sexual partners. Newborns of mothers with genital herpes are at great risk of acquiring infection during vaginal delivery. Some patients with genital herpes suffer significant anxiety because of their infection.

Syphilis. Syphilis has been recognized as a clinical entity since the European pandemics of the fifteenth century. The manifestations of syphilis are diverse and may simulate a variety of other disease states. There are over 25,000 new cases of syphilis reported annually in the US. Although syphilis is a far less common cause of genital lesions than are other STDs, its prompt diagnosis is crucial because of the sequelae of the untreated disease and because it is a curable infection. In addition, with the recognition of penicillinase-producing *N. gonorrhoeae* and chlamydial urogenital infections, the use of antibiotics other than penicillin for the treatment of venereal diseases may result in incubation stage syphilis going untreated, yielding an increase in the number of individuals with syphilis.

The causative agent of syphilis is *Treponema pallidum*, a spirochete. It is transmitted by direct contact of an infectious lesion with mucous membranes or abraded skin. Sexual intercourse is the usual mode of transmission, though kissing or biting may occasionally be responsible.

The primary stage of syphilis develops at the site of inoculation after an incubation period that averages about 3 weeks (range of 10–90 days). The chancre is usually a single, nontender sore ranging in size from a few millimeters to 2 cm in diameter. The lesion appears as an eroded papule whose edge is raised and indurated. It has a clean base with a serous rather than purulent exudate. The lesion is usually painless and without erythema and most often does not bleed when scraped.

Chancres are more often identified in the male, where the common locations include the glans, shaft, foreskin, and meatus. The lesions are less frequently identified in women where, although they may occur externally, cervical and intravaginal sites are also common. The anorectal area has been increasingly recognized as the primary site of inoculation in homosexual males. Even without treatment, the chancre heals spontaneously 3–6 weeks after its appearance, leaving no trace or, at most, an atrophic scar.

The secondary stage of syphilis appears approximately 6 weeks after the primary lesion (range 2 weeks to 6 months). The manifestations of secondary syphilis are varied, but the most common lesions develop in the skin. They tend to be widespread and symmetric in distribution, and frequently involve the genitalia, palms, and soles. The lesions

are most frequently papulosquamous but may be macular, maculopapular, pustular, or annular. The rash is rarely pruritic, but its appearance may simulate pityriasis rosea, psoriasis, or tinea versicolor.

In the anogenital region, condyloma lata may be present. These consist of moist, flat-topped, pale-colored papules or plaques that are usually multiple. Involvement of the oral and genital mucosa may appear as painless, dull, erythematous patches or silvery gray superficial erosions (mucous patches). The skin and mucous membrane lesions of secondary syphilis are all highly infectious.

More than half of the patients with secondary syphilis have an influenza-like syndrome, with fever, malaise, anorexia, and myalgia. Generalized lymphadenopathy with firm, nontender nodes is characteristic of the secondary stage. Alopecia of the scalp, eyelashes, or eyebrows may be present. Rare manifestations of secondary syphilis include iritis, nephritis, hepatitis, meningitis, and osteomyelitis. The manifestations of the secondary stage resolve with or without therapy in 4–12 weeks. The skin lesions heal without scarring.

Following the secondary stage, the patient enters the latent phase, during which there are no clinical signs or symptoms of the disease except for a reactive serology. Tertiary (or late) syphilis develops in approximately one third of untreated infected individuals.

Condyloma Acuminata (Venereal or Genital Warts). Condyloma acuminata are common, sexually transmitted lesions of the anogenital region. The etiologic agent is a papilloma virus which is morphologically identical to but antigenically distinct from the virus causing the common cutaneous wart, verruca vulgaris. Nearly two thirds of sexual partners of patients with condyloma acuminata develop warts after an incubation period of about 3 months (range 1½–8 months). The lesions developing in the anal or genital area are usually multiple, discrete, pink to brown colored, and verrucous or papillary. The warts may enlarge and appear confluent, forming a cauliflower-like mass. Warts regress spontaneously or persist for years.

Molluscum Contagiosum. Molluscum contagiosum is a common pediatric skin infection caused by a member of the poxvirus group. Recently, it has been recognized as a sexually transmitted disease in adolescents and adults. The incubation period ranges from 2 to 7 weeks. Unlike the virus of venereal warts, molluscum contagiosum tends to infect the normal skin of the lower abdominal wall, pubis, and inner thighs and not the genitalia and mucous membranes. The typical lesions are discrete pearly papules, 2–10 mm in diameter, with a central umbilication from which a caseous material is expressible. There is no surrounding erythema. Usually there are 2–10 lesions in the genital region. There are no associated local or systemic manifestations. The lesions spontaneously resolve within 12 months or persist for years.

Scabies. Scabies is a superficial skin infestation caused by the mite, *Sarcoptes scabiei*. Uncommonly recognized prior to the 1960s, scabies has now risen to epidemic proportions throughout the world. The mite is transmitted by close personal contact with an infected person. Occasionally, the scabies mite that infests dogs may be spread to man.

The clinical manifestations of scabies depend to some extent on the host's immune responsiveness (sensitization). Following an initial exposure to scabies, symptoms develop after a 2–6 week incubation period, while persons who have been previously infected develop symptoms 1–4 days after repeat exposure. The main symptom of scabies is intense pruritus, which is worse at night. The classic finding of a linear burrow up to 10 mm in length, produced by the female mite as it travels through the skin, is infrequently identified. Individual and grouped erythematous

papules are the lesions most commonly seen, though papulovesicular and nodular lesions also occur. Chancriform lesions may occur on the penis. The genitalia, buttocks, and thighs are the sites most commonly involved after sexual transmission. However, frequently there is spread to the typical nongenital sites, including the interdigital webs, flexor surfaces of the wrists and elbows, anterior axillary folds, umbilicus, and legs. Excoriation and secondary bacterial infection often confuse the clinical findings.

Pediculosis Pubis (Pubic Lice). In the sexually transmitted disease clinics of New York City, pediculosis pubis was the fourth most commonly encountered venereal disease in 1978. The crab louse, *Phthirus pubis*, is usually transmitted by sexual contact but can also be acquired from sleeping in the same bed with an infected person. The louse is 1–3 mm in length and is large enough to be seen with the naked eye. It is a translucent gray insect that may be difficult to identify unless it is filled with blood from a recent meal. The crab louse is not known to transmit any systemic infection.

Itching in the genital region is the most frequent complaint, although, on occasion, the patient will have noticed the nits (eggs) or lice. Some infected persons have no complaints. Physical examination of the genital skin may reveal pruritic erythematous papules or pathognomonic maculae caeruleae. The latter are asymptomatic blue macules, 0.5–3.0 cm in diameter, that do not blanch on pressure. Scratching may result in excoriated lesions and secondary bacterial infection. The lice may be identified crawling along the hair shaft near the skin. The nits are oval, opalescent structures approximately 1 mm long, which are tightly adherent to the hair shaft.

Lymphogranuloma Venereum. Lymphogranuloma venereum (LGV) is a systemic sexually transmitted disease caused by *C. trachomatis* serotypes LGV I, II, and III. LGV is endemic in tropical and subtropical regions of Asia, Africa, and South America. Less than 500 cases per year are reported in the US. LGV is recognized 3 times more frequently in men than in women, and the highest incidences in the US are among lower socioeconomic groups in the Southeast, in male homosexuals, and in travelers returning from endemic regions.

After an incubation period of about 10 days (range of 3 days to 3 weeks), a primary genital lesion is noticed in about one third of heterosexual men and less frequently in women and homosexual men. The primary lesion is an evanescent, painless papule, vesicle, or ulcer, which heals spontaneously in a few days. Two to eight weeks after exposure, painful regional lymphadenopathy develops (secondary stage), and it is at this time when patients most often present for evaluation. With anorectal involvement, diarrhea and tenesmus occur, and endoscopy reveals a granulomatous proctocolitis. Concurrent with the lymphadenitis, a variety of constitutional symptoms, such as fever, malaise, myalgia, nausea, and vomiting, may be present. Untreated, the patient enters the tertiary stage.

Granuloma Inguinale. Granuloma inguinale (Donovanosis) is a chronic granulomatous disease usually involving the genitalia, caused by the agent *Calymmatobacterium granulomatis*. It is rare in the US but common in tropical and subtropical regions. The genital lesion initially appears as a papule that erodes into an ulcer. The ulcers are painless, have an exuberant granulomatous appearance, bleed easily on contact, and show slow progressive enlargement. Despite the name, inguinal involvement occurs in less than 10% of cases.

Chancroid. Chancroid is an ulcerative genital infection caused by *Haemophilus ducreyi*. Although the disease is common in Asia, less than 1,000 cases per year are reported in the US. Chancroid is most often recognized clinically in noncircumcised, nonwhite males. After an incubation period averaging 5 days (range 1–14 days), the primary lesion begins as an inflamed macule that rapidly progresses through vesicular and pustular stages to a ragged ulcer (soft chancre). The ulcers range in size from 1 mm to 2 cm in diameter, may be sngle or multiple, and are painful, with an erythematous, nonindurated, and undermined border. The base of the ulcer is covered with a necrotic exudate and bleeds easily when abraded.

Differential Diagnosis

History. The evaluation of the patient with genital lesions should begin with obtaining a history of sexual activity in terms of most recent intercourse, frequency, sexual practices, and any known infections in the sexual partner(s). Determination of a specific etiology based on an estimated incubation period is difficult to establish because of the broad overlap among the entities under consideration and the inability to ascertain during which sexual encounter exposure occurred. The emotional stress or physical trauma of the most recent intercourse may be the trigger for reactivation of genital herpes rather than exposure to the virus itself. Incubation periods of up to several months for primary and secondary syphilis, condyloma acuminata, and molluscum contagiosum further complicate the determination.

Trauma should be considered in the differential diagnosis of genital edema or abrasions that are noted within hours after vigorous or repeated intercourse or masturbation. Contact allergy to spermicides, vaginal douches, or other topical preparations may repeatedly produce local swelling, rash, and pruritus within hours to days after each sexual encounter.

Symptoms associated with the genital lesion may narrow the differential diagnosis. Genital herpes and chancroid are painful, whereas the lesions of syphilis, primary LGV, granuloma inguinale, molluscum contagiosum, and condyloma acuminata are painless. Pruritus is the main complaint of patients with scabies and pubic lice, as well as in the prodome of some with genital herpes. With the exception of primary genital herpes and secondary syphilis, fever or constitutional symptoms are rarely present in uncomplicated sexually transmitted disease. A prior episode of similar genital lesions should strongly suggest genital herpes. Many of the infections run their course in days to weeks. However, molluscum contagiosum, condyloma acuminata, scabies, and pubic lice may be present for months. Pearly penile papules (papillae corona glandis) are a normal anatomic variant that may first appear in adolescence and are commonly misdiagnosed as venereal warts.

Physical Examination. Both the dermatologic lesions encountered with specific sexually transmitted diseases (Table 11) and other physical findings as they relate to particular etiologic agents have been described above. The degree of overlap of such findings often precludes reliance upon the physical examination in the determination of a specific diagnosis. However, the physical examination is most often helpful in narrowing the range of diagnostic possibilities and may at times yield a definitive diagnosis. For instance, single lesions are usually noted in primary syphilis and primary LGV, whereas multiple lesions are generally present in the other conditions.

Particular attention should be paid to regional lymph node involvement. Tender inguinal adenopathy occurs in almost all patients with primary and half the patients with recurrent genital herpes. The initial lesion of LGV usually goes unnoticed, but the painful inguinal and femoral adenitis is the complaint that brings most patients to medical attention. Fifty percent of patients with chancroid develop unilateral painful inguinal adenitis, which may either resolve or progress to rupture and drainage. Painless, firm, nonsuppurative, bilateral inguinal adenopathy develops in most patients with primary syphilis. Nontender, mild enlargement of the inguinal nodes may also be present in patients with scabies or pubic lice when scratching has resulted in a superficial secondary bacterial infection. Inguinal adenopathy accompanies uncomplicated gonococcal urethritis in about 5% of patients. Granuloma inguinale produces a subcutaneous inguinal granuloma (pseudobubo) that progresses to a superficial granulomatous ulcer in less than 10% of patients but does not primarily involve the lymph nodes.

A variety of nonvenereal infections and noninfectious conditions may also involve the inguinal nodes. Streptococcal and staphylococcal infections of the lower extremities are frequent causes of inguinal lymphadenopathy or adenitis. Cat-scratch disease, bubonic plague, tularemia, and mycobacterial infection are uncommon diseases that may involve the inguinal lymph glands. Other disorders that may affect the inguinal lymph nodes alone or as a part of a diffuse lymphadenopathy are described in Chapter 16.

Laboratory Procedures. For several of the sexually transmitted diseases, such as genital herpes, molluscum contagiosum, or condyloma acuminata, the history and physical appearance of the genital lesions are sufficiently characteristic for a diagnosis to be made on clinical grounds alone. Not infrequently, however, the clinical picture is ambiguous, and laboratory studies are required to make the diagnosis. In suspected herpetic infection, a variety of laboratory techniques can be utilized to demonstrate the virus. The lesions can be cultured directly. Intact vesicles should be unroofed prior to obtaining a specimen. A Tzanck preparation of the base of the lesion can be prepared and stained with Giemsa or Wright stain in search of multinucleate giant cells or stained with fluorescein-conjugated antibodies for the detection of herpes simplex viral antigens. Cervical Pap smears may also demonstrate the presence of herpes virus. Serology is currently of no value in diagnosing genital herpes.

Laboratory confirmation of syphilis can be accomplished by darkfield microscopic examination of specimens obtained from genital or cutaneous lesions and by serology. Because of the frequency of chancres with an atypical appearance, any genital lesion that cannot be unquestionably diagnosed as some specific entity (e.g., genital herpes, trauma) should be examined for the presence of spirochetes. Oral lesions cannot be directly examined because of the normal presence of saprophytic treponema that are indistinguishable from *T. pallidum*. Specimens may be aspirated from enlarged regional lymph nodes. On darkfield microscopy, *T. pallidum* has the characteristic appearance of a corkscrewlike organism. Positive findings on darkfield examination allow for an unequivocal diagnosis of syphilis. However, a negative examination does not rule out syphilis, since the treponemes may be too few to be identified or may have been altered by systemic or topical treatment, or the lesion may already be healing.

The two main types of serologic techniques used in the diagnosis of syphilis are the nontreponemal (VDRL, RPR, Kolmer, Wassermann) and treponemal (FTA-ABS, MHA-TP, TPI) tests (Table 12). The non-

treponemal tests identify nonspecific reaginic antibodies that react with a nontreponemal antigen. The VDRL is easy to perform, inexpensive, reproducible, and quantitative, and is thus a good screening test. However, the VDRL may be negative in early primary or late syphilis. If dilutions are performed to exclude the prozone phenomenon, it will always be positive in secondary syphilis. Low titer, false positive VDRLs are frequent (Table 13), mandating the use of a specific treponemal test to confirm the diagnosis of syphilis. In patients with treated pri-

TABLE 13. FALSE POSITIVE VDRL

Acute	Chronic
Acute viral infections, e.g., hepatitis, infectious mononucleosis, varicella, measles, viral pneumonia	Intravenous drug abuse
	Aging
	Leprosy
	Malignancy
	Systemic lupus erythematosus
Severe bacterial infections, e.g., pneumonia, endocarditis, scarlet fever	Nonvenereal treponematoses
Pregnancy	
Smallpox vaccination	
Malaria	

TABLE 12. SENSITIVITY OF DIAGNOSTIC TESTS IN SYPHILIS

	Stage of Infection			
	Primary	Secondary	Latent or Tertiary	Response to Treatment
Nontreponemal tests, e.g., VDRL	70%	100%	70%	Treatment of primary or secondary stage results in seronegativity within 2 yrs
Treponemal tests, e.g., FTA-ABS	85%	100%	97%	Patient may remain seropositive despite adequate therapy

mary syphilis, the VDRL titer should decline and become negative within 1 year. In treated secondary syphilis, the VDRL should become negative within 2 years. The treatment of syphilis of more than 1 year's duration may result in a decline of the VDRL to a stable but low level positivity.

The treponemal tests are generally more difficult to perform and not readily quantitative. The FTA-ABS, which is representative of these tests, is rarely falsely positive except in patients with systemic lupus erythematosus. It is positive in all treponemal infections, including the nonsyphilitic spirochetes causing pinta and yaw. The FTA-ABS is somewhat more sensitive for the identification of primary syphilis than is the VDRL. Once positive, the treponemal tests may remain positive for life despite treatment.

Condyloma acuminata are usually diagnosed on clinical grounds, although occasionally biopsy may be required to exclude other conditions. The clinical diagnosis of molluscum contagiosum can be confirmed by the presence of intracytoplasmic molluscum inclusion bodies on a biopsy of the lesion or a Giemsa-stained preparation of the caseous material. Scabetic infection can be confirmed microscopically by the demonstration of the mite or its eggs in a biopsy of the lesion or a scraping, under mineral oil, of a fresh, unexcoriated papule.

The clinical diagnosis of LGV may be confirmed by the recovery of *C. trachomatis* from the adenitis, by seroconversion, or by a single high titer in the LGV complement fixation serology. The Frei skin test is no longer used because it is both insensitive and nonspecifically positive. The diagnosis of granuloma inguinale is confirmed by a Wright- or Giemsa-stained smear or biopsy of the lesion demonstrating intracytoplasmic Donovan bodies. Definitive diagnosis of chancroid can be accomplished by demonstrating gramnegative coccobacilli in a specimen obtained from either the undermined border of an ulcer or from an aspirate of a bubo. In addition, *H. ducreyi* can be cultured from either site.

Management

Herpes. A variety of topical treatments has been promoted for primary genital herpes, but only acyclovir has been demonstrated to significantly accelerate healing (Table 14). The duration of symptoms and of viral shedding is also reduced by acyclovir, but the rate of subsequent recurrent genital herpes is not. Topical acyclovir has little if any effect on the course of an episode of recurrent genital herpes and is not licensed for use in this condition. Intravenous acyclovir has recently been approved for the treatment of initial episodes of genital herpes. However, at present its use should be limited to the immunocompromised host or the patient with particularly severe disease.

During an acute episode, patients should be advised to wear loosely fitting clothing and to keep the area dry. Warm sitz baths several times per day may help to relieve discomfort. Because of the association with cervical cancer, women with genital herpes should have an annual Pap smear. If pregnant, they should inform their obstetrician of their condition so that he may make special plans for monitoring and/or delivery.

Syphilis. Penicillin remains the drug of choice for treatment of syphilis unless allergy requires the use of an alternate regimen. Following therapy, patients with either primary or secondary syphilis should have a repeat VDRL every 2–3 months until negative. Persistent positivity of the VDRL of greater than 1 year in primary or 2 years in secondary suggests either reinfection, inadequate initial treatment, or biologic false positive reactions. Consultation with an infectious diseases specialist should be obtained for patients whose VDRLs are persistently positive and for those with syphilis of greater than 1 year's duration.

Condyloma Acuminata. Condyloma acuminata of the genital skin may be treated with topical application of podophyllin to the warts, taking care to avoid the surrounding

TABLE 14. TREATMENT OF SEXUALLY TRANSMITTED DISEASES THAT PRESENT AS GENITAL LESIONS

Disease	Treatment
Genital herpes simplex	Acyclovir ointment* 5%, apply to lesions q3h 6 times/day for 7 days (wear rubber gloves)

Syphilis
  Early (primary, secondary, and latent syphilis of less than 1 year's duration)
	Benzathine penicillin 2.4 million units IM once
	    or
	Procaine penicillin 600,000 units/day IM for 8 days
	Patients allergic to penicillin:
	    Tetracycline HCl† 500 mg qid po for 15 days
	        or
	    Erythromycin 500 mg qid po for 15 days

Late (more than 1 year's duration)	Benzathine penicillin 2.4 million units IM weekly for 3 weeks
	    or
	Procaine penicillin 600,000 units/day IM for 15 days
	Patients allergic to penicillin:
	    Tetracycline HCl† 500 mg qid po for 30 days
	        or
	    Erythromycin 500 mg qid po for 30 days

Condyloma acuminata
  External genital and perianal warts
	Podophyllin‡ 10%–25% in tincture of benzoin topically applied to lesion and washed off in 4 hours; repeat weekly for 4 weeks
	Alternatives
	    Surgical excision
	    Cryotherapy
	    Electrosurgery

Vaginal, cervical, intra-urethral, and intra-anal warts	Any of the nonpodophyllin alternatives
Molluscum contagiosum	Curettage or Cryotherapy

Pediculosis pubis§,‖	Pyrethrin 0.3% with piperonyl butoxide (RID and others) applied topically and washed off after 10 min
	    or
	Gamma benzene hexachloride 1%‡ (Lindane, Kwell, and others) shampoo: work thoroughly into hair for 4 min, then rinse
	    or
	Gamma benzene hexachloride 1%‡ cream or lotion: rub into skin and hair, wash off 12 hr later

Scabies‖	Gamma benzene hexachloride 1%‡ cream or lotion applied to skin in thin layer from chin down and rubbed in thoroughly, wash off in 12 hr
	    or
	Crotamiton 10% cream or lotion applied to skin from chin down, repeat 24 hr later, wash off 48 hr after initial application
	    or
	Sulfur 6% in petrolatum applied to skin from chin down nightly for 3 nights, bathe before each application and 24 hr after last treatment

(*continued*)

TABLE 14 (*Continued*)

Disease	Treatment
Lymphogranuloma venereum¶	Tetracycline HCl† 500 mg qid po for 21 days
	or
	Doxycycline† 100 mg po bid for 21 days
	or
	Erythromycin 500 mg po qid for 21 days
	or
	Sulfisoxazole 1 g po qid for 21 days
Chancroid	Trimethoprim-sulfamethoxazole‡ 2 tablets (or one DS tablet) bid for 14 days
	or
	Erythromycin 500 mg po qid for 14 days
	or
	Tetracycline HCl† 500 mg po qid for 14 days
Granuloma inguinale	Initial therapy:
	Tetracycline HCl† 500 mg po qid for 21 days
	or
	Ampicillin 500 mg po qid for 12 weeks
	For initial therapy failures:
	Chloramphenicol 500 mg po q8h for 21 days
	or
	Gentamicin 1 mg/kg IM bid for 21 days

*Acyclovir is not approved for recurrent genital herpes and is not recommended for pregnant women.
†Not recommended for pregnant women and children less than 8 years old.
‡Not recommended for pregnant women.
§Retreatment is indicated if lice are found or eggs are seen at the hair–skin junction 7 days after initial treatment.
‖Clothing, towels, and bed linen should be washed and/or dried on the hot cycle or dry cleaned.
¶Fluctuant nodes should be aspirated through adjacent areas of healthy, noninvolved skin.

normal tissue. Cryotherapy, electrosurgery, or surgical removal is recommended during pregnancy, for warts on mucosal surfaces, or for podophyllin treatment failures.

Other Conditions. The treatment of choice for molluscum contagiosum is simple curettage of the lesion; cryotherapy is an alternative. Pyrethrin with piperonyl butoxide is the least toxic topical agent for treatment of pubic lice. Lindane may also be used. Crotamiton, sulfur in petrolatum, and lindane are all effective against scabies. Both LGV and granuloma inguinale can be treated with tetracycline. Trimethoprim-sulfamethoxazole is the drug of choice for chancroid.

RECTAL PAIN AND DISCHARGE (PROCTITIS)

Definition of the Problem
Infectious diarrhea has traditionally been associated with the ingestion of contaminated food or water and, occasionally, with nonvenereal person to person transmission. Recently, the bacterial and protozoal agents causing diarrhea have been demonstrated to be sexually transmissible. Studies of male homosexuals have found that these infections are commonly acquired via analingus, though transmission may also occur from a fecally contaminated penis in passive oral-genital and anal-genital sex. Proctologic com-

plications of passive anal intercourse include infectious, traumatic, and allergic proctitis. Hepatitis B has been demonstrated to be transmitted by sexual contact, and evidence of infection is very common in the homosexual community. It has also been recognized that hepatitis A is more frequent among homosexual men than controls and that infection correlates with frequent oral-anal intercourse. Collectively these disorders have been referred to as the "gay bowel syndrome." However, it is the pattern of sexual activity, i.e., frequent anonymous sexual partners and the opportunity for fecal contamination or rectal penetration, and not the sexual orientation per se that puts one at risk for acquisition of these infections.

Etiology (Table 15)

The clinical characteristics of the diarrheal illnesses and hepatitis are identical to the manifestations of the infection acquired via a nonvenereal route. (See Chapters 7 and 14.) Proctitis is most often caused by *N. gonorrhoeae* and *herpes simplex,* but infection with

TABLE 15. ETIOLOGIC AGENTS OF SEXUALLY TRANSMITTED ENTERIC DISEASES

Proctitis	Diarrheal Syndromes	Other
N. gonorrhoeae	*Entamoeba histolytica*	Hepatitis A virus
C. trachomatis	*Dientamoeba fragilis*	Hepatitis B virus
Herpes simplex	*Giardia lamblia*	
T. pallidum	*Salmonella* spp.	
Shigella spp.	*Shigella* spp.	
Campylobacter spp.	*Campylobacter* spp.	
Entamoeba histolytica		
Trauma		
Allergy		

other agents is being seen with increasing frequency.

Differential Diagnosis

Other than a history of receptive anal intercourse, there is little to differentiate the various causes of proctitis on the basis of history and physical examination. Proctitis may be asymptomatic or may cause severe anorectal pain, itching, and burning accompanied by tenesmus, hematochezia, and a mucopurulent rectal discharge. The clinical illness may simulate idiopathic ulcerative colitis or Crohn's disease. Traumatic proctitis may be suspected if the patient described anal penetration by a fist or foreign body. Allergic reaction should be considered if the patient uses scented or colored lubricants for anal intercourse and rectal cultures are negative, or if the proctitis is unresponsive to antibiotic therapy.

Anoscopic examination reveals ulcerations, friability, or cobblestoning of the mucosa. Herpetic proctitis may be associated with a lumbosacral radiculomyelopathy manifested by paresthesias in the buttocks, urinary difficulties, or erectile dysfunction. The determination of specific etiology depends on laboratory studies. Rectal discharge should be gram stained to identify gonococcal infection. Bacterial cultures for *N. gonorrhoeae, Shigella* species, and *Campylobacter* species, viral culture for herpes simplex, cultures for *C. trachomatis,* stools for parasitic examination, and a VDRL should all be obtained. Rectal biopsy in herpetic proctitis may reveal the characteristic multinucleate giant cells. Biopsies showing granulomatous involvement of the rectum, indistinguishable from Crohn's disease, have been reported with chlamydial proctitis.

Management

Specific antimicrobial therapy should be directed by the results of laboratory studies. Conventional drug regimens should be employed for infections with *Entamoeba histo-*

lytica, Dientamoeba fragilis, Giardia lamblia, Shigella species, and *Campylobacter* species. The treatment protocols described previously for urethral chlamydial infection and syphilis should be employed for anorectal disease. Gonococcal proctitis in men is best managed with either aqueous procaine penicillin 4.8 million units IM plus 1.0 g probenecid or 2.0 g spectinomycin IM. The use of either a tetracycline or ampicillin/amoxicillin results in unacceptably high failure rates. At present, there is no specific treatment for herpetic proctitis.

Patients with a suggestive history and negative rectal cultures for *N. gonorrhoeae* and other pathogenic organisms should receive a 10-day trial of tetracycline 500 mg qid prior to initiating steroid therapy for presumed idiopathic ulcerative proctitis or Crohn's disease of the rectum. Stool softeners should be prescribed to decrease the discomfort of defecation. The patient should be advised to abstain from passive rectal intercourse until the inflammation resolves. Consultation with a gastroenterologist or infectious diseases specialist should be sought for patients with severe, recurrent, or persistent disease.

ACQUIRED IMMUNODEFICIENCY SYNDROME (AIDS)

Since 1979 an epidemic of Kaposi's sarcoma and opportunistic infections have appeared in homosexual young men. The population at risk has now expanded to include heterosexual drug abusers, hemophiliacs, and Haitians. A prodrome of persistent generalized lymphadenopathy and weight loss has often preceded the unusual illnesses. The infections have included *Pneumocystis carinii* pneumonia, disseminated cryptococcal and mycobacterial infections, invasive candidiasis, chronic ulcerative herpes simplex, and toxoplasmosis.

The mortality rate within 2 years of diagnosis exceeds 50%. Several immunologic abnormalities have been identified, including hypergammaglobulinemia, lymphopenia, and a reversed helper-inducer T cell to suppressor T cell ratio (T_H/T_S).

The etiology of this syndrome is currently unknown. However, the leading hypothesis is that there is an infectious agent that is transmissible through sexual contact or blood products. The recent recognition of immunodeficiency in infants whose parents belong to one of the above risk groups and in the female sexual partners of men with AIDS supports this theory. This problem is now the subject of much basic and clinical research. In the near future, AIDS will likely be added to the expanding list of sexually transmitted diseases.

BIBLIOGRAPHY

General

Centers for Disease Control: Sexually transmitted diseases treatment guideline 1982. Morbid Mortal Weekly Rep 31:33S, 1982

Mandell GL, Douglas RG, Bennett JE (eds): Principles and Practice of Infectious Diseases. New York, Wiley, 1979

Zelnik M, Kantner JF: Sexual activity, contraceptive use and pregnancy among metropolitan-area teenagers: 1971–1979. Fam Plann Perspect 12:230, 1980

Urethritis

Bowie WR: Urethritis and infections of the lower urogenital tract. Urol Clin North Am 7:17, 1980

Felman YM, Nikitas JA: Nongonococcal urethritis: a clinical review. JAMA 245: 381, 1981

Jacobs NF, Kraus SJ: Gonococcal urethritis in men: clinical and laboratory differentiation. Ann Intern Med 82:7, 1975

Epididymitis

Berger RE, Alexander ER, Harnisch JP, et al.: Etiology, manifestations, and therapy of acute epididymitis: Prospective study of 50 cases. J Urol 121:750, 1979

Sufrin G: Acute epididymitis. Sex Transm Dis 8:132, 1981

Vaginitis

Altchek A: Vulvovaginitis, vulvar skin disease, and pelvic inflammatory disease. Pediatr Clin North Am 28:397, 1981

Demetriou E, Emans SJ, Masland RP Jr: Dysuria in adolescent girls: Urinary tract infection or vaginitis? Pediatrics 70:299, 1982

Rein MF: Current therapy of vulvovaginitis. Sex Transm Dis 8:316, 1981

Spiegel CA, Amsel R, Eschenbach D, et al.: Anaerobic bacteria in nonspecific vaginitis. N Engl J Med 303:601, 1980

Acute Salpingitis

Holmes KK, Eschenbach DA, Knapp JS: Salpingitis: Overview of etiology and epidemiology. Am J Obstet Gynecol 138:893, 1980

Jacobson L: Differential diagnosis of acute pelvic inflammatory disease. Am J Obstet Gynecol 138:1006, 1980

Shafer MAB, Irwin CE, Sweet RL: Acute salpingitis in the adolescent female. J Pediatr 100:399, 1982

Genital Lesions

Brown ST, Weinberger J: Molluscum contagiosum: Sexually transmitted disease in 17 cases. J Am Vener Dis Assoc 1:35, 1974

Brown ZA, Kern ER, Spruance SL, et al.: Clinical and virologic course of herpes simplex genitalis. West J Med 130:414, 1979

Corey L, Nahmias AJ, Guinan ME, et al.: A trial of topical acyclovir in genital herpes simplex virus infections. N Engl J Med 306:1313, 1982

Felman YM, Nikitas JA: Condyloma acuminata. NY State J Med 79:1747, 1979

Jaffe HW: The laboratory diagnosis of syphilis. Ann Intern Med 83:846, 1975

Proctitis

Quinn TC, Corey L, Chaffee RG, et al.: The etiology of anorectal infections in homosexual men. Am J Med 71:395, 1981

Cross-Reference to *Pediatrics,* 17th ed.

THIRTY-EIGHT

Precocious Puberty

S. Hahm

Precocious puberty is the appearance of symptoms and signs of puberty earlier than is expected. The age of onset of puberty in normal children varies widely; in the United States the average age is 11–12 years in girls and 12–13 years in boys, but it is not unusual for sexual development to begin as early as 8 years in girls and 9 years in boys, especially when there is a family pattern of early adolescence.

Most frequently, precocious puberty in children is idiopathic, i.e., not due to a demonstrable organic endocrine disorder. However, careful evaluation should be done in each case. Even if no organic disorder is found initially, the children should have periodic follow-up examinations.

Definition

Precocious puberty is defined as the appearance of symptoms and signs of puberty before the age of 8 years in girls or before the age of 9 years in boys. Puberty is also considered precocious in girls whose menarche occurs before the age of 9 years.

Sexual precocity is referred to as *isosexual* if it is appropriate for the child's phenotype and *heterosexual* if it is at variance with the child's phenotype, i.e., virilization of the female or feminization of the male child.

Etiology

Precocious puberty can be divided into true precocious puberty, pseudoprecocious puberty, and incomplete precocious puberty (Table 1). Precocious puberty may result from disorders of the gonads, the adrenal cortex, or the brain. Precocious puberty is encountered more than twice as frequently in females as in males.

True Precocious Puberty

In true precocious puberty sexual development is always isosexual and, eventually, complete. In addition to premature onset of secondary sexual characteristics there is also an increase in the size of the gonads, due to premature activation of the hypothalamic-pituitary system. Pituitary gonadotropins cause gonadal development and maturation, and eventually gametogenesis (ovulation or spermatogenesis) will occur.

Onset may be at any age, even in the first year of life. Occasionally, vaginal bleeding is the initial manifestation, particularly in the McCune-Albright syndrome, but many girls do not menstruate until 4 years or more after the onset of puberty.

True precocious puberty accounts for approximately 90% of the cases of isosexual precocity in girls. In 80–90% of these cases, it is termed idiopathic or cryptogenic, since no

TABLE 1. CLASSIFICATION OF THE MOST COMMON ETIOLOGIES OF PRECOCIOUS PUBERTY

True Precocious Puberty—Isosexual
  Idiopathic (cryptogenic)
    Sporadic
    Familial
  Cerebral
    Tumors of central nervous system: glioma, ependymoma, hamartoma, teratoma, pinealoma
    Congenital anomalies: septo-optic dysplasia or other midline defect
    Hydrocephalus
    Postinfectious: encephalitis, meningitis, brain abscess
    Trauma
    Specific syndromes: McCune-Albright syndrome (polyostotic fibrous dysplasia), neurofibromato-
      sis, tuberous sclerosis, untreated hypothyroidism
Pseudoprecocious Puberty
  Gonadotropin-producing tumors—isosexual: chorioepithelioma, teratoma, hepatoma, hepato-
    blastoma
  Steroid-producing lesions—isosexual or heterosexual
    Gonad
      Ovary: granulosa-theca cell tumor, luteoma or follicular cyst, arrhenoblastoma
      Testis: Leydig cell tumor
    Adrenal
      Congenital adrenal hyperplasia
      Tumor
      Bilateral hyperplasia with Cushing syndrome
  Exogenous: estrogen, androgen, chorionic gonadotropin
Incomplete Precocious Puberty
  Premature thelarche
  Premature pubarche

obvious cause can be found, although EEG changes are sometimes found suggesting a possible functional disturbance. In boys the cerebral type of true precocious puberty accounts for a high proportion of cases. The idiopathic type is unusual.

The differentiation between idiopathic precocious puberty and that due to brain lesions is often difficult or even impossible. Therefore, the diagnosis of the idiopathic type can be made only by exclusion of all other causes and careful continuing evaluation.

Idiopathic Precocious Puberty. Precocious puberty is called idiopathic when examination, laboratory tests, and follow-up fail to re-veal any organic endocrine abnormality. The exact mechanism for a premature activation of the hypothalmic/pituitary/gonadal system is not known.

Gonads develop and mature in response to pituitary gonadotropin and produce gonadal steroids. Sexual development may be complete, with gametogenesis (ovulation or spermatogenesis) and menstruation, or it may be incomplete, with isolated breast development or sexual hair as the only finding. However, physical examination often does not help in differentiating true from pseudo-precocious puberty. In boys, increased testicular size suggests true precocious puberty, but this finding is not always reliable. At the beginning of puberty, testicular size may not have increased, even though histologic examination will reveal Leydig cell hyperplasia (Table 2).

Plasma levels of gonadotropin and gonadal steroids are usually elevated. Ovulation or spermatogenesis occurs frequently in idiopathic true precocious puberty but rarely in precocious puberty due to intracranial lesions. It does not occur in pseudoprecocious puberty (see below). Ovulation is demonstrated when luteal activity is seen (increased plasma progesterone and urine pregnanediol or a progesterone effect on vaginal smear). Sperm can be found in the first morning voided urine in boys. However, repeated testing for gonadotropin or gonadal steroids may be necessary to rule out the diagnosis of true precocious puberty, since they may fluctuate widely at the onset of puberty. Sleep studies on an overnight urine collection for gonadotropin may help in the diagnosis.

True precocious puberty is usually associated with a rapid rate of growth and advanced bone age, although the degree will vary depending on duration. Not infrequently, subtle abnormalities of EEG have been reported, and skull x-rays are normal. Even in the absence of any neurologic abnormality, a CT scan should be performed, particularly in boys.

The clinical course is extremely variable; maturity may be reached either rapidly or slowly. In some cases the manifestations remain stationary or even regress, only to resume development later. In general, sexual development follows the usual pattern, but variation in the sequence of the developmental stages may occur, e.g., vaginal bleeding may be the first symptom.

Most cases of idiopathic precocious puberty occur sporadically, particularly in girls, and a clear genetic pattern is not evident. Familial forms account for only a few cases. An autosomal dominant form occurs almost exclusively in boys and is transmitted usually through the father.

TABLE 2. DIAGNOSTIC CONSIDERATIONS ON THE BASIS OF PHYSICAL EXAMINATION

Physical Examination	Diagnostic Considerations
Measurements	
Height	True precocious puberty or pseudoprecocious puberty is associated with rapid growth; growth rate remains normal for age in incomplete precocious puberty; slow growth may suggest hypothyroidism.
Weight	Obesity or cachexia may suggest hypothalamic dysfunction; obesity may also suggest hypothyroidism or Cushing syndrome
↑ Head circumference	Hydrocephalus
↑ Blood pressure	May be elevated in Cushing syndrome or virilizing adrenal hyperplasia
Pulse	Slow pulse may suggest presence of intracranial lesion or hypothyroidism
General appearance	
Stigmatized face	Congenital anomalies of central nervous system
General habits	Incomplete precocious puberty should maintain juvenile habitus
Skin	
Acne, seborrhea	Excessive androgen secretion
Striae (purple)	Cushing syndrome
Café au lait spots, smooth edged	Neurofibromatosis

(*continued*)

TABLE 2 (Continued)

Physical Examination	Diagnostic Considerations
Skin	
Café au lait spots, irregular edged	McCune-Albright syndrome
Depigmented lesions, shagreen patch, sebaceous adenoma of the face	Tuberous sclerosis
Dry and cool	Hypothyroidism
Muscular development	
Increased	Consider virilizing disorder
Dental development	
Delayed	Consider hypothyroidism
Thyroid gland	
Palpable	May suggest primary hypothyroidism; it also becomes easily palpable normally in early adolescence
Sexual development	
Female	
Isolated breast development without other estrogen effect; areola-flat, immature; vaginal mucosa bright red, not moist, little or no discharge	Premature thelarche or early true precocious puberty or early estrogen-producing tumor
With other estrogen effect, areola development > 12 mm in diameter, puffy, presence of Montgomery follicles, pigmentation; labia minora, increase in size and bluish red color; vaginal mucosa change, dull, paler gray-pink, moist, may have discharge	Estrogen-producing tumor or true precocious puberty or exogenous estrogen
Breast development may be merely excessive adipose tissue in obese girls	
Isolated pubic hair or axillary hair	Premature pubarche or first sign of true precocious puberty or virilizing disorder
With virilizing signs: clitoris enlargement, rugation and pigmentation of labia majora	Virilizing disorder
Combined estrogen and androgen effects, i.e., breast development and sexual hair	True precocious puberty or occasionally estrogen-producing ovarian tumor; very rarely, feminizing adrenal tumor
Male	
Isolated pubic hair or axillary hair	Premature pubarche, early true precocious puberty, or masculinizing disorder

(continued)

TABLE 2 (*Continued*)

Physical Examination	Diagnostic Considerations
Sexual development	
Male	
With external genitalia development, increase in length and circumference of the penis, scrotal change (pigmentation, rugation, wrinkling, or thinning)	True precocious puberty or masculinizing disorder; not in premature pubarche
Testes size and consistency	
Infantile	Premature pubarche or adrenal hyperplasia or tumor or early true precocious puberty or early gonadotropin-producing tumor
Unilateral enlargement	Unilateral testicular tumor or could represent initial asymmetry early in true precocious puberty
Bilateral enlargement	True precocious puberty or gonadotropin-producing tumor or aberrant adrenal tissue in congenital adrenal hyperplasia
Abdomen	
Tenderness, increase in size, ascites or palpable mass	Suggest ovarian tumor or adrenal tumor or gonadotropin-producing tumor
Large liver	Gonadotropin-producing hepatic tumor (seen only in males)
Rectal examination	
Increased uterine size for age	Uterine size will increase in response to estrogen; true precocious puberty or estrogen-producing tumor
Adnexal mass	Ovarian tumor
Gonadotropin-producing tumor, such as presacral teratoma, may be palpable on rectal examination	
Neurologic examination	
Mental or motor impairment	Positive findings suggest intracranial lesion
Eye—funduscropic and visual field by perimetry	
Optic nerve atrophy or papilledema, defect in visual field	Prompt to suspicion of intracranial lesion
Chorioretinitis	Intrauterine infection

Cerebral Precocious Puberty. Cerebral types of precocious puberty are due to a variety of disorders involving the cerebral-hypothalamic-pituitary system. In hamartoma and some cases of McCune-Albright syndrome, hypersecretion of gonadotropin-releasing factor has been demonstrated.

Tumors, Congenital Anomalies, Hydrocephalus, Infection, and Trauma. Tumors in or adjacent to the hypothalamus, pineal gland, or optic chiasm, such congenital anomalies as septo-optic dysplasia or other midline defect, hydrocephalus, and infections have been associated with premature activation of the pituitary-gonadal system. Pinealoma as a cause of precocious puberty has been reported only in males. Hypothalamic hamartomas usually cause early onset of sexual development with rapid progression. They sometimes even presents at birth or are associated with compulsive laughing seizures and visual or neurologic signs, depending on the size and location of the tumor.

A thorough neurologic examination is essential, as is visual field evaluation by perimetry. An EEG is an essential part of the initial evaluation. Skull radiographs may show an enlarged sella, evidence of increased intracranial pressure, or intracranial calcification. CT scan and other radiographic studies may be ordered by the neurologist. A neurosurgeon should be consulted promptly when there are findings suggestive of a space-occupying lesion.

McCune-Albright Syndrome. The McCune-Albright syndrome, which occurs sporadically, probably represents a congenital defect in hypothalamic function. A characteristic triad consists of precocious puberty, irregularly edged café au lait skin lesions, and multiple bony lesions called "polyostotic fibrous dysplasias." In this syndrome, true precocious puberty occurs mostly in females. Other endocrine disturbances, such as acromegaly, gigantism, Cushing syndrome, or hyperthyroidism, may be present.

Neurofibromatosis. Precocious puberty has been observed in association with optic or hypothalamic gliomas in neurofibromastosis. This disease is inherited as an autosomal dominant and is usually diagnosed on the basis of a characteristic skin lesion larger than five smooth-edged café-au-lait spots. Patients may have neurologic manifestations, such as mental retardation and a seizure disorder. Neurofibromas are not present at birth but develop later in childhood, arising in the CNS or other organs.

Tuberous Sclerosis. Tuberous sclerosis is another dominantly inherited neurocutaneous syndrome which may produce precocious puberty. The characteristic skin manifestations are depigmented ash-leaf lesions, sebaceous adenomas of the face (acneiform lesions), and shagreen patches. Mental retardation is common, as are seizures, with hypsarrhythmia (infantile spasm) being the most characteristic. Retinal lesions may be seen. Tumors can occur in various organs, and asymptomatic family members may have the characteristic skin lesions.

Untreated Hypothyroidism. Sexual precocity and hypothyroidism are a rare association, with the hypothyroidism usually being severe and easily diagnosed. Patients of both sexes may have galactorrhea, and girls may menstruate. Unlike other types of precocious puberty, there is retarded linear growth and skeletal maturation. Regression in sexual development follows treatment of the hypothyroidism.

Pseudoprecocious Puberty

Pseudoprecocious puberty refers to early sexual development without activation of the hypothalamic pituitary gonadal system. The gonads do not mature, and spermatogenesis or ovulation does not occur. Pseudoprecocious puberty may be either isosexual or heterosexual.

Gonadotropin-producing Tumor. Gonadotropin-producing tumors are rare in children and an unusual cause of pseudoprecocious puberty. They usually are highly malignant. The tumor produces HCG and compounds with LH activity, which then stimulate gonadal secretion causing isosexual precocity. In boys, there may be bilateral testicular enlargement as in true precocious puberty. Differentiation is possible, since positive assay for the beta-HCG is seen with gonadotropin-producing tumors.

Steroid-producing Lesion. Steroid-producing lesions of the gonad or the adrenal cortex induce only secondary sex characteristics, which may be either isosexual or heterosexual. The gonads do not develop or mature.

Ovarian Tumors. Ovarian tumors are rare in children, accounting for only 1–2% of girls with precocious puberty. The most common type is a granulosa-theca cell tumor, but luteomas or follicular cysts are also seen. Though ovarian tumors are usually benign in children, they cause rapidly progressing isosexual maturation. Of interest and importance is that estrogen-producing tumors induce not only estrogen effects but occasionally may cause growth of pubic hair and even axillary hair for unknown reasons. If vaginal bleeding occurs, it is usually irregular. Rarely, it is regular, mimicking cyclic ovulatory bleeding, which can be mistaken for true precocious puberty. A careful abdominal-rectal examination should be done in all girls with precocious puberty. Ultrasonography is helpful when evaluating uterine size and adnexal masses and should be performed in all girls with isosexual precocity even in the absence of a palpable mass.

Once the tumor is removed, the sexual development usually disappears. Follow-up estrogen measurements are done to detect recurrence of the tumor.

Virilizing ovarian tumors, such as arrhenoblastoma, are extremely rare in children children and need to be differentiated from an adrenal source.

Testicular Tumor, Leydig Cell Tumor. This is a rare cause of isosexual precocious puberty. The tumor is usually benign and presents with a unilateral enlarged testis with an infantile contralateral testis. When this is seen, the physician should think of the possibility of a testicular tumor. Sexual development disappears after its removal.

Congenital Adrenal Hyperplasis (CAH). This inherited defect in steroid biosynthesis is the most common cause of pseudoprecocious puberty in males and heterosexual precocity in females. Virilization in the female is due most commonly to 21-hydroxylase deficiency, but it may also be caused by 11-hydroxylase deficiency and 3-β ol dehydrogenase deficiency. Only 21-hydroxylase deficiency and 11-hydroxylase deficiency will cause masculinization in the male. Complete salt-losing type of 21-hydroxylase deficiency and 3-β ol dehydrogenase deficiency usually present with ambiguous genitalia at birth in the female or with severe dehydration and shock (salt-losing crisis) in infancy in either sex. Nonsalt-losing type (incomplete form) of 21-hydroxylase deficiency and 11-hydroxylase deficiency may present with late onset of virilization or masculinization.

Any virilized girl should be evaluated. In boys, since these disorders cause isosexual precocity (masculinization), differentiation from other causes of precocious puberty is more difficult. Family history of a similarly affected sibling, a consanguineous marriage, death of an infant sibling, or a short adult male family member with a history of sexual precocity are helpful clues.

Adrenal Tumor—Adenoma or Carcinoma. In these disorders, clinical and hormonal findings are very similar to those in congenital adrenal hyperplasia. In adrenal carcinoma, abdominal x-rays may show calcifications. Ultrasonography may show a unilateral mass with atrophy of the contralateral adrenal gland. Differentiation between congenital adrenal hyperplasia and adrenal tumor can be made by a dexamethasone suppression test. Elevated androgens will be suppressed by dexamethasone in CAH but not with adrenal tumor.

Feminizing adrenal tumors are extremely rare.

Bilateral Adrenal Hyperplasia with Cushing's Syndrome. Cushing's syndrome may be associated with early sexual development, isosexual in boys and heterosexual in girls, when excess androgen secretion is present along with signs of cortisol hypersecretion, cushingoid face, hypertension, truncal obesity, and purple striae.

Pseudoprecocious Puberty Due to Exogenous Hormone. This cause of premature development of breast (estrogen) or sexual hair (androgen) is often overlooked. A careful family and environmental history may reveal ingestion of hormonal medications, absorption through contact with hormone-containing cosmetics or ointments, or iatrogenic use of hormone (e.g., human chorionic gonadotropin for cryptorchidism).

Dark pigmentation of the areolae, the linea alba, or inguinal creases may be more characteristic of exogenous hormone, especially stilbestrol. In most cases, physical examination does not help the differentiation from an estrogen-producing tumor. Laboratory tests may reveal increased estrogen levels with suppressed gonadotropin levels. However, because most ingested estrogens are synthetic, frequently a discrepancy will be found between clinical estrogen effect and plasma estrogen level.

Incomplete Precocious Puberty.

Incomplete precocious puberty refers to development of breasts or of sexual hair without development of other secondary sexual characteristics. It includes premature thelarche or premature pubarche.

Premature Thelarche. Premature thelarche is isolated breast development without other signs of sexual development. It occurs most commonly at the age of 1–2 years, though it may occur at any time. Frequently, the breast tissue represents neonatal breast enlargement due to maternal estrogen. Occasionally, it may be merely excessive adipose tissue, easily distinguished by palpation. No other evidence of estrogen effect, such as external genital development, occurs. The uterus and ovaries remain infantile in size, and the growth rate and skeletal maturation are normal for the chronologic age. The breast enlargment usually regresses within 2–3 years but may persist until the onset of puberty, usually occurring at normal age limits.

Premature thelarche has been thought to be due to inappropriate sensitivity of breast tissue to physiologic levels of estrogen, but it may be associated with transient hypersecretion of estrogen because slightly elevated estrogen levels can sometimes be demonstrated at the time of onset.

A vaginal smear is a single inexpensive rapid method to determine estrogen effect. Since surface epithelial cells of the vagina change under the stimulus of endogenous or exogenous estrogen, lack of effect is consistent with premature thelarche. It is important to differentiate premature thelarche from early true precocious puberty or early signs of an estrogen-producing tumor. When the most likely diagnosis is premature thelarche, the patient and the parents can be reassured and told that most likely puberty will occur at the usual age. However, to verify the diagnosis periodic follow-up at 3–4 month intervals is necessary to assess the growth rate and to detect additional features of precocious puberty or developing neurologic signs.

Premature Pubarche (Adrenarche). Premature pubarche is isolated premature growth of pubic hair or, on occasion, axillary hair. It is more frequent in girls and more often seen in children with brain damage. It is usually seen in prepubertal children (age 4–6 years) but may begin as early as the neonatal period. The remainder of pubertal development will begin at the usual age and progress normally. It may be the first sign of true precocious puberty, for in 20% of normal girls pubarche, rather than breast development, is the first sign of adolescence.

In order to rule out a virilizing disorder, a careful examination for other signs of excess androgen should be done. No other signs of sexual development and no other signs of virilization should be present. Accelerated growth rate or advanced bone age is usually not present.

The etiology of premature pubarche is unknown. Possibly, unusual endorgan sensitivity to normal physiologic levels of adrenal androgens may be the cause. Occasionally, however, slightly elevated adrenal adrogen levels may be found in association with slightly advanced skeletal maturation. Gonadotropin levels are within the normal prepubertal range.

Hormonal evaluation to rule out a virilizing disorder (late onset congenital adrenal hyperplasia or virilizing adrenal or ovarian tumor) should be done routinely at the initial evaluation (Table 2) in all girls with isolated premature growth of sexual hair before the diagnosis of premature pubarche is made. Prolonged follow-up observation is necessary, as in premature thelarche.

Differential Diagnosis

Careful history and physical exmination will help the physician to select those laboratory tests most likely to be helpful in the differential diagnosis. Every child with precocious sexual development needs to be evaluated promptly and thoroughly. This means referral to an endocrinologist for further evaluation and follow-up. Any child with possible true precocious puberty should have a thorough neurologic examination by a neurologist. Visual fields should be evaluated by perimetry.

It is often impossible to differentiate between idiopathic and cerebral true precocious puberty during the initial evaluation, since neurologic signs may not become evident until later. Prolonged observation with repeated examinations is necessary to exclude an organic lesion.

History

A careful and detailed history should be taken regarding the onset, progress, associated complaints, past history, use of tonics, vitamins, or medications, possible accidental exposure, and family history. Important questions in the history of a child with signs or symptoms suggesting precocious puberty should include:

- What is the presenting complaint: true isosexual or heterosexual premature development? If there is isolated heterosexual development, such as pubic hair in girls, one must consider the possibility of a virilizing disorder. If a child presents with isolated vaginal bleeding, the possibility of a foreign body, infection, or trauma must be considered. Vaginal bleeding must be distinguished from urinary tract bleeding. Regular cyclic menstruation occurs only in true precocious puberty. Estrogen-producing ovarian tumors usually will cause irregular breakthrough bleeding.
- What was the age of onset? What was the progression of symptoms and signs? If breast development was present since birth, it should be remembered that neonatal breast development due to maternal estrogen can persist for more than 6 months of the postnatal period. Neonatal onset of sexual development strongly suggests the possibility of congenital adrenal hyperplasia (isosexual in male, heterosexual in female) or of a hypothalamic hamartoma (true precocious puberty). A very sudden onset and rapid progression of sexual characteristics suggests an organic lesion. This must be identified and dealt with promptly.
- Are there associated complaints? If there is abdominal pain or an abdominal mass, an ovarian tumor must be included in the dif-

ferential diagnosis. Are there symptoms suggestive of hypothalamic dysfunction, such as polyphagia, polydipsia, polyuria, impaired temperature regulation, obesity, cachexia, unusual crying or laughing? Are there symptoms of increased intracranial pressure, such as headache, nausea, vomiting, or blurred vision? Is there a recent change in personality, behavior, or school work? These symptoms and signs may be associated with an intracranial lesion.

- Is there a history of a fracture or of a limp? If so, McCune-Albright syndrome must be considered.
- Is there a recent spurt in growth? If a growth spurt is present, excess hormone production is likely to be present due to either true precocious puberty or pseudoprecocious puberty. Incomplete precocious puberty (premature thelarche or premature pubarche) does not usually induce rapid growth.
- Is there early tooth eruption? Dental development usually correlates with chronologic age in isosexual precocity. Delayed dental development may suggest hypothyroidism.
- Are there symptoms suggestive of hypothyroidism, such as poor appetite, constipation, cold intolerance, short stature, or slow growth?
- Is there any possibility of accidental exposure to hormones? Is the mother taking birth control pills which the child might have ingested accidentally? Are any estrogen-containing cosmetics, ointment, or vitamins available to the child? Grandparents, babysitters, and visitors should also be included in the inquiries. Has the child received androgen-containing drugs? Is there a history of human chorionic gonadotropin administration (iatrogenic)? Could the type of work the parents do possibly cause contamination from their clothes?
- Is there a history of developmental delay or seizures? The presence of mental retardation or a seizure disorder may be indicative

of cerebral dysfunction as a cause of precocious development.

- Is there any significant past illness that could possibly cause precocious puberty?
  1. Maternal infection during pregnancy, such as rubella or toxoplasmosis, has been associated with true precocious puberty.
  2. Birth trauma or other perinatal insults can cause hypothalamic dysfunction.
  3. CNS infections (meningitis, encephalitis) may be associated with precocity.
  4. Past significant head trauma can also be a possible cause.
- Is there a history of early maturation in the family? What are the ages of menarche of mother and female siblings? At what age did the father begin to shave? At what age were final heights achieved? The family history may be helpful, e.g., a tendency toward the early onset of puberty in a constitutional form or of an autosomal dominant father-son transmission. It should be remembered that a positive family history does not rule out the possibility of an organic lesion.
- Is there a history of consanguineity, early infant death, or a short adult with early sexual development? Is there a history of salt craving or recurrent diarrhea and vomiting? These facts suggest the diagnosis of congenital adrenal hyperplasia.

Physical Examination

When the child is first seen, the full picture of sexual maturity usually has not developed. Therefore, it is important to attempt to differentiate pure androgen effects from combined estrogen and androgen effects, which lead to different major diagnostic considerations. In addition, one should be able to differentiate virilizing signs (e.g., development of the scrotum or labia majora, development of the penis, enlargement of the clitoris, excessive muscle development) from normal adrenal androgen effects (e.g., pubic hair, seborrheic change of the skin) in order to rule

TABLE 3. DIFFERENTIAL DIAGNOSIS ON THE BASIS OF THE HISTORY, PHYSICAL EXAMINATION, AND LABORATORY EVALUATION IN FEMALES WITH ISOSEXUAL PRECOCITY

History and Physical Examination	Vaginal Smear for Estrogen Effect	E2	FSH/LH	BA	Most Probable Diagnosis	Further Work-up
		Initial Work-up				
		Plasma				
Breast only No other estrogen signs (e.g., areola or external genitalia development), no other sexual development	Negative	$\rightarrow$	$\rightarrow$	$\rightarrow$	Premature thelarche	None
Breast and $\pm$ sexual hair Other estrogen signs usually present but may not be present at early period	Positive	$\uparrow$	$\uparrow$	$\uparrow$	True precocious puberty	Skull x-ray EEG Neurologic and eye examination
	Positive	$\uparrow\uparrow$	$\rightarrow,\downarrow$	$\uparrow$	Estrogen-producing tumor, usually ovary, rarely adrenal	Ultrasound Plasma progesterone Urine pregnanediol
	Positive	$\uparrow$	$\rightarrow/\uparrow\uparrow$	$\uparrow$	Gonadotropin-producing tumor	Plasma β-HCG
	Positive	$\uparrow,\rightarrow$	$\rightarrow,\downarrow$	$\rightarrow$	Exogenous	Careful history
With palpable abdominal mass	Positive	$\uparrow\uparrow$	$\rightarrow,\downarrow$	$\uparrow$	Ovarian tumor	Ultrasound and other radiographic studies
Hypothyroidism $\pm$	Positive	$\uparrow$	$\uparrow$	$\downarrow,\rightarrow$	True precocious puberty associated with hypothyroidism	Plasma—TSH, T_4, T_3, prolactin

BA, bone age, E2, estradiol; T_3, triiodothyronine; T_4, thyroxine.

TABLE 4. DIFFERENTIAL DIAGNOSIS ON THE BASIS OF THE HISTORY, PHYSICAL EXAMINATION, AND LABORATORY EVALUATION IN FEMALES WITH HETEROSEXUAL PRECOCITY

| History and Physical Examination | Initial Work-up | | | | | | | Most Probable Diagnosis | Further Work-up |
| | Plasma | | | | Urine | | | | |
	T	DHEA	17OHP	FSH/LH	17KS	P_3	BA		
Pubic hair and/or axillary hair No signs of excess androgen (virilization)	→	→,sl. ↑	→	→	→,sl. ↑	→	→,sl. ↑	Premature pubarche	None
	→	→, ↑	→	↑	→, ↑	→	↑	True precocious puberty	Skull x-ray EEG Neurologic and eye examination
Pubic hair and/or axillary hair Other signs of excess androgen (virilization), often present but may be absent at early period	↑	↑ ↑	↑ ↑	→, ↓	↑ ↑	↑	↑	*Congenital adrenal hyperplasia	Dexamethasone test, suppressible
	→, ↑	↑ ↑	→, ↑	→, ↓	↑ ↑	→, ↑	↑	Adrenal tumor (adenoma, carcinoma)	Dexamethasone test, nonsuppressible, Sonographic and other radiographic studies
	↑ ↑	→, ↑	→	→, ↓	↑ ,→	→	↑	Virilizing ovarian tumor	Sonographic and other

DHEA, dehydroepiandrosterone; 17OHP, 17-hydroxyprogesterone; 17KS, 17-ketosteroids; P_3, pregnanetriol; T, testosterone.
*Some variations in hormonal finding depending on the type: Testosterone not usually elevated in 3βol dehydrogenase, 17OH progesterone or urinary P_3 only modestly elevated in 11-hydroxylase deficiency and usually not elevated in 3βol dehydrogenase, DHEA, and 17OHP characteristic for 21 hydroxylase deficiency. Further hormonal study in the plasma and urine necessary for specific enzyme block.

TABLE 5. DIFFERENTIAL DIAGNOSIS ON THE BASIS OF THE HISTORY, PHYSICAL EXAMINATION, AND LABORATORY EVALUATION IN MALES

History and Physical Examination	Testicular Size	Initial Work-up Plasma				Urine	
		T	DHEA	17OHP	FSH/LH	17KS	P₃
Pubic hair and/or axiliary hair No other masculinizing sign	Infantile	→	→,sl, ↑	→	→	→,sl, ↑	→
Pubic hair and/or axiliary hair Other masculinizing sign (e.g., penile growth, scrotal change) usually present but may not be present at early period	Infantile	↑	↑ ↑	↑ ↑	→,↓	↑ ↑	↑
	Infantile	↑,→	↑ ↑	→,↑	→,↓	↑ ↑	→,↑
	Unilateral enlargement	↑ ↑	↑	→	→,↓	↑,→	→
	Bilateral enlargement	↑	↑	→	↑	↑	→
		↑	↑	→	→/↑ ↑	↑	→
		↑	↑ ↑	↑ ↑	→,↓	↑ ↑	↑
With hypothyroidism ± galactorrhea	Bilateral enlargement	↑	↑	→	↑	↑	→

out a virilizing disorder. Table 2 summarizes the significant positive physical findings.

Laboratory Investigation

The laboratory evaluation of the child with precocious puberty is outlined in Tables 3, 4, and 5.

Initial work-up by an endocrinologist should include serum and urine hormone analysis, a bone age, and skull radiographs. In girls with isosexual precocity, estrogen effects can be assessed rapidly by vaginal cytology. If elevated estrogen levels are present without concomitantly elevated gonatotropin levels, ultrasonographic and other imaging studies are indicated to determine the presence of an estrogen-producing tumor. In girls with heterosexual precocity, adrenocortical and gonadal steroid levels should be measured to differentiate premature adrenarche from congenital adrenal hyperplasia or an androgen-producing tumor. Adrenal androgens and their urinary metabolites may be slightly elevated to early pubertal levels in some children with premature adrenarche.

Gonadotropin levels may still be within the prepubertal range in early true precocious puberty. Documentation of a nocturnal rise of gonadotropins is evidence of true precocious puberty. Gonadotropin response to luteinizing hormone-releasing hormone (LHRH) analog stimulation will be pubertal in true precocious puberty but will not differ from that of normal prepubertal children in incomplete precocious puberty.

Children who have elevated androgen levels should be fully evaluated promptly. Specific adrenal hormones (17-OH progesterone, deoxycorticosterone, deoxycortisol, androgens) and the urinary metabolites of these steroids are usually elevated in children with congenital adrenal hyperplasia and are easily suppressed by glucocorticoid administration (dexamethasone suppression test). When the initial baseline levels do not give adequate information, these children may need to have an ACTH stimulation test to detect this late onset form of congenital adrenal hyperplasia. Androgen-producing tumors cause significant elevations of an-

BA	Most Probable Diagnosis	Further Work-up
→,sl, ↑	Premature pubarche	None
↑	Congenital adrenal hyperplasia	Dexamethasone test, suppressible
↑	Adrenal tumor	Dexamethasone test, nonsuppressible, Sonographic and other radiographic study
↑	Testicular tumor	
↑	*True precocious puberty	Skull x-ray, EEG, Neurologic and eye examination, CT scan
↑	*Gonadotropin-producing tumor	Plasma β-HCG Urine pregnancy test
↑	CAH with aberrant adrenal tissue	Dexamethasone test, suppressible
→, ↓	True precocious puberty associated with hypothyroidism	Plasma—TSH, T_4, T_3, prolactin

*Testicular size may be infantile or asymmetric at early period.

drogens, which are usually not suppressible by glucocorticoid administration.

The beta-HCG assay will differentiate an ectopic gonadotropin tumor from true precocious puberty. The child with true precocious puberty should be evaluated for an intracranial lesion for which CT scan may be helpful.

Accelerated bone maturation indicates either true or pseudoprecocious puberty, although slightly advanced bone age (compatible with height age) can be seen in premature adrenarche. With precocity due to hypothyroidism, the bone age will be retarded or similar to the chronologic age.

MANAGEMENT

All children with precocious puberty should also be evaluated by an endocrinologist. Children with suspected true precocious puberty should be referred to a neurologist. Even after the initial evaluation, continuous evaluation of growth and sexual development and repeat hormone measurements are necessary in order to confirm the initial diagnosis.

Precocious puberty will cause a premature growth spurt in association with accelerated skeletal maturation, and early epiphyseal closure will lead to ultimate short stature. In the majority of children with precocious puberty, skeletal maturation is advanced but not to the same degree as sexual maturation, differing from normal puberty where height age, bone age and sexual developmental stage are identical. In true precocious puberty the course is extremely variable; it may progress slowly, or sexual maturation may be completed rapidly. Precocious puberty due to a definable intracranial lesion usually progresses rapidly.

Proper psychologic management of the patient and the family is of great importance. Since psychosexual and social maturation age correlate with chronologic age and not with the stage of sexual development, patients usually have an infantile attitude toward their own sexuality. Personality and behavior disorders may be caused by parental reactions to the patient's physical changes. The child should be treated as normal, i.e., according to his chronologic age. A straightforward explanation of the physical changes and their causes combined with earlier than usual sexual education may be helpful. Counseling should be offered to the whole family, patient, parents, and siblings.

Normal adolescence will occur at the usual time in children with premature thelarche or premature pubarche. Reassurance and follow-up visits are all that is required.

In idiopathic true precocious puberty, attempts have been made with drug therapy (e.g., medroxyprogesterone acetate, cyproterone acetate) to prevent the secretion or peripheral effect of gonadotropin. These drugs are primarily used to prevent menstruation in very young children. These drugs have been found to cause arrest or regression in sexual development but have not been able to prevent accelerated linear growth and skeletal maturation. In addition, these drugs are associated with suppression of the pituitary-adrenal system and other undesirable side effects. Drug therapy needs critical evaluation before it can be recommended. Recent work with LHRH suggests that it may prove to be the specific therapy for idiopathic true precocious puberty.

With a defined lesion, surgical removal is the choice of treatment whenever possible, and sexual development will usually regress. Treatment of hypothyroidism or suppressive replacement therapy in congenital adrenal hyperplasia will also cause regression of development. However, if skeletal maturation is greater than 11–12 years in children with adrenal hyperplasia or tumor or gonadal tumor, regression may either not occur or occur only transiently, followed by true precocious puberty. In these cases the hypothalamic-pituitary system has already matured, and removal of the inhibitory influence of peripheral sexual steroids will cause activation of this system. Use of LHRH in these cases may also lead to regression of development as in isolated idiopathic true precocious puberty.

SUMMARY

Precocious puberty requires an understanding of normal to evaluate problems properly. Any child who presents with premature sexual development should have a thorough evaluation to identify a possible organic disorder. If no organic abnormality is found, the parents can be reassured, but continuous periodic observation is mandatory to be certain that the diagnosis is correct. Reassessments should include growth velocity, changes in sexual development, bone age, and repeated hormonal measurements when necessary. Repeat careful neurologic examinations are also essential. In addition to medical follow-up, continued psychologic support for both child and parents is necessary.

BIBLIOGRAPHY

Barnes ND, Hayle AB, Ryan RJ: Sexual maturation in juvenile hypothyroidism. Mayo Clin Proc 48:849, 1973

Beas F, Vargas L, Spada RP, Merchadi N: Pseudoprecocious puberty in infants caused by dermal ointments containing estrogens. J Pediat 75:127, 1969

Boyar RM, Finkelstein JD, David R, et al.: Twenty-four hour patterns of plasma luteinizing hormone and follicle-stimulating hormone in sexual precocity. N Engl J Med 289:282, 1093

Cook CD, McArthur JD, Berenberg W: Pseudoprecocious puberty in girls as a result of estrogen ingestion. N Engl J Med 248:671, 1953

Crowley WT Jr, Comite F, et al.: Therapeutic use of pituitary desensitization with a long-acting LHRH agonist: a potential new treatment for idiopathic precocious puberty. J Clin Endocrinol Metab 52:370, 1981

Eberlein WB, Bongiovanni AM, Jones IT, et al.: Ovarian tumors and cysts associated with sex precocity. J Pediatr 57:484, 1960

Hampson JG, Money J: Idiopathic sex precocity in female. Psychosom Med 17:16, 1955

Harwood-Nash DC, Breckbill DL: Computed tomography in children: A new diagnostic technique. J Pediatr 89:343, 1976

Hung W, Milhorat TH, Nelson KB, August GP: Sexual precocity as the only sign of a brain tumor in a 9 year old boy. Am J Dis Child 121:524, 1971

Jenner MR, Kelch RP, Kaplan SL, et al.: Hormonal changes in puberty. IV. Plasma estradiol, LH and FSH in prepubertal children, pubertal female, and in precious puberty, premature thelarche, hypogonadism and in a child with a feminizing ovarian tumor. J Clin Endocrinol Metab 34:521, 1972

Judge DM, Kulin HE, Page R, et al.: Hypothalamic hamartoma: A source of luteinizing hormone-releasing factor in precocious puberty. N Engl J Med 296:6, 1977

Kulin HE, Moore RG Jr, Santrier SJ: Circadian rhythm in gonadotropin excretion in prepubertal and pubertal children. J Clin Endocrinol Metab 42:770, 1976

Lightner ES, Penny R, Frasier SD: Growth hormone excess and sexual precocity in polyostotic fibrous dysplasis (McCune-Albright's syndrome) evidence for abnormal hypothalamic function. J Pediatr 87:922, 1975

Liu N, Grumbach MM, DeNapoli RA, Morishima A: Prevalence of electroencephalographic abnormalities in idiopathic precocious puberty and premature pubarche. J Clin Endocrinol Metab 25:1296, 1965

Loop JD: Precocious puberty, pneumoencephalography demonstrating a hamartoma in the absence of cerebral symptoms. N Engl J Med 271:409, 1964

McArthur JW, Toll GD, Russfield AB, et al.: Sexual precocity attributable to ectopic gonadotropin secretion by hepatoblastoma. Am J Med 54:390, 1973

Money J, Hampson JG: Idiopathic sex precocity in male. Psychosom Med 17:1, 1955

Radfar N, Ansusingha K, Kenny FM: Circulating bound and free estradiol and estrone during normal growth and development in premature thelarche and isosexual precocity. J Pediatr 89:719, 1976

Reiter EO, Kaplan SL, Conte FA, Grumbach MM: Responsivity of pituitary gonadotropes to luteinizing hormone-releasing factor in idiopathic precocious puberty, precocious thelarche, precocious adrenarche, and in patients treated with medroxyprogesterone acetate. Pediatr Res 9:111, 1975

Root AD: Endocrinology of puberty. II. Aberrations of sexual maturation. J Pediatr 83:187, 1973

Sizonenko PC: Preadolescent and adolescent, endocrinology and physiology and physiopathology. II. Hormonal changes during abnormal pubertal development. Am J Dis Child 132:797, 1978

Weinberger L, Grant FC: Precocious puberty and tumors of the hypothalamus. Arch Intern Med 67:762, 1941

Wilkins L: The Diagnosis and Treatment of Endocrine Disorders in Childhood and Adolescence, 3rd ed Springfield, IL, Thomas, 1965

Cross-reference to *Pediatrics,* 17th ed.

Index